Poc...
to Bre...
Recto...
THE KIDNEY

Medical Library

Queen's University Belfast
Tel: 028 9063 2500
E-mail: med.issue@qub.ac.uk

For due dates and renewals:

QUB borrowers see 'MY ACCOUNT' at
http://library.qub.ac.uk/qcat
or go to the Library Home Page

HPSS borrowers see 'MY ACCOUNT' at
www.honni.qub.ac.uk/qcat

This book must be returned not later
than its due date but may be recalled
earlier if in demand

Fines are imposed on overdue books

Pocket Companion to Brenner & Rector's THE KIDNEY

SEVENTH EDITION

Michael R. Clarkson, M.B., M.R.C.P.I.

Instructor in Medicine, Harvard Medical School;
Instructor in Medicine, Renal Division, Department of Medicine,
Brigham and Women's Hospital, Boston, Massachusetts

Barry M. Brenner, M.D., A.M. (Hon.), D.Sc. (Hon.), D.M.Sc. (Hon), M.D. (Hon.), Dipl. (Hon.), F.R.C.P. (Lond., Hon.)

Samuel A. Levine, Professor of Medicine, Harvard Medical School;
Director Emeritus, Renal Division, and Senior Physician,
Department of Medicine, Brigham and Women's Hospital, Boston,
Massachusetts

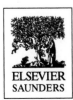

ELSEVIER
SAUNDERS

01205205

ELSEVIER
SAUNDERS

The Curtis Center
170 S Independence Mall W 300E
Philadelphia, Pennsylvania 19106

POCKET COMPANION TO BRENNER & RECTOR'S THE KIDNEY
SEVENTH EDITION   0-7216-0559-1
Copyright © 2005, Elsevier Inc. All rights reserved.

NOTICE

Medicine is an ever-changing field. Standard safety precautions must be followed,
but as new research and clinical experience broaden our knowledge, changes
in treatment and drug therapy may become necessary or appropriate. Readers
are advised to check the most current product information provided by the
manufacturer of each drug to be administered to verify the recommended dose,
the method and duration of administration, and contraindications. It is the
responsibility of the licensed prescriber, relying on experience and knowledge
of the patient, to determine dosages and the best treatment for each individual
patient. Neither the publisher nor the author assumes any liability for any
injury and/or damage to persons or property arising from this publication.

Acquisitions Editor: Susan F. Pioli
Assistant Editor: Laurie Anello
Production Manager: David Saltzberg

Printed in the United States of America

Last digit is the print number: 9 8 7 6 5 4 3 2 1

3 MAY 2005

To sharing the inherent elegance
of
renal pathophysiology and clinical nephrology
with physicians
of
today and tomorrow.

Contents

Preface

Given the dramatic expansion in the number of patients being treated for chronic kidney disease and end-stage renal failure over the past three decades a working knowledge of renal medicine is a prerequisite for the practicing physician. Nephrology is often perceived as being among the more challenging and complex areas of internal medicine, and the major nephrology textbooks can appear daunting at first glance to the uninitiated. Therefore, in designing this concise first edition of *Pocket Companion to Brenner & Rector's The Kidney* we have endeavored to provide a readily accessible and current source of information on clinical renal disease for medical students, residents, renal fellows, primary care physicians, internists, pediatricians and urologists, and trainees in these specialties. To ensure that the text meets the requirement of the busy clinician, we have chosen the most clinically relevant chapters from *Brenner & Rector's The Kidney* and distilled the essence of the pathophysiologic, diagnostic, and treatment issues pertaining to the practice of clinical nephrology. The goal of the *Pocket Companion* is not to replace the main textbook but rather to provide a source of immediate clinical information at the bedside and to act as a starting point for further in-depth reading of *Brenner and Rector's The Kidney* and its companion volumes *Therapy in Hypertension and Nephrology*, *Acute Renal Failure*, *Dialysis and Transplantation*, *Hypertension*, and *Acid-Base and Electrolyte Disorders*.

We wish to express our sincere gratitude to the professional staff at Elsevier and in particular to Susan Pioli for her encouragement, guidance, and support.

I

Approach to the Patient with Renal Disease

Clinical Assessment of the Patient with Kidney Disease

1

ACUTE RENAL FAILURE

Acute renal failure (ARF) is defined as a sudden decrease in kidney function (hours to weeks). The distinction between acute and chronic kidney disease is an important factor in the management of the patient with renal failure (Table 1–1). Early manifestations of renal failure vary and depend in part on context and underlying cause (Table 1–2).

History

The history should initially focus on two key areas: renal hypoperfusion and nephrotoxins.

Table 1–1: Differentiation of Acute from Chronic Kidney Disease

History	Long-standing history suggests chronic kidney disease
Renal osteodystrophy	Radiographic evidence of osteitis fibrosa cystica, osteomalacia suggest chronic kidney disease
Renal size (length)	
Small kidneys (e.g., <9 cm)	Chronic kidney disease
Normal (9–12 cm)	Acute kidney disease
Enlarged kidneys (>12 cm)	Human immunodeficiency virus nephropathy
	Diabetic nephropathy
	Amyloidosis
	Autosomal dominant polycystic kidney disease
	Tuberous sclerosis
	Obstructive nephropathy
Renal biopsy	Histologic diagnosis

Table 1–2: Presentations of Renal Failure

Symptomatic presentation	Musculoskeletal
General	• Muscle weakness
• Fatigue	• Periarticular or
• Weakness	articular pain
	• Bone pain
Cardiovascular	
• Hypertension	Genitourinary
• Pulmonary congestion	• Hematuria
• Cough	• Dysuria
• Dyspnea	
• Hemoptysis	Cutaneous
	• Pruritus
Neurologic	• Necrosis
• Encephalopathy	• Vasculitis
• Seizure	• Bruising
• Peripheral neuropathy	
	Asymptomatic
Gastrointestinal	presentation
• Anorexia	• Hypertension
• Nausea	• Proteinuria
• Vomiting	• Hematuria
• Abdominal pain	• Abnormal renal
• Bleeding	imaging findings

A meticulous review of the medical record should include a careful search for ischemic and nephrotoxic insults. Common causes of volume depletion such as vomiting, diarrhea, excessive sweating, burns, and renal salt wasting (e.g., diabetic ketoacidosis) must be investigated. Evidence of "effective" circulating volume depletion should also be evaluated (e.g., congestive heart failure or cirrhosis). A history of recent trauma with or without overt blood loss or muscle trauma should raise the possibility of ischemia, myoglobin-induced tubular necrosis, or both. Fever, rash, and joint pains are associated with lupus nephritis, vasculitides, endocarditis, drug allergy, and infectious diseases that cause intrinsic acute renal failure. A history of dyspnea or hemoptysis may be a sign of pulmonary vasculitis but typically results from pulmonary edema due to volume overload. Obstructive uropathy and acute inflammation of the kidney can cause painful stretching of the renal capsule. Upper quadrant pain is also a sign of acute renal infarction (e.g., renal artery emboli). Prominent neurologic signs are often observed in thrombotic thrombocytopenic purpura, toxic nephropathies, and poisonings. Constitutional and nonspecific symptoms, such as malaise, weakness, fatigue, anorexia, nausea, and vomiting, are common in patients with ARF but do not alone establish an underlying diagnosis.

A history of nephrotoxin exposure is an extremely important component of the evaluation of a patient with ARF. Both endogenous and exogenous toxins can cause renal failure (Table 1–3). A thorough review of the patient's history and medical record for evidence of nephrotoxin exposure is essential. The potential toxicity of over-the-counter drugs and poisons should be considered in all patients in whom the cause of ARF is not readily apparent. Endogenous toxins include myoglobin, hemoglobin, uric acid, paraproteins, and calcium-phosphorus complexes. Tumor lysis, usually occurring in patients with bulky abdominal lymphomas, can be caused by acute uric acid nephropathy or deposition of calcium and phosphorus and can lead to severe, even anuric ARF. Cancers, including solid tumors and lymphoma, may also cause intrinsic renal failure as a result of hypercalcemia or tumor infiltration.

A history of the color and volume of the patient's urine as well as the pattern of urination can be useful in some settings. For example, abrupt anuria suggests urinary obstruction or vascular obstruction due to renal artery emboli or atherosclerotic occlusion of the aortorenal bifurcation. A history of gradually diminishing

Table 1–3: Nephrotoxins Reported to Cause Acute Renal Failure

Endogenous substances
- Myoglobin
- Uric acid
- Calcium phosphorus
- Light chains
- Atheroemboli

Exogenous substances
Antibiotics
- Aminoglycosides
- Penicillins
- Cephalosporins
- Fluoroquinolones
- Sulfa drugs
- Pentamidine

Continued

Table 1–3: (cont'd)

- Foscarnet
- Cidofovir
- Acyclovir

Angiotensin-converting enzyme inhibitors
Angiotensin II receptor 1 antagonists
Analgesics and nonsteroidal anti-inflammatory drugs
Acetaminophen
Aspirin
Nonselective cyclooxygenase inhibitors
Cyclooxygenase-2 inhibitors
Calcineurin inhibitors

- Cyclosporin
- Tacrolimus

Chemotherapeutic agents

- Cisplatin
- Mitomycin C
- Methotrexate
- Cytosine arabinoside
- Interleukin-2

Reverse transcriptase inhibitors

- Indinavir
- Stavudine

Mannitol
Immunomodulatory agents

- Interferon-α
- Therapeutic immunoglobulins

Radiocontrast agents
Heavy metals and poisons

- Mercury
- Arsenic
- Cadmium
- Lead
- Ethylene glycol

Antidepressants and anticonvulsants

- Citalopram (Celexa)
- Phenytoin
- Carbamazepine

urine output may indicate urethral stricture or in an older man bladder outlet obstruction due to prostate enlargement. Gross hematuria in the setting of ARF suggests acute glomerulonephritis or ureteral obstruction by tumor, blood clots, or sloughed renal papillae.

Physical Examination

The physical examination can provide many clues to the underlying cause of and potential therapy for ARF.

Skin

Petechiae, purpura, and ecchymoses suggest inflammatory or vascular causes of kidney failure. Cutaneous infarcts may result from embolic phenomena, and cutaneous vasculitis manifesting as palpable purpura occurs in patients with septic shock, atheroembolic disease, systemic vasculitis, and infective endocarditis.

Eye

Eye manifestations include uveitis (interstitial nephritis and necrotizing vasculitis), ocular muscle paralysis (ethylene glycol poisoning and necrotizing vasculitis), signs of severe hypertension, atheroembolic lesions, Roth spots (endocarditis), and cytoid bodies (cotton-wool exudates are seen in acute lupus nephritis). Conjunctivitis can be a result of vasculitis or drug toxicity or a manifestation of end-stage renal disease (ESRD) ("red eyes of renal failure"), the latter being due to conjunctival calcium deposition.

Cardiovascular and Volume Status

Meticulous assessment of cardiovascular and volume status is the most important aspect in the diagnosis and initial management of ARF. Evidence for volume depletion, including orthostatic hypotension, dry mucous membranes, and decreased skin turgor, as well as signs of sepsis, congestive heart failure, and cardiac tamponade, should be sought in patients with low blood pressure or overt hypotension. However, often it is difficult to assess the volume status from physical findings alone, and in some patients it may be necessary to place a central venous catheter or pulmonary artery catheter to measure right heart pressures, cardiac output, and systemic vascular resistance. If severe hypertension is present, ARF may be due to malignant nephrosclerosis (e.g., scleroderma), glomerulonephritis, or atheroembolic disease. Cardiac murmurs are associated with endocarditis or atrial myxoma, which can cause ARF due to fulminant glomerulonephritis. A pericardial friction rub in a patient with newly diagnosed renal failure may be a sign of impending cardiac tamponade and is an indication for emergency dialysis. In this situation, progressive hypotension is dramatic but blood pressure can be temporarily stabilized by a rapid intravenous bolus infusion of fluids.

Abdomen

Abdominal examination may reveal a palpable bladder (urinary obstruction). Also, tenderness in the upper quadrants can be associated with ureteral obstruction or renal infarction. Ascites may be observed in fulminant hepatic failure, severe nephrotic syndrome, and Budd-Chiari syndrome, all of which are associated with ARF. Abdominal bruit evokes the diagnosis of severe atherosclerotic disease, which can engender renal failure from renal artery stenosis, thrombosis of the aortorenal bifurcation, or atheroembolic renal disease. A flank mass can be a sign of renal obstruction from tumor or retroperitoneal fibrosis. In addition, a tense distended abdomen in a patient who has just undergone surgery raises the possibility of abdominal compartment syndrome.

Extremities

Examination of the extremities for signs of edema, evidence of tissue ischemia, muscle tenderness (e.g., rhabdomyolysis causing myoglobinuric renal failure), and arthritis (e.g., systemic lupus erythematosus) may provide clues to the diagnosis of renal failure.

Neuropsychiatric Features

Neuropsychiatric abnormalities range from signs of uremic encephalopathy (e.g., confusion, somnolence, stupor, coma, and seizures) to focal neurologic abnormalities in specific diseases such as the vasculitides. Cranial nerve palsies can be seen in patients with ethylene glycol poisoning or vasculitides. Altered and changing mental status is common in thrombotic microangiopathies and systemic atheroembolism.

Urinalysis

The urinalysis is essential in the evaluation of ARF (Table 1–4). An abnormal urinary sediment strongly suggests intrarenal kidney failure. Reddish brown urine or "Coca-Cola" urine is characteristic of acute glomerulonephritis, myoglobinuria, and hemoglobinuria. Bilious urine in patients with combined liver and renal disease appears yellow-brown owing to bile pigments.

Qualitative assessments for proteinuria and heme pigment are helpful in identifying glomerulonephritis, interstitial nephritis, and toxic and infectious causes of tubular necrosis. Microscopic examination of urine sediment after centrifugation is extremely helpful for differentiating prerenal from intrarenal causes of kidney failure. The urine sediment in acute tubular necrosis (ATN)

Table 1–4: Urine Tests in the Differential Diagnosis of Acute Renal Failure

Diagnosis	Urinalysis	Urine-to-Plasma Osmolality	UNa (mEq/L)	Fractional Excretion of Na
Prerenal	Normal	>1.0	<20	<1.0
Acute tubular necrosis	Granular casts, epithelial cells	≤1.0	>20	>1.0
Interstitial necrosis	RBCs WBCs, ± eosinophils, granular casts	≤1.0	>2.0	>1.0
Glomerulonephritis	RBCs, RBC casts, marked proteinuria	>1.0	<20	<1.0
Vascular disorders	Normal or RBCs, proteinuria	>1.0	<20	<1.0
Postrenal	Normal or RBCs, casts, pyuria	<1.0	>20	>1.0

RBC, red blood cell; UNa, urine sodium concentration; WBC, white blood cell.

typically has granular "muddy" casts and renal tubular cells. Interstitial nephritis is often accompanied by pyuria, microhematuria, and eosinophiluria. Glomerulonephritis is heralded by hematuria and red blood cell casts. In addition, granular casts, fat globules, and oval fat bodies may be seen in glomerulopathies associated with heavy proteinuria. Uric acid crystals suggest ATN associated with acute uric acid nephropathy from tumor lysis syndrome. Calcium oxalate crystals may be present in ethylene glycol poisoning with ARF due to nephrocalcinosis, and acetaminophen crystals may be observed in acute acetaminophen poisoning.

Blood Tests

Increases in blood urea nitrogen (BUN) and serum creatinine (Cr) levels are hallmarks of renal failure. The normal BUN/Cr ratio of 10:1 is usually maintained in cases of intrinsic ARF. The ratio is usually elevated (>20/1) in prerenal conditions and in some patients with obstructive uropathy. Also, in patients with significant upper gastrointestinal bleeding, the BUN/Cr ratio may increase further as digested blood proteins are absorbed and metabolized by the liver. The BUN/Cr ratio may be reduced in liver failure, malnutrition, and rhabdomyolysis. The serum creatinine level begins to rise within 24 to 48 hours in patients with ARF after renal ischemia, atheroembolization, or exposure to radiocontrast medium—three major diagnostic possibilities in patients undergoing emergency cardiac or aortic angiography and surgery. Creatinine levels typically peak at 7 to 10 days in ischemic ATN and resolve within the next 7 to 14 days in the absence of further ischemic or nephrotoxic insults. These rapid changes are in marked contrast to the delayed elevation in serum creatinine levels (commencing at 7 to 10 days) that is characteristic of many tubule epithelial cell toxins (e.g., aminoglycosides and cisplatin).

Additional diagnostic clues can be gleaned from routine biochemical and hematologic tests. Hyperkalemia, hyperphosphatemia, hypocalcemia, and increased concentrations of serum uric acid and creatine kinase (CK3 isoenzyme) suggest a diagnosis of rhabdomyolysis. A similar biochemical profile in association with ARF after cancer chemotherapy, but with higher levels of uric acid, a urine uric acid-to-creatinine ratio greater than 1, and normal or marginally elevated creatine kinase, is typical of acute urate nephropathy and tumor lysis syndrome. Severe hypercalcemia of any cause can induce ARF. Widening of the serum anion gap (concentration of Na^+ – that of HCO_3^- + Cl^-) and of the osmolal gap (measured serum osmolality – calculated osmolality) is a clue to diagnosis of ethylene glycol toxicity. Severe anemia in the absence of hemorrhage may reflect the presence of hemolysis, multiple myeloma, or thrombotic microangiopathy. Other laboratory findings suggestive of thrombotic microangiopathy include thrombocytopenia, dysmorphic red blood cells on a peripheral blood smear, a low circulating haptoglobin level, and an increased circulating level of lactate dehydrogenase. Systemic eosinophilia suggests allergic interstitial nephritis but may also be a prominent feature in other diseases, such as atheroembolic disease and polyarteritis nodosa, particularly the Churg-Strauss variant. Depressed complement levels and high titers of antiglomerular basement membrane antibodies, antineutrophil cytoplasmic antibodies, antinuclear antibodies, circulating immune complexes, or cryoglobulins are useful diagnostic indicators in patients with suspected glomerulonephritis or vasculitis.

Urine Chemistry Evaluation

Urine electrolyte measurement in a patient with ARF is performed to test functional integrity of the renal tubules. The single most informative test is the fractional excretion of sodium (FENa), which is defined as follows:

$$\text{FeNa} = \frac{\text{Urine Na} \times \text{Plasma Cr}}{\text{Urine Cr} \times \text{Plasma Na}} \times 100$$

In prerenal azotemia, the FENa is usually less than 1%, and in ATN, it is usually greater than 1%. The FENa is typically less than 1% in patients with acute glomerulonephritis, because tubular function remains intact with increased, rather than decreased, proximal tubular sodium reabsorption. Also, FENa is most accurate for differentiating prerenal from intrarenal ARF when it is determined in the patient with hypotension and oliguria. Because of these limitations, FENa alone should not be used in assessing the cause of ARF.

The urine-to-plasma osmolality ratio (U/P Osm) is another useful test of tubular function in the setting of ARF. With intact tubular function, the urinary osmolality exceeds plasma osmolality three- to fourfold, whereas when tubules are damaged and concentrating capacity is impaired, urine is isosthenuric to plasma. Therefore, a U/P Osm value of 1 or less is consistent with ATN, and a value greater than 1 is consistent with a pre-renal cause. If the amount of urine is scant and the sample volume is low, routine urinalysis is the best diagnostic test. Diagnosis of acute uric acid nephropathy can be substantiated by a urine uric acid-to-urine creatinine ratio greater than 1.

Assessing Urine Output

- *Anuria*: Urine output less than 100 mL/day.
- *Oliguric renal failure*: Urine output of 100 and 400 mL/day.
- *Nonoliguric renal failure*: Urine output greater than 400 mL/day.

In patients with suprapubic discomfort and an obviously distended bladder or in patients with a history of declining urine output or documented oliguria, a bladder catheter should be temporarily placed to relieve or rule out bladder outlet obstruction. Measurement of subsequent daily urine output is important for management of patients.

Fluid Challenge

In patients with a suspected prerenal cause of renal failure from significant intravascular volume depletion, an intravenous infusion of normal saline may be helpful. In prerenal ARF, a fluid challenge should improve renal blood flow with correction of renal failure and increased urine output. This maneuver usually consists of an infusion of 1 to 2 L of normal saline administered over 2 to 4 hours, depending on the clinical judgment of the treating physician. Close and careful bedside monitoring of vital signs, physical findings, and urine output is required. Failure of this maneuver to improve vital signs and urine output can help point to intrarenal or postrenal causes of renal failure. Caution must be exercised during fluid challenge because of the potential for producing pulmonary edema in patients with congestive heart failure or intrarenal failure, conditions which do not respond to volume expansion. Therefore, the rate of fluid challenge should be adjusted, and the patient should be carefully and repeatedly examined to reduce the risk of precipitating pulmonary edema according to the discretion of the treating physician.

IMAGING

Renal Ultrasonography and Doppler Flow Scanning

Ultrasonography should be performed whenever urinary tract obstruction is considered in the differential diagnosis of ARF. The test is readily available, noninvasive, accurate, reliable, and very reproducible. In some cases, such as ureteral encasement by tumor or fibrosis, ureteral and renal pelvis dilatation may not be detected by ultrasonography. Increased echogenicity of renal parenchyma is a common and nonspecific indicator of intrinsic renal disease. In some cases of ATN, renal parenchymal echogenicity may be normal. Absence of renal blood flow on Doppler scanning suggests complete thrombosis of the renal circulation.

Nuclear Scanning

Radionuclide imaging with ^{99m}Tc-labeled diethylenetriamine-pentaacetic acid or ^{131}I-labeled iodohippurate (^{131}I-Hippuran) can be used to assess renal blood flow and tubular function. Unfortunately, a marked delay in tubular excretion of nuclide occurs in both prerenal and intrarenal diseases; thus, this technique is of little value in the evaluation of most patients with ARF.

Computed Tomography and Magnetic Resonance Imaging

Computed tomography or magnetic resonance imaging may be useful in detecting parenchymal renal disease and obstructive uropathy. However, these modalities are of limited value and in most cases do not provide more information than Doppler flow scanning.

Renal Angiography

A renal angiogram is helpful in patients with ARF due to vascular disorders, including renal artery stenosis with ARF from angiotensin-converting enzyme inhibition, renal artery emboli, and aortic atherosclerosis with acute aortorenal occlusion, as well as in cases of systemic necrotizing vasculitides such as polyarteritis nodosa and Takayasu arteritis. However, due to contrast nephrotoxicity this modality has largely been replaced by duplex ultrasonography and magnetic resonance angiography in the evaluation of ARF.

Renal Biopsy

When clinical, biochemical, and noninvasive imaging studies are insufficient for diagnosis and management of ARF, a renal biopsy should be considered. Some studies show that the findings on biopsy in the setting of ARF are often unexpected. Renal biopsy is considered the "gold standard" for diagnostic accuracy in ARF, but in clinical practice, it is not often performed. An exception is biopsy of a renal transplant, which is performed relatively commonly in patients with ARF because of the need to exclude transplant rejection as the cause. Patients presenting with the clinical syndrome of rapidly progressive glomerulonephritis should undergo renal biopsy unless there is an overt contraindication. This condition is considered a medical emergency because effective kidney-preserving therapy may be available and should be instituted as soon as possible.

CHRONIC KIDNEY DISEASE

A greater appreciation for the prevalence of chronic kidney disease (CKD) in the population has resulted in improvements in identification and diagnosis of chronic kidney diseases leading to progressive renal failure and ESRD. The most common causes of CKD leading to ESRD are diabetes mellitus, hypertension, glomerulonephritis, and cystic kidney disease, which together account for 90% of all new cases of CKD. Patients with CKD typically present with nonspecific symptoms or are referred to a nephrologist because of an abnormal blood test or urinalysis. The key initial step in the evaluation of kidney disease is the differentiation of acute from chronic renal failure (see Table 1–1).

A careful history and thorough physical examination combined with routine laboratory testing and imaging are usually sufficient to differentiate between acute and chronic renal failure and can usually direct additional appropriate investigations to facilitate a diagnosis. Once this has been accomplished, further evaluation is needed to establish the following:

- The degree of renal impairment (determination of glomerular filtration rate [GFR])
- The presence of risk factors for progression
- Evaluation of comorbid cardiovascular risk factors
- Evaluation of secondary comorbidities (hyperparathyroidism/ anemia)
- Review of medication (avoid nephrotoxins/adjust dosages to GFR)

Kidney disease progresses toward the end stage in most patients with CKD. Several interventions have been demonstrated to slow the progression of renal disease, and late referral to a nephrologist is independently associated with worse patient outcomes. Therefore, early recognition, referral, and appropriate intervention are of paramount importance in slowing or preventing the development of ESRD.

Establishing Chronicity of Disease

Clinical History
In most patients with CKD symptoms have been present for months or years. No specific blood or urine test unequivocally differentiates acute from chronic kidney disease. Historical pointers to the presence of CKD include a history of urinary tract infections, passage of kidney stones, and nocturia. In advanced disease a common early sign of uremic encephalopathy is sleep disturbance and in particular reversal of the sleep-wake cycle. Subsequent loss of short-term memory, difficulty concentrating, and episodes of confusion occur as the disease approaches end stage, although the prescription of centrally acting medications (e.g., benzodiazepines) may precipitate such symptoms at a higher GFR. Because patients may be unaware of these abnormalities, the history should be supplemented by interviewing a family member whenever possible.

Specific inquiry should be routinely made about risk factors for CKD, including hypertension, diabetes mellitus, congestive heart failure, previous episodes of acute renal failure, known or suspected hepatitis B or C infection, and rheumatologic diseases. A previous history of urologic disorders or procedures may provide clues to the detection and diagnosis of obstructive and reflux nephropathies and congenital anomalies of the urinary tract. Abnormal findings on a urinalysis conducted as part of an entrance examination for an educational institution, military service, or other purposes should also be elicited by direct questioning. The presence of back pain or bone pain, particularly in an older patient with CKD, should raise the possibility of malignancy, especially multiple myeloma. A history of exposure to nephrotoxins is critical for establishing causes of CKD. Nephrotoxins take many forms, including prescription medication, over-the-counter drugs, and environmental substances. A long-standing history of ingestion of combination analgesic agents (e.g., phenacetin, acetaminophen, or aspirin) is important in establishing the diagnosis of analgesic nephropathy. Environmental exposure to lead, arsenic, mercury, or silicon or ingestion of certain herbal remedies (e.g., slimming regimens containing aristolochic acid) can lead to the diagnosis of CKD. Exposure to cancer chemotherapeutic agents, herbal remedies, lithium in patients with bipolar disorders, and cyclosporin in recipients of solid organ transplants can cause CKD. A history of recurrent urinary tract infection with flank pain, fever, polyuria, and nocturia suggests chronic pyelonephritis.

A family pedigree should be constructed for all patients to aid identification of autosomal dominant (e.g., autosomal dominant polycystic kidney disease), sex-linked (e.g., Fabry disease) and autosomal recessive (e.g., medullary cystic disease) diseases. A family history of anemia and sickle cell disease is important, particularly in African-American patients. A complete family history also has relevance for more common diseases, including diabetes and hypertension, because CKD arising from these conditions aggregates in families; indeed, up to 50% of patients will have one family member with CKD.

Physical Examination

The skin should be examined for excoriations due to uremic pruritus, which are often seen on the back, torso, and lower extremities. Vitiligo and periungual fibromas may be seen in tuberous sclerosis. Neurofibromas may be a clue to renal disease caused by underlying renal artery stenosis in patients with neurofibromatosis. Hyperpigmented macules in the pretibial skin are often observed in patients with cryoglobulinemic disease, and livedo reticularis may be observed in those with atherosclerotic ischemic nephropathy. A general sallow appearance (urochromic pallor) of the skin is also a common finding in patients with advanced CKD. Funduscopic examination may demonstrate vascular findings, such as microaneurysms and proliferative retinopathy characteristic of diabetic retinopathy. Arteriolar narrowing, arteriovenous nicking, hemorrhage, and exudates consistent with hypertension are also common. Less common findings that are more difficult to demonstrate on routine examination are anterior lenticonus and retinal flecks characteristic of Alport syndrome. Angioid streaks may be present in patients with Fabry disease. Ocular palsy may be present in patients with vasculitides (e.g., Wegener granulomatosis), and diffuse conjunctivitis is a sign of calcium-phosphorus deposition in CKD with secondary hyperparathyroidism.

High-tone sensorineural hearing loss is overt in about 50% of patients with Alport syndrome. Nasal and oropharyngeal ulcers may be present in those with active lupus nephritis. The presence of a perforated nasal septum should raise the suspicion for Wegener granulomatosis. Examination for carotid bruit as a manifestation of underlying atherosclerosis may also provide a clue to the presence of ischemic nephropathy as a cause of CKD.

Assessment of the cardiovascular and volume status is essential, because abnormal findings may require early and rapid intervention before completion of the evaluation for CKD. Cardiopulmonary examination for signs of volume overload is essential for the evaluation and management of CKD, because volume overload contributes to the development of hypertension, and many patients have will have developed hypertensive heart disease by the time of presentation (left ventricular hypertrophy and heart failure). Cardiac murmurs may be present in patients with endocarditis or atrial myxoma associated with glomerulonephritis.

Abdominal examination should include a search for palpable kidneys, as observed in polycystic kidney disease and tuberous sclerosis. A flank mass can be found in patients with retroperitoneal fibrosis, lymphoma, or other tumors that can obstruct the ureters. A palpable bladder or enlarged prostate gland suggests chronic urinary outlet obstruction. Musculoskeletal examination, including examination for edema, should be performed. Synovial thickening in the small joints of the hands may be seen in systemic lupus erythematosus and rheumatoid arthritis, both of which may be associated with CKD. Neurologic signs in patients with CKD include peripheral sensorimotor neuropathy and central nervous system manifestations. Generalized muscle weakness and diminished deep tendon reflexes are common.

Urinalysis

Urinalysis is not particularly useful for differentiating acute from chronic kidney disease. Similar findings, such as pyuria, hematuria, and proteinuria, can be seen in the two disorders. The presence of oval fat bodies in the urine, signifying high-grade proteinuria, implies a glomerular disease, as does the presence of dysmorphic red blood cells. Calcium oxalate crystals may be seen in the urine of patients with hereditary or secondary forms of oxalosis causing kidney disease. The presence of calcium phosphate and sodium urate crystals may signify previous stone disease as a cause of CKD. Triple phosphate crystals may suggest recurrent urinary tract infection and staghorn calculi as causes of CKD. As described later, proteinuria is an important finding in any patient with CKD.

Renal Osteodystrophy

Radiographic evidence for renal osteodystrophy is present in CKD but not in ARF. Elevated plasma parathyroid hormone concentrations can be present in both acute and chronic kidney disease but is not sufficient evidence for the diagnosis of osteodystrophy. Radiographs of the shoulders, ribs, hands, and pelvis illustrating signs of osteitis fibrosa cystica strongly suggest CKD; this finding is rarely if ever observed in ARF. A possible exception may be a patient with parathyroid adenoma in whom severe primary hyperparathyroidism may induce hypercalcemic ARF.

Renal Mensuration

The most sensitive and specific test for establishing the chronicity of kidney disease is measurement of renal size. Currently, renal ultrasonography is the technique of choice. The finding of small kidneys (i.e., small relative to body size) on renal ultrasonography is a reliable indicator of CKD. However, it is important to note that kidney size varies from individual to individual and between evaluation methods (e.g., computed tomography versus ultrasonography). In contrast to the finding of small kidneys as a sign of CKD, the finding of normal-size or large kidneys is a sensitive but not specific sign of acute kidney disease. That is, patients with acute kidney disease have normal or enlarged kidneys; however, normal or enlarged kidneys are also observed in many forms of CKD including human immunodeficiency virus nephropathy, diabetic nephropathy, and autosomal dominant polycystic kidney disease

Renal Biopsy

Renal biopsy is the most definitive method for differentiating acute from chronic kidney disease. A biopsy is used to establish the diagnosis, determine a treatment regimen, and collect prognostic information, and in some patients (e.g., those with systemic lupus erythematosus) track the clinical course of CKD. Histologic findings of chronicity include glomerulosclerosis, tubular atrophy, and interstitial fibrosis. The last finding is the best indicator of chronicity and best prognosticator of long-term outcome. Renal biopsy is a low-risk procedure in stable patients with CKD, including elderly patients.

Risk Factors for Chronic Kidney Disease

It is now recognized that a number of factors increase the risk for development of CKD (Table 1–5). Among the strongest factors associated with increased risk for CKD are diabetes mellitus and hypertension. Currently, nearly 50% of new cases of ESRD occur in diabetic patients and 27% in hypertensive patients. Additional clinical factors associated with increased risk for CKD are autoimmune disease, chronic systemic infection, urinary tract infection, obstruction of the urinary tract, cancer, family history, reduced renal mass, low birth weight, drug exposure, ethnicity, and recovery after ARF. Certain ethnic minorities have a markedly higher risk for CKD, including African Americans, Mexican Americans, Native Americans, Asians, and Pacific Islanders. Cigarette smoking has also been linked with development of CKD, as has dyslipidemia.

Definition and Staging of Chronic Kidney Disease

Chronic kidney disease is defined as kidney damage with or without decreased GFR, manifested as either pathologic abnormalities or markers of kidney damage, including abnormalities in

Table 1–5: Risk Factors for Chronic Kidney Disease

Established Risk Factors
  Age
  Sex (male predilection)
  Race (African American, Hispanic, Native American)
  High blood pressure
  Diabetes mellitus
  Proteinuria
  Family history of kidney disease
  Smoking
  Atherosclerosis
  Exposure to nephrotoxins such as analgesics, aristolochic acid, heavy metals
  Dyslipidemia
  Reduced nephron number at birth
  Recurrent urinary tract infection

composition of blood or urine, abnormalities in renal imaging findings, and a GFR less than 60 mL/min/1.73 m². Staging of CKD is based on an estimate of overall renal function by GFR (Table 1–6). Patients with CKD have an increased risk for both progression to ESRD and cardiovascular morbidity and mortality due to risk factors common to both progression of kidney disease and cardiovascular disease including diabetes, hypertension, and dyslipidemia. Therefore, management of risk factors is paramount in this patient population.

For further discussion of the evaluation of the GFR in CKD and evaluation and management of proteinuria, please see Chapter 2, Laboratory Assessment of Renal Disease: Clearance, Urinalysis, and Kidney Biopsy. For further discussion of the management of the patient with established CKD, please refer to the following relevant chapters: Chapter 24, Essential Hypertension; Chapter 28, Cardiovascular Aspects of Chronic Kidney Disease; Chapter 20, Diabetic Nephropathy; Chapter 30, Renal Osteodystrophy; Chapter 31, Nutritional Therapy in Renal Disease; and Chapter 27, Hematologic Consequences of Renal Disease.

Table 1–6: Staging of Chronic Kidney Disease

Stage	Description	Estimated GFR*	Evaluation Plan
	At increased risk	>90	Screening CKD in risk reduction
1	Kidney damage with normal or increased GFR	≥90	Diagnose and treat cause, slow progression, evaluate risk of cardiovascular disease
2	Kidney damage with mild decrease in GFR	60–89	Estimate progression
3	Moderate decrease in GFR	30–59	Evaluate and treat complications
4	Severe decrease in GFR	15–29	Prepare for renal replacement therapy
5	Kidney failure	<15	Initiate renal replacement therapy

*GFR = 186 • SCr$^{-1.154}$ • Age$^{-0.203}$ (0.742 for female and/or 1.210 for African Americans).

CKD, chronic kidney disease; GFR, glomerular filtration rate; SCr, serum creatinine level.

Laboratory Assessment of Kidney Disease: Clearance, Urinalysis, and Kidney Biopsy

2

DETECTION AND DIAGNOSIS OF KIDNEY DISEASE

No single test of the glomerular filtration rate (GFR) is ideally suited for every clinical application. Rather, the goal should be to select the most accurate and precise test to answer the question being addressed in the safest, most cost-effective, and most convenient manner possible in the population being studied. In clinical practice, tests of GFR are most commonly used for the following:

1. Screening for the presence of kidney disease.
2. Measuring disease progression to determine prognosis and effects of therapy.
3. Confirming the need for treatment of end-stage renal disease with dialysis or transplantation.
4. Estimating renal clearance of drugs to guide dosing.

The cost and inconvenience of 24-hour creatinine clearance determinations and radionuclide measurements of GFR ordinarily preclude their use for these screening purposes. Therefore, measurements of serum urea and creatinine have most often been used to screen for the presence of significant renal impairment.

Serum Creatinine

Serum creatinine is probably the most widely used indirect measure of GFR; its popularity is attributable to convenience and low cost. Creatinine is a metabolic product of creatine and phosphocreatine, which are both found almost exclusively in muscle. Thus, creatinine production is proportional to muscle mass and varies little from day to day. Age- and sex-associated differences in creatinine production are largely attributable to differences in muscle mass. Because production of creatinine is constant, the serum creatinine level depends on the rate of clearance, which mainly reflects the GFR. Unfortunately, serum creatinine is very insensitive to substantial declines in GFR early in the course of renal disease when enhanced tubular secretion can maintain the serum creatinine within the "normal" range. In addition, failure to consider variations in creatinine production due to differences in muscle mass often leads to misinterpretation of serum creatinine levels. This confusion may be compounded by the use of standard normal ranges for serum creatinine levels that appear on routine laboratory reports. For example, a serum creatinine value that occurs in the normal range may indicate an acceptable GFR in a young, healthy individual. However, the same serum creatinine value in an elderly individual could indicate a twofold reduction in GFR because of a comparably smaller muscle mass. Failure to remember the potential effects of tubular secretion on serum creatinine, especially in a patient with reduced kidney function, may lead the clinician to believe that kidney function is better than it actually is.

Creatinine Clearance

GFR is traditionally measured as the renal clearance of a particular substance, or marker, from plasma. The *clearance* of an indicator substance is the amount removed from plasma divided by the average plasma concentration over the time of measurement. If one assumes that there is no extrarenal elimination, tubular reabsorption, or tubular secretion of the marker, then GFR can be calculated as follows:

$$GFR = \frac{U \times V}{P \times T}$$

where U is the urine concentration of creatinine, V is the urine volume, and P is the average plasma concentration of creatinine over the time (T) of the urine collection. Measuring the creatinine clearance rate obviates some of the problems of using the serum creatinine concentration as a marker of GFR. Differences in steady-state creatinine production due to differences in muscle mass that affect serum creatinine level should not affect creatinine clearance. However, the reliability of the creatinine clearance measurement is greatly diminished by variability in tubular secretion of creatinine and by the inability of most patients to accurately collect timed urine samples. Prolonged storage of the urine sample can also introduce error because high temperature and low urine pH enhance the conversion of creatine to creatinine in stored urine. Therefore, urine samples should be refrigerated, and the urine creatinine level should be measured without undue delay.

Cimetidine-Enhanced Creatinine Clearance

In clinical studies, cimetidine, which blocks tubular secretion of creatinine, substantially improves the creatinine clearance estimate of GFR in patients with mild to moderate renal impairment. A cimetidine-enhanced creatinine clearance measurement requires little additional cooperation from the patient than is needed for a standard creatinine clearance measurement. Although it is not as accurate as other more costly methods for measuring GFR, the cimetidine-enhanced creatinine clearance measurement is a cost-effective alternative in many clinical situations.

Serum Creatinine Formulas to Estimate Kidney Function

Many attempts have been made to mathematically transform or correct the serum creatinine value so that it may more accurately reflect GFR (Table 2–1). The most widely used formula is that developed by Cockcroft and Gault. However, the formula does not take into account differences in creatinine production between individuals of the same age and sex or even in the same individual over time, and it systematically overestimates GFR in individuals who are obese or edematous. Moreover, it does not account for extrarenal elimination, tubular handling, or inaccuracies in the laboratory measurement of creatinine that can contribute to error in the serum creatinine estimate of GFR. Despite these drawbacks, use of the Cockcroft-Gault formula has remained widespread because of its readily available parameters and relative simplicity. In some clinical studies outpatient 24-hour urine collections and timed creatinine clearances offered no more precision than the Cockcroft-Gault formula.

Based on the results of isotopically measured GFR determinations from the Modification of Diet in Renal Disease (MDRD) study, the investigators derived a formula for estimating GFR using readily measurable clinical variables (see Table 2–1). The formula, sometimes referred to as the *MDRD equation*, uses serum chemistry values (creatinine, urea, and albumin) and patient characteristics (age, sex, and race) and gives a more accurate

Table 2–1: Formulas for Estimating Glomerular Filtration Rate Using Serum Creatinine and Other Clinical Parameters

Cockcroft-Gault formula

$$\text{Estimated creatinine clearance} = \frac{(140-\text{age})(\text{weight in kg})}{72 \times \text{PCr}} (\times 0.85 \text{ for women})$$

MDRD equation

$$\text{GFR} = 170 \times \text{PCr}^{-0.999} \times \text{Age}^{-0.176} \times \text{BUN}^{-0.170} \times \text{Alb}^{-0.318}$$

If the subject is black, multiply by 0.762. If the subject is female multiply by 0.762. To convert the Cockcroft-Gault formula to SI units simply omit the multiplication factor 72 from the denominator. Online calculation of the MDRD equation is available at http://www.nephron.com.

Alb, serum albumin (g/dL); BUN, blood urea nitrogen (mg/dL); PCr, plasma creatinine (mg/dL).

estimation of the GFR than the Cockcroft-Gault formula, at least in patients with moderate to advanced renal insufficiency. Despite concerns about the applicability of this equation to individuals not included in the MDRD trial (those with normal kidney function, elderly persons, and kidney transplant recipients), the National Kidney Foundation, as stated in their K/DOQI guidelines, considers the MDRD equation to be a reliable measure for GFR in adults. Online calculation of the MDRD equation is available at http://nephron.com

Plasma Urea

Urea is not an ideal marker of GFR, and the plasma urea concentration alone is a poor measure of GFR. The plasma urea, or blood urea nitrogen (BUN), concentration is affected by a number of factors other than alterations in GFR. Increased plasma levels caused by greater production are seen with elevated dietary protein intake, gastrointestinal bleeding, and tetracycline use. On the other hand, reduced levels of plasma urea can be seen in patients who abuse alcohol and have chronic liver disease. With a molecular weight of 60 D, urea is freely filtered at the glomerulus. However, it can be readily reabsorbed, and the amount of tubular reabsorption is variable. In states of actual or effective intravascular volume depletion, urea reabsorption, can be substantial.

Urea Clearance

Because of tubular urea reabsorption, renal urea clearance usually underestimates GFR. Urea clearance can be as little as one half or less of the GFR as measured by other techniques. However, the degree of underestimation of glomerular filtration is less in patients with markedly reduced kidney function, and because creatinine clearance overestimates GFR in this setting, a mean of creatinine and urea clearance has been suggested as a reasonable estimate of GFR in patients with advanced chronic kidney disease (CKD).

Radionuclide and Radiocontrast Markers of Glomerular Filtration Rate

Several radionuclide-labeled markers and unlabeled radiocontrast markers of GFR can be used in either renal or plasma clearance studies. Estimating GFR by plasma clearance of a single intravenous bolus injection of an indicator is convenient and has been used more often than constant infusion or renal clearance techniques. Basically, renal clearance is measured as the plasma clearance, or the amount of indicator injected divided by the integrated area of the plasma concentration curve over time. This requires a single bolus injection of the marker and at least two to three timed blood samples. The most widely used agents are technetium (Tc)-radiolabeled diethylenetriaminepentaacetic acid (^{125m}Tc-DTPA, and ^{99m}Tc-DTPA), radioiodinated iodohippurate (Hippuran), ^{123}I-*ortho*-iodohippurate, and ^{99m}Tc-mercaptoacetyltriglycine. The measurement of plasma clearance can also be achieved without plasma sampling. A gamma camera positioned over the kidneys can be used to measure renal elimination of a radioactive indicator. However, GFR determination obtained through quantitative renal imaging is not as precise as that determined through plasma sampling. The advantage of quantitative renal imaging is that additional information pertaining to the anatomy of kidney function can be obtained. Indeed, the "split function" or relative contribution to total GFR from each kidney can be calculated. This information can be important in the evaluation of some patients with renal vascular disease and can be crucial in certain circumstances (e.g., in deciding whether or not to carry out a unilateral nephrectomy).

All radionuclide markers are radioactive, and this feature has begun to erode their acceptance by patients and to mandate close monitoring by regulatory agencies. The actual amount of radiation delivered to a patient is less than the amount any patient receives while undergoing most standard radiologic procedures. However, the isotope is concentrated in the urine, so that exposure of the urinary collecting system may be greater. To alleviate this potential problem, patients are advised to maintain high fluid intake with high urine volume after the procedure. In an effort to avoid the use of radiolabeled compounds, techniques have been developed to use unlabeled radiocontrast agents to measure GFR. Radiocontrast agents have low molecular weight (600 to 1600 D), are not protein bound, are eliminated from plasma mainly by glomerular filtration, and can be measured by high-performance liquid chromatography. The main disadvantages of high-performance liquid chromatography are the expense, time, and labor needed to carry out the assay. A rapid and convenient method has been developed to measure relatively low concentrations of iodine with the use of x-ray fluorescence, and the method has been applied to the measurement of the plasma clearance of the radiocontrast agent iohexol.

URINALYSIS

Color

Urine may be almost colorless if the output is high and the concentration is low. Cloudy urine is generally the result of the presence of phosphates (usually normal) or leukocytes and bacteria (usually abnormal). Black urine is seen in alkaptonuria. Acute intermittent porphyria often causes dark urine. A number of exogenous chemicals and drugs can make urine green, but green urine may also be associated with *Pseudomonas* bacteriuria and urine bile pigments. The most common cause of red urine is hemoglobin. Red urine in the absence of red blood cells usually indicates either free hemoglobin or myoglobin. Finally, red-orange urine due to rifampin is one of the better-known drug effects.

Specific Gravity

Specific gravity is a convenient and rapidly obtained indicator of urine osmolality. It can be measured accurately with a refractometer or a hygrometer or more crudely estimated with a dipstick. The dipstick contains a polyionic polymer with binding sites saturated with hydrogen ions. The release of hydrogen ions when they are competitively replaced with urinary cations causes a change in the pH-sensitive indicator dye. Specific gravity values measured by dipstick tend to be falsely high at a urine pH value of less than 6 and falsely low if the pH is greater than 7. The effects of albumin, glucose, and urea on urine osmolality are not reflected by changes in the dipstick specific gravity. The normal range for specific gravity is 1.003 to 1.030, but values decrease with age as the kidney's ability to concentrate urine decreases. Self-monitoring of urine specific gravity may be useful for stone-forming patients, who benefit from maintaining a dilute urine.

Urine pH

Urine pH is usually measured with a reagent test strip. Most commonly, the double indicators methyl red and bromthymol blue are used in the reagent strips to give a broad range of colors at different pH values. In conjunction with other specific urine and plasma measurements, urine pH is often invaluable in diagnosing systemic acid-base disorders. By itself, however, urine pH provides little useful diagnostic information. The normal range for urine pH is 4.5 to 7.8. A very alkaline urine (pH > 7) suggests infection with a urea-splitting organism. Prolonged storage can lead to overgrowth of urea-splitting bacteria and a high urine pH. However, diet (vegetarian), diuretic therapy, vomiting, gastric suction, and alkali therapy can also cause a high urine pH. Low urine pH (pH < 5) is seen most commonly in metabolic acidosis. Acid urine is also associated with the ingestion of large amounts of meat.

Bilirubin and Urobilinogen

Only conjugated bilirubin is passed into the urine. Thus, the result of a reagent test for bilirubin is typically positive in patients with obstructive jaundice or jaundice due to hepatocellular injury, whereas it is usually negative in patients with jaundice due to hemolysis. In patients with hemolysis, however, the urine urobilinogen result is often positive. Reagent test strips are very sensitive to bilirubin, detecting as little as 0.05 mg/dL. False-positive test results for urine bilirubin can occur if the urine is contaminated with stool. Prolonged storage and exposure to light can lead to false-negative results.

Leukocyte Esterase and Nitrites

Dipstick screening for urinary tract infection has been recommended for high-risk individuals, but the issue is controversial. The esterase method relies on the fact that esterases released from lysed urine granulocytes cause a dye change on the strip. The result is usually interpreted as negative, trace, small, moderate, or large. In urine that is allowed to stand indefinitely, greater lysis of leukocytes occurs and a more intense reaction is seen. False-positive results can occur with vaginal contamination.

High levels of glucose, albumin, ascorbic acid, tetracycline, cephalexin, or cephalothin or large amounts of oxalic acid can inhibit the dye reaction.

Urinary bacteria convert nitrates to nitrites. The latter induce a dye change on the strip. Results are usually interpreted as positive or negative. High specific gravity and the presence of ascorbic acid may interfere with the test. False-positive results are common and may be due to low urine nitrate levels resulting from low dietary intake. It may take up to 4 hours to convert nitrate to nitrite, so inadequate bladder retention time can also cause false-negative results. Prolonged storage of the sample can lead to degradation of nitrites, another source of false-negative results. Finally, several potential urinary pathogens such as *Streptococcus faecalis*, other gram-positive organisms, *Neisseria gonorrhoeae*, and *Mycobacterium tuberculosis* do not convert nitrate to nitrite. Retrospective analysis of the available data suggests that the pairing of tests for both esterase and nitrates is the most accurate approach to screening for infection. However, when the likelihood of infection is high (e.g., when signs and symptoms are present), negative results on both tests are still inadequate to exclude infection. These tests, in combination with other clinical information, may be more useful in situations in which the likelihood of infection is low.

Glucose

Reagent strip measurement of the urine glucose level, once used to monitor diabetic therapy, has been almost completely replaced by more reliable methods that measure fingerstick blood glucose level. Most reagent strips detect levels of glucose as low as 50 mg/dL. Because the renal threshold for glucose is generally 160 to 180 mg/dL, the presence of detectable urine glucose indicates blood glucose values in excess of 210 mg/dL. Large quantities of ketones, ascorbate, and pyridinium metabolites may interfere with the color reaction, and urine peroxide contamination can cause false-positive results. Nevertheless, the appearance of glucose in the urine is a specific indicator of high serum glucose levels.

Ketones

Ketones (acetoacetate and acetone) are generally detected with the nitroprusside reaction. Ascorbic acid and phenazopyridine can give false-positive reactions. β-Hydroxybutyrate (often 80% of total serum ketones in ketosis) is not normally detected by the nitroprusside reaction. Ketones can appear in the urine, but not in serum, with prolonged fasting or starvation. Ketones may also be observed in the urine in alcoholic or diabetic ketoacidosis.

Hemoglobin and Myoglobin

Hematuria and contamination of the urine with menstrual blood produce a positive reaction on dipstick urinalysis. Myoglobin, oxidizing contaminants, and povidone iodine can cause false-positive reactions. Free hemoglobin is filtered at the renal glomerulus and thus appears in the urine when the capacity for plasma protein binding with haptoglobin is exceeded. Some of the hemoglobin is catabolized by the proximal tubules. The principle cause of increased serum and urine free hemoglobin levels is hemolysis. Rhabdomyolysis, on the other hand, yields myoglobin. A positive dipstick test result for hemoglobin in the absence of red blood cells in the urine sediment suggests either hemolysis or rhabdomyolysis.

Protein

Normal Physiology
The upper limit of normal total urine protein excretion in healthy adults is 150 to 200 mg/day. The upper limit of normal albumin excretion is 30 mg/day. Most urinary protein consists of Tamm-Horsfall protein, a glycoprotein that is formed on the epithelial surface of the thick ascending limb of the loop of Henle and early distal convoluted tubule. Disruption of the glomerular capillary wall barrier can lead to the filtration of a large amount of high molecular weight plasma proteins that overwhelm the limited capacity for tubular reabsorption and cause protein to appear in the urine, resulting in *glomerular proteinuria*. Another cause of proteinuria is tubular damage or dysfunction that inhibits the normal resorptive capacity of the proximal tubule, resulting in *tubular proteinuria* that generally consists of lower molecular weight proteins.

Techniques to Measure Urine Protein
Total protein concentration in urine can be rapidly estimated with chemically impregnated plastic strips. Most dipstick reagents contain a pH-sensitive colorimetric indicator that changes color when negatively charged proteins bind to it. However, positively charged proteins are less readily detected. Positively charged immunoglobulin light chains (myeloma), for example, may escape urine dipstick detection even when large amounts are

present in the urine. A very high urine pH (>7) can also give false-positive results, as can contamination of the urine with blood. The dipstick technique is sensitive to very small urine protein concentrations (the lower limit of detection is 10 to 20 mg/dL). However, at these low levels, the major constituent of urine protein may be Tamm-Horsfall protein, particularly when the urine volume is low and the concentration is high. When urine volume is high and the urine is maximally dilute, however, a relative large amount of protein can go undetected. Indeed, total protein excretion approaching 1 g/day may not be detected if urine output is high. Screening methods have been developed to measure albumin concentrations low enough to detect albumin excretion rates that are abnormal but are below the level of detection with standard reagent strips (i.e., in the microalbuminuria range, see later). In general, these albumin reagent strip tests are more sensitive than standard dipsticks, but they also have a relatively high rate of false-positive results.

Urine albumin concentrations can be quantified more accurately by a number of techniques including radioimmunoassay, immunoturbidimetry, laser nephelometry, or enzyme-linked immunosorbent assay. Protein can be measured in random samples, in timed or untimed overnight samples, or in 24-hour collections. Inaccurate urine collection is probably the greatest source of error in quantifying protein excretion in timed collections, particularly 24-hour collection. The adequacy of collection can be judged by performing a simultaneous measurement of urine creatinine excretion. For men aged 20 to 50 years, the normal range of creatinine excretion is 20 to 25 mg/kg/day (0.18 to 0.22 mmol/kg/day), and for women of the same age it is 15 to 20 mg/kg/day (0.13 to 0.18 mmol/kg/day). These values decline with age so that the normal ranges are approximately 20% to 25% lower in patients older than 60 years of age.

In an effort to correct for problems arising from variability in urine volume and concentration, many investigators have used the protein-to-creatinine or albumin-to-creatinine ratio in random or timed urine collections. There is a high degree of correlation between 24-hour urine protein excretion and protein-to-creatinine ratios in random, single-voided urine samples in patients with a variety of kidney diseases (i.e., a protein-to-creatinine ratio of 3 mg/mg indicates a protein excretion rate of 3 g/24 hr). Protein-to-creatinine ratios have been shown to predict declining kidney function in patients with nondiabetic CKD and are useful as both screening devices and as longitudinal tests for following the level of proteinuria. Although protein-to-creatinine or albumin-to-creatinine ratios may be more quantitative than a simple dipstick screening procedure, their use has a number of limitations. For example, obtaining protein-to-creatinine or albumin-to-creatinine ratios on first-void morning samples may underestimate 24-hour protein excretion because of the reduction in proteinuria that normally occurs at night. Storage time and temperature may also affect albumin levels in urine, and specimens should be analyzed as soon as possible after collection. Urine creatinine concentration is extremely variable, so that very different ratios can be obtained in individuals with similar protein excretion rates. Despite these limitations, the urine protein-to-creatinine or albumin-to-creatinine ratio may be useful, especially in individuals for whom urine collection is difficult or impossible.

Applications of Urine Protein Measurement

SCREENING FOR KIDNEY DISEASE   Although urine protein measurement can be used to assist in the diagnosis of kidney disease and to assess disease progression and response to therapy (discussed later), it is most commonly used as a screening test. Microalbuminuria is currently defined as urine albumin excretion of 30 to 300 mg/day and appears to be an important risk factor for end-organ damage in patients with diabetes or hypertension. In most studies showing a relationship between microalbuminuria and end-organ damage, 24-hour quantitative techniques have been used to measure urine albumin excretion. As alluded to earlier, these techniques are cumbersome and prone to error. To overcome these problems, an albumin-to-creatinine ratio in an untimed urine specimen can be used. A value greater than 30 mg/g (or 0.03 mg/mg) suggests that albumin excretion is greater than 30 mg/day and therefore that microalbuminuria is probably present. Indeed, albumin-to-creatinine ratios have been shown to predict the subsequent development of overt kidney disease.

The appropriate manner in which to use various tests to screen for kidney disease in the general population has not been extensively investigated. Because the number of false-positive results of dipstick tests for protein excretion is high, a positive result should probably be followed by tests designed to more accurately quantitate urine protein excretion. However, in some clinical circumstances, the likelihood that a positive dipstick test result for urine protein excretion indicates CKD is so low that the screening test should be repeated at a later date before more costly quantitation procedures are undertaken. Fever can cause tubular and glomerular proteinuria that usually disappears when the fever resolves. Congestive heart failure and seizures can also cause transient proteinuria. Light or strenuous exercise is often associated with urine protein excretion that resolves spontaneously. Posture can cause a rise in urine protein excretion in otherwise normal individuals. Postural proteinuria usually does not exceed 1 g/24 hr. It is usually diagnosed through detection of protein excretion during the day that is absent in a first-void morning sample. Patients with postural proteinuria have been shown to have an excellent long-term prognosis.

DIAGNOSIS AND PROGNOSIS Proteinuria can be caused by systemic overproduction (e.g., multiple myeloma with Bence Jones proteinuria), tubular dysfunction (e.g., Fanconi syndrome), or glomerular dysfunction. It is important to identify patients in whom the proteinuria is a manifestation of substantial glomerular disease as opposed to patients who have benign transient or postural (orthostatic) proteinuria.

Isolated proteinuria is a mild transient proteinuria that typically accompanies physiologically stressful conditions, including fever, exercise, and congestive heart failure.

Orthostatic proteinuria is defined by the absence of proteinuria while the patient is in a recumbent posture and its appearance during upright posture, especially during exercise. It is most common in adolescents. The total amount of protein excretion in a 24-hour period is generally less than 1 g. The diagnosis is made by comparing the protein excretion in two 12-hour urine collections, one recumbent and one during ambulation. Importantly, patients should be recumbent for at least 2 hours before their ambulatory collection is completed to avoid the possibility of contamination of the "recumbent" collection by urine formed during ambulation. The diagnosis of orthostatic proteinuria requires that protein excretion during recumbency be less than 50 mg during those 8 hours. Patients should be followed on an annual basis until the proteinuria resolves, and the long-term prognosis is typically excellent.

Fixed proteinuria is present whether the patient is upright or recumbent. The proteinuria disappears in some patients, whereas others have a more ominous glomerular lesion that portends an adverse long-term outcome. The prognosis depends on the persistence and severity of the proteinuria. If proteinuria disappears, it is less likely that the patient will develop hypertension or a reduced GFR. These patients must be evaluated periodically for as long as the proteinuria persists.

Plasma cell dyscrasias can produce monoclonal proteins, immunoglobulin, free light chains, and combinations of these.

Light chains are filtered at the glomerulus and may appear in the urine as Bence Jones protein. The detection of urine immunoglobulin light chains can be the first clue to a number of important clinical syndromes associated with plasma cell dyscrasias that involve the kidney. Unfortunately, urine immunoglobulin light chains may not be detected by reagent strip tests for protein. However, plasma cell dyscrasias may also manifest as proteinuria or albuminuria when the glomerular deposition of light chains causes disruption of the normally impermeable capillary wall. The diagnosis of a plasma cell dyscrasia can be entertained when a tall, narrow band on electrophoresis suggests the presence of a monoclonal γ-globulin or immunoglobulin light chain. However, monoclonal proteins are best detected with serum and urine immunoelectrophoresis.

Formed Elements

Urine Microscopy Methods

A midstream, "clean-catch" specimen should be collected when possible; the patient should be instructed to retract the foreskin or labia. A high urine concentration and a low urine pH help preserve formed elements. Thus, a first-void morning specimen, which is most likely to be acidic and concentrated, should be used whenever possible. Strenuous exercise and bladder catheterization can cause hematuria, and urine specimens collected to detect hematuria should not be obtained under these conditions. Urine should be examined as soon as possible after collection to avoid lysis of the formed elements and bacterial overgrowth. The specimen should not be refrigerated, because lowering the temperature causes the precipitation of phosphates and urates.

It is helpful to first measure the urine specific gravity and pH to judge the density of formed elements according to the concentration and acidity of the specimen. Specimens from concentrated and acidic urine may be expected to have a greater density of formed elements than dilute and alkaline specimens from the same patients. Urine should be centrifuged at approximately 2000 rpm for 5 to 10 minutes. The supernatant should be carefully poured off, the pellet resuspended by gentle agitation, and a drop placed on a slide under a coverslip.

Most commonly, urine is examined with an ordinary bright-field microscope. However, polarized light can be used to identify anisotropic crystals, and phase-contrast microscopy can enhance the contrast of cell membranes (×400).

Hematuria

Gross hematuria may first be detected as a change in urine color. Microscopic hematuria can be identified by dipstick methodology, microscopic examination, or both. Even when the urine is red or when a dipstick screening test result is positive, the sediment should be examined to determine whether red blood cells are present. The presence of other pigments, such as free hemoglobin and myoglobin, can masquerade as hematuria. An occasional red blood cell can be seen in normal individuals, but generally only one or two cells per high-power field are seen. The differential diagnosis of hematuria is broad but for practical purposes can be categorized as originating in either the upper or lower urinary tract. Hematuria that is accompanied by red blood cell casts, marked proteinuria, or both is most likely of glomerular origin. Red blood cells originating in glomeruli have been reported to have a distinctive dysmorphic appearance that is most readily seen with phase-contrast microscopy.

The differential diagnosis of hematuria is broad (Table 2–2). Kidney vascular causes include arterial and venous thrombosis, arteriovenous malformations, arteriovenous fistula, and the nutcracker syndrome (compression of the left renal vein between the aorta and superior mesenteric artery). Most patients undergoing anticoagulant therapy who have hematuria can be found to have an underlying cause, especially if the hematuria is macroscopic. However, excessive anticoagulation or other coagulopathies can themselves be associated with hematuria.

A reasonable approach to the patient with asymptomatic hematuria is to first obtain a thorough history and perform a complete physical examination. Red blood cell casts, significant proteinuria, or both may suggest a glomerular source for the hematuria. For the patient in whom glomerular proteinuria is likely, a kidney biopsy may yield the diagnosis. If the source of proteinuria is not evident from the history, physical examination, or urinalysis, renal ultrasonography is probably a reasonable next step. In the young patient (e.g., younger than 40 years) in whom renal ultrasonography findings are normal and who otherwise has a low risk for uroepithelial malignancy, the next step can be 24-hour urine collection to exclude hypercalciuria and hyperuricuria. If the urinalysis tests are normal, it is reasonable to observe the patient without further evaluation. However, some patients may wish to undergo kidney biopsy to better understand the prognosis. Patients who are older than 40 years, have risk factors for uroepithelial malignancies or both should undergo an intravenous pyelogram and possibly cystoscopy, in addition to renal ultrasonography.

Table 2–2: Common Sources of Hematuria

Vascular
- Coagulation abnormalities
- Excessive anticoagulation
- Arterial emboli or thrombosis
- Arteriovenous malformation
- Arteriovenous fistula
- Nutcracker syndrome
- Renal vein thrombosis
- Loin-pain hematuria syndrome (vascular?)

Glomerular
- IgA nephropathy
- Thin basement membrane diseases (including Alport syndrome)
- Other causes of primary and secondary glomerulonephritis

Interstitial
- Allergic interstitial nephritis
- Analgesic nephropathy
- Renal cystic diseases
- Acute pyelonephritis
- Tuberculosis
- Renal allograft rejection

Uroepithelium
- Malignancy
- Vigorous exercise
- Trauma
- Papillary necrosis
- Cystitis/urethritis/prostatitis (usually caused by infection)
- Parasitic diseases (e.g., schistosomiasis)
- Nephrolithiasis or bladder calculi

Multiple sites or source unknown
- Hypercalciuria
- Hyperuricosuria
- Sickle cell disease

Leukocyturia

More than one white cell per high-power field can be considered abnormal. The differential diagnosis of leukocyturia is broad. The presence of proteinuria or casts suggests a glomerular source. Most often, leukocytes in the urine are polymorphonuclear. However, it should not be assumed that all urinary leukocytes are neutrophils. The presence of non-neutrophil white blood cells in the urine, for example, eosinophils, can sometimes be an important diagnostic clue. Although the true sensitivity and specificity of urinary eosinophils for detecting different clinical kidney diseases are unclear, eosinophiluria has been associated with a variety of other renal diseases including acute interstitial nephritis, infection, acute tubular necrosis, atheroembolism, and glomerulonephritis.

Other Cells

It is difficult to identify the origin of cells that are neither leukocytes nor red blood cells without special stains. Squamous epithelial cells are probably the most common; these are shed from the bladder or urethra and are rarely pathologic. Renal tubular cells may appear whenever tubular damage has occurred. Transitional epithelial cells are rare but may be seen in patients with collecting system infections or neoplasia.

Urine Fat

In the absence of contamination, urinary lipids are almost always pathologic. Lipids usually appear as free fat droplets or oval fat bodies. They have a distinctive appearance but are most readily seen under polarized light as doubly refractile "Maltese crosses." Urinary lipids are most commonly associated with proteinuria and are particularly common in patients with the nephrotic syndrome. Urine fat can also be seen in bone marrow or fat embolization syndromes.

Casts

Casts are cylindrical bodies that are several-fold larger than leukocytes and red blood cells. They form in distal tubules and collecting ducts where Tamm-Horsfall glycoprotein precipitates and entraps cells present in the urinary space. Dehydration and the resulting increased tubular fluid concentration favor the formation of casts. The differential diagnosis of cast formation is aided by considering the type of cast found. Hyaline or finely granular casts can be seen in normal individuals and provide little useful diagnostic information. Cellular casts are generally more helpful. Red blood cell casts are distinctive and indicate glomerular disease. White blood cell casts are most commonly associated with interstitial nephritis but can also be seen in glomerulonephritis. Casts made up of renal tubular epithelial cells are always indicative of tubular damage. Coarsely granular casts often result from the degeneration of different cellular casts and their presence is usually pathologic, but nonspecific. Waxy casts are also nonspecific. They are believed to result from the degeneration of cellular casts and, thus, can be seen in a variety of kidney diseases. Pigmented casts usually derive their distinctive color from bilirubin or hemoglobin and are found in hyperbilirubinemia or hemoglobinuria, respectively.

Crystals and Other Elements

A large variety of crystals can be seen in the urine sediment. Most result from urine concentration, acidification, and ex vivo cooling of the sample and have little pathologic significance. However, an experienced observer can gain useful information about patients with microhematuria, nephrolithiasis, or toxin ingestion by examining a freshly voided, warm specimen. For example, a large number of calcium oxalate crystals suggest ethylene glycol toxicity when seen in the right clinical setting. Calcium oxalate crystals are uniform, small, double pyramids that often appear as crosses in a square. Calcium phosphate crystals, on the other hand, are usually narrow rectangular needles, often clumped in a flower-like configuration. Uric acid crystals are reddish brown and rectangular or rhomboidal and are also often seen in flower-like clumps. Calcium magnesium ammonium pyrophosphate (so-called triple phosphate) crystals form domed rectangles that take on the appearance of coffin lids.

Microorganisms

The most common cause of bacteria in the urine is contamination, particularly in specimens that have been improperly collected. The concomitant presence of leukocytes, however, suggests infection. Fungal elements can also be seen, especially in women. Like bacteria, fungi can be contaminants or pathogens. The most common protozoan seen in the urine is *Trichomonas vaginalis*. Urinary parasites are generally not seen in the urine sediment. In Africa and the Middle East, however, *Schistosoma haematobium* is common.

KIDNEY BIOPSY

Indications

At present, no specific clinical indications mandate the use of a kidney biopsy, and its utility must be taken in the context of the patients' needs in terms of diagnosis, prognosis, and therapy. Nonetheless, there are clinical settings in which kidney biopsy is likely to be useful. These include the following.

Nephrotic Syndrome

A renal biopsy is indicated for the investigation of all cases of the nephrotic syndrome with two exceptions:

- Children with the idiopathic nephrotic syndrome. Minimal change glomerulopathy, which is sensitive to steroid therapy, accounts for nearly 80% of cases of the syndrome in children.

- Diabetic patients for whom the history and urinalysis are consistent with a diagnosis of diabetic nephropathy (e.g., diabetes mellitus for > 10 years, inactive urinary sediment, and normal renal ultrasound studies).

Non-nephrotic Proteinuria

The value of renal biopsy in the setting of lesser degrees of proteinuria (< 2 g) is less certain. Many of these patients will have either focal segmental glomerulosclerosis or membranous nephropathy. However, at this degree of proteinuria, immunosuppressive treatment would not be contemplated and nonspecific measures to reduce proteinuria (angiotensin-converting enzyme inhibition) can be instituted without reference to renal histologic findings. Indications to proceed with a biopsy include evidence of a fall in the GFR, worsening proteinuria, or evidence of a systemic process (e.g., vasculitis, systemic lupus erythematosus, or multiple myeloma).

Nephritic Syndrome/Rapidly Progressive Glomerulonephritis

In patients with clinical and urinary sediment findings consistent with either the nephritic syndrome or rapidly progressive glomerulonephritis, a kidney biopsy provides invaluable information for determining the treatment options and prognosis. Some authorities have suggested that the clinical presentation of rapidly progressive glomerulonephritis in the setting of circulating antineutrophil cytoplasmic or anti–glomerular basement membrane antibodies is sufficient grounds to initiate immunosuppressive therapy. However, at present most clinicians consider the finding of circulating antineutrophil cytoplasmic or anti–glomerular basement membrane antibodies not sufficient alone to initiate therapy in the absence of histologic confirmation.

Isolated Hematuria

Patients with isolated hematuria should be closely evaluated to exclude extrarenal causes such as uroepithelial malignancy in patients with known risk factors or age older than 40 years. The underlying differential diagnosis of isolated hematuria in this setting includes thin basement membrane disease and immunoglobulin A nephropathy. In the absence of proteinuria, most clinicians forgo renal biopsy because the prognosis is typically excellent.

Post-transplantation Biopsy

Biopsy of the transplanted kidney has been established as an important diagnostic and therapeutic technique in the management of patients in whom rejection of the kidney allograft is suspected. It has become particularly important in an era when the differential diagnosis of decreased allograft function includes nephrotoxicity from the immunosuppressive drugs that are most commonly used. Two cores (obtained with a 15-gauge needle) are needed to avoid missing moderate or severe acute rejection in 10% of patients. Although the most common diagnosis resulting from kidney allograft biopsy is acute rejection, biopsies also play a role in determining the cause of proteinuria and chronic allograft dysfunction. Biopsy findings, particularly the amount of interstitial fibrosis, are useful in predicting the long-term function of the transplanted kidney independent of the underlying cause of kidney damage.

Other Indications

There does not appear to be any indication for a kidney biopsy in patients with chronic, end-stage renal failure, and biopsy in this setting is probably associated with a higher risk of complications. In patients with acute renal failure in whom no obvious cause for rapid deterioration in kidney function can be found, kidney biopsy may be indicated. Biopsy in this setting appears valuable mostly for those few patients with acute allergic interstitial nephritis, in whom a course of corticosteroids may be of benefit. Acute renal failure without the typical clinical presentation caused by cholesterol emboli has been more commonly observed in older patients with atherosclerotic disease, presenting a diagnostic challenge. Because some of these patients may regain kidney function after prolonged intervals, closer attention to kidney function during dialysis is appropriate. However, a clear-cut case for the utility of a kidney biopsy for diagnosis, prognosis, or therapy has not been made in patients with acute renal failure.

Patient Preparation

Before biopsy, the patient should be evaluated for conditions that may raise the risk or worsen the consequences of complications. Postbiopsy bleeding can necessitate nephrectomy, and the consequences of this complication are obviously greater in patients with only one functioning kidney. The use of 18-gauge, automated needles and direct ultrasonographic visualization has reduced the risk of biopsy, and biopsy of a solitary kidney is no longer absolutely contraindicated. Most clinicians consider the biopsy of a very small, shrunken kidney to be ill-advised.

Because bleeding is the major complication of biopsy, a platelet count, prothrombin time, and partial thromboplastin time (and possibly a bleeding time if the patient is uremic) should be obtained in all patients before biopsy. The most commonly encountered abnormality is a prolonged bleeding time caused by uremic platelet dysfunction. This can be reversed by the use of 0.3 mcg of 1-deamino-8-D-arginine vasopressin/kg body weight diluted in saline and infused slowly over 15 to 30 minutes. Salicylates or nonsteroidal anti-inflammatory drugs should be discontinued for at least 1 week before and after biopsy. For patients with a bleeding diathesis or those undergoing anticoagulation for a thromboembolic disorder, the accepted approach is not clear. Guidelines devised for the management of patients receiving anticoagulation therapy before and after elective surgery are of uncertain relevance to a kidney biopsy, a closed procedure in which the level of hemostasis cannot be determined. Suspending anticoagulation or treating the diathesis is feasible, although many investigators recommend open biopsy with direct visualization of the kidney. Alternatively, transjugular kidney biopsy has been successfully performed in some institutions. Significant anemia that would substantially increase the risk of bleeding should be corrected before a kidney biopsy is performed. Uncontrolled hypertension can raise the risk of bleeding after biopsy. Therefore, it is advisable to control blood pressure before the procedure is undertaken (<140/80 mm Hg). Having the patient void immediately before the biopsy may help reduce the risk of inadvertent puncturing of the bladder. Because a major complication of biopsy can require surgical intervention, it may be advisable to carry out the procedure with the patient fasting to reduce the potential risks of vomiting and aspiration during anesthesia induction. However, these risks must be weighed against the risk of hypoglycemia in diabetic patients and the rarity of complications requiring surgical intervention.

Needle Selection

With automated, spring-loaded biopsy devices significantly larger samples can be collected than with manual devices using comparable gauged needles. There is a significant correlation between needle gauge and sample size, with 14-gauge needles providing the largest number of glomeruli per core and, thus, the greatest diagnostic success compared with 16-gauge and 18-gauge needles. The complication rates for the three types of needles are not significantly different.

Complications

Microscopic hematuria occurs in virtually in all patients, whereas gross hematuria occurs in less than 10% of patients.

The presence of uncontrolled hypertension or azotemia increases the risk of overt hematuria. It usually resolves spontaneously in 48 to 72 hours, although in approximately 0.5% of patients, it persists for 2 to 3 weeks. Transfusions are necessary in 0.1% to 3% of patients. Surgery for persistent bleeding is required in less than 0.3% of patients. Perinephric hematomas occur commonly but are usually clinically silent. In 1% to 2% of patients, perinephric hematoma manifests as flank pain and swelling associated with signs of volume contraction and a decrease in hematocrit. Rarely, these hematomas can become infected, requiring antibiotic therapy and surgical drainage. Less common complications of kidney biopsy include arteriovenous fistulas, aneurysms, and infection. A number of unusual complications of kidney biopsy have been reported, including ileus, lacerations of other abdominal organs, pneumothorax, ureteral obstruction, and dissemination of carcinoma. The mortality rate is approximately 0.12%.

Radiologic Assessment of the Kidney

3

In the last two decades, spurred by the explosive growth of technology, the approach to imaging of the kidneys has undergone significant change. These developments have improved renal diagnostic evaluation, facilitated interventional approaches for diagnosis and treatment, and refined the assessment of therapeutic results. To derive the most benefit from this vast array of imaging options, to avoid duplication, and to achieve the best results efficiently, one must understand the advantages and limitations of each modality.

ACUTE RENAL FAILURE

Although renal obstruction is an uncommon cause of acute renal failure (ARF) (<5% of cases), it is potentially curable and can be surgically corrected if it is identified early. Therefore, it is imperative that it be excluded in patients with ARF. It is difficult to identify urinary obstruction clinically; therefore, radiologic evaluation is necessary. In the past intravenous contrast studies were used, but the nephrotoxic effects of radiocontrast media and a poor diagnostic yield led to the widespread use of ultrasonography (US).

Ultrasonography

US is accurate in detecting hydronephrosis; its sensitivity is estimated to be 90% to 100%. *Hydronephrosis* is a descriptive term that denotes dilation of the collecting system. It may be caused by obstruction, high-output urine flow, or nonobstructive conditions such as vesicoureteral reflux, postobstructive renal atrophy, and congenital megacalyces. Although the morphologic display is excellent on US, the detection of hydronephrosis is not pathognomonic of urinary tract obstruction, and the severity of hydronephrosis does not always correlate with the severity of renal failure. In addition hydronephrosis may not be apparent early in the course (<24 hours) of acute obstructive nephropathy.

Computed Tomography

Although US is the principal modality for evaluation of obstructive nephropathy in patients with ARF, computed tomography (CT) is advantageous when the use of US is technically limited. The dilated, fluid-filled renal pelvis and proximal ureter can be clearly demonstrated on nonenhanced CT scans, and scrutiny of sequential transverse sections allows identification of the site of ureteral obstruction, whether it is due to a stone, neoplasm, or fibrosis. Retroperitoneal or pelvic tumors and ureteral calculi are reliably demonstrated by CT. If residual renal function is present, contrast-enhanced scans show the pattern of a delayed and prolonged nephrogram familiar from conventional urography, albeit at the risk of inducing contrast nephropathy.

Magnetic Resonance Imaging

A significant advance in uroradiologic imaging is magnetic resonance urography (MRU). MRU is useful for evaluating both the dilated and the nondilated urinary tract, even in patients with impaired renal function. An injection of furosemide (Lasix) combined with gadolinium administration is important for increased excretion and good distribution of contrast media in the collecting system to improve image quality. A sufficient urographic effect is regularly obtained up to a serum creatinine level of 2 mg/dL. An advantage of MRU is the ability to evaluate the cause of obstruction when it cannot be determined with intravenous urography (IVU) because a high-grade obstruction prevents contrast excretion. MRU can also demonstrate collecting system morphology independent of excretory function. MRU has allowed diagnosis of a dilated urinary tract and determination of the level of obstruction with sensitivity and specificity of 100%.

Because urine has a low signal intensity on T1-weighted images, ureteral dilation and renal pelvic dilation can be readily seen on these images. The distended ureter can be differentiated from other structures, and the site of the obstruction can be located by evaluating sequential contiguous images. In addition, it is possible to detect infected urine in the dilated collecting system. The presence of pus changes urine characteristics on T1-weighted images: infected urine has a higher than normal signal intensity. The cause of an obstruction—pelvic tumor, lymphadenopathy, or retroperitoneal fibrosis—can also be identified. The appearance of the obstructed kidney varies, depending on the "age" of the obstruction. With acute or subacute obstruction, the kidney may appear normal, or the tissue contrast between the cortex and medulla on T1-weighted images may decrease. With chronic obstruction, however, it is no longer possible to differentiate the cortex from the medulla. The kidney is often smaller, and the cortex demonstrates decreased signal intensity on T2-weighted images.

MEDICAL RENAL DISEASE

The role of radiology in diagnosing medical renal disease is limited. Because IVU studies may trigger acute on chronic renal failure and are limited by insufficient contrast excretion in chronic kidney disease, they do not have any role in the evaluation of a patient with chronic kidney disease. US and CT are helpful to the extent that they demonstrate morphologic findings, such as symmetrically small kidneys or altered echogenicity (on US), both of which indicate pathologic changes. Magnetic resonance imaging (MRI) demonstrates loss of corticomedullary differentiation as an indicator of renal disease, but this finding, too, is nonspecific.

Ultrasonography

Diagnostic US allows the assessment of kidney size and cortical thickness and evaluation of cortical echogenicity. Cortical echogenicity can be graded as normal (grade 0) when it is less than that of the adjacent liver. It is judged as grade I when the amplitude of the cortical echoes equals that of the liver, grade II when it is greater than that of the liver but less than that of the renal sinus, and grade III when the echogenicity of the renal parenchyma is markedly increased and approaches that of renal sinus fat. A significant correlation has been found between cortical echogenicity and the prevalence of global sclerosis, focal tubule atrophy, and the number of hyaline casts per glomerulus. Although cortical echogenicity corresponds to the severity of histopathologic changes, it does not allow specific pathologic diagnosis.

Computed Tomography

The role of CT in the evaluation of medical renal disease, like that of US, is limited to the demonstration of morphologic findings, including symmetrically small kidneys, often with abundant hilar fat. CT is helpful in the evaluation of patients with medical renal disease who routinely receive hemodialysis and therefore have an increased risk for both benign (cystic metaplasia) and malignant renal neoplasms. Poor renal function hampers CT diagnosis by negating the benefit of contrast enhancement.

Magnetic Resonance Imaging

MRI demonstrates a number of abnormalities associated with a variety of medical renal diseases, but these findings are also nonspecific. Although loss of corticomedullary differentiation is a sensitive indicator of renal disease, it is a nonspecific finding and provides no information on the cause of the renal damage. In addition to renal parenchymal disease, conditions such as renal vein thrombosis (RVT), diffuse infiltrative involvement in leukemia, and, rarely, lymphoma may cause loss of the corticomedullary boundary.

RENAL VEIN THROMBOSIS

RVT is a recognized, but often silent, complication of the nephrotic syndrome. Renal venography is considered the definitive study for the diagnosis of RVT. Selective renal venography, however, is an invasive and costly procedure not suitable for screening an asymptomatic population with a high risk for RVT. Cross-sectional imaging modalities—Doppler US, contrast-enhanced CT, and MRI—have largely replaced invasive venography. With cross-sectional imaging modalities, the diagnosis of this condition depends on the demonstration of a widened renal vein containing the thrombus, thrombus extension into the inferior vena cava, ipsilateral renal enlargement, thickened Gerota fascia, and formation of pericapsular venous collaterals. Although the accuracy of CT for diagnosing RVT is excellent, it requires the use of iodinated contrast medium and hence has an associated risk of contrast nephropathy not observed with either Doppler US or contrast-enhanced magnetic resonance venography. The US findings indicative of RVT are a swollen, rounded kidney and relatively hypoechoic parenchyma compared with the normal renal parenchyma. Contrast-enhanced magnetic resonance venography is emerging as an excellent imaging modality in this setting.

RENAL HYPERTENSION

The role of gray-scale US in renovascular hypertension is limited to evaluation of kidney size. With Doppler US, evaluation of renal artery stenosis is possible, although results vary. If the proximal renal arteries are not identified with color-flow Doppler US, normal velocity and morphology of the waveform obtained from intrarenal arteries make it possible to rule out renal artery occlusion and most severe stenoses (reduction in luminal diameter > 80%). Although a good correlation has been reported between renal hilar Doppler US and angiographic findings in the diagnosis of renal artery stenosis, a number of limitations exist. Doppler US is operator dependent, and for a substantial proportion of patients, especially obese ones, it is technically inadequate. Furthermore, the value of this modality is limited in the presence of multiple renal arteries, distal arterial stenoses, and renal artery occlusion, which are sources of false-negative diagnoses. Considering its strengths and limitations, US appears to have limited value in screening of hypertensive patients for renal artery stenosis.

Helical CT and multidetector helical CT angiography are now often used in this setting. CT angiography has more than 90% sensitivity and specificity for identifying renal artery stenoses, and angiography data can be reconstructed to provide three-dimensional visualization of the renal vessels. Because it requires iodinated contrast medium, CT angiography has limited value in patients with impaired renal function.

Gadolinium-enhanced three-dimensional magnetic resonance angiography (MRA) is a reliable and well-established technique for identification of renal artery stenosis. An advantage of MRA is that it uses gadolinium-chelate contrast medium rather than an iodinated medium. Several studies have shown that MRA can detect renal artery stenosis with sensitivity and specificity of more than 90%. MRA also has the potential to depict collateral vessels in patients with renal artery occlusion. Because it is the most accurate technique for detecting proximal renal artery stenoses, MRA is most useful for patients with stenoses at the ostium or proximal artery. MRA also can be used to evaluate patients with fibromuscular dysplasia; however, because these patients may have distal renal artery stenosis, this modality may be less useful for evaluating fibromuscular dysplasia than for evaluating atherosclerotic lesions.

Captopril renography can detect renal artery stenoses greater than 50% with sensitivity and specificity as high as 90% in screened populations of hypertensive patients. This technique uses computer-assisted quantitative evaluation of a technetium-99m renogram augmented by administration of 25 to 50 mg of oral captopril. The action of captopril, an angiotensin-converting enzyme inhibitor, can unmask renal artery stenosis, which may appear normal on standard renograms. Intra-arterial digital subtraction angiography (DSA) has now been perfected and is performed as an outpatient procedure with smaller catheters and half the dose of contrast material used in conventional angiography. This makes the procedure safer and less painful. Furthermore, selective injection of renal arteries allows better demonstration of detail. The definitive diagnostic procedure for renal hypertension is arterial DSA, plus assays of venous renin when appropriate. Owing to the invasive nature and expense of DSA, however, most institutions reserve this modality for (1) patients in whom noninvasive tests are not diagnostic or (2) when transluminal angioplasty is being contemplated. When a stenosis is deemed significant, angioplasty and stenting can be performed during the same procedure. (For a further discussion of this topic see Chapter 24, Renovascular Hypertension and Ischemic Nephropathy.)

INFECTIONS

Intravenous Urography

In renal infection, IVU may show enlargement of the kidney, a striated nephrogram, delayed excretion of contrast material, and either a spidery appearance of the collecting system (due to interstitial edema) or a dilated collecting system (when a urinary obstruction is also present). Calyceal distortion due to stricture has been reported in patients with renal tuberculosis. Despite these findings, IVU is not a sensitive modality for evaluating renal infection, and 75% of patients with proven renal infection have been reported to have normal IVU findings.

Ultrasonography

The sonographic appearance of renal inflammatory disease is not specific, varying with the type of infection. Although renal enlargement with relatively hypoechoic parenchyma has been reported in acute pyelonephritis, gray-scale sonography is a relatively poor modality for identifying this condition. In focal pyelonephritis (bacterial nephritis), the sonogram may demonstrate localized areas of decreased or heterogeneous echogenicity indistinguishable from the appearance of tumor. A perinephric abscess may be seen as an anechoic or hypoechoic region, with or without internal echoes, but sterile and pyogenic perinephric fluid collections cannot be consistently distinguished with US. In patients with acquired immunodeficiency syndrome, renal US may show increased cortical echogenicity, hydronephrosis, nephromegaly, and focal abnormalities due to infection, neoplasm, or infarct.

Computed Tomography

The presence and extent of parenchymal or perinephric infection are detected most accurately with contrast-enhanced CT. CT is helpful in detecting intrarenal abscess and in assessing for the presence and extent of perinephric effusion or abscess. Diffuse pyelonephritis, focal pyelonephritis, and renal abscesses produce a spectrum of CT abnormalities related to the extent of parenchymal edema, distribution of inflammation, and severity of functional impairment. Pyelonephritis produces renal enlargement, nonuniform enhancement, and delayed excretion of contrast material. Striated collections of gas may be seen in the renal parenchyma, and perinephric fluid collections may be detected. Focal pyelonephritis produces wedge-shaped areas of low attenuation in both nonenhanced and enhanced images. These wedge-shaped lesions are irregularly margined, lobar in distribution, and typically unilateral.

Renal abscesses appear as irregularly shaped focal masses that are thick walled, are of heterogeneous attenuation, and have central low-density fluid and gas collections. Penetration of the renal capsule with formation of a perinephric abscess manifests on CT as the appearance of a collection of mixed fluid density and soft tissue density that surrounds and sometimes deforms the kidney. Gas within a perinephric collection indicates bacterial infection, extensive tissue necrosis, or previous diagnostic instrumentation. Perinephric fluid may be seen to be confined by bridging septa within the perinephric fascia. In this situation, CT can facilitate accurate percutaneous positioning of drainage catheters.

Magnetic Resonance Imaging

The MRI appearance of a kidney involved in an infectious process depends on the amount and distribution of renal edema. In severe pyelonephritis, the kidney is swollen and the corticomedullary differentiation is no longer visible. In focal pyelonephritis, the lobar areas of lower signal intensity may be seen extending through the medulla to the cortex and obscuring corticomedullary contrast. Renal abscesses appear as somewhat ill-defined masses, usually of low signal intensity on T1-weighted images and increased heterogeneous signal intensity on T2-weighted images, but signal intensity can vary with the underlying pathologic process and the content of fluid, protein, and debris. Because abscesses may be indistinguishable from "complicated" cysts or from solid neoplasms on MRI, the specific diagnosis depends on the clinical findings and biopsy. MRI remains the test of choice to evaluate renal abscesses in patients with renal failure or an allergy to iodine contrast media.

CALCULI

Calcifications in the kidney are classified according to anatomic distribution: cortical calcifications, medullary calcifications (nephrocalcinosis), and calculi in the urinary collecting system (urolithiasis).

Plain Film and Intravenous Urography

In the routine workup of a patient with renal colic, about 85% of urinary calculi contain calcium and are, therefore, visualized on plain films. However, overlying bowel gas and rib cartilage calcification make interpretation difficult. Although IVU is still used for the diagnosis of obstruction by urinary calculus, nonenhanced CT is the initial examination of choice in many institutions because of its high sensitivity for identifying hydronephrosis and the ability to demonstrate small renal and ureteral stones.

Ultrasonography

In obstructive uropathy due to nephrolithiasis, US studies demonstrate hydronephrosis and may show the calculus itself. The sensitivity of US for detecting renal calculi is superior to that of abdominal radiography but less than that of nonenhanced CT. Its accuracy for determining stone size is limited, and it should not be used to monitor the status of renal stones. US is less sensitive for detecting ureteral calculi, although stones can be seen in the proximal and mid-ureter. Obstructive calculi are most commonly located at the ureteropelvic or ureterovesical junctions, and assessment of these sites with US requires experience and expertise. At least moderate distention of the urinary bladder is necessary for evaluation of the distal ureter. When US is used for the diagnosis of renal calculi, it is important to remember that findings may be misleading when there is obstruction without hydronephrosis. For example, hydronephrosis may be absent if the obstruction is early or partial or if forniceal rupture has resulted in urinary decompression. Therefore, normal US findings in the presence of clinical symptoms that suggest calculous obstruction should not preclude further evaluation.

Computed Tomography

Unenhanced helical CT is superior to excretory urography for investigating suspected ureterolithiasis and is now considered the test of choice for evaluating patients with suspected renal colic. (The exception would be a pregnant patient for whom US or MRU is preferred.) Nonenhanced CT spares the patient the risks associated with intravenous contrast material and, with the advent of multidetector CT, can be completed in less than 5 minutes. CT is more sensitive than IVU for detecting a calculus, regardless of its size, location, or chemical composition. For the detection of obstructing ureteral calculi in patients with flank pain, the sensitivity of CT has been shown to be 100% and specificity to be 100% also, with 100% positive and 97% negative predictive values.

Nearly all ureteric stones can be visualized, regardless of their composition, size, or location. Even previously described "radiolucent" stones consisting of pure uric acid, xanthine, and cystine are visible on CT because their attenuation is significantly greater than that of soft tissue. Only two types of stones may not be visible on CT: pure matrix stones, which account for less than 1% of all stones, and stones of pure indinavir, which have been described in patients with human immunodeficiency virus disease. However, with the use of CT secondary findings suggestive of an obstructing stone, including hydronephrosis, perinephric or periureteral stranding, and renal enlargement may be seen, even if the stone is one of the rare radiolucent variety.

When no calculus is found, CT often provides the additional advantage of detecting extraurinary tract disease that is responsible for the symptoms, such as appendicitis, diverticulitis, or a perforated viscous. One disadvantage of unenhanced CT is that a higher radiation dosage is used than with conventional IVU.

Magnetic Resonance Imaging

MRU is a viable alternative for the assessment of ureteric obstruction, especially during pregnancy, when US is not diagnostic, or for patients who are allergic to iodinated contrast media. Several studies have demonstrated accuracy and sensitivity values for MRU of up to 100% for detecting both urinary tract dilation and level of obstruction and excellent correlation with results of excretory urography.

MRI is not sensitive for the detection of small calcifications, including small calculi, limiting its usefulness in the detection of nephrocalcinosis and nephrolithiasis. Calculi may be evident, however, if their foci of signal void are large enough or if they lie adjacent to tissue of relatively high signal intensity. Filling defects in the collecting system are nonspecific on MRU, because calculi, blood clot, surgical clips, debris, and tumors may have the same appearance. MRU has also been found useful for the detection and depiction of duplex renal systems, including ureteral duplication.

RENAL MASSES

Renal Cysts

Benign cortical cysts are the most common renal masses. They may be solitary or numerous, and although they are often asymptomatic, they may cause pain by stretching the renal capsule. Intracystic hemorrhage or infection can also produce pain or fever.

Ultrasonography
A lesion is considered a benign simple cyst when the following US findings are observed:

- No internal echoes (anechoic cyst) are seen.
- All the walls of the cyst are smooth and sharply defined.
- Acoustic enhancement beyond the posterior wall of the cyst is proportional to the fluid content (the single most important finding).
- A narrow band of acoustic shadowing is seen beyond the outer margin.

If these criteria are met, no further studies are necessary to characterize the mass. If, however, the results of US are technically suboptimal or if the mass is characterized as intermediate or has the characteristics of a solid lesion, CT is indicated. However, if there are contraindications to CT or if CT findings remain indeterminate, MRI can be performed.

Computed Tomography

A renal mass can confidently be called a simple cyst when it meets the following CT criteria:

- It has a homogeneous attenuation value near that of water.
- Its wall is so thin that it is nearly indiscernible.
- It is sharply delineated from surrounding renal parenchyma.
- Its fluid contents do not increase in attenuation value after intravenous infusion of contrast medium by more than 10 Hounsfield units (HU).

If the fluid contents of the cyst are of higher density or if the cyst is irregularly shaped with thickened or calcified walls, it may be a complicated renal cyst or a solid tumor. Such lesions require further diagnostic evaluation, especially when clinical symptoms such as pain and hemorrhage raise the possibility of renal tumor. Percutaneous cyst aspiration and biopsy may be performed with CT guidance, and if a solid renal mass is detected, CT is helpful in evaluating the anatomic extent of the lesion. CT is sensitive or specific in the detection of superinfected cysts. However, a thick-walled cystic mass associated with perinephric stranding, in the proper clinical setting, would suggest the diagnosis of superinfected cyst. This scenario would warrant close follow-up to exclude cystic renal cell carcinoma.

Magnetic Resonance Imaging

On MRI, simple renal cysts appear as clearly defined, rounded masses of homogeneous signal intensity (low on T1-weighted images and high on T2-weighted images). Once a cyst is complicated by either hemorrhage or infection, the MR signal usually becomes heterogeneous and nonspecific. Calcification within the walls of a complicated cyst may cause wall thickening, but, unlike CT findings, MRI findings are nonspecific and do not clearly identify calcifications. In complicated cysts, benign disease cannot be differentiated from malignant disease, nor is it possible to distinguish between cystic and solid lesions. MRI has demonstrated utility in the workup of the native kidneys in patients with renal transplants, many of whom have acquired cystic disease. MRI is more sensitive than US and is preferred over CT, which exposes the patient to potentially nephrotoxic contrast material.

Polycystic Kidney Disease

See Chapter 19, Cystic Diseases of the Kidney.

Solid Renal Masses

Although US is excellent for detecting renal cysts, it is considerably less accurate for detecting solid lesions, and its use can be limited by technical factors including patient body habitus and the skill of the person conducting the examination. It is insufficient to recommend US for the detection of solid renal lesions; the best modality for this purpose is CT, which is more sensitive in the detection of small (<3 cm) renal masses but also now has the capability to categorize inflammatory, neoplastic, and various cystic lesions through utilization of arterial, corticomedullary, nephrographic, and excretory phase imaging.

Overall, MRI has an accuracy similar to that of CT for detection and characterization of renal masses. Because of its operator dependence, relatively long scan time, and expense, however, MRI is usually reserved for patients with impaired renal function, for patients in whom use of contrast material is contraindicated, or for further assessment when CT findings are equivocal, especially for differentiating between a complicated cyst and cystic or hypovascular renal cell carcinoma.

Renal Cell Carcinoma

Imaging has an important role in the determination of the type of surgery required: nephron-sparing, simple nephrectomy, or radical nephrectomy. Because surgery is the only effective therapy and because survival depends on local and distant extent, precise staging is critical for preoperative planning and prognosis.

Helical CT is the imaging modality of choice for staging renal cell carcinoma. Because nephron-sparing surgery is becoming more common as renal cell cancers are detected earlier and, therefore, when they are smaller, the utility of preoperative CT has increased, especially with respect to three-dimensional volume rendering. This adjunct to routine imaging delineates the renal tumor as well as normal and complex renal anatomy before surgery, and the relationship of the tumor to the collecting system, allowing determination of resectability of the mass. The CT appearance of renal cell carcinoma varies with tumor size and vascularity. Detection of small lesions is facilitated by rapid-sequence scanning techniques during administration of contrast material, because abnormal enhancement may be evident even when renal contours are normal. Renal cell carcinomas tend to have a solid growth pattern, attenuation values of 20 HU or more, and an increase in attenuation values of at least 10 HU after administration of contrast medium. Nonuniform enhancement is characteristic, but after administration of the contrast medium, renal cell carcinomas typically appear less dense than surrounding renal tissue. Metastases to the lungs, the mediastinum, and the liver are readily recognized, but demonstration of renal vein and inferior vena cava tumor thrombus requires contrast enhancement. Typically, tumor thrombi enlarge the renal vein and inferior vena cava and cause their density to be nonuniform.

Although CT has been the study of choice for staging of renal cell carcinoma, MRI has comparable accuracy. Combined transverse and sagittal MRI planes are optimal for evaluating venous anatomy and the normal tissue–tumor interfaces. The particular advantages of MRI staging are determination of the origin of the mass, evaluation of vascular patency, detection of perihilar lymph node metastases, and evaluation of direct tumor invasion to adjacent organs. MRI is also a sensitive tool for determining the extent of tumor thrombus (seen as abnormal signal intensity within the renal vein or inferior vena cava) and for demonstrating invasion of the wall of the inferior vena cava. For assessing thrombus extension into the renal vein or inferior vena cava, MRI has replaced venography.

EVALUATION OF RENAL TRANSPLANTS

US is an essential component of the management of renal transplants and is commonly utilized, usually in the setting of increased serum creatinine values but also with pain, hematuria, and abnormal urine output. US is also the method of choice for guiding percutaneous biopsy of the transplant to exclude rejection, although CT must occasionally be used, if the graft cannot be visualized sonographically for technical reasons, including overlying bowel. Color-flow Doppler US provides accurate information about renal perfusion, providing a valuable noninvasive test for diagnosis of vascular tree abnormalities. US not only gives a global assessment of the intraparenchymal vasculature but also confirms patency of the main renal artery and vein and the iliac vessels to which they are anastomosed.

US is important in the diagnosis and management of perigraft fluid collections, including hematoma, lymphocele, and urinoma, and in the detection of post-transplant lymphoproliferative disorder, which can manifest as a hilar mass. Unfortunately, two common entities, allograft rejection and acute tubular necrosis, cannot be reliably distinguished on US, which is not accurate enough to obviate biopsy. Both can be associated with an elevated resistive index, and for reliable distinction between the two, histologic evaluation via biopsy must be obtained.

Color-flow Doppler US has been shown to be valuable in evaluating post-transplantation renal artery stenosis, with sensitivity of 100% and specificity of 86%. Therefore, most patients do not require angiography. An elevated resistive index has been suggested as a risk marker for chronic allograft nephropathy in one clinical trial. This finding awaits confirmation in other studies.

Obstruction of the renal transplant remains an important reversible cause of allograft dysfunction, requiring prompt diagnosis to prevent long-term graft damage. When the serum creatinine value rises, US is the initial test acquired to investigate the causes of graft dysfunction, including obstruction, which is usually manifested by hydronephrosis. US is very sensitive in the detection of hydronephrosis, but it cannot be used to assess the functional significance and cannot differentiate between obstruction and vesicoureteral reflux as the cause of hydronephrosis. For this, mercaptoacetyltriglycine diuretic renography may be used. However, acute tubular necrosis, dehydration, or very poor renal function may cause false-positive results.

II

Disturbances in Control of Body Fluid Volume and Composition

Control of Extracellular Fluid Volume and the Pathophysiology of Edema Formation

4

CONTROL OF EXTRACELLULAR FLUID VOLUME

The volume of extracellular fluid (ECF) is maintained within narrow limits in normal human subjects, despite day-to-day variations in dietary intake of salt and water. The ECF is divided between two separate compartments: the intravascular or plasma volume compartment and the extravascular or interstitial compartment. The relationship of ECF volume and, in particular, the volume of the plasma compartment to overall vascular capacitance determines fundamental indices of cardiovascular performance such as mean arterial blood pressure and left ventricular filling volume. Given the rigorous defense of ECF sodium concentration, mediated mainly by osmoregulatory mechanisms concerned with external water balance, the quantity of Na^+ rather than the concentration determines the volume of the ECF compartment. Changes in total body water content alter the serum Na^+ concentration and osmolality but contribute little to determining the volume of the ECF. At a given steady state, total daily Na^+ intake and excretion are equal. Acute deviations from a preexisting steady state, caused by an alteration in Na^+ intake or extrarenal excretion, result in an adjustment in renal Na^+ excretion. This adjustment in renal Na^+ excretion occurs as a result of a new total body Na^+ content and ECF volume, and the aim is to restore the preexisting steady state. Alternatively, an alteration in the capacitance of the extracellular compartment can also result in an adjustment in renal Na^+ excretion, the aim of which is to restore the preexisting relationship of volume to capacitance. It is clear that the operation of such a system for Na^+ homeostasis requires the following:

- Sensors that detect changes in ECF volume relative to vascular and interstitial capacitance
- Effector mechanisms that ultimately modify the rate of Na^+ excretion by the kidney to meet the demands of volume homeostasis

Volume Receptors

Volume detectors are located at several locations throughout the body, including the cardiopulmonary and arterial baroreceptors, as well as renal, central nervous system, and hepatic sensors. Each compartment can be viewed as reflecting a unique characteristic of overall circulatory function, such as cardiac filling, cardiac output, renal perfusion, or fluid transudation into the interstitial space. Sensors within each compartment monitor a physical parameter (e.g., stretch or tension) that serves as an index of circulatory function within that compartment. These signals are then transduced via neural and hormonal signals to the efferent limb of the integrated homeostatic response system. In addition to its role as a major effector target responding to signals indicating the need for adjustments in Na^+ excretion, the kidney participates in the afferent limb of volume homeostasis. In the kidney the volume sensors are found in the juxtaglomerular apparatus of the afferent arteriole. Signals from this site affect volume homeostasis primarily via modulation of the renin-angiotensin-aldosterone axis (RAAS) and intrarenal hemodynamics such that alteration in the ECF results in adjustments in physical forces governing tubule Na^+ handling. In contrast, the effects of cardiopulmonary and neural receptors are mediated primarily through the actions of natriuretic peptides and the sympathetic nervous system.

Effector Mechanisms

The major renal effector mechanisms defending against changes in volume status include the RAAS, sympathetic nervous system, and natriuretic peptides and intrarenal factors (tubuloglomerular feedback).

Renin-Angiotensin-Aldosterone Axis

The RAAS plays a major role in the regulation of ECF volume homeostasis. Renin release from the kidney is enhanced in situations that compromise extracellular volume homeostasis, such as loss of blood volume, reduced ECF volume, "effective" circulating volume depletion (heart failure or cirrhosis), diminished salt intake, and hypotension. Renin release accelerates the generation of angiotensin II, which has multiple actions: it raises the blood pressure by arterial vasoconstriction; it promotes efferent arteriolar vasoconstriction within the kidney, thus maintaining the glomerular filtration rate (GFR); it triggers enhanced proximal tubule Na^+ and H_2O absorption; and it promotes aldosterone release, which, in turn, induces Na^+ retention in the distal tubule.

Sympathetic Nervous System
Sympathetic nervous system activity is enhanced in the setting of actual or effective volume depletion and is normally suppressed in states of ECF expansion. In addition to the well-described effects on systemic hemodynamics (vasoconstriction and increased cardiac contractility), activation of the sympathetic nervous system results in direct enhancement of proximal tubule Na^+ reabsorption, as well as indirect effects on distal Na^+ handling mediated via activation of the RAAS.

Vasopressin
Release of arginine vasopressin (AVP) occurs in response to a threat to intracellular fluid volume (osmotic stimulus) or to diminished ECF volume (nonosmotic volume stimulus). AVP enhances water permeability and reabsorption in the medullary collecting duct, but it also increases Na^+ reabsorption in the thick ascending limb and cortical collecting duct. It also is a potent vasoconstrictor and in terms of overall volume homeostasis, the predominant influence of AVP in response to perceived ECF depletion results indirectly from water accumulation or blood pressure changes.

Natriuretic Peptides
Atrial natriuretic peptide (ANP), an endogenous 28-amino acid residue peptide of cardiac origin, has been the most extensively studied member of the natriuretic peptide family, which contains at least two other members: brain natriuretic peptide and C-type natriuretic peptide. ANP is released in response to atrial stretch that occurs in the setting of volume overload. At the renal level, ANP increases the GFR and the filtered load of Na^+ via an elevation of glomerular capillary hydrostatic pressure that results from a combination of efferent arteriolar constriction and afferent arteriolar dilatation. ANP antagonizes reabsorption of Na^+ mediated by angiotensin II, and it directly inhibits Na^+ reabsorption in the inner medullary collecting duct.

Tubuloglomerular Feedback
Modest changes in GFR that accompany volume expansion and depletion are not sufficient to explain the accompanying adjustments in urinary Na^+ excretion. Rather, local intrarenal factors, acting at the level of the coupling of tubule reabsorption to glomerular filtration, are responsible for regulating urinary Na^+ excretion, responding to afferent limb signals that are responsive to volume perturbation. The mechanisms mediating tubuloglomerular feedback are beyond the scope of this text but include changes in hydrostatic and oncotic pressure within the peritubular capillaries, alterations in flow-related proximal reabsorption of Na^+, and changes in Na^+ handling in the loop of Henle. The net result of these changes is enhanced Na^+ excretion in states of ECF volume expansion and vice versa.

EXTRACELLULAR FLUID VOLUME DEPLETION

Etiology

Volume contraction can result from water and salt loss from either renal or nonrenal sources.

Renal Losses
The most common renal cause of ECF volume depletion is Na^+ wasting due to diuretic use. This is most often observed with loop diuretic use and is more common in the elderly, in whom the homeostatic responses to volume contraction are impaired. The combination of a loop diuretic and the thiazide diuretic metolazone causes a brisk diuresis that is frequently associated with volume depletion in clinical practice. Other causes of renal Na^+ wasting include osmotic diuresis (hyperglycemia, mannitol administration, and postobstructive diuresis), primary renal salt wasting syndromes (Bartter syndrome and medullary cystic kidney disease) and secondary renal salt wasting syndromes (aldosterone deficiency). Free-water loss generally does not induce hypovolemia unless the losses are severe (>10 L/day) and the patient is denied free access to free water and hypernatremic hypovolemia ensues.

Gastrointestinal Losses
The amount of gastrointestinal secretions exceeds several liters per day of electrolyte-rich fluid, most of which is reabsorbed. Volume depletion is commonly observed if significant amounts of gastrointestinal secretions are either lost (vomiting, osmotic diarrhea, or nasogastric suction) or their secretion is increased

(secretory diarrhea) in the absence of adequate water and electrolyte repletion.

Hemorrhage

Hemorrhage from any site can lead to life-threatening volume depletion. Excluding traumatic blood loss, common causes encountered in clinical practice include variceal hemorrhage and bleeding from a peptic ulcer.

Sequestration

Sequestration of fluid into the third spaces, if severe, can cause ECF volume depletion. Commonly encountered clinical scenarios include intestinal obstruction, pancreatitis, crush injury, peritonitis, and hip fracture.

Dermal and Respiratory Losses

Sweat fluid is typically hypotonic with respect to the plasma; hence, enhanced losses in the setting of fever, exercise, or a warm climate trigger thirst mechanisms to prevent net free water loss. If dermal losses are exaggerated (>3 L/day) and water and salt repletion is not appropriate, then volume depletion can ensue. Transdermal volume losses are markedly increased in the setting of burns and require substantial fluid and electrolyte repletion.

Clinical Manifestations of Volume Depletion

The historical enquiry should focus on potential causes of volume depletion including diuretic use, vomiting, diarrhea, or polyuria. The symptoms of volume contraction are typically nonspecific but can include postural dizziness, thirst, or a craving for salt. Despite the frequency of this clinical presentation, the diagnosis of volume depletion by physical examination can be difficult even for the experienced clinician. The physical manifestations of volume depletion are variable, and the absence of physical findings does not preclude the diagnosis.

Body Weight

A rapid decline in body weight is a key finding in the evaluation of the patient with volume contraction, particularly elderly patients in whom other physical signs are often highly unreliable. The change in body weight not only aids in the diagnosis of volume depletion but can also help guide therapy.

Skin and Mucous Membranes

Volume depletion is classically associated with a loss of normal skin turgor over the forearm or thigh. However, due to a loss of the inherent elastic tone of skin with aging, loss of skin turgor is an unreliable clinical sign in older subjects. Dryness of the mucous membranes is also associated with ECF volume contraction but can represent mouth breathing.

Jugular Venous Pressure
When hypovolemia is suspected, the jugular venous pulse is best assessed with the patient lying recumbent at a lower angle than normal (20 to 35 degrees) with the head tilted away from the examiner. At this angle the jugular venous pulse should be visible in the euvolemic patient, arising between the two heads of the sternocleidomastoid muscle. Absence of a jugular venous pulse suggests low right-sided filling pressures consistent with ECF contraction.

Arterial Blood Pressure
Overt hypotension is typically only observed in severe volume depletion and may be associated with the signs and symptoms of peripheral hypoperfusion such as oliguria, clammy extremities, and confusion. Less profound ECF volume deficits may be elicited by checking for postural hypotension.

Diagnosis of Volume Depletion

Hemodynamic Monitoring
Intravascular hemodynamic monitoring is often required in the critically ill patient in whom clinical clues of volume status are often conflicting. Measurements of intravascular volume status include central venous pressure (CVP), which reflects right heart filling pressures, and pulmonary capillary wedge pressure (PCWP), which reflects left ventricular filling pressures. Measurement of the latter is not usually performed unless measurements of other hemodynamic parameters are required (e.g., cardiac output or systemic vascular resistance). Under normal circumstances the CVP reflects the PCWP and can be used as a surrogate marker of left-sided filling pressures. When the CVP is in the low-normal range, the response to a fluid volume challenge can further help define the intravascular filling status. Situations in which the CVP does not reflect the PCWP include isolated right heart failure (cor pulmonale) or pure left-sided heart failure. In these settings PCWP may provide a more accurate index of the optimal left ventricular filling pressure.

Serum Indices
Analysis of blood biochemistry is useful in the determination of ECF volume status based on knowledge of the normal

physiologic response to volume contraction outlined above. Volume depletion leads to enhanced proximal tubule salt and water retention, and this in turn causes passive reabsorption of urea, leading to a rise in the normal blood urea nitrogen-to-creatinine ratio from a normal level of 10:1 to greater than 20:1. Factors that alter urea generation independent of renal clearance can affect the reliability of this index. The nonosmotic release of vasopressin can trigger a modest decrement in the serum Na^+ concentration, whereas hemoconcentration (high hematocrit) may result from plasma volume contraction. Analysis of the acid-base status can also further aid in the diagnosis of the cause of the volume-contracted state. A hypochloremic metabolic alkalosis is characteristic of volume depletion due to diuretic use, vomiting, or nasogastric suctioning. In contrast, diarrhea can lead to heavy losses of bicarbonate-rich fluids with secondary NaCl retention by the kidney, leading to a hyperchloremic metabolic acidosis.

Urine Indices

In volume-depleted patients sodium is avidly reabsorbed in the renal tubule and urine with a Na^+ concentration greater than 10 mEq/L and a high specific gravity is excreted. The fractional excretion of Na^+ (FENa), which relates Na^+ clearance to creatinine clearance is a more sensitive urine test to diagnose ECF volume depletion. Creatinine is reabsorbed to a much smaller extent than Na^+ in volume depletion. Consequently, patients with volume depletion typically have a FENa of less than 1% (often <0.01%), whereas the FENa is usually greater than 1% in euvolemic patients. The FENa may be greater than 1% in patients with prerenal azotemia who are receiving diuretics or in those with a metabolic alkalosis (in which Na^+ is excreted with HCO_3^- to maintain electroneutrality). In the latter situation, the urine Cl^- is a better index of intravascular volume status with a level less than 20 mEq/L suggesting ECF volume contraction.

Management of Volume Depletion

The management of volume depletion is discussed in Chapter 9, Acute Renal Failure.

PATHOPHYSIOLOGY OF EDEMA FORMATION

Generalized edema formation, the clinical hallmark of ECF volume expansion, represents the accumulation of excessive fluid in the interstitial compartment and is invariably associated with renal Na$^+$ retention. It occurs most commonly in response to congestive heart failure (CHF), cirrhosis with ascites, and the nephrotic syndrome.

Local Mechanisms in Interstitial Fluid Accumulation

The balance of Starling forces prevailing at the arteriolar end of the capillary (Δ hydraulic pressure > Δ oncotic pressure) favors the net filtration of fluid into the interstitium. Net outward movement of fluid along the length of the capillary is associated with an axial decrease in the capillary hydraulic pressure and an increase in the plasma colloid osmotic pressure such that the net balance of forces favors fluid movement back into the capillary at the distal end of the capillary bed. In some tissues, the local transcapillary hydraulic pressure gradient continues to exceed the opposing colloid osmotic gradient throughout the length of the capillary bed so that filtration occurs along its entire length. In such capillary beds, a substantial volume of filtered fluid must return to the circulation via lymphatics.

The appearance of generalized edema implies one or more disturbances in microcirculatory hemodynamics associated with expansion of the ECF volume: increased venous pressure transmitted to the capillary, unfavorable adjustments in precapillary and postcapillary resistances, or lymphatic flow inadequate to drain the interstitial compartment and replenish the intravascular compartment. Generalized edema implies substantial renal Na$^+$ retention. Indeed, the volume of accumulated interstitial fluid required for clinical detection of generalized edema (>2 to 3 L) necessitates that all states of generalized edema are associated with expansion of ECF volume and hence with body-exchangeable sodium content. Therefore, it can be concluded that all states of generalized edema reflect past or ongoing renal Na$^+$ retention.

Renal Sodium Retention and Edema Formation in Congestive Heart Failure

CHF is a clinical syndrome in which the heart is unable to satisfy the requirements of peripheral tissues for oxygen and other nutrients. This happens most commonly in the setting of a decrease in cardiac output (low-output CHF), but it may also occur when cardiac output is increased, such as in patients with an arteriovenous fistula, hyperthyroidism, or beriberi (high-output CHF). In both situations, the kidney responds in a similar manner, by avidly retaining Na$^+$ and water despite expansion of the ECF volume.

cirrhosis, a volume-independent stimulus for renal Na^+ retention is envisioned. Possible mediators include adrenergic reflexes activated by hepatic sinusoidal hypertension and increased systemic concentrations of an unidentified antinatriuretic factor as a result of impaired liver metabolism.

It is likely that neither the underfilling nor the overflow theory can account exclusively for all of the observed derangements in volume regulation in cirrhosis. Rather, it is possible that elements of the two concepts may occur simultaneously or sequentially in patients with cirrhosis. There is evidence to suggest that, early in cirrhosis, intrahepatic hypertension caused by hepatic venous outflow block signals primary renal Na^+ retention with consequent intravascular volume expansion. Whether at this stage underfilling of the arterial circuit consequent to vasodilatation also applies remains to be determined. Because of the expansion of the intrathoracic venous compartment at this stage, plasma ANP levels rise. The rise in ANP levels is sufficient to counterbalance the renal Na^+-retaining forces; however, it does so at the expense of an expanded intravascular volume with the potential for overflow ascites. The propensity for accumulation of volume in the peritoneal compartment and in the splanchnic bed results from altered intrahepatic hemodynamics. With progression of disease, disruptions of intrasinusoidal Starling forces and loss of volume from the vascular compartment into the peritoneal compartment occur. These events, coupled with other factors such as portosystemic shunting, hypoalbuminemia, and vascular refractoriness to pressor hormones, lead to underfilling of the arterial circuit, without the necessity for measurable underfilling of the venous compartment. This underfilling of the circulation may attenuate further increases in ANP levels and promote the activation of antinatriuretic factors. Whether the antinatriuretic factors activated by underfilling are the same as or different from those that promote primary renal Na^+ retention in early disease remains to be determined. At this later stage of disease, increased levels of ANP may not be sufficient to counterbalance antinatriuretic influences. It should be noted that in early cirrhosis salt retention is isotonic and is accompanied by ECF expansion and normonatremia. However, with advancing cirrhosis, defective water excretion supervenes, resulting in hyponatremia, which reflects combined ECF and intracellular fluid space expansion. However, impaired water excretion and hyponatremia in cirrhotic patients with ascites is a marker of the severity of the same accompanying hemodynamic abnormalities that initiate Na^+ retention and eventuate in hepatorenal failure. The pathogenesis is primarily related to nonosmotic stimuli for release of vasopressin, acting together with additional factors such as renal prostaglandins and impaired distal sodium delivery. For a further discussion of the clinical aspects of diuretic use in cirrhosis see Chapter 33, Diuretics.

Renal Sodium Retention and Edema Formation in the Nephrotic Syndrome

Edema is the most common presenting symptom of patients with the nephrotic syndrome. Various theories for the cause of nephrotic edema have been proposed. Hypovolemia as a consequence of reduced plasma oncotic pressure has long been considered the proximal cause of salt and water retention by the kidney. Enhanced tubular sodium reabsorption is considered to be a function of multiple mediator systems responding to the "perceived volume depletion" with activation of the RAAS, sympathetic nervous, and vasopressor systems. Whether plasma volume is low or high is unclear from the literature, although it is reasonable to assert that hypoproteinuria results in a fall in the plasma oncotic pressure and the movement of fluid into the interstitial space. Several factors mitigate this phenomenon. Normally, the transcapillary oncotic pressure gradient (plasma oncotic pressure minus interstitial oncotic pressure) acts synergistically to retain fluid within the vascular space. In normal patients, colloid osmotic pressure in the plasma is approximately 26 mm Hg. The interstitial oncotic pressure may be as high as 10 to 15 mm Hg because of the filtration of albumin across the capillary wall. In nephrotic patients, the interstitial oncotic pressure may decrease to as low as 2.6 mm Hg in the lower leg. The fall in interstitial oncotic pressure functions as a protecting factor in hypoproteinemic patients. There may be a consequent parallel decline in interstitial oncotic pressure, matching the fall in plasma oncotic pressure and minimizing the change in the transcapillary gradient. Thus, there would be a smaller change in the transcapillary gradient and a reduced drive of fluid shifting from the vascular compartment into the interstitium. Other factors that limit the amount of fluid movement into the interstitium include compliance of the interstitium in most tissues and increased lymphatic fluid flow. Excessive dietary salt ingestion or the administration of saline to hypoproteinemic patients results in a rapid fall in the transcapillary oncotic pressure gradient and subsequent substantial edema.

Although evidence supports the underfilling hypothesis of edema formation, recent studies suggest that the salt and water retention characteristic of the nephrotic syndrome occurs as a primary renal phenomenon rather than as a response to perceived intravascular volume depletion. The overfill hypothesis suggests that primary renal salt retention is the cause of edema in patients with nephrotic syndrome. Supportive evidence for this theory comes from the finding that the plasma volume is expanded in the nephrotic syndrome and the finding that many adults with the nephrotic syndrome are hypertensive, both of which argue against hypovolemia and, in fact, suggest hypervolemia. Other persuasive evidence is the finding that levels of ANP and plasma renin activity in patients with the nephrotic syndrome are equivalent to those of normal subjects ingesting a usual amount of sodium in their diet, suggesting that renal sodium retention in nephrosis is probably a consequence of primary renal sodium retention rather than a consequence of plasma hormone effects on the kidney.

Certain important issues should be considered when decisions about management of edema in the nephrotic syndrome are made. In some patients, the edema only causes minimal discomfort, but in others the edema causes substantial morbidity. The goal should be to have a slow resolution of edema. In all instances, the institution of rapid diuresis resulting in hypovolemia and, at times, hypotension must be avoided. Dietary restriction of sodium intake has been the mainstay of therapy in the treatment of nephrotic edema. Patients with nephrosis have sodium avidity and the amount of sodium in the urine may be as low as 10 mmol/day.

Consequently, it is virtually impossible to lower the sodium intake to these levels. It is more useful to suggest mild sodium restriction. Mild diuretics, including thiazide diuretics, may be sufficient in many patients with mild edema. Potassium-sparing diuretics, such as triamterene, amiloride, or spironolactone, are useful for patients in whom hypokalemia becomes a clinical problem. However, their use is limited in patients with renal insufficiency. Furosemide and other loop diuretics are typically used for moderate to severe nephrotic edema. Whereas the high-protein content of tubular fluid was once thought to inhibit furosemide and other loop diuretics by binding to them, new data suggest that urinary protein binding does not affect the response to furosemide. Metolazone may be effective when used alone or in combination with loop diuretics (i.e., furosemide) in patients with refractory nephrotic edema. In patients treated with diuretics, episodes of profound volume depletion may occur. The resultant peripheral vasoconstriction, tachycardia, orthostatic hypotension, and, at times, oliguria and renal insufficiency usually resolve with cessation of the diuretic and rehydration. Albumin infusions transiently increase plasma volume and are most useful in patients with profound volume depletion. Unfortunately, because of the rapid excretion of the infused albumin within 48 hours, the utility of this approach is short lived and may result in transient development of pulmonary edema. In extreme cases of marked edema and especially pulmonary edema, usually in the setting of reduced GFR, filtration using either intermittent or continuous extracorporeal dialysis is useful. For a further discussion of the clinical aspects of diuretic use in the nephrotic syndrome see Chapter 33, Diuretics.

Idiopathic Edema and Capillary Leak

Idiopathic edema is a disorder characterized by fluid retention that cannot be attributed to the known causes or pathogenic mechanisms of edema formation. Although the etiology of this syndrome has not yet been clarified, it is clear that idiopathic edema is overwhelmingly more common in women. It is important to distinguish this disorder from excessive estrogen-stimulated Na^+ and fluid retention associated with the premenstrual state (cyclic or premenstrual edema), diabetes mellitus, or hypothyroidism. A hallmark of idiopathic edema is the observation that most of the affected patients retain Na^+ and water in the upright posture but diurese in the recumbent position. There is considerable evidence that affected patients have a decreased plasma volume, which is seen with stimulation of antinatriuretic and antidiuretic effector mechanisms in the upright position. The relative importance of secondary hyperaldosteronism in sustaining the progressive weight gain in this disorder is highlighted by the observation that treatment with angiotensin-converting enzyme inhibitors often results in weight loss and symptomatic improvement. A subpopulation of patients with idiopathic edema have been reported to develop edema while receiving diuretic agents. It is assumed that in these patients salt-retaining mechanisms overcompensate for the direct effects of the drug. However, it is possible that K^+ depletion, a common complication of chronic diuretic therapy, in itself contributes to edema formation. Overall the effects of diuretic therapy in this setting are unclear, and patients are best treated by salt restriction.

Acid-Base Disorders

5

The diagnosis and management of acid-base disorders in acutely ill patients requires an accurate and timely interpretation of the laboratory parameters associated with any specific acid-base disorder. Appropriate interpretation requires simultaneous measurement of serum electrolytes and arterial blood gases, as well as an appreciation by the clinician of the physiologic adaptations and compensatory responses that occur with specific acid-base disturbances.

The acid-base status of the body is tightly controlled to maintain pH within a normal range of 7.35 to −7.45. Primary changes in serum concentrations of fixed acid or base lead to either metabolic acidosis or alkalosis and are reflected in the serum HCO_3^- concentration, whereas primary changes in partial pressure of arterial carbon dioxide ($Paco_2$) lead to either respiratory acidosis or alkalosis. The patient with an acid-base disorder is usually seriously ill, and the often complex presentation of these disorders requires a methodical approach to both diagnosis and management.

METABOLIC DISORDERS

Metabolic Acidosis

Metabolic acidosis is characterized by a fall in both the blood pH and the serum HCO_3^- concentration and is normally accompanied by a compensatory respiratory alkalosis (Table 5–1). It develops as the result of a marked increase in endogenous production of acid (such as lactic acid and ketoacids), loss of HCO_3^- stores (diarrhea or renal tubular acidosis [RTA]), or progressive accumulation of endogenous acids (renal failure).

Table 5–1: Acid-Base Abnormalities and Appropriate Compensatory Responses for Simple Disorders

Primary Acid-Base Disorders	Primary Defect	Effect on pH	Compensatory Response	Expected Range of Compensation	Limits of Compensation
Respiratory acidosis	Alveolar hypoventilation ($\uparrow$ P_{CO_2})	$\downarrow$	$\uparrow$ Renal HCO_3^- reabsorption ($\uparrow$ HCO_3^-)	Acute Δ [HCO_3^-] = 1 mEq/L for each $\uparrow$$\Delta P_{CO_2}$ of 10 mm Hg Chronic Δ [HCO_3^-] = +4 mEq/L for each $\uparrow$$\Delta P_{CO_2}$ of 10 mm Hg	[HCO_3^-] = 38 mEq/L [HCO_3^-] = 38 mEq/L
Respiratory alkalosis	Alveolar hyperventilation ($\downarrow$ P_{CO_2})	$\uparrow$	$\downarrow$ Renal HCO_3^- reabsorption ($\downarrow$ HCO_3^-)	Acute Δ [HCO_3^-] = –2 mEq/L for each $\downarrow$$\Delta$ P_{CO_2} of 10 mm Hg Chronic Δ [HCO_3^-] = 5 mEq/L for each $\downarrow$$\Delta$ P_{CO_2} of 10 mm Hg	[HCO_3^-] = 45 mEq/L [HCO_3^-] = 15 mEq/L
Metabolic acidosis	Loss of HCO_3^- or gain of H^+ ($\downarrow$ HCO_3^-)	$\downarrow$	Alveolar hyperventilation to $\uparrow$ pulmonary CO_2 excretion ($\downarrow$ P_{CO_2})	[P_{CO_2}] = 1.5 [HCO_3^-] + 8 ± 2 P_{CO_2} = last 2 digits of pH × 100 P_{CO_2} = 15 + [HCO_3^-]	P_{CO_2} = 15 mm Hg
Metabolic alkalosis	Gain of HCO_3^- or loss of H^+ ($\uparrow$ HCO_3^-)	$\uparrow$	Alveolar hyperventilation to $\downarrow$ pulmonary CO_2 excretion ($\uparrow$ P_{CO_2})	P_{CO_2} = + 0.6 mm Hg for Δ [HCO_3^-] of 1 mEq/L P_{CO_2} = 15 + [HCO_3^-]	P_{CO_2} = 55 mm Hg

P_{CO_2}, partial pressure of carbon dioxide.
Adapted from Bidani A, DuBose TD Jr: Cellular and whole body acid-base regulation. In Arieff AI, DeFronzo RA (eds): *Fluid, Electrolyte, and Acid-Base Disorders*, 2nd ed. New York, Churchill Livingstone, 1995, p. 95.

The Anion Gap

The anion gap (AG) serves a useful role in the differential diagnosis of metabolic acidoses and should always be calculated:

$$AG = Na^+ - (Cl^- + HCO_3^-)$$

The AG represents the unmeasured anions that are normally present in serum and unaccounted for by the serum electrolytes measured on the electrolyte panel. The normal value is 9 ± 3 mEq/L. The unmeasured anions normally present in serum include anionic proteins (principally albumin), PO_4^{3-}, SO_4^{2-}, and organic anions. When acid anions, such as acetoacetate and lactate, are produced endogenously in excess and accumulate in the extracellular fluid (ECF), the AG increases above the normal value. This is referred to as a *high AG acidosis*. A metabolic acidosis with a normal AG (*hyperchloremic or non-AG acidosis*) suggests that HCO_3^- has been effectively replaced by Cl^-. A modest increase in the AG may also be caused by a decrease in unmeasured cations (severe hypocalcemia) or an increase in the effective anionic charge of albumin (alkalemia). A modest decrease in the AG can be generated by an increase in unmeasured cations (e.g., paraprotein in multiple myeloma), a decrease in unmeasured anions (e.g., hypoalbuminemia), or a decrease in the effective anionic charge on the albumin due to acidosis. In general, each decline in serum albumin by 1 g/dL, from the normal value of 4.5 g/dL, decreases the expected AG by 2.5 mEq/L.

Hyperchloremic (Normal Anion Gap) Metabolic Acidoses

The diverse clinical disorders that may result in a hyperchloremic metabolic acidosis are outlined in Table 5–2. Because reduced serum HCO_3^- and elevated Cl^- concentrations may also occur in chronic respiratory alkalosis, it is important to confirm the acidemia by measuring arterial pH. Most disorders in this category are caused by four conditions:

- Loss of bicarbonate from the kidney (proximal RTA)
- Inappropriately low renal acid excretion (distal RTA or renal failure)
- Loss of bicarbonate from the gastrointestinal tract (diarrhea, ureteral diversion, or ileostomy)
- Rapid dilution of the serum HCO_3^- by saline ("expansion acidosis") or ingestion of an inorganic acid other than HCl

PROXIMAL RENAL TUBULAR ACIDOSIS The first phase of acidification by the nephron involves reabsorption of most filtered HCO_3^- by the proximal convoluted tubule. If the capacity of the proximal tubule is reduced, increased HCO_3^- delivery overwhelms

Table 5–2: Clinical Causes of High Anion Gap and Normal Anion Gap Acidosis

High Anion Gap Acidosis	Normal Anion Gap Acidosis

Ketoacidosis
  Diabetic ketoacidosis
    (acetoacetate)
  Alcoholic (β-hydroxybutyrate)
  Starvation
	Gastrointestinal loss of HCO_3^-
	  (negative urine anion gap)
	  Diarrhea
	  Fistulae external
	Renal loss of HCO_3^- or failure
	  to excrete NH_4^+ (low net
	  acid excretion = positive
	  urine anion gap)

Lactic acid acidosis
  L-Lactic acid acidosis
    (type A and B)
  D-Lactic acid acidosis
Toxins
  Ethylene glycol
  Methyl alcohol
  Salicylate
	Proximal renal tubular
	  acidosis
	Acetazolamide
	Classical distal renal tubular
	  acidosis (low serum K^+)
	Generalized distal renal
	  tubular defect (high
	  serum K^+)
	Miscellaneous
	  NH_4Cl ingestion
	  Sulfur ingestion
	  Dilutional acidosis

the distal nephron, and bicarbonaturia ensues, net acid excretion ceases, and metabolic acidosis follows. Enhanced Cl^- reabsorption, stimulated by ECF volume contraction, results in a hyperchloremic form of chronic metabolic acidosis. With progressive metabolic acidosis, the filtered HCO_3^- load declines progressively. As the serum HCO_3^- concentration decreases, the absolute amount of HCO_3^- entering the distal nephron eventually reaches a level approximating the distal HCO_3^- delivery in normal individuals. At this point, the quantity of HCO_3^- entering the distal nephron can be reabsorbed completely, and the urine pH declines. A new steady state, in which acid excretion equals acid production, then prevails, typically at a serum HCO_3^- concentration of 15 to 18 mEq/L, so the systemic acidosis is not progressive. Therefore, in proximal RTA, in the steady state the serum HCO_3^- concentration is low, and the urine pH is acidic (<5.5). With bicarbonate therapy, the amount of bicarbonate in the urine increases, and the urine pH becomes alkaline. Most cases of proximal RTA occur as part of generalized proximal tubule dysfunction with glycosuria, generalized aminoaciduria, hypercitraturia, and phosphaturia, often referred to as the Fanconi syndrome (see Chapter 16, Toxic Nephropathy, and Chapter 18, Inherited Disorders of the Renal Tubule). The diagnosis of proximal RTA relies initially on the documentation of a chronic hyperchloremic metabolic acidosis with an acid urine pH, which both reverse upon correction of the serum HCO_3^- concentration to near normal.

CLASSIC (HYPOKALEMIC) DISTAL RENAL TUBULE ACIDOSIS   The characteristic feature of this entity is an inability to acidify the urine maximally (to pH < 5.5) in the setting of systemic acidosis. The defect in acidification by the collecting duct impairs NH_4^+ and titratable acid excretion and results in a positive acid balance (net HCO_3^- loss), hyperchloremic metabolic acidosis, and volume depletion. Hypercalciuria and hypocitraturia occur, favoring the development of nephrolithiasis and nephrocalcinosis. Osteomalacia may occur as a result of Ca^{2+}, Mg^{2+}, and PO_4^{3-} wasting.

Classic distal RTA may occur as an inherited defect (primary distal RTA) or as a result of chronic transplant nephropathy, chronic pyelonephritis, hyperglobulinemic states, medullary sponge kidney, and nephrotoxin exposure (e.g., amphotericin B, toluene, or lithium carbonate). The diagnosis can be confirmed by excluding nonrenal losses of HCO_3^- (urine AG, see later) and by the inability to lower the urine pH to less than 5.4 in response to an oral ammonium chloride load.

HYPERKALEMIC DISTAL RENAL TUBULAR ACIDOSIS   The coexistence of hyperkalemia and hyperchloremic acidosis suggests a generalized dysfunction of distal tubule physiology in which urinary ammonium excretion is invariably depressed and renal function is often compromised. Although hyperchloremic metabolic acidosis and hyperkalemia commonly occur in advanced renal insufficiency, hyperkalemia that is disproportionate to the reduction in glomerular filtration rate suggests hyperkalemic distal RTA (e.g., diabetic nephropathy or tubulointerstitial diseases). The transtubular potassium gradient (TTKG) is useful for estimating the appropriateness of the distal tubular response to hyperkalemia. The TTKG is defined as follows:

$$TTKG = \frac{[K]_u / [K]_p}{U / P_{osm}}$$

where u and p reflect the ion concentration in the urine and plasma respectively, and osm is osmolality.

The value is usually low in patients with this disorder (<8), indicating that the collecting tubule is not responding appropriately to the prevailing hyperkalemia. In such patients, dysfunction of both potassium and acid secretion by the collecting tubule occurs and can be attributed either to hypoaldosteronism or to tubule resistance to the effects of aldosterone. In patients presenting with this constellation of findings, an evaluation of the renin-aldosterone system is indicated. A suggested classification of the clinical disorders associated with hyperkalemia and defects in acidification is summarized in Table 5–3.

ACIDOSIS OF EARLY GLOMERULAR INSUFFICIENCY The metabolic acidosis in early renal failure (glomerular filtration rate [GFR], 20 to 30 mL/min) is hyperchloremic in nature but converts to the normochloremic, high AG variety as renal insufficiency progresses and the GFR falls below 15 mL/min. The principal defect in net acid excretion in patients with a reduced GFR is not an inability to secrete H^+ in the distal

Table 5–3: Disorders Associated with Hyperkalemic Distal Renal Tubular Acidosis

Mineralocorticoid Deficiency	Mineralocorticoid Resistance
Primary mineralocorticoid deficiency	Drugs that interfere with Na^+ channel function in CCT
Addison disease	Amiloride
Bilateral adrenalectomy	Triamterene
Adrenal hemorrhage or carcinoma	Trimethoprim
Congenital enzymatic defects	Pentamidine
Chronic idiopathic hypoaldosteronism	Drugs that interfere with Na^+, K^+-ATPase in CCT
Heparin in critically ill patient	Cyclosporine
ACE inhibitors and AT1 receptor antagonists	Drugs that inhibit aldosterone effect on CCT
Secondary mineralocorticoid deficiency	Spironolactone
Hyporeninemic hypoaldosteronism	Eplerenone
Diabetic nephropathy	Disorders associated with tubulointerstitial nephritis and renal insufficiency
Tubulointerstitial nephropathies	Lupus nephritis
Nephrosclerosis	Methicillin nephrotoxicity
Nonsteroidal anti-inflammatory agents	Obstructive nephropathy
Acquired immunodeficiency syndrome	Kidney transplant rejection
IgM monoclonal gammopathy	Sickle cell disease

ACE, angiotensin-converting enzyme; AT1, angiotensin II type 1; CCT, cortical collecting duct.

nephron, but rather an inability to produce or to excrete NH_4^+. The acidosis of chronic renal insufficiency is typically stable over long periods, despite the fact that net acid excretion is significantly less than the acid load from diet and metabolism. To a large extent, alkaline salts from bone buffer the positive acid load. Over the long term this can contribute to the bone disease of chronic renal insufficiency and may warrant correction of the acidosis by alkali therapy.

GASTROINTESTINAL HCO_3^- LOSS   Loss of gastrointestinal fluids distal to the pylorus results in the loss of large quantities of HCO_3^-. Because diarrheal stools and pancreaticobiliary juices contain a higher concentration of HCO_3^- than serum does, volume depletion and metabolic acidosis develop. The volume depletion triggers NaCl reabsorption in the renal tubule; thus, the HCO_3^- that was lost is replaced by a Cl^- anion, resulting in a hyperchloremic metabolic acidosis. An unusual variant of this disorder is seen in cases of ureterocolonic diversion. In this setting, if the urine is not rapidly expelled from the colon, then luminal Cl^- exchanges for serum HCO_3^-, resulting in a hyperchloremic metabolic acidosis.

URINE ANION GAP IN THE DIAGNOSIS OF HYPERCHLOREMIC METABOLIC ACIDOSIS   The urine anion gap (UAG) can help distinguish between gastrointestinal and renal HCO_3^- losses. Because urinary NH_4^+ excretion is typically low in RTA and high in patients with diarrhea, the level of urinary NH_4^+ excretion in metabolic acidosis can be assessed indirectly by calculating the UAG:

$$UAG = [UNa^+ + UK^+] - [UCl^-]$$

In chronic metabolic acidosis of nonrenal origin, the expected response by the kidney is to increase ammonium production and excretion. Because NH_4^+ can be assumed to be present if the sum of the major cations ($Na^+ + K^+$) is less than the sum of major anions in urine, a negative UAG (usually in the range of −20 to −50 mEq/L) can be taken as evidence of nonrenal HCO_3^- losses (diarrhea). Urine estimated in this manner to contain little or no NH_4^+ has more $Na^+ + K^+$ than Cl^- (i.e., the UAG is positive), suggests a renal mechanism for the hyperchloremic acidosis, such as in classic distal RTA (hypokalemia) or hypoaldosteronism with hyperkalemia.

High Anion Gap Metabolic Acidoses
The addition to the body fluids of an acid load in which the attendant non-Cl^- anion is not excreted rapidly results in the development of a high AG acidosis (see Table 5–2). The normochloremic

acidosis is maintained as long as the anion that was part of the original acid load remains in the blood. This may occur if the anion does not undergo glomerular filtration (e.g., uremic acid anions), if the anion is filtered but is readily reabsorbed (e.g., ketoacids or lactate), or if, because of alterations in metabolic pathways, the anion cannot be utilized (e.g., ketoacidosis and L-lactic acidosis).

LACTIC ACIDOSIS Lactate is generated from pyruvate when glucose undergoes anaerobic glycolysis. The normal basally produced lactate is rapidly cleared from the serum by the liver (70%) and kidney (30%). Accumulation of lactic acid in the blood results either from enhanced generation, decreased clearance, or, more typically, a combination of both. This leads to a reduction in serum HCO_3^- concentration, with an equivalent increase in the AG. The causes of lactic acidosis can be classified as follows: type A, which results from tissue hypoperfusion or acute hypoxia, or type B, which results from an inability of tissue to utilize oxygen. Type A lactic acidosis is common in the setting of shock (hypovolemic, septic, or cardiogenic), in which tissue ischemia accelerates lactate production and simultaneously decreases lactate utilization by the liver and kidney. Conditions (without tissue hypoxia) that predispose an individual to type B L-lactic acidosis include hepatic failure; inborn errors of metabolism (glucose 6-phosphatase deficiency); toxins such as ethylene glycol, methanol, and cyanide; and drugs including metformin and nucleoside analogs. Type A lactic acidosis is usually suspected on clinical grounds and can be confirmed either by measuring the serum lactate concentration or by excluding ketoacidosis and intoxications. Lactate concentrations are mildly increased in various nonpathologic states (e.g., during exercise or with use of nucleoside analog), but the magnitude of the elevation is generally small. In practical terms, a lactate concentration greater than 4 mEq/L (normal is 1 mEq/L) is considered pathologic. Importantly, if the cause of the acidosis is removed, then the accumulated lactate can be rapidly recycled to generate an equimolar amount of HCO_3^-.

D-LACTIC ACIDOSIS D-Lactate is the isomer of L-lactate produced by humans and is produced by bacteria in the intestine, from which it can be absorbed into the circulation. D-Lactic acidosis has been described in patients with bowel obstruction, jejunal bypass, short bowel, or ischemic bowel disease. The unifying finding in these disorders is that ileus or stasis is associated with overgrowth of gut flora and is often exacerbated by a high-carbohydrate diet. D-Lactate is not measured by the typical laboratory determination that is used to measure the L-isomer.

KETOACIDOSIS   Diabetic ketoacidosis (DKA), a common cause of high AG acidosis, is caused by increased fatty acid metabolism and the accumulation of ketoacids (acetoacetate and β-hydroxybutyrate) as a result of insulin deficiency. DKA is usually seen in insulin-dependent (type 1) diabetes mellitus in association with cessation of insulin use or an intercurrent illness that increases insulin requirements temporarily and acutely (e.g., infection, gastroenteritis, pancreatitis, or myocardial infarction). The accumulation of ketoacids accounts for the increment in the AG and is accompanied most often by evidence of hyperglycemia (glucose > 300 mg/dL or 17 mmol/L). Compared with alcoholic ketoacidosis (AKA), described next, DKA is characterized by a higher serum glucose concentration, a lower ratio of β-hydroxybutyrate to acetoacetate, and a lower ratio of lactate to pyruvate.

Some chronic alcoholics, especially binge drinkers, who discontinue solid food intake while continuing alcohol consumption develop AKA (also known as β-hydroxybutyric acidosis) when alcohol ingestion is curtailed abruptly. Usually the onset of vomiting and abdominal pain with dehydration leads to cessation of alcohol consumption before presentation to the hospital. The metabolic acidosis may be severe, but it is accompanied by only modestly deranged glucose levels, which are usually low but may be slightly elevated. Insulin levels are low and levels of triglyceride, cortisol, glucagon, and growth hormone are increased. The net result of this deranged metabolic state is ketosis. The acidosis is predominantly caused by the increased levels of ketones, which exist predominantly in the form of β-hydroxybutyrate because of the altered redox state induced by the metabolism of alcohol. Rarely, lactic acidosis is also present.

DRUG AND TOXIN-INDUCED ACIDOSIS   Adult patients with salicylate intoxication usually have pure respiratory alkalosis or mixed respiratory alkalosis–metabolic acidosis. Only part of the increase in the AG is due to the increase in the serum salicylate concentration. A toxic salicylate level of 100 mg/dL would account for an increase in the AG of only 7 mEq/L. High ketone concentrations and lactic acid production also contribute.

Under most physiologic conditions, Na^+, urea, and glucose generate the osmotic pressure of blood. Serum osmolality is calculated according to the following equation:

$$Osmolality = 2[Na^+] + [glucose]/18 + [BUN]/2.8$$

The calculated and determined osmolalities should agree to within 10 to 15 mOsm/kg. If the measured osmolality exceeds the calculated osmolality by more than 15 to 20 mOsm/kg in the setting of a high AG metabolic acidosis then this suggests that a toxic alcohol is present. Ingestion of ethylene glycol, commonly used in antifreeze, leads to an osmolar gap with a high AG metabolic acidosis attributable to ethylene glycol metabolites, especially oxalic acid and glycolic acid. Lactic acid production also increases as a result of a toxic depression in the reaction rates of the citric acid cycle and an altered intracellular redox state. Methanol (wood alcohol) ingestion also causes metabolic acidosis in addition to severe optic nerve and central nervous system manifestations resulting from its metabolism to formic acid from formaldehyde. Lactic acids and ketoacids, as well as other unidentified organic acids, may contribute to the acidosis.

UREMIA   Advanced renal insufficiency eventually converts the hyperchloremic acidosis, discussed earlier, to a typical high AG acidosis. Poor filtration, together with continued reabsorption of as yet poorly identified uremic organic anions, contributes to the pathogenesis of this metabolic disturbance. Uremic acidosis, which classically has an insidious onset, is not usually evident until the GFR declines to less than 15 mL/min. The HCO_3^- concentration rarely falls below 15 mEq/L, and the AG rarely exceeds 20 mEq/L. Numerous studies have demonstrated that the acid retained by patients with chronic renal disease is buffered by alkaline salts derived from bone, which results in significant loss of bone tissue. Despite significant retention of acid (up to 20 mEq/day), the serum HCO_3^- concentration does not decrease further, indicating participation of buffers outside the extracellular compartment.

Metabolic Alkalosis

Metabolic alkalosis is a primary acid-base disturbance that is manifested as alkalemia (elevated arterial pH) together with an increase in $PaCO_2$ as a result of compensatory alveolar hypoventilation (see Tables 5–1 and 5–4). A rise in the serum HCO_3^- concentration requires either exogenous administration of HCO_3^- or a net acid loss from the kidney or gastrointestinal tract. The maintenance of a metabolic alkalosis thereafter represents a failure of the kidneys to eliminate HCO_3^- at the normal capacity. Therefore, in assessing a patient with metabolic alkalosis, two questions must be considered:

1. What is the source of alkali gain (or acid loss) that generated the alkalosis (see Table 5–4)?

Table 5–4: Causes of Metabolic Alkalosis

Exogenous HCO_3^- loads	**ECV expansion,**
Acute alkali administration	**hypertension, K^+**
Milk-alkali syndrome	**deficiency, and**
Effective extracellular	**hypermineralocorticoidism**
volume (ECV) contraction,	*Associated with high renin*
K^+ deficiency, and	Renal artery stenosis
secondary hyperreninemic	Accelerated hypertension
hyperaldosteronism	Renin-secreting tumor
Gastrointestinal origin	Estrogen therapy
Vomiting	*Associated with low renin*
Gastric aspiration	Primary aldosteronism
Congenital chloridorrhea	Adrenal enzymatic defects
Villous adenoma	Cushing syndrome or disease
Renal origin	*Other*
Diuretics	Licorice
Edematous states	Carbenoxolone
Posthypercapnic state	Liddle syndrome
Recovery from lactic	
acidosis or ketoacidosis	
Nonreabsorbable anions	
such as penicillin	
Mg^{2+} deficiency	
K^+ depletion	
Bartter syndrome	
Gitelman syndrome	

2. What renal mechanisms are operating to prevent the excretion of excess HCO_3^-?

Maintenance of a Metabolic Alkalosis
Maintenance of a metabolic alkalosis occurs if one of the following two mechanisms is operative:

1. Cl^- deficiency (volume depleted). Cl^- deficiency, often with concurrent hypokalemia, leads to a fall in GFR or enhanced proximal fractional HCO_3^- reabsorption or both. The associated secondary hyperreninemic hyperaldosteronism stimulates H^+ secretion in the collecting duct, further worsening the acid-base disturbance. These disorders are characterized by a low rate of urinary Cl^- excretion (<20 mEq/L). The alkalosis may be corrected by administration of NaCl and K^+. Causes include vomiting, Cl^--losing diarrhea, nasogastric suctioning, diuretic use, and posthypercapneic states.

2. Hypermineralocorticoidism (volume expanded). In this setting the stimulation of distal H^+ secretion is sufficient to reabsorb the increased filtered HCO_3^- load of metabolic alkalosis and to overcome the decreased proximal HCO_3^- reabsorption caused by ECF expansion. These disorders are characterized by a normal rate of urinary Cl^- excretion (>20 mEq/L) and are not responsive to NaCl administration. Causes include hyperaldosteronism, Cushing syndrome, exogenous corticosteroids, Bartter syndrome, alkali loading, and profound K^+ depletion.

RESPIRATORY DISORDERS

Respiratory Acidosis

Respiratory acidosis occurs as the result of severe pulmonary disease, respiratory muscle fatigue, or depressed ventilatory control (Table 5–5). The increase in $PaCO_2$ caused by reduced alveolar ventilation is the primary abnormality leading to acidemia. In acute respiratory acidosis, there is an immediate compensatory elevation (due to cellular buffering mechanisms) in the HCO_3^- concentration, which increases by 1 mEq/L for every 10 mm Hg increase in $PaCO_2$. In chronic respiratory acidosis (>24 hours), renal adaptation is achieved, and the HCO_3^- increases by 4 mEq/L for every 10 mm Hg increase in $PaCO_2$ (see Table 5–1). The serum bicarbonate does not usually increase more than 38 mEq/L, however. The clinical features of respiratory acidosis vary according to severity, duration, underlying disease, and the presence or absence of accompanying hypoxemia. A rapid increase in $PaCO_2$ may result in anxiety, dyspnea, confusion, psychosis, and hallucinations and may progress to coma. Lesser degrees of dysfunction in chronic hypercapnia include sleep disturbances, loss of memory, daytime somnolence, and personality changes. Coordination may be impaired, and motor disturbances such as tremor, myoclonic jerks, and asterixis may develop. The sensitivity of the cerebral vasculature to the vasodilating effects of CO_2 can cause headaches and other signs that mimic increased intracranial pressure, such as papilledema, abnormal reflexes, and focal muscle weakness. The causes of respiratory acidosis are displayed in Table 5–5 (*right column*).

Respiratory Alkalosis

Alveolar hyperventilation decreases $PaCO_2$ and increases the HCO_3^--to-$PaCO_2$ ratio, thus increasing pH (alkalemia).

Table 5–5: Causes of Respiratory Acid-Base Disorders

Alkalosis	Acidosis
Central nervous system stimulation	Central
Pain	Drugs (anesthetics,
Anxiety, psychosis	morphine, sedatives)
Fever	Stroke
Cerebrovascular accident	Infection
Meningitis, encephalitis	Airway
Tumor	Obstruction
Trauma	Asthma
Hypoxemia or tissue hypoxia	Parenchyma
High altitude, $\downarrow$PaCO$_2$	Emphysema, chronic
Pneumonia, pulmonary edema	obstructive pulmonary
Aspiration	disease
Severe anemia	Pneumoconiosis
Drugs or hormones	Bronchitis
Pregnancy, progesterone	Acute respiratory distress
Salicylates	syndrome
Nikethamide	Barotrauma
Stimulation of chest receptors	Mechanical ventilation
Hemothorax	Hypoventilation
Flail chest	Permissive hypercapnia
Cardiac failure	Neuromuscular
Pulmonary embolism	Poliomyelitis
Miscellaneous	Kyphoscoliosis
Septicemia	Myasthenia
Hepatic failure	Muscular dystrophies
Mechanical hyperventilation	Multiple sclerosis
Heat exposure	Miscellaneous
Recovery from metabolic acidosis	Obesity
	Hypoventilation

Nonbicarbonate cellular buffers respond by consuming HCO$_3^-$. Hypocapnia develops whenever a sufficiently strong ventilatory stimulus causes CO$_2$ output in the lungs to exceed its metabolic production by tissues. Serum pH and HCO$_3^-$ concentration vary proportionately with PaCO$_2$ over a range from 40 to 15 mm Hg. The relationship between the pH and PaCO$_2$ is about +0.01 pH unit for each 1 mm Hg fall in the PaCO$_2$ and that for the serum HCO$_3^-$ concentration is −0.2 mEq/L. Beyond 2 to 6 hours, sustained hypocapnia is further compensated for by a decrease in renal ammonium and titratable acid excretion and a reduction in filtered HCO$_3^-$ reabsorption. The full expression of renal adaptation may take several days and depends on normal volume status and renal function. The effects of respiratory alkalosis vary according to duration and severity, but in general they are primarily those of the underlying disease. A rapid decline in $PaCO_2$ can cause dizziness, mental confusion, and seizures, even in the absence of hypoxemia, as a consequence of reduced cerebral blood flow. Cardiac rhythm disturbances may occur in patients with coronary artery disease as a result of changes in oxygen unloading by blood due to a left shift in the hemoglobin-oxygen dissociation curve (Bohr effect). Acute respiratory alkalosis causes minor intracellular shifts of sodium, potassium, and phosphate and reduces serum-free calcium by increasing the protein-bound fraction. Hyperventilation usually results in hypocapnia. The finding of normocapnia and hypoxemia may herald the onset of rapid respiratory failure and should prompt an assessment to determine whether the patient is becoming fatigued. The causes of respiratory alkalosis are outlined in Table 5–5.

TREATMENT OF ACID-BASE DISORDERS

Treatment of Metabolic Acidosis: General Concepts

The goal of therapy in a metabolic acidosis is the reversal of the underlying cause (e.g., use of insulin for DKA or restoration of tissue perfusion in type A lactic acidosis). If this is not possible, then alkali administration may be considered. It has been emphasized that treatment of a metabolic acidosis with alkali therapy should be reserved for severe acidemia only (pH < 7.2). This dictum is clearly incorrect in situations in which the patient has no "potential HCO_3^-" in serum. Potential HCO_3^- can be estimated from the increment in the AG (ΔAG = patient's AG – 10). Next it must be established whether the acid anion in serum is metabolizable (i.e., β-hydroxybutyrate, acetoacetate, or lactate) or nonmetabolizable (e.g., anions that accumulate in chronic renal failure). The latter variety requires normal renal function and renal ammoniagenesis to replenish the HCO_3^- deficit, a slow and often unpredictable process. Therefore, patients who have no AG (hyperchloremic acidosis), a small AG (mixed hyperchloremic and AG acidosis), or a high AG that is attributable to a nonmetabolizable anion with renal insufficiency should receive alkali therapy to increase the serum HCO_3^- concentration slowly into the range of 20 to 22 mEq/L. In acute life-threatening metabolic acidosis, once the blood pH falls below 7.20, the decrease in myocardial contractility predisposes the patient to congestive heart failure; therefore, a pH of 7.20 is a reasonable therapeutic end point. Intravenous HCO_3^- should be given in amounts that increase the pH to this value. There is no fixed dose to achieve this goal, and a reasonable estimated starting dose is as follows:

Serum $[HCO_3^-] > 10$ mEq/L:
    Dose in mEq = Desired $\Delta HCO_3^- \times$ [body weight (kg) $\times$ 0.5]

or

Serum $[HCO_3^-] < 10$ mEq/L:
    Dose in mEq = Desired $\Delta HCO_3^- \times$ [body weight (kg) $\times$ 0.8]

The need for the two equations results from the increasing volume of distribution of HCO_3^- as acidemia worsens. It is necessary to monitor serum electrolytes hourly during the course of therapy for these disorders so that treatment can be modified as needed, especially because the serum K^+ concentration may decline precipitously as the pH increases.

Treatment of Lactic Acidosis
The basic principle and only effective form of therapy for lactic acidosis is correction of the underlying condition that is initiating the disruption in normal lactate metabolism. In type A lactic acidosis, cessation of acid production through improved tissue oxygenation, restoration of the circulating fluid volume, improvement or augmentation of cardiac function, resection of ischemic tissue, or amelioration of sepsis is necessary in many cases. Alkali therapy is generally advocated for acute, severe acidemia (pH < 7.1) to improve inotropy and lactate utilization. However, administration of $NaHCO_3$ in large amounts may depress cardiac performance and exacerbate the acidemia. The accumulation of lactic acid may be relentless and may necessitate use of ultrafiltration or dialysis, which can simultaneously deliver HCO_3^-, remove lactate, and correct fluid and electrolyte abnormalities. If the underlying cause can be remedied, blood lactate will be reconverted to HCO_3^-. The HCO_3^- derived from lactate conversion and any new HCO_3^- generated by renal mechanisms during acidosis or from exogenous alkali therapy are additive and may result in an overshoot alkalosis.

Treatment of Diabetic Ketoacidosis
Insulin administration and correction of extracellular volume and K^+ deficits are the cornerstones of the treatment of DKA. Administration of alkali is not usually required except in cases of severe acidemia (pH < 7.1) when myocardial depression may hamper tissue perfusion. In less severe acidosis administration of

alkali can result in an overshoot alkalosis once the accumulated ketoacids are recycled into HCO_3^- after insulin administration. Occasionally a patient may develop a substantial normal AG acidosis due to urinary loss of ketoacid anions with Na^+ or K^+ that may benefit from alkali administration. Starvation and alcoholic ketoacidosis largely self-correct with caloric intake; however, care should be taken to ensure that K^+, PO_4^{3-}, and Mg^{2+} levels are monitored and supplemented as required.

The treatment of salicylate and toxic alcohol ingestion are reviewed in Chapter 39, Extracorporeal Treatment of Poisoning.

Treatment of Hyperchloremic Acidosis

Correction of the chronic metabolic acidosis associated with a hypokalemic distal RTA can be achieved with approximately 1 to 3 mEq/kg of oral HCO_3^-/day. In growing children, endogenous acid production is higher and between 2 and 5 mEq/kg/day may be required to maintain normal growth. Severe hypokalemia and metabolic acidosis can occur in some patients under extreme circumstances and may require immediate intravenous therapy. Because increases in the systemic pH with alkali therapy may worsen the hypokalemia, intravenous potassium replacement should begin before alkali administration. In proximal RTAs, the magnitude of the bicarbonaturia at normal or near-normal HCO_3^- concentrations requires that large amounts of HCO_3^- be administered. At least 10 to 30 mEq/kg/day of HCO_3^- or its metabolic equivalent (citrate) is required to maintain the serum HCO_3^- concentration at normal levels. Large supplements of K^+ are often necessary because of the kaliuresis induced by high distal HCO_3^- delivery when the serum HCO_3^- concentration is normalized. Thiazides have proved useful for diminishing the therapeutic requirements for HCO_3^- supplementation by causing ECF contraction to stimulate proximal HCO_3^- absorption. In hyperkalemic distal RTA, treatment should be focused on correction of the hyperkalemia, restoration of euvolemia, adequate alkali therapy, administration of loop diuretics, and dietary potassium restriction. In severe hypoaldosteronism, the effect of loop diuretics can be augmented significantly by administration of small doses of mineralocorticoid. Fludrocortisone should be used cautiously, however, and should be avoided if the patient has hypertension or congestive heart failure.

Although the uremic acidosis and the hyperchloremic acidosis of chronic kidney disease are rarely severe, the progressive dissolution of bone by acidosis warrants treatment to maintain the

HCO_3^- concentration higher than 20 mEq/L. This can be accomplished by administration of relatively modest amounts of alkali (1 to 1.5 mEq/kg/day). If hyperkalemia is present, furosemide (60 to 80 mg/day) should be added. An occasional patient may require chronic sodium polystyrene sulfonate (Kayexalate) therapy orally (15 to 30 g/day in 70% sorbitol).

Treatment of Metabolic Alkalosis

The first aim of treatment is to remove the underlying stimulus for HCO_3^- generation. If primary hypermineralocorticoidism is present, cessation of excess mineralocorticoid elaboration or antagonism of mineralocorticoid action reverses the alkalosis. Likewise, increased H^+ loss from the stomach can be prevented by the use of H_2-receptor blockers or proton pump inhibitors and loss from the kidneys can be prevented by the discontinuation of diuretics. The second aspect of treatment is removal of the factors that sustain HCO_3^- reabsorption, such as ECF contraction or K^+ deficiency. Although K^+ deficits should be repaired, sodium chloride therapy is usually sufficient to reverse the alkalosis if ECF contraction exists. Unusual cases, termed saline resistant, are associated with marked K^+ deficits (>1000 mEq), Mg^{2+} deficiency, Bartter syndrome, or primary autonomous mineralocorticoid states, as listed in Table 5–4. Therapy in these patients must be focused on correcting the underlying pathophysiologic problem. If warranted by associated conditions that preclude infusion of saline (such as a mixed metabolic alkalosis and respiratory acidosis in chronic obstructive pulmonary disease or congestive heart failure), accelerated renal HCO_3^- loss can be achieved by the administration of the carbonic anhydrase inhibitor acetazolamide (250 mg twice a day). The use of dilute hydrochloric acid (0.1 N HCl), although effective, can be dangerous and can result in brisk hemolysis. Acidification can be achieved with oral ammonium chloride, which should be avoided in the presence of liver disease. Finally, hemodialysis with a custom dialysate that is lower in HCO_3^- and higher in Cl^- can be effective when renal function is impaired.

Treatment of Respiratory Acid-Base Disorders

The treatment of respiratory acidosis depends on its severity and rate of onset. Acute respiratory acidosis can be life-threatening, and measures to reverse the underlying cause should be taken simultaneously with restoration of adequate alveolar ventilation to relieve severe hypoxemia and acidemia. Temporarily, this may necessitate tracheal intubation and assisted mechanical ventilation. Oxygen should be carefully titrated in patients with severe chronic obstructive pulmonary disease and chronic CO_2 retention who are breathing spontaneously. When oxygen is used injudiciously, these patients may experience progression of the respiratory acidosis. Aggressive and rapid correction of hypercapnia should be avoided, because the falling $PaCO_2$ may provoke the same complications that are noted with acute respiratory alkalosis (i.e., cardiac arrhythmias, reduced cerebral perfusion, and seizures). The $PaCO_2$ should be lowered gradually in chronic respiratory acidosis, with the aim of restoring the $PaCO_2$ to baseline levels while at the same time providing sufficient chloride and potassium to enhance the renal excretion of bicarbonate.

Chronic respiratory acidosis is often difficult to correct, but general measures focused on maximization of lung function; cessation of smoking; use of oxygen, bronchodilators, corticosteroids, and diuretics; and physiotherapy can help some patients and can forestall further deterioration. Respiratory stimulants may prove useful in selected patients, particularly if they appear to have hypercapnia out of proportion to the level of lung function. The treatment of respiratory alkalosis is primarily focused on alleviation of the underlying disorder. Respiratory alkalosis is rarely life-threatening, and direct measures to correct it will be unsuccessful if the stimulus remains unchecked.

DIAGNOSIS OF ACID-BASE DISORDERS: A STEPWISE APPROACH

Step 1: Obtain arterial blood gas and electrolyte values simultaneously. Both pH and $PaCO_2$ from an arterial blood sample are measured, but the reported HCO_3^- concentration is a calculated figure. Therefore, it should be compared with the measured HCO_3^- concentration (total CO_2) obtained on the electrolyte panel. The two values should agree to within 2 or 3 mEq/L. If these values do not agree, the clinician should suspect that the samples were not obtained simultaneously or that a laboratory error is present.

Step 2: Define the major acid-base disorder that exists. There are two broad types of acid-base disorders: acidosis, characterized by a low pH, and alkalosis, characterized by a high pH. The concentration of HCO_3^- in serum should be examined to determine whether or not the observed change in pH can be accounted for by the change in serum HCO_3^- concentration (see Table 5–1). This process should then be repeated for the $PaCO_2$.

The most commonly encountered clinical disturbances are simple acid-base disorders due to primary derangement of either the serum HCO_3^- concentration alone or the $PaCO_2$ alone.

Step 3: Determine whether a mixed acid-base disturbance exists. In more complicated clinical situations, especially in severely ill patients, a mixed acid-base disturbance may be observed. It is important to understand that the finding of a normal pH does not preclude the existence of a mixed acid-base disorder; close attention should be paid to the measured HCO_3^- and $PaCO_2$ values, even if the pH is normal, when an acid-base disorder is suspected on clinical grounds. To appreciate and recognize a mixed acid-base disturbance, it is important to understand the physiologic compensatory responses that occur in the simple acid-base disorders. Primary respiratory disturbances invoke secondary metabolic responses, and primary metabolic disturbances evoke a predictable respiratory response (see Table 5–1). The levels of HCO_3^- and the $PaCO_2$ change in the same direction in simple acid-base disorders—increased HCO_3^- + increased $PaCO_2$ or decreased HCO_3^- + decreased $PaCO_2$. Any change in the opposite direction suggests a mixed disorder. After determining that the direction of change of the compensatory response is appropriate, one should determine whether the magnitude of the compensatory response is appropriate. An inappropriate change, either too small or too great, suggests a mixed disorder. The expected change and limits of the compensatory response to simple acid-base disorders are outlined in Table 5–1.

Step 4: Calculate the Anion Gap. All evaluations of acid-base disorders should include a simple calculation of the AG (see below). Modest increases in the AG may be seen in volume depletion and metabolic alkalosis; however an AG greater than 20 signifies the presence of a metabolic acidosis regardless of the pH or serum HCO_3^- concentration. If one assumes that the serum albumin is within the normal range, for each milliequivalent per liter change in the AG (ΔAG), there should be an approximately equal and opposite change in the serum HCO_3^- concentration (ΔHCO_3^-). If ΔAG is greater than ΔHCO_3^-, then the presence of a metabolic acidosis with a superimposed metabolic alkalosis or chronic respiratory acidosis is suggested, whereas if ΔAG is less than ΔHCO_3^-, then the coexistence of non-AG (hyperchloremic) metabolic acidosis or a chronic respiratory alkalosis is suggested.

Step 5: Review the clinical history, physical examination, and other laboratory data. For correct diagnosis of a simple or mixed acid-base disorder, it is imperative that a careful history be obtained. The most common causes of acid-base disorders should be kept in mind for the differential diagnosis while one searches for clues that may suggest the specific type of disturbance. For example, a patient with chronic renal failure would be expected to have metabolic acidosis, whereas a patient with chronic vomiting would be expected to have metabolic alkalosis.

Step 6: Make the diagnosis and initiate treatment if required. With the stepwise approach outlined previously one should be able to establish the diagnosis. The decision of whether to treat the acid-base disorder depends on the severity of the acid-base disturbance or its potential for acute and chronic sequelae.

Disorders of Potassium Balance

6

The diagnosis and management of potassium disorders require an understanding of the underlying physiology of potassium homeostasis. In this chapter aspects of the physiology of potassium homeostasis judged to be immediately relevant to a bedside understanding are reviewed; a more detailed review is provided in Chapter 10, Control of Potassium Excretion in *Brenner and Rector's The Kidney*.

NORMAL POTASSIUM BALANCE

Despite the variation in daily intake (30 to 110 mmol/day), homeostatic mechanisms precisely maintain serum K^+ levels between 3.5 and 5 mmol/L. In a healthy individual at steady state, the entire daily intake of potassium is excreted (urine 90%, stool 10%). More than 98% of total body potassium is intracellular, located mainly in muscle, and buffering of extracellular K^+ by this large intracellular pool plays a crucial role in the regulation of serum K^+ levels. The rapid exchange of intracellular K^+ with extracellular K^+ is accomplished by overlapping and synergistic regulation of a number of cellular and renal transport pathways.

Potassium Transport Mechanisms

The intracellular accumulation of K^+ against its electrochemical gradient is an energy-consuming process, mediated primarily by the Na^+,K^+-activated adenosine triphosphatase (Na^+,K^+-ATPase) enzyme, which exchanges three intracellular Na^+ ions for two extracellular K^+ ions. Changes in skeletal muscle Na^+,K^+-ATPase activity and abundance are major determinants of the capacity for extrarenal K^+ homeostasis. Hypokalemia induces a marked decrease in Na^+,K^+-ATPase activity and muscle K^+ content, helping to maintain the serum K^+ within the normal range. In contrast, hyperkalemia due to potassium loading is associated with adaptive *increases* in Na^+,K^+-ATPase activity and muscle K^+ content.

Factors Affecting Internal Distribution of Potassium

Several hormones and physiologic conditions have acute effects on the distribution of K^+ between the intracellular and extracellular space.

Insulin
Insulin promotes a fall in serum K^+ by stimulating the uptake of K^+ by the liver, skeletal muscle, and fat.

Sympathetic Nervous System
Uptake of K^+ by liver and muscle is stimulated through β_2-adrenergic receptors and is largely independent of changes in circulating insulin. In contrast to β-adrenergic stimulation, α-adrenergic agonists impair the ability to buffer increases in K^+.

Acid-Base Status
It has long been thought that acute disturbances in acid-base equilibrium result in changes in the K^+ level, such as the fact that alkalemia shifts K^+ into cells, whereas acidemia is associated with K^+ release from the cells. Despite the complexities of changes in K^+ homeostasis associated with various acid-base disorders, a few general observations can be made. Induction of metabolic acidosis by infusion of mineral acids (NH_4^+/Cl^- or H^+/Cl^-) consistently increases serum K^+, whereas organic acidosis fails to increase serum K^+ in most cases. Metabolic alkalosis induced by sodium bicarbonate infusion usually results in a modest reduction in the plasma K^+ level. Respiratory alkalosis reduces the serum K^+ concentration by a magnitude comparable to that of metabolic alkalosis. Acute respiratory acidosis increases the serum level of K^+; however, the absolute increase is smaller than that induced by metabolic acidosis from inorganic acids.

Renal Potassium Excretion

Potassium Secretion in the Distal Nephron
Renal potassium excretion is determined by regulated secretion in the principal cells of the cortical collecting duct (CCD). Apical Na^+ entry through the amiloride-sensitive epithelial Na^+ (ENaC) channel results in the generation of a lumen-negative potential difference in the CCD, which drives passive K^+ exit through apical K^+ channels. A critical consequence of this relationship is that K^+ secretion depends on delivery of adequate

luminal Na^+ to the distal convoluted tubule and CCD. Basolateral exchange of Na^+ and K^+ is mediated by a Na^+, K^+-ATPase, which provides the driving force for Na^+ entry and K^+ exit at the apical membrane. Several subpopulations of apical K^+ channels exist in the CCD, most prominently a small-conductance channel and a large-conductance, Ca^{2+}-activated, 150-pS ("maxi-K") channel. The higher density and higher open probability of the small-conductance channel suggest that it probably mediates K^+ secretion under baseline conditions. In contrast, flow-dependent K^+ secretion is thought to be mediated by an apical, voltage-gated, calcium-sensitive maxi-K channel.

Regulation of Renal Renin and Adrenal Aldosterone
Modulation of the renin-angiotensin-aldosterone axis has profound clinical effects on K^+ homeostasis. Renin secretion by juxtaglomerular cells within the afferent arteriole in response to various stimuli including decreased Cl^- delivery to the macula densa, renal hypoperfusion, and heightened renal sympathetic tone ultimately results in aldosterone release from the adrenal gland by means of angiotensin II. Hyperkalemia is also an independent and synergistic stimulus for aldosterone release from the adrenal gland although dietary K^+ loading is less potent perhaps than dietary NaCl restriction in increasing circulating aldosterone.

Control of Potassium Secretion: Aldosterone,
K^+ Intake, and Vasopressin
Aldosterone and downstream effectors of this hormone have clinically relevant effects on K^+ excretion, and the ability to excrete K^+ is modulated by systemic aldosterone levels. Aldosterone mediates its K^+ loss by inducing a marked increase in the density of apical ENaC channels in the CCD, thus increasing the driving force for apical K^+ excretion. Other factors favoring K^+ excretion include enhanced dietary K^+ intake and a brisk urine flow rate in the distal nephron segment.

Urinary Indices of Potassium Excretion
A widely used surrogate to measure distal tubule K^+ excretion is the transtubule K^+ gradient (TTKG), which is defined by the following equation:

$$TTKG = \frac{[K^+]_{urine} \times Osm_{blood}}{[K^+]_{blood} \times Osm_{urine}}$$

Water absorption may be an important determinant of the absolute K^+ concentration in the final urine, hence, the use of a ratio of urine-to-plasma osmolality. The expected values of the TTKG are less than 3 in the presence of hypokalemia and more than 7 to 8 in the presence of hyperkalemia. The TTKG may be less useful in patients ingesting diets with changing K^+ and mineralocorticoid intake. There is, however, a linear relationship between serum aldosterone and the TTKG, suggesting that it provides a rough approximation of the ability to respond to aldosterone with a kaliuresis. Moreover, determination of urinary electrolytes provides a measurement of urinary Na^+, which can determine whether significant prerenal stimuli are limiting distal Na^+ delivery and thus K^+ excretion.

CONSEQUENCES OF HYPERKALEMIA AND HYPOKALEMIA

Hypokalemia

Excitable Tissues: Muscle and Heart
Hypokalemia is a risk factor for ventricular and atrial arrhythmias especially in those with other risk factors including preexisting heart disease or use of digoxin or antiarrhythmic medication. ECG changes include broad flat T waves, ST depression, and QT prolongation. Hypokalemia, often accompanied by hypomagnesemia, is a very important cause of the long QT syndrome, alone or in combination with drug toxicity or with the inherited long QT syndromes. In muscle, hypokalemia impairs membrane depolarization, resulting in muscle weakness that can progress to paralysis in severe cases.

Renal Consequences
Short-term K^+ restriction in healthy humans and in patients with essential hypertension induces Na^+ retention and hypertension. Correction of hypokalemia is particularly important in hypertensive patients treated with diuretics because the cardiovascular benefits of diuretic agents are blunted by hypokalemia. Polyuria may result from a vasopressin-resistant defect in urinary concentrating ability. Hypokalemic nephropathy can cause end-stage renal disease, mostly in patients with long-standing hypokalemia due to eating disorders or laxative abuse.

Hyperkalemia

Excitable Tissues: Muscle and Heart
Hyperkalemia constitutes a medical emergency largely because of its effect on the heart. Classically, the ECG manifestations in

Table 6–1: Approximate Relationship Between Hyperkalemic Electrocardiographic Changes and Serum Potassium Levels

Serum K⁺ Levels	ECG Abnormality
Mild hyperkalemia (5.5–6.5 mmol/L)	Tall peaked T waves with narrow base, best seen in precordial leads
Moderate hyperkalemia (6.5–8.0 mmol/L)	Peaked T waves
	Prolonged PR interval
	Decreased amplitude of P waves
	Widening of QRS complex
Severe hyperkalemia (>8.0 mmol/L)	Absence of P wave
	Intraventricular blocks, fascicular blocks, bundle-branch blocks, QRS axis shift
	Progressive widening of the QRS complex
	Sine wave pattern (sinoventricular rhythm), ventricular fibrillation, asystole

Data from Mattu A, Brady WJ, Robinson DA: Electrocardiographic manifestations of hyperkalemia. *Am J Emerg Med* 18:721-729, 2000.

hyperkalemia progress as shown in Table 6–1. However, these changes are variable and not always observed. Patients undergoing dialysis and patients with chronic renal failure may not demonstrate ECG changes, perhaps because of concomitant abnormalities in serum Ca^{2+}. Hyperkalemia rarely manifests with ascending paralysis.

Renal Consequences
Hyperkalemia has a significant effect on the ability to excrete acidic urine because of interference with the urinary excretion of ammonium (NH_4^+).

HYPOKALEMIA

Hypokalemia (K⁺ < 3.6 mEq/L) in clinical practice is usually mild, with K⁺ levels in the 3 to 3.5 mmol/L range, but in up to 25% of patients, it can be moderate to severe (<3 mmol/L) and is associated with increased in-hospital mortality. It is a common problem in patients receiving thiazide diuretics (50%) for hypertension.

Spurious Hypokalemia

Delayed sample analysis can cause spurious hypokalemia due to cellular uptake. Rarely, patients with profound leukocytosis due to acute leukemia are seen with artifactual hypokalemia caused by time-dependent uptake of K^+ by the large white blood cell mass.

Redistribution and Hypokalemia

Administered insulin is a frequent cause of iatrogenic hypokalemia. Alterations in the activity of the endogenous sympathetic nervous system can cause hypokalemia in several settings, including alcohol withdrawal, acute myocardial infarction, and head injury. β_2-Agonists and the xanthines are powerful activators of cellular K^+ uptake and hypokalemia may complicate the therapy of asthma and the use of tocolytics during labor. Occult sources of sympathomimetics, such as pseudoephedrine and ephedrine in cough syrup or dieting agents, are an overlooked cause of hypokalemia.

Hypokalemic Periodic Paralysis

Hypokalemic periodic paralysis (type I and II) is a genetic disorder characterized by reversible attacks of paralysis with hypokalemia that are typically precipitated by rest after exercise and meals rich in carbohydrate. Although the induction of endogenous insulin by carbohydrate meals is thought to reduce serum K^+ levels, insulin can precipitate paralysis in hypokalemic periodic paralysis in the absence of significant hypokalemia. Patients with thyrotoxic periodic paralysis typically present with weakness of the extremities and limb girdles. Attacks may be precipitated by rest and carbohydrate-rich meals and almost never occur during vigorous activity. Clinical signs and symptoms of hyperthyroidism are not always present. Hypokalemia is profound, ranging between 1.1 and 3.4 mol/L, and is frequently accompanied by hypophosphatemia and hypomagnesemia. Treatment involves high-dose propranolol (3 mg/kg), which rapidly reverses the metabolic disturbances. Of note, aggressive K^+ replacement can result in hyperkalemia in this setting.

Nonrenal Potassium Loss

The loss of K^+ from skin is typically low, with the exception of extreme physical exertion. Direct gastric loss of K^+ due to vomiting or nasogastric suctioning is typically minimal, but the ensuing hypochloremic alkalosis results in persistent kaliuresis due to secondary hyperaldosteronism and bicarbonaturia.

Intestinal loss of K^+ due to diarrhea is an important cause of hypokalemia, and it may be associated with a non-anion gap metabolic acidosis with a negative urinary anion gap (consistent with an intact ability to increase NH_4^+ excretion).

Renal Potassium Loss

Drugs
Diuretics are an important cause of hypokalemia because of their ability to increase distal flow rate and distal delivery of Na^+. Thiazides generally cause more hypokalemia than loop diuretics, despite their lower natriuretic efficacy. Other drugs associated with hypokalemia due to kaliuresis include high doses of penicillin-related antibiotics, which are thought to increase obligatory K^+ excretion by acting as nonreabsorbable anions in the distal nephron. K^+ and magnesium wasting can result from tubule toxins, including gentamicin, cisplatin, amphotericin, foscarnet, and ifosfamide. Aggressive replacement of magnesium is obligatory in the treatment of combined hypokalemia and hypomagnesemia, because successful K^+ replacement depends on treatment of the hypomagnesemia.

Hyperaldosteronism
Primary and secondary forms of hyperaldosteronism lead to increased angiotensin II and aldosterone and may be associated with hypokalemia. Causes of secondary hyperaldosteronism include renal artery stenosis and paraneoplastic or renin-secreting renal tumors. Primary hyperaldosteronism may be genetic or acquired. The two major forms of isolated primary hyperaldosteronism are denoted familial hyperaldosteronism type I (FH-I, also known as glucocorticoid-remediable hyperaldosteronism) and familial hyperaldosteronism type II (FH-II). Symptoms in patients with FH-II are clinically indistinguishable from those of patients with sporadic forms of primary hyperaldosteronism due to bilateral adrenal hyperplasia. FH-I usually causes hypertension and typically presents at an early age; the severity of hypertension varies, such that some affected individuals are normotensive. FH-I is caused by a fusion of the adrenocorticotropic hormone–responsive 11β-hydroxylase promoter to the coding region of aldosterone synthase. Aldosterone levels are modestly elevated and regulated solely by adrenocorticotropic hormone. The diagnosis can be confirmed by a dexamethasone suppression test.

Acquired causes of primary hyperaldosteronism include aldosterone-producing adenomas, primary or unilateral adrenal hyperplasia, idiopathic hyperaldosteronism due to bilateral adrenal hyperplasia, and adrenal carcinoma. Aldosterone-producing adenomas and idiopathic hyperaldosteronism account for close to 60% and 40%, respectively, of cases of diagnosed hyperaldosteronism. Because surgery can be curative in patients with aldosterone-producing adenomas, adequate differentiation of these tumors from idiopathic hyperaldosteronism is critical; this may require adrenal imaging and adrenal venous sampling. However, hypokalemia is not a universal feature of primary hyperaldosteronism because compensatory mechanisms can return the serum K^+ to the normal range. Hypokalemia may also occur with systemic increases in glucocorticoids. In Cushing syndrome the incidence of hypokalemia is 10%.

Syndromes of Apparent Mineralocorticoid Excess

In the classic form of apparent mineralocorticoid excess (AME), recessive loss-of-function mutations in the gene *(HSD11B2)* for 11β-hydroxysteroid dehydrogenase-2 cause a defect in the peripheral conversion of cortisol to the inactive glucocorticoid cortisone. Because the mineralocorticoid receptor has equivalent affinity for aldosterone and cortisol, in patients with AME, the unregulated mineralocorticoid effect of glucocorticoids results in hypertension, hypokalemia, and metabolic alkalosis, with suppressed plasma renin activity and aldosterone. Pharmacologic inhibition of 11β-hydroxysteroid dehydrogenase-2 by glycyrrhetinic or glycyrrhizinic acid, contained in licorice, and carbenoxolone is also associated with hypokalemia and AME.

Liddle Syndrome, Bartter Syndrome, and Gitelman Syndrome

These important genetic disorders resulting in hypokalemia are discussed in Chapter 18, Inherited Disorders of the Renal Tubule.

Magnesium Deficiency

Magnesium deficiency results in refractory hypokalemia, particularly if the serum Mg^{2+} concentration is less than 0.5 mg/dL (0.22 mmol/L). Mg^{2+} deficiency often accompanies hypokalemia, in part because the causative renal tubule disorders (e.g., aminoglycoside nephrotoxicity) may cause both kaliuresis and magnesium wasting. Magnesium depletion inhibits muscle Na^+,K^+-ATPase activity triggering K^+ efflux from muscle and cardiac myocytes promoting a secondary kaliuresis and depletion of intracellular myocardial K^+ stores. This phenomenon is particularly important in patients with cardiac disease on diuretics and digoxin. In such patients, hypokalemia and arrhythmias respond to correction of magnesium deficiency and potassium supplementation.

Differential Diagnosis of Chronic Hypokalemia

The most common causes of chronic, diagnosis-resistant hypokalemia are Gitelman syndrome, surreptitious vomiting, and diuretic abuse. Patients with hypokalemia caused by eating disorders may have a constellation of associated symptoms and signs, including dental erosion and depression. Hypokalemic patients with bulimia have an associated metabolic alkalosis, with an obligatory natriuresis accompanying the loss of bicarbonate; the urinary Cl^- level is typically less than 10 mmol/L. Urinary excretion of Na^+, K^+, and Cl^- is high in patients who abuse diuretics. Marked variability in urinary electrolytes is an important clue for diuretic abuse, which can be verified with urinary drug screens. Nephrocalcinosis is very common in furosemide abuse because of the increase in urinary calcium excretion. The differentiation of Gitelman syndrome from Bartter syndrome is discussed in Chapter 18.

TREATMENT OF HYPOKALEMIA

The goals of therapy in hypokalemia are as follows:

- Prevention of life-threatening conditions
- Replacement of the K^+ deficit
- Diagnosis and correction of the underlying cause
- Avoidance of rebound hyperkalemia

The urgency of therapy depends on the severity of hypokalemia, associated conditions, and the rate of decline in the serum K^+ level. Although replacement is usually limited to patients with a true deficit, it should be considered in patients with hypokalemia due to redistribution (e.g., hypokalemic periodic paralysis) when serious complications such as muscle weakness, rhabdomyolysis, and cardiac arrhythmias are present or imminent.

The goal is to raise the serum K^+ to a safe range rapidly and then to replace the remaining deficit at a slower rate over days to weeks. In the absence of abnormal K^+ redistribution, the serum K^+ concentration drops by approximately 0.3 mmol/L for every 100 mmol reduction in total body stores. The treatment of asymptomatic patients with borderline or low normal serum K^+ concentrations is controversial, but supplementation is recommended in patients with serum K^+ levels lower than 3 mmol/L. In high-risk patients (i.e., those with cardiac or severe hepatic disease), serum K^+ concentrations should be maintained above 4 mmol/L. In patients with mild-to-moderate hypertension, potassium supplementation should be considered when the serum K^+ concentration falls below 3.5 mmol/L.

Potassium chloride is the most widely administered salt, because in most patients, hypokalemia results from renal K^+ wasting due to metabolic alkalosis, which usually results from selective chloride losses induced by losses through upper gastrointestinal secretion or diuretic use. In these patients, replacing chloride along with K^+ is essential in treating the alkalosis and preventing further K^+ loss. Slow-release forms are more palatable and better tolerated; however, they have been associated with gastrointestinal ulceration and bleeding. Potassium phosphate is indicated when phosphate deficit accompanies K^+ depletion (e.g., diabetic ketoacidosis). Potassium bicarbonate or its precursors should be considered in patients with hypokalemia and metabolic acidosis (e.g., diarrheal conditions or renal tubular acidosis).

Rapid correction of hypokalemia through oral supplementation is possible; 125 to 165 mmol of K^+ as a single oral dose can increase the serum K^+ concentration by approximately 2.5 to 3.5 mmol/L in 60 to 120 minutes. If the patient is experiencing life-threatening signs and symptoms of hypokalemia, however, intravenous infusion of K^+ should be administered acutely. Concentrations of KCl of up to 400 mmol/L (40 mmol in 100 mL of normal saline) have been used in this setting under continuous ECG monitoring. These solutions are best given through a large central vein; the femoral vein is preferable as it avoids acute local increases in the concentration of K^+ with deleterious effects on cardiac conduction. To avoid venous pain, irritation, and sclerosis, concentrations of more than 60 mmol/L should not be given through a peripheral vein. The maximum rate of administration should be 10 to 20 mmol/hr, although rates of 40 to 60 mmol/hr (for a short period) have been used in patients with life-threatening conditions. In patients with combined severe hypokalemia and hypophosphatemia (e.g., diabetic ketoacidosis), intravenous K^+ phosphate can be used. However, this solution should be infused at a rate of less than 50 mmol over 8 hours to prevent the risk of hypocalcemia and metastatic calcification.

In addition to potassium supplementation, strategies to minimize K^+ losses including minimizing the dose of non–K^+-sparing diuretics, restricting Na^+ intake, and using a combination of non–K^+-sparing and K^+-sparing medications (e.g., angiotensin-converting enzyme inhibitors, angiotensin receptor blockers, K^+-sparing diuretics, and β-blockers). The use of a K^+-sparing diuretic is of particular importance in hypokalemia resulting from primary hyperaldosteronism and related disorders, such as Liddle syndrome and AME because K$^+$ supplementation alone may be ineffective in this setting. It is important to measure the magnesium level and correct hypomagnesemia in all patients with hypokalemia (see earlier). The risk of overcorrection or rebound hyperkalemia in redistribution hypokalemia is high and may result in fatal arrhythmias. When increased sympathetic tone or increased sympathetic response is thought to play a dominant role (e.g., thyrotoxic periodic paralysis, theophylline overdose, and acute head injury), the use of nonspecific β-adrenergic blockade with propranolol generally avoids this complication.

Hyperkalemia

Hyperkalemia is usually defined as a potassium level of 5.5 mmol/L or higher. In most hospitalized patients, the cause of hyperkalemia is multifactorial, with reduced renal function, medications, older age, and hyperglycemia being the most common contributing factors.

Pseudohyperkalemia

Factitious hyperkalemia or pseudohyperkalemia is an artifactual increase in the serum K$^+$ concentration caused by fist clenching and tourniquet use during venepuncture. Severe thrombocytosis or leukocytosis may increase the measured K$^+$ concentration due to release from these cellular elements. In addition, acute anxiety may provoke a respiratory alkalosis and hyperkalemia due to redistribution.

Excess Potassium Intake and Tissue Necrosis

Hyperkalemia is uncommon in the absence of a defect in distal tubule secretion usually combined with a reduction in glomerular filtration rate. However, increased intake of even small amounts of K$^+$ may provoke hyperkalemia in susceptible patients such as those with renal impairment and hyporeninemic hypoaldosteronism. Occult sources of K$^+$ must also be considered, including salt substitutes and alternative medicines. Iatrogenic causes include simple over-replacement with KCl or administration of a potassium-containing medication, such as K$^+$-penicillin, to a susceptible patient. Hyperkalemia often complicates rhabdomyolysis due to the enormous store of K$^+$ in muscle, and this condition is further compounded by the fall in glomerular filtration rate triggered by pigment-mediated acute tubule necrosis. Massive releases of K^+ and other intracellular contents may also occur as a result of acute tumor lysis.

Redistribution and Hyperkalemia

Several different mechanisms can induce efflux of intracellular K^+, resulting in hyperkalemia. Increases in serum K^+ due to hypertonic mannitol and saline are generally attributed to a "solvent drag" effect as water moves in response to the osmotic gradient. Similarly patients that are diabetic are prone to severe hyperkalemia in response to intravenous hypertonic glucose in the absence of coadministered insulin. Succinylcholine depolarizes muscle cells, resulting in a rapid but usually transient hyperkalemia. The use of this agent is contraindicated in patients who have sustained thermal trauma, neuromuscular injury, mucositis, or prolonged immobilization in an intensive care unit setting, because efflux is enhanced in these patients and can result in significant hyperkalemia. Digoxin inhibits Na^+,K^+-ATPase and impairs the uptake of K^+ by skeletal muscle, such that digoxin overdose can result in hyperkalemia. β-Blockers cause hyperkalemia, in part by inhibiting cellular uptake and through hyporeninemic hypoaldosteronism induced by inhibition of renal renin release and adrenal aldosterone release.

Reduced Renal Potassium Excretion

Hypoaldosteronism
Acquired hyperreninemic hypoaldosteronism has been described in critical illness, type 2 diabetes, amyloidosis, and metastasis of carcinoma to the adrenal gland. Heparin also reduces the adrenal aldosterone response to angiotensin II and hyperkalemia, resulting in hyperreninemic hyperaldosteronism.

Most primary adrenal insufficiency is caused by autoimmunity in Addison disease or in the context of a polyglandular endocrinopathy. The risk of hyperkalemia in patients with Addison disease is only 50% to 60%, reflecting the importance of aldosterone-independent modulation of K^+ excretion by the CCD. Adrenal insufficiency also occurs in renal amyloidosis, the antiphospholipid syndrome (adrenal infarction) and human immunodeficiency virus disease. Although adrenal involvement in human immunodeficiency virus disease is usually subclinical, adrenal insufficiency may be precipitated by stress, drugs such as ketoconazole that inhibit steroidogenesis, or the acute withdrawal of steroid agents such as megestrol.

Inherited causes of hypoaldosteronism include X-linked adrenal hypoplasia congenita, which presents with primary adrenal failure and hyperkalemia either shortly after birth or much later in childhood; lipoid congenital adrenal hyperplasia, a severe autosomal recessive syndrome characterized by impaired synthesis of mineralocorticoids, glucocorticoids, and gonadal steroids and the classic, salt-wasting form of congenital adrenal hyperplasia due to 21-hydroxylase deficiency. Isolated deficits in aldosterone synthesis with hyperreninemia may also be caused by loss-of-function mutations in aldosterone synthase.

Hyporeninemic Hypoaldosteronism
Hyporeninemic hypoaldosteronism is a very common predisposing factor for hyperkalemia. It is associated with diabetes mellitus, older age, and renal insufficiency. Classically, patients have suppressed plasma renin activity and aldosterone levels, which cannot be activated by furosemide administration or sodium restriction. Approximately 50% have an associated acidosis, with reduced renal excretion of NH_4^+, a positive urinary anion gap, and urine pH less than 5.5. See Chapter 5, Acid-Base Disorders.

Acquired Tubule Defects and Potassium Excretion
Unlike hyporeninemic hypoaldosteronism, hyperkalemic distal renal tubular acidosis is associated with a normal or increased aldosterone level or plasma renin activity or both. Urine pH in these patients is greater than 5.5, and they are unable to increase acid or K^+ excretion in response to furosemide or fludrocortisone. Classic causes include systemic lupus erythematosus, sickle cell anemia, and amyloidosis.

Hereditary Tubule Defects and Potassium Excretion
These include pseudohypoaldosteronism and Gordon syndrome. See Chapter 18, Inherited Disorders of the Renal Tubule.

Medication-Related Hyperkalemia

Nonsteroidal Anti-inflammatory Drugs
Hyperkalemia is a well-recognized complication of nonsteroidal anti-inflammatory drugs. Nonsteroidal anti-inflammatory drugs cause hyperkalemia by a variety of mechanisms including the following:

- Decreased glomerular filtration rate and increased sodium retention
- Decreased distal delivery of Na^+ and reduced distal flow rate

- Indirect inhibition of the flow-activated apical maxi-K channel in the CCD (prostaglandin-dependent)
- Hyporeninemic hypoaldosteronism
- Blunting of the adrenal response to hyperkalemia (prostaglandin-dependent)

Of note, cyclooxygenase-2 inhibitors are equally likely to cause hyperkalemia.

Cyclosporine and Tacrolimus

Cyclosporine and tacrolimus cause hyperkalemia by a variety of mechanisms including hyporeninemic hypoaldosteronism, inhibition of the apical secretory K^+ channels in the distal nephron, and basolateral Na^+-K^+-ATPase.

Amiloride-Sensitive Epithelial Sodium Ion Channel Inhibition

Inhibition of apical ENaC activity in the CCD by amiloride and other K^+-sparing diuretics predictably results in hyperkalemia. Amiloride is structurally similar to the antibiotics trimethoprim and pentamidine, which also inhibit ENaC and can cause significant hyperkalemia even with standard doses. Risk factors for hyperkalemia due to normal doses of trimethoprim include renal insufficiency and hyporeninemic hypoaldosteronism.

Angiotensin-Converting Enzyme Inhibitors and Mineralocorticoid and Angiotensin Antagonists

Hyperkalemia is a predictable and common effect of angiotensin-converting enzyme inhibition and antagonism of the mineralocorticoid receptor. The adrenal release of aldosterone due to an increased K^+ concentration depends on an intact adrenal-renal angiotensin system; this response is abrogated by systemic angiotensin-converting enzyme inhibitors and angiotensin receptor blockers.

TREATMENT OF HYPERKALEMIA

Most occurrences of hyperkalemia result from K^+ accumulation due to a combination of renal insufficiency and impaired distal K^+ excretion. Therefore, K^+ elimination is the overriding goal. However, on occasion, K^+ redistribution is the underlying problem, and the clinical approach is focused on achieving intracellular translocation of K^+ rather than K^+ loss because this may result in rebound hypokalemia (e.g., diabetic ketoacidosis).

The management of hyperkalemia is based on the severity of the hyperkalemia and/or the presence of ECG evidence of cardiac toxicity or clinical signs of hyperkalemia. Severe hyperkalemia (serum K^+ = 8 mmol/L or serum K^+ > 6.5 with ECG changes other than peaked T waves) is a medical emergency and requires urgent intervention. Given the limitations of ECG changes as a predictor of cardiac toxicity, patients with moderate hyperkalemia (K^+ = 6.5 mmol/L) in the absence of ECG changes or symptomatic patients (muscle weakness) should also receive prompt mdical intervention.

Urgent management of severe hyperkalemia includes a 12-lead electrocardiogram, admission to the hospital, and continuous ECG monitoring. The treatment of hyperkalemia is generally divided into three categories:

1. Antagonism of the cardiac effects of hyperkalemia
2. Rapid reduction in K^+ by redistribution into cells
3. Removal of K^+ from the body

The necessary measures to treat the underlying conditions causing hyperkalemia should be undertaken to minimize the factors that are contributing to hyperkalemia and to prevent future episodes. Dietary restriction (usually 60 mEq/day) with emphasis on the K^+ content of total parenteral nutrition solutions and enteral feeding products (typically 25 to 50 mmol/L) and adjustment of medications and intravenous fluids are necessary; hidden sources of K^+, such as intravenous antibiotics, should not be overlooked. Asymptomatic patients with lower levels of hyperkalemia can be managed with a combination of withdrawal of aggravating factors (angiotensin-converting enzyme I, adrenergic receptor blockers, K^+-sparing diuretics, nonsteroidal anti-inflammatory drugs, and volume depletion), short-term administration of cation-exchange resins and loop diuretics, and dietary modification.

Antagonism of Cardiac Effects

Intravenous calcium raises the action potential threshold and reduces excitability without changing the resting membrane potential and reverses the depolarization blockade that occurs with hyperkalemia. Calcium is available as calcium chloride or calcium gluconate (10-mL ampules of 10% solutions) for intravenous infusion. Calcium gluconate is less irritating to the veins and can be used through a peripheral intravenous line; calcium chloride can cause tissue necrosis if it extravasates and requires a central line.

The recommended dose is 10 mL of 10% calcium gluconate (3 to 4 mL of calcium chloride), infused intravenously over 2 to 3 minutes and under continuous ECG monitoring. The effect of the infusion starts in 1 to 3 minutes and lasts 30 to 60 minutes. The dose should be repeated if there is no change in ECG findings or if they recur after initial improvement. Of note, calcium should be used with extreme caution in patients taking digoxin, because hypercalcemia potentiates the cardiotoxic effects of digoxin. In such patients the infusion should proceed over 20 to 30 minutes to avoid hypercalcemia.

Redistribution of Potassium into Cells

Insulin and Glucose
Insulin lowers the serum K^+ concentration by shifting K^+ into cells. The effect is reliable, dose dependent, and effective, even in patients with chronic renal failure and end-stage renal disease. The recommended dose is 10 units of regular insulin administered intravenously, in 50 mL of 50% dextrose. The effect of insulin on the K^+ level begins in 10 to 20 minutes, peaks at 30 to 60 minutes, and lasts for 4 to 6 hours. The expected fall in serum K^+ concentration should be 0.5 to 1.2 mmol/L, and the dose can be repeated as necessary. Hypoglycemia may occur in up to 75% of patients. Therefore, a continuous infusion of 10% dextrose at 50 to 75 mL/hour and close monitoring of the blood glucose levels are recommended after administration of the bolus insulin/dextrose dose. In hyperglycemic patients with glucose levels of greater than 300 mg/dL, insulin may be administered without glucose, but this should be followed by close monitoring of serum glucose levels.

β_2-Adrenergic Agonists
Albuterol, a selective β_2-agonist, is the most widely used agent and both intravenous and nebulized forms are effective. The recommended dose for intravenous administration is 0.5 mg of albuterol in 100 mL of 5% dextrose, given over 10 to 15 minutes. The K^+-lowering effect starts in few minutes, is maximal at about 30 to 40 minutes, and lasts for 2 to 6 hours. It reduces serum K^+ levels by approximately 0.9 to 1.4 mmol/L. The recommended dose for inhaled albuterol is 10 to 20 mg of nebulized albuterol in 4 mL of normal saline, inhaled over 10 minutes. Its effects start at 30 minutes, peak at 90 minutes, and last for 2 to 6 hours. Inhaled albuterol reduces serum K^+ levels by approximately 0.5 to 1 mmol/L. Importantly, up to 40% of patients with end-stage renal disease exhibit no response to the K^+-lowering effect of albuterol, and albuterol should not be used as a single agent in patients with end-stage renal disease. It should be used with caution in patients with ischemic heart disease.

Sodium Bicarbonate

The role of bicarbonate in the acute treatment of hyperkalemia is increasingly being challenged. The effect of combining bicarbonate with either insulin-glucose or with albuterol has been studied, and no convincing benefit in terms of lowering of the serum K^+ has been demonstrated. Potential adverse effects include a reduction in ionized calcium levels and volume overload. As a result, the routine administration of bicarbonate, especially as a single agent, has no role in the acute treatment of hyperkalemia. One exception may be the management of patients with severe acidemia.

Removal of Potassium

Diuretics

Diuretics have a relatively modest effect on urinary K^+ excretion in patients with chronic renal failure. However, they are useful in correcting chronic hyperkalemia in patients with the syndrome of hyporeninemic hypoaldosteronism and selective renal K^+ secretory problems (e.g., after transplantation or administration of trimethoprim). In patients with impaired renal function, oral diuretics with the highest bioavailability and the least renal metabolism (e.g., torsemide and bumetanide) minimize the chance of accumulation and toxicity.

Mineralocorticoids

Fludrocortisone may be useful in treating chronic hyperkalemia in patients with hypoaldosteronism with or without hyporeninism, and patients with end-stage renal disease patients undergoing hemodialysis who have interdialytic hyperkalemia. The recommended dose is 0.1 to 0.3 mg/day. In patients with end-stage renal disease undergoing hemodialysis, this regimen reduces serum K^+ by up to 0.5 to 0.7 mmol/L. Close monitoring of blood pressure and weight after initiation of these medications is prudent, especially in patients without end-stage renal disease.

Cation Exchange Resins

Sodium polystyrene sulfonate (Kayexalate) exchanges Na^+ for K^+ in the gastrointestinal tract. To prevent constipation and to facilitate the passage of the resin through the gastrointestinal tract, sorbitol may be administered concomitantly. The current recommended dose is 15 to 30 g of powder in water or, preferably, 70% sorbitol one to four times daily. It can take from 4 to 24 hours for the full effect to occur. Therefore, this approach should be used only in conjunction with other measures in the treatment of acute hyperkalemia. Sodium polystyrene sulfonate can be administered rectally as a retention enema in patients who are unable to take or tolerate the oral form. The recommended dose is 30 to 50 g of resin every 6 hours administered as a warm (i.e., body temperature) emulsion in 100 mL of 20% dextrose in water after an initial cleansing enema (i.e., body temperature tap water) and through a rubber tube secured at about 20 cm from the rectum and well into the sigmoid colon. The emulsion should be introduced by gravity, flushed with an additional 50 to 100 mL of non–sodium-containing fluid, retained for at least 30 to 60 minutes, and followed by a cleansing enema (250 to 1000 mL of body temperature tap water). Ischemic colitis and perforation have been reported, but their incidence is minimized by avoiding direct colonic administration with sorbitol and the pre- and postadministration cleansing enemas. This complication can also occur with oral administration of sodium polystyrene sulfonate in sorbitol, although the incidence tends to be much lower. Other potential complications, although rare, include reduction of serum calcium, volume overload, and iatrogenic hypokalemia.

Dialysis
Both continuous hemodiafiltration and peritoneal dialysis can remove significant amounts of K^+ over a 24-hour period. However, hemodialysis is the preferred mode when rapid correction of an acute hyperkalemic episode is desired in patients. Typical clinical settings include the patient with end-stage renal disease, failure of conservative measures to control severe hyperkalemia, and massive K^+ release (e.g., rhabdomyolysis). Hemodialysis removes approximately 30 to 50 mmol of K^+/hr with the greatest decline in serum K^+ levels (1.2 to 1.5 mmol/L) occurring during the first hour. Dialysates with a lower K^+ concentration are more effective in reducing serum K^+ levels. However, a rapid decline in serum K^+ is associated with an increased incidence of cardiac arrhythmias. Therefore, dialysates with a very low K^+ concentration (0 or 1 mmol/L) should be used cautiously, particularly in high-risk patients (e.g., those who use digoxin; have a history of arrhythmia, coronary artery disease, left ventricular hypertrophy, or hypertension; and are older). A rebound increase in serum K^+ can occur after hemodialysis. This phenomenon can be especially marked in patients with massive release from devitalized tissues (e.g., tumor lysis or rhabdomyolysis).

Pathophysiology of Water Metabolism

7

Disorders of body fluids are among the most commonly encountered problems in the practice of clinical medicine, in large part because many different disease states can potentially disrupt the finely balanced mechanisms that control the intake and output of water and solute. Because body water is the primary determinant of the osmolality of the extracellular fluid, disorders of water metabolism can be broadly divided into hyperosmolar disorders, in which there is a deficiency of body water relative to body solute, and hypo-osmolar disorders, in which there is an excess of body water relative to body solute. Because sodium is the main constituent of plasma that determines osmolality, these disorders are typically characterized by hypernatremia and hyponatremia, respectively.

Osmolality is defined as the concentration of all of the solutes in a given weight of water and is expressed as units either of osmolality (milliosmoles of solute per kilogram of water, [mOsm/kg H_2O]) or osmolarity (milliosmoles of solute per liter of water [mOsm/L H_2O]). The total solute concentration can be estimated by summing the concentrations of all individual ions and other solutes. Plasma osmolality can be measured directly (freezing point) or calculated using the formula:

$$P_{osm} \text{ (mOsm/kg } H_2O) = 2 \times \text{plasma } [Na^+] \text{ (mEq/L)}$$
$$+ \text{ glucose (mg/dL)/ 18}$$
$$+ \text{ blood urea nitrogen (mg/dL)/2.8}$$

The total osmolality of plasma is not always equivalent to the "effective" osmolality, because the latter is a function of the relative solute permeability properties of the membranes separating the intracellular fluid (ICF) and extracellular fluid (ECF) compartments. Solutes that cannot freely traverse cell membranes (e.g., Na^+ and mannitol) are restricted to the ECF compartment and are effective solutes, because they create osmotic pressure gradients across cell membranes, leading to osmotic movement of water from the ICF to the ECF compartments. Solutes that are permeable to cell membranes (e.g., urea, ethanol, and methanol) are ineffective solutes, because they do not create osmotic pressure gradients across cell membranes and therefore are not associated with such water shifts. Glucose is usually an ineffective solute; however, under conditions of impaired cellular uptake (e.g., insulin deficiency), it becomes an effective extracellular solute. The importance of this distinction between total and effective osmolality is that only the effective solutes in plasma are determinants of whether clinically significant hyperosmolality or hypo-osmolality is present. An example is uremia: A patient with a urea concentration that has increased by 30 mEq/L will have a corresponding 30 mOsm/kg H_2O elevation in plasma osmolality, but the effective osmolality will remain normal because the increased urea is proportionally distributed across both the ECF and ICF. In contrast, a patient whose plasma Na^+ concentration has increased by 15 mEq/L will also have a 30 mOsm/kg H_2O elevation of plasma osmolality, because the increased cation must be balanced by an equivalent increase in plasma anions. However, in this case, the effective osmolality will also be elevated by 30 mOsm/kg H_2O because the Na^+ and accompanying anions will largely remain restricted to the ECF owing to the relative impermeability of cell membranes to Na^+ and other univalent ions. Thus, elevations of solutes such as urea, unlike elevations in plasma Na^+ concentrations, do not cause cellular dehydration, and consequently do not activate mechanisms that defend body fluid homeostasis by acting to increase body water stores.

CONTROL OF PLASMA OSMOLALITY

Arginine Vasopressin Synthesis and Secretion

Arginine vasopressin (AVP) is a nonapeptide that is synthesized in the hypothalamus. As implied by its name, *arginine vasopressin* causes constriction of blood vessels, but the pressor effect occurs only at concentrations many times those required to produce antidiuresis and is probably of no physiologic or pathologic importance in humans except under conditions of severe hypotension and hypovolemia. AVP is produced by the *posterior pituitary gland* in response to a rise in serum osmolality. It effects antidiuresis by binding to AVP V_2 receptors in the collecting duct of the kidney, which results in increased water permeability through the insertion of the aquaporin-2 water channel into the apical membranes of collecting tubule principal cells.

This leads to enhanced reabsorption of water, which lowers the plasma osmolality toward the normal range. In healthy adults, the osmotic threshold for AVP secretion ranges from 275 to 290 mOsm/kg H_2O (averaging $\approx$280 to 285 mOsm/kg H_2O). A rise in plasma osmolality of as little as 1% is sufficient to trigger AVP release, and maximal antidiuresis is achieved after increases in plasma osmolality of only 5 to 10 mOsm/kg H_2O above the threshold for AVP secretion. However, many factors can alter either the sensitivity or the set point of the osmoregulatory system for AVP secretion. Other nonosmotic causes of AVP release include actual or effective circulating volume depletion, nausea, hypoglycemia, stress, and a variety of drugs (Table 7–1).

Thirst

Thirst is the body's defense mechanism to increase water consumption in response to a perceived water deficit. However, most fluid ingestion is determined by influences such as meal-associated fluid intake, taste, or psychosocial factors rather than true thirst. In healthy adults, an increase in effective plasma

Table 7–1: Drugs and Hormones That Affect Vasopressin Secretion

Stimulatory	*Inhibitory*
Acetylcholine	Norepinephrine
Nicotine	Fluphenazine
Apomorphine	Haloperidol
Morphine (high doses)	Promethazine
Epinephrine	Oxilorphan
Isoproterenol	Butorphanol
Histamine	Opioid agonists
Bradykinin	Morphine (low doses)
Prostaglandin	Alcohol
β-Endorphin	Carbamazepine
Cyclophosphamide IV	Glucocorticoids
Vincristine	Clonidine
Insulin	Muscimol
2-Deoxyglucose	Phencyclidine
Angiotensin II	?Phenytoin
Lithium	
Corticotropin-releasing factor	
Naloxone	
Cholecystokinin	
?Chlorpropamide	
?Clofibrate	

osmolality of only 2% to 3% above basal levels produces a strong desire to drink. The absolute level of plasma osmolality at which a person develops a conscious urge to seek and drink water is called the *osmotic thirst threshold*. It varies appreciably among individuals but averages approximately 295 mOsm/kg H_2O. Of physiologic significance is the fact that this level is above the osmotic threshold for AVP release and approximates the plasma osmolality at which the maximal concentration of the urine is normally achieved.

HYPERNATREMIA

Hypernatremia, defined as a plasma Na^+ level greater than 146 mEq/L, implies a deficiency of total body water relative to total body sodium. When a patient with either hypo- or hypernatremia is treated, it is important to understand the following key concept:

> Total body Na^+ stores are a major factor determining ECF volume status; however, the measured serum Na^+ reflects only the *concentration* of sodium within the ECF. Analysis of the serum Na^+ without reference to the physical examination or other laboratory indices of volume status gives no information regarding a patient's ECF volume status.

Therefore, hypernatremia *does not* imply total body sodium overload (i.e., ECF volume overload), rather it implies a deficiency of water relative to total body Na^+ stores. The patient with hypernatremia may be hypovolemic or euvolemic or have ECF volume expansion, and clinical determination of the volume status is attained by evaluating factors including the physical examination (e.g., blood pressure and skin turgor), laboratory findings (e.g., blood urea nitrogen-to-creatinine ratio), and hemodynamic parameters (e.g., central venous pressure).

Hypernatremia rarely develops in patients who have free access to water because the hyperosmolar-induced thirst sensation triggers avid water ingestion that returns the serum osmolality to normal or near normal. When access to free water is limited, which may occur in critically ill patients, infants, and patients with dementia, then either free water losses in excess of Na^+ losses (diarrhea or osmotic diuresis), free water losses alone (diabetes insipidus), or augmented Na^+ intake without sufficient free water (hypertonic feedings or $NaHCO_3$ administration) can lead to the development of hypernatremia. Because Na^+ is the principle determinant of serum osmolality, hypernatremia is associated with a rise in serum osmolality, which causes fluid to exit brain cells, causing cell shrinkage and a variety of neurologic sequelae. Depending on the speed of onset of the hypernatremia, these include restlessness, anxiety, confusion, coma, and seizures (see later).

Management of the Patient with Hypernatremia

The approach to the patient with documented hypernatremia includes the following key steps:

1. Determination of total body Na$^+$ stores (i.e., ECF volume status)
2. Identification of the underlying cause of the water deficit
3. Calculation of total body water deficit and ongoing free water losses
4. Correction of the volume disturbance if present
5. Correction of the water deficit with specific regard to the risk of cerebral edema from overly rapid correction

Hypovolemic Hypernatremia

Hypovolemic hypernatremia implies renal or extrarenal losses of sodium that are outweighed by a greater loss of free water. Extrarenal losses can be caused by increased dermal losses (e.g., burns or sweating) or more commonly by diarrhea (e.g., lactulose administration). Extrarenal losses can be distinguished from renal losses by examining the urine chemistry values. In the former setting, the kidney avidly reabsorbs Na$^+$ and water, leading to the excretion of concentrated urine with urine Na$^+$ concentration [U_{Na^+}] less than 10 mEq/L. In contrast, primary renal salt and water losses (water > salt), such as those that may occur during an osmotic diuresis (mannitol, postobstruction, or hyperglycemia), are characterized by the excretion of isotonic or hypotonic urine (U_{osm} < 300 mOsm/L) and U_{Na^+} greater than 20 mEq/L.

Euvolemic Hypernatremia

Euvolemic hypernatremia implies a disorder of urinary concentration related to either the absence of AVP or a resistance to the actions of AVP within the principle cells in the distal tubule. The common causes of euvolemic hyponatremia are discussed in the following.

Central Diabetes Insipidus
Central diabetes insipidus (DI) is caused by inadequate secretion of AVP from the posterior pituitary gland in response to

Table 7–2: Etiology of Hypotonic Polyuria

Central diabetes insipidus
    Congenital (congenital malformations; autosomal dominant:
        arginine vasopressin [AVP]–neurophysin gene mutations)
    Drug/toxin-induced (ethanol, diphenylhydantoin, snake venom)
    Granulomatous (histiocytosis, sarcoidosis)
    Neoplastic (craniopharyngioma, meningioma, pituitary tumor,
        metastases)
    Infectious (meningitis, tuberculosis, encephalitis)
    Inflammatory/autoimmune (lymphocytic
        infundibuloneurohypophysitis)
    Trauma (neurosurgery, deceleration injury)
    Vascular (cerebral hemorrhage/infarction, brain death)
    Idiopathic
Osmoreceptor dysfunction
    Granulomatous (histiocytosis, sarcoidosis)
    Neoplastic (as above)
    Vascular (anterior communicating artery aneurysm/ligation,
        intrahypothalamic hemorrhage)
Idiopathic
Increased AVP metabolism
    Pregnancy
Nephrogenic diabetes insipidus (DI)
    Congenital
    Drug-induced (demeclocycline, lithium, cisplatin, methoxyflurane)
    Hypercalcemia
    Hypokalemia
    Infiltrating lesions (sarcoidosis, amyloidosis)
    Vascular (sickle cell anemia)
    Mechanical (polycystic kidney disease, bilateral obstruction)
    Solute diuresis (glucose, mannitol, sodium, radiocontrast dyes)
    Idiopathic
Primary polydipsia
    Psychogenic (schizophrenia, obsessive-compulsive behavior)
    Dipsogenic (downward resetting of thirst threshold: idiopathic
        or similar lesions as in central DI)

osmotic stimulation. In most cases this is due to destruction of the neurohypophysis by a variety of acquired or congenital anatomic lesions (Table 7–2). Familial central DI, an autosomal dominant disorder, is caused by mutations in the gene that encodes the AVP-neurophysin precursor. Idiopathic forms of AVP deficiency may represent autoimmune destruction of the neurohypophysis. AVP antibodies have been seen in the serum of as many as one third of patients with idiopathic DI and two thirds of those with Langerhans cell histiocytosis X, but not in patients with DI caused by tumors.

Osmoreceptor Dysfunction

The primary osmoreceptors that control AVP secretion and thirst are located in the anterior hypothalamus. Lesions of this region cause hyperosmolality through a combination of impaired thirst and osmotically stimulated AVP secretion— "adipsic hypernatremia." Most instances of osmoreceptor dysfunction are due to the same types of lesions that can cause simple central DI, but in this case they are located, or extend, more anteriorly in the hypothalamus. One lesion that is unique to this disorder is an anterior communicating cerebral artery aneurysm. Spontaneous or postsurgical infarction of the region of the hypothalamus containing the osmoreceptor cells can lead to this disorder.

Gestational Diabetes Insipidus

A relative deficiency of plasma AVP due to the action of the circulating enzyme oxytocinase/vasopressinase normally produced by the placenta to degrade circulating oxytocin can trigger gestational diabetes insipidus.

Nephrogenic Diabetes Insipidus

Resistance to the antidiuretic action of AVP due to a defect within the kidney is commonly referred to as nephrogenic DI. Nephrogenic DI can be an inherited disorder or may be caused by a variety of drugs, diseases, and metabolic disturbances, among them lithium, hypokalemia, and hypercalcemia (see Table 7–2). Inherited causes of nephrogenic DI are discussed in Chapter 18, Inherited Disorders of the Renal Tubule.

Clinical Manifestations of Diabetes Insipidus

The cardinal clinical symptoms of DI are polyuria and polydipsia. Clinical manifestations of hyperosmolality can be divided into the signs and symptoms produced by dehydration, which are largely cardiovascular, and those caused by the hyperosmolality itself, which are predominantly neurologic and reflect brain dehydration as a result of osmotic water shifts out of the central nervous system. Severe water depletion can lead to cardiovascular manifestations of hypertonic dehydration including hypotension and azotemia resulting from renal hypoperfusion. More commonly, symptoms of hyperosmolality predominate, with neurologic manifestations ranging from nonspecific symptoms such as irritability and cognitive dysfunction to more severe manifestations of *hypertonic encephalopathy* such as disorientation, a decreased level of consciousness, seizures, focal neurologic deficits, and cerebral infarction. The length of time over which hyperosmolality develops can markedly affect clinical symptomatology.

Rapid development of severe hyperosmolality is often associated with marked neurologic symptoms, whereas gradual development over several days or weeks generally causes milder symptoms.

Hypervolemic Hypernatremia

Patient with hypervolemic hypernatremia typically have received an exogenous Na^+ load. Examples of this include the administration of hypertonic intravenous sodium bicarbonate to a patient with a metabolic acidosis or the administration of excess NaCl to an infant.

Treatment of Hypernatremia

Rapid development of severe hyperosmolality is often associated with marked neurologic symptoms, whereas gradual development over several days or weeks generally causes milder symptoms. In chronic hypernatremia the brain counteracts osmotic shrinkage by increasing the intracellular content of solutes. The net effect of this process is protection of the brain against excessive shrinkage during sustained hyperosmolality. However, once the brain has adapted by increasing its solute content, rapid correction of the hyperosmolality can trigger cerebral edema. To reduce the risk of central nervous system damage from protracted exposure to severe hyperosmolality, in most cases, the free water administration in the first 24 hours should include an estimation of ongoing water loss plus only 50% of the estimated water deficit (see later). Further correction to a normal plasma osmolality should be spread over the next 24 to 72 hours to avoid triggering of cerebral edema. This is especially important in children, because several studies have indicated that limiting correction of hypernatremia to a maximal rate of no greater than 0.5 mmol/L/hr prevents the occurrence of symptomatic cerebral edema with seizures. In addition, the possibility of associated thyroid or adrenal insufficiency should also be kept in mind, because patients with central DI caused by hypothalamic masses can have associated deficiencies of anterior pituitary function. Acute hypernatremia with associated neurologic signs can be corrected over a shorter time period (<24 hours).

Hypovolemic Hypernatremia

Restoration of the ECF volume is the primary therapeutic maneuver in hypovolemic hypernatremia. This is accomplished with 0.9% NaCl, which is relatively hypotonic compared with the serum in the patient with hypernatremia. Once euvolemia is established and ongoing losses (Na^+ + water) are accounted for, any residual hypernatremia can be managed with 5% dextrose or 0.45% NaCl as outlined for the management of euvolemic hyponatremia.

Euvolemic Hypernatremia
The total body water deficit in a hypernatremic patient can be estimated using the following formula:

$$\text{Total body water deficit} = 0.6 \times \text{Premorbid weight} \times (1 \times 140/[\text{Plasma Na}^+])$$

This above formula does not take into account ongoing water losses. Therefore, frequent serum and urine electrolyte determinations should be made, and the administration rate of oral water or intravenous 5% dextrose in water should be adjusted accordingly.

Specific Management Issues
CENTRAL DIABETES INSIPIDUS   Patients with central DI should be treated with intranasal or oral desmopressin (Table 7–3). Treatment must be individualized to determine the optimal dosage and dosing interval. Usually a satisfactory schedule can be achieved with modest doses, and the maximum dosage needed is rarely greater than 0.2 mg orally or 20 mcg (two sprays) given two to three times daily. In selected patients, chlorpropamide may lower the required desmopressin dose.

The patient with acute postsurgical central DI is sometimes treated only with intravenous fluid replacement for a period before the institution of antidiuretic hormone therapy to minimize the risk of cerebral edema. Postoperatively, desmopressin may be given parenterally in a dose of 1 to 2 mcg subcutaneously,

---

Table 7–3: Therapies for the Treatment of Diabetes Insipidus

Water
Antidiuretic agents
   Arginine vasopressin (Pitressin)
   1-Deamino-8-D-arginine vasopressin (desmopressin, DDAVP)
Antidiuresis-enhancing agents
   Chlorpropamide
   Prostaglandin synthetase inhibitors (indomethacin, ibuprofen,
      tolmetin)
Natriuretic agents
   Thiazide diuretics
   Amiloride

intramuscularly, or intravenously. A prompt reduction in urine output should occur, and the duration of its antidiuretic effect is generally 6 to 12 hours. The urine osmolality and serum Na^+ concentration must be checked every several hours during the initial therapy and then at least daily until stabilization or resolution of the DI. It is generally advisable to allow some return of the polyuria before administration of subsequent doses of desmopressin because postoperative DI is often transient. The clinical management of acute traumatic DI after injuries to the head is similar to that of postsurgical DI, except that the possibility of anterior pituitary insufficiency must also be considered in such cases, and the patient should be given stress doses of hydrocortisone (100 mg intravenously every 8 hours) until anterior pituitary function can be definitively evaluated.

OSMORECEPTOR DYSFUNCTION The long-term management of osmoreceptor dysfunction syndromes requires a thorough search for a potentially treatable cause in conjunction with the use of measures to prevent recurrence of dehydration. The mainstay of management is education of the patient and family about the importance of continuously regulating fluid intake in accordance with hydration status. This regulation can be done most efficaciously by establishing a daily schedule of water intake based on changes in body weight regardless of the patient's thirst.

GESTATIONAL DIABETES INSIPIDUS The treatment of choice for gestational diabetes insipidus is desmopressin, because it is not destroyed by oxytocinase/vasopressinase and appears to be safe for both mother and child.

NEPHROGENIC DIABETES INSIPIDUS By definition, nephrogenic DI is resistant to the effects of AVP. Some patients with nephrogenic DI can be treated by eliminating the drug (e.g., lithium) or disease (e.g., hypercalcemia) responsible for the disorder. For many others, the only practical form of treatment at present is to restrict sodium intake and administer a thiazide diuretic either alone or in combination with a prostaglandin synthetase inhibitor or amiloride. When combined with dietary sodium restriction, thiazides cause modest hypovolemia. This stimulates isotonic proximal tubular solute reabsorption and diminishes solute delivery to the more distal diluting site. Another advantage of amiloride is that it decreases lithium entrance into cells in the distal tubule, and because of this may have a preferable action for the treatment of lithium-induced nephrogenic DI. Although desmopressin is generally not effective in nephrogenic DI, a few patients may have partial responses to AVP or desmopressin, with increases in urine osmolality after much higher doses of these agents than are typically used to treat central DI (e.g., 6 to 10 mcg), and it is generally worth a trial of desmopressin at these doses to ascertain whether this is a useful therapy in selected patients.

Hypervolemic Hypernatremia

The principle therapeutic intervention in hypervolemic hypernatremia is induction of a natriuresis with a loop diuretic such as furosemide. Patients with end-stage renal disease may require hemodialysis. Care must be taken to avoid overly rapid rates of correction, as may occur when furosemide and hypotonic fluids are administered simultaneously.

HYPO-OSMOLAR DISORDERS

Hyponatremia (plasma Na^+ concentration < 130 mEq/L) is one of the most common electrolyte disorders encountered in clinical medicine. As reviewed in the introduction to this chapter, changes in plasma Na^+ concentrations are usually associated with comparable changes in plasma osmolality. When the "measured" osmolality exceeds the calculated osmolality by more than 10 mOsm/kg H_2O, an *osmolar gap* is said to be present. This occurs in two circumstances: (1) with a decrease in the water content of serum, and (2) on addition of a solute other than urea or glucose to the serum. A decrease in the water content of serum is usually due to its displacement by excessive amounts of protein or lipids, as may occur in severe hyperglobulinemia or hyperlipidemia. The hyponatremia associated with normal osmolality has been termed *factitious hyponatremia* or *pseudohyponatremia*. The most common causes of pseudohyponatremia are primary or secondary hyperlipidemic disorders. It has been estimated that the plasma Na^+ concentration declines by 1 mEq/L for every 4.6 g/L of plasma lipids. Plasma protein elevations greater than 10 g/dL, as seen in multiple myeloma or macroglobulinemia, can also cause pseudohyponatremia. The second setting in which an osmolar gap occurs is the presence in plasma of an exogenous low-molecular-weight substance such as ethanol, methanol, ethylene glycol, or mannitol. As discussed previously, in the presence of relative insulin deficiency, glucose does not penetrate cells readily and remains in the ECF. As a consequence, it draws water from the cellular compartment, causing cell shrinkage, and this translocation of water commensurately decreases the extracellular concentration of Na^+. In this setting, therefore, the plasma Na^+ concentration may be low while plasma osmolality is high. For every 100 mg/dL (5.5 mmol/L) rise in plasma glucose, the osmotic shift of water causes plasma Na^+ concentration to drop by 1.6 to 2.4 mEq/L. Similar "translocational" hyponatremia occurs with mannitol or maltose or with the absorption of glycine during transurethral prostate resection, as well as in gynecologic and orthopedic procedures. However, when the plasma solute is readily permeable (e.g., urea, ethylene glycol, methanol, or ethanol), it enters the cell and so does not establish an osmotic gradient for water movement. There is no cellular dehydration despite the hypertonic state, and the plasma Na^+ concentration remains unchanged.

Etiology of Hyponatremia

In approaching the hyponatremic patient, the physician's first task is to ensure that hyponatremia is not a consequence of the causes of pseudohyponatremia as discussed (Fig. 7–1). Thereafter, an assessment of ECF volume provides a useful working classification of hyponatremia because it can be associated with decreased, normal, or high total body sodium:

1. Hyponatremia with ECF volume depletion
2. Hyponatremia with excess ECF volume
3. Hyponatremia with normal ECF volume

Hyponatremia with Extracellular Fluid Volume Depletion

Patients with hyponatremia who have ECF volume depletion have sustained a deficit in total body Na^+ that exceeds the deficit in water. If sufficiently severe, volume depletion is a potent stimulus to AVP release. Although hyponatremia in this setting involves depletion of body solutes, a concomitant failure to excrete water is critical to the process. An examination of the urinary Na^+ concentration (U_{Na^+}) is helpful in assessing whether the fluid losses are renal or extrarenal in origin. A U_{Na^+} less than 20 mEq/L reflects the normal renal response to volume depletion and suggests an extrarenal source of fluid loss (e.g., gastrointestinal, burns, or sequestration). Hypovolemic hyponatremia in patients with a U_{Na^+} greater than 20 mEq/L points to the kidney as the source of the fluid losses.

Diuretic-induced hyponatremia accounts for a significant proportion of symptomatic hyponatremia in hospitalized patients. It occurs almost exclusively with thiazide rather than loop diuretics, most likely because the former have no effect on urine concentrating ability but the latter do. Risk factors include

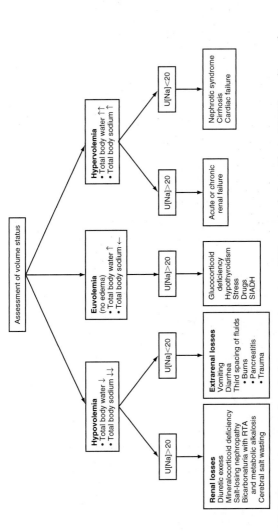

Figure 7–1. Diagnostic approach to the hyponatremic patient. RTA, renal tubular acidosis; SIADH, syndrome of inappropriate antidiuretic hormone secretion. (Modified from Halterman R, Berl T: Therapy of dysnatremic disorders. In Brady H, Wilcox C (eds): *Therapy in Nephrology and Hypertension.* Philadelphia, WB Saunders, 1999, p. 256.)

female sex and older age. Diuretics can cause hyponatremia by a variety of mechanisms: (1) volume depletion, which enhances AVP release and decreases fluid delivery to the diluting segment; or (2) a direct effect of diuretics on the diluting segment. Salt-losing nephropathy with hypovolemic hyponatremia may occur in the following settings: advanced renal insufficiency, interstitial nephropathy, medullary cystic kidney disease, polycystic kidney disease, or partial urinary obstruction. It has long been recognized that adrenal insufficiency is associated with impaired renal water excretion and hyponatremia. This diagnosis should be considered in the volume-contracted hyponatremic patient whose urinary Na^+ concentration is not low, particularly when the serum K^+, blood urea nitrogen, and creatinine levels are elevated. Cerebral salt wasting is a rare syndrome seen primarily in patients with subarachnoid hemorrhage; it leads to renal salt wasting and volume contraction.

Hyponatremia with Excess Extracellular Fluid Volume

Many edematous states are associated with hyponatremia. These patients have an increase in total body Na^+ content, but the rise in total body water exceeds that of Na^+. With the exception of renal failure and ongoing diuretic use, these states are characterized by avid Na^+ retention ($U_{Na^+} < 10$ mEq/L).

Congestive Heart Failure
Advanced congestive heart failure is associated with hyponatremia due to excess water retention. This is mediated by a combination of decreased delivery of tubule fluid (i.e., Na^+) to the distal nephron and increased release of AVP in response to the decrement in effective blood volume sensed by aortic and carotid sinus baroreceptors.

Hepatic Failure
Patients with advanced cirrhosis and ascites often present with hyponatremia as a consequence of their inability to excrete a water load. This process results from a decrement in effective arterial volume (splanchnic venous pooling, decreased plasma oncotic pressure, or peripheral vasodilatation), leading to avid Na^+ and water retention.

Nephrotic Syndrome
The incidence of hyponatremia in the nephrotic syndrome is lower than that in either congestive heart failure or cirrhosis, most likely as a consequence of the higher blood pressure, higher glomerular filtration rate, and more modest impairment

in Na^+ and water excretion than those in the other groups of patients. Because lipid levels are often elevated, a direct measurement of plasma osmolality should be performed.

Renal Failure
Hyponatremia with edema can occur with either acute or chronic renal failure due an inability to excrete an ingested water load.

Hyponatremia with Normal Extracellular Fluid Volume

Syndrome of Inappropriate Antidiuretic Hormone Secretion
CLINICAL CHARACTERISTICS Patients with the syndrome of inappropriate antidiuretic hormone secretion (SIADH) are hypo-osmolar while excreting urine that is less than maximally dilute (>50 mOsm/kg H_2O). However, the development of hyponatremia with dilute urine (<100 mOsm/kg H_2O) should raise suspicion for a primary polydipsic disorder. U_{Na^+} is usually greater than 20 mEq/L, but it may be low in patients with the syndrome who are receiving a low-sodium diet. Before the diagnosis of SIADH is made, other causes for decreased diluting capacity, such as renal, pituitary, adrenal, thyroid, cardiac, or hepatic disease, must be excluded. In addition, nonosmotic stimuli for AVP release, particularly hemodynamic derangements (e.g., due to hypotension, nausea, or drugs), need to be ruled out. The measurement of an elevated level of AVP confirms the clinical diagnosis. It must be noted, however, that most patients with SIADH have AVP levels in the "normal" range (up to 10 pg/mL), but the presence of any AVP is abnormal in the hypo-osmolar state.

The causes of SIADH fall into three general categories: (1) malignancies, (2) pulmonary disease, and (3) central nervous system disorders. It has been increasingly recognized that an idiopathic form is common in elderly patients. Of the tumors that cause SIADH secretion, bronchogenic carcinoma, particularly small cell lung cancer, is the most common. It appears that patients with bronchogenic carcinoma have higher plasma AVP levels in relation to plasma osmolality, even if they do not manifest full-blown SIADH. In view of the potential to treat patients with this tumor, it is important that patients with unexplained SIADH be fully investigated and evaluated for the presence of this malignancy.

Glucocorticoid Deficiency
There is considerable evidence for an important role for glucocorticoids in the abnormal water excretion of adrenal insufficiency.

The water excretory defect of anterior pituitary insufficiency, and particularly corticotropin deficiency, is associated with elevated AVP levels and corrected by physiologic doses of glucocorticoids.

HYPOTHYROIDISM Hypothyroidism is associated with the development of hyponatremia that can be reversed by treatment with thyroid hormones. Both decreased delivery of filtrate to the diluting segment and persistent secretion of AVP, alone or combination, have been proposed as mechanisms responsible for the defect.

Postoperative Hyponatremia
The incidence of hospital-acquired hyponatremia is high in postoperative patients ($\approx 4\%$). Most affected patients appear to be clinically euvolemic and have measurable levels of AVP in their circulation. Although this condition occurs primarily as a consequence of administration of hypotonic fluids, a decrease in serum Na^+ can occur in this high AVP state, even when isotonic fluids are given. A subgroup of postoperative patients—almost always premenstrual women—can develop catastrophic neurologic events, often accompanied by seizures and hypoxia.

Strenuous Exercise
There is increasing recognition that strenuous exercise, such as that performed in military service and during marathons or triathlons, can cause hyponatremia that is often symptomatic. Excessive prehydration and consumption of water during exercise, coupled with high loss of electrolytes through sweat and the use of nonsteroidal anti-inflammatory drugs, are the most likely risk factors.

Pharmacologic Agents
Table 7–4 shows drugs that are associated with development of hyponatremia.

CHLORPROPAMIDE The incidence of hyponatremia may be as high as 7%, but severe hyponatremia (<130 mEq/L) occurs in 2% of patients treated with chlorpropamide. As noted earlier, the drug exerts its action primarily by potentiating the renal action of AVP.

CARBAMAZEPINE Carbamazepine possesses antidiuretic properties. The incidence of hyponatremia in carbamazepine-treated patients is approximately 5%. The hyponatremia is mediated by enhanced AVP release, enhancement sensitivity to the hormone's action, and decreased sensitivity of the vasopressin response to osmotic stimulation.

Table 7–4: Drugs Associated with Hyponatremia

Antidiuretic hormone analogs
  Desmopressin acetate
  Oxytocin
Drugs that enhance arginine vasopressin (AVP)
  Chlorpropamide
  Clofibrate
  Carbamazepine, oxycarbazepine
  Vincristine
  Nicotine
  Narcotics (μ-opioid receptors)
  Antipsychotics, antidepressants
  Ifosfamide
Drugs that potentiate renal action of AVP
  Chlorpropamide cyclophosphamide
  Nonsteroidal anti-inflammatory drugs
  Acetaminophen
Drugs that cause hyponatremia by unknown mechanisms
  Haloperidol
  Fluphenazine
  Amitriptyline
  Thioridazine
Selective serotonin reuptake inhibitors
  Ecstasy (amphetamine-related)

Data from Berl T, Schrier RW: Disorders of water metabolism. In Schrier RW (ed): *Renal and Electrolyte Disorders*, 6th ed. Philadelphia, Lippincott Williams & Wilkins, 2003.

PSYCHOTROPIC DRUGS A large number of psychotropic drugs have been associated with hyponatremia, and they are often implicated to explain water intoxication in psychotic patients. Recently, an increasing number of cases of amphetamine (Ecstasy)-related hyponatremia have been described. Likewise the antidepressants fluoxetine and sertraline can trigger hyponatremia. Elderly patients appear to be particularly susceptible, with an incidence as high as 22% to 28%. The tendency for these drugs to cause hyponatremia is further compounded by their anticholinergic effect.

ANTINEOPLASTIC DRUGS Vincristine exerts a direct neurotoxic effect on the hypothalamic microtubule system, which then alters normal osmoreceptor control of AVP release. The mechanism of the diluting defect that results from cyclophosphamide administration is not fully understood. The importance of anticipating potentially severe hyponatremia in cyclophosphamide-treated patients who are vigorously hydrated to avert urologic complications cannot be overstated.

Symptoms
Most patients with hyponatremia are asymptomatic. The manifestations are variable and occur only at a serum Na^+ concentration less than 125 mmol/L. The manifestations of hyponatremia are usually neuropsychiatric and include lethargy, psychosis, and seizures, designated hyponatremic encephalopathy. In its severe form hyponatremic encephalopathy can cause brainstem compression, leading to pulmonary edema and hypoxemia. Elderly persons and young children with hyponatremia are most likely to develop symptoms. It has also become apparent that neurologic complications occur more often in menstruating women. The degree of clinical impairment is related not to the absolute measured level of lowered serum Na^+ concentration but to both the rate and the extent of the drop in ECF osmolality. The observed central nervous system symptoms are most likely related to the cellular swelling and cerebral edema that result from acute lowering of ECF osmolality, which leads to movement of water into cells. In fact, such cerebral edema occasionally causes herniation. The increase in brain water is, however, much less marked than would be predicted from the decrease in tonicity were the brain to operate as a passive osmometer. After the onset of hyponatremia, there is a prompt loss of both electrolytes and organic osmolytes from brain cells. The rate at which the brain restores the lost electrolytes and osmolytes when hyponatremia is corrected is of great pathophysiologic importance. Na^+ and Cl^- concentrations recover quickly and may even overshoot. However, the reaccumulation of osmolytes is considerably delayed, giving rise to the potential for cerebral dehydration upon correction of the serum Na^+ concentration.

Treatment
The treatment strategy should be guided by the volume status of the patient, the severity of symptoms, and the estimated duration of illness rather than by the plasma Na^+ level alone. In view of the devastating neurologic consequences that can be associated with acute symptomatic hyponatremia, it has been suggested that rapid correction (1 to 2 mEq/L/hr) is indicated for patients in this setting until seizures subside. Potential risks of this approach include the development of central pontine myelinolysis. Factors that predispose patients to central pontine myelinolysis include the chronicity of the hypo-osmolar state, the rate of correction, and possibly the absolute change in serum

Na$^+$ concentration. A general estimate of the sodium deficit is provided by the following formula:

$$\text{Sodium deficit} = (\text{Desired [Na}^+] - \text{Measured [Na}^+]) \times (0.6) (\text{Weight in kilograms})$$

It is essential to understand, however, that changes in free water excretion induced by NaCl administration or diuretic use can alter the free water excretion rate such that the rate of change in serum sodium may differ substantially from that predicted by this equation. Therefore repeated measurement of the serum Na$^+$ and U$_{Na^+}$ levels and urine output is essential to help guide therapy and avoid central pontine myelinolysis.

HYPOVOLEMIC HYPONATREMIA   Isotonic NaCl (0.9%) should be administered to patients with hypovolemic hyponatremia. Importantly, if isotonic saline is administered to patients with SIADH whose U$_{osm}$ is greater than 300 mOsm/L, worsening hyponatremia will result. This occurs because the patient with SIADH is in Na$^+$ balance. Therefore, all of the administered Na$^+$ will be excreted; however, it will be excreted in hypertonic urine and free H$_2$O will be retained.

NORMOVOLEMIC HYPONATREMIA   If the patient is asymptomatic, the cornerstone of treatment is water restriction. In practical terms, however, severe water restriction is difficult to enforce for prolonged periods, especially in the outpatient setting. Pharmacologic agents that antagonize AVP action and maneuvers that increase solute excretion have allowed patients with SIADH to drink more water. The agent most commonly used is demeclocycline at doses between 600 and 1200 mg/day. This treatment restores the serum Na$^+$ concentration (S$_{Na^+}$) to a normal level within 5 to 14 days, permitting unrestricted water intake. A nonpharmacologic alternative to the treatment of these patients involves an increase in solute intake and excretion. Because the level of urine concentration is more or less fixed in many patients with SIADH, any fluid intake above insensible losses plus electrolyte-free water excretion (which can be a negative figure) will cause the S$_{Na^+}$ to fall. Therefore the following guide to therapy has been proposed:

(U$_{Na^+}$ + U$_{K^+}$)/S$_{Na^+}$	Water restriction
>1	<500 mL/day
1	750 mL/day
<1	1000 mL/day

HYPERVOLEMIC HYPONATREMIA   Fluid restriction with or without loop diuretic therapy is the treatment of choice for patients with hypervolemic hyponatremia. Dialysis may be required to normalize the S_{Na^+} in patients with advanced chronic kidney disease or end-stage renal disease.

SYMPTOMATIC HYPONATREMIA   If the patient is symptomatic, then rapid correction of euvolemia can be achieved by administration of hypertonic saline (3% NaCl) containing 513 mEq of Na^+/L. The rate of administration required to raise the S_{Na^+} concentration to 120 mEq/L, at a rate not to exceed 1 mEq/L hr, can be derived from the preceding formula. For example, a 70-kg man with a S_{Na^+} of 110 mEq/L would require the following:

$$\text{Sodium deficit} = (120 - 110) \times (0.6)(70) = 420 \text{ mEq}$$

Given that 3% NaCl contains 513 mEq of Na^+/L one would administer 0.8 L of 3% NaCl over 10 hours at a rate of 80 ml/hr. If the desired rate of correction was 0.5 mEq/L/hr, then the rate of infusion would be halved. Patients with symptomatic hypovolemic hyponatremia may be managed with 0.9% NaCl at a correspondingly higher rate of infusion. It is important to emphasize that these figures do not take into account ongoing urinary losses of either Na^+ or water. The figure derived from this formula should be considered a rough estimate, and in the symptomatic patient undergoing hypertonic saline therapy, hourly monitoring of the serum Na^+ is mandatory to minimize the risk of osmotic brain injury.

Polyuria and Primary Polydipsia

There are two different definitions of polyuria. The second one illustrates the importance of analyzing data on the basis of the prevailing stimulus and knowing the expected renal response to an abnormal plasma Na^+ concentration (P_{Na^+}):

- *Nonphysiologic definition:* In adults consuming a typical Western diet, polyuria is present when the urine volume is very noticeable or inconvenient—typically greater than 3 L/day.
- *Physiologic definition:* The urine volume is compared with values expected for the same provocative stimulus. Hence, polyuria is present when the urine volume is higher than expected. Under this definition polyuria can be present when the urine volume is much less than 3 L/day in one setting and not present when the urine volume is 4 L/day in another setting.

For example, when the P_{Na^+} is in the high-normal range, water must be conserved so vasopressin will be released and cause the U_{osm} to be as high as possible. A typical osmole excretion rate is 600 to 900 mOsm/day in an adult and the maximum U_{osm} is approximately 1200 mOsm/kg H_2O. Therefore, in this setting the expected minimum urine volume would be 0.5 L/day (600 ÷ 1200). Now, if this patient had an impaired renal concentrating ability (e.g., a maximum U_{osm} of 600 mOsm/kg H_2O), then the patient's minimum urine volume would be 1 L/day when vasopressin acts (i.e., 600 ÷ 600). In this latter circumstance, the 1 L/day urine output is twice the expected minimum value, indicating polyuria due to an impaired renal concentrating ability. This example illustrates the error of using data gathered in one population (subjects consuming their usual diet) to define a condition such as polyuria in a population with a much lower osmole excretion rate (subjects consuming a low-protein and low-salt diet). In contrast, in a patient with a 24-hour U_{osm} of 80 mOsm/kg H_2O and a P_{Na^+} of 131 mmol/L, a urine output of 4 L should not be considered to be polyuric. The urine volume is inappropriately low because in most adults the U_{osm} can be lowered to close to 50 mOsm/kg H_2O when vasopressin is maximally suppressed, as should occur in the setting of hyponatremia. The basis for this patient's diminished diluting capacity could be a very low level, but not absence, of vasopressin because this hormone was released in response to nonosmotic stimuli (see earlier).

Differential Diagnosis of Polyuria

Use the following stepwise approach to diagnose polyuria:

1. 24-hour collection to confirm either a *water diuresis* or an *osmotic diuresis*
   —water diuresis = urine volume greater than 50 mL/kg body weight and osmolality less than 250 mOsm/kg H_2O
   —osmotic diuresis = urine volume greater than 50 mL/kg body weight and osmolality greater than 300 mOsm/kg H_2O
   A spot urine osmolality measurement may suffice in many cases. The major causes of an osmotic diuresis are sodium, glucose, urea, and mannitol. These are easily distinguished by routine urinalysis and urine chemistry values.

2. If the U_{osm} is less than 250 mOsm/kg H_2O and the P_{Na^+} is less than 140, then the diagnosis is probably primary polydipsia. If the P_{Na^+} is greater than 140, then a submaximally concentrated urine (i.e., urine osmolality < 800 mOsm/kg H_2O) strongly suggests the diagnosis of DI.

3. Distinguish between central and nephrogenic DI: Administer desmopressin 1 to 2 mcg subcutaneously or intravenously. A significant increase in urine osmolality within 1 to 2 hours after injection indicates central DI, whereas an absent response indicates renal resistance to the effects of AVP and, therefore, nephrogenic DI.

Interpretational difficulties can arise because the water diuresis produced by AVP deficiency in central DI produces a washout of the renal medullary concentrating gradient. Therefore, the initial increases in urine osmolality in response to administered desmopressin may be blunted in central DI. Generally, increases of urine osmolality greater than 50% reliably indicate central DI and responses of less than 10% indicate nephrogenic DI, but responses between 10% and 50% are less certain and indeterminate.

Primary Polydipsia

Excessive fluid intake also causes hypotonic polyuria and, by definition, polydipsia. Many different names have been used to describe excessive fluid intake, but *primary polydipsia* remains the best descriptor because it does not presume any single cause for the increased fluid intake. Primary polydipsia is often due to a severe mental illness, in which case it is called *psychogenic polydipsia*. However, primary polydipsia can also be caused by an abnormality in the osmoregulatory control of thirst, in which case it has been termed *dipsogenic diabetes insipidus*. These patients have no overt psychiatric illness and invariably attribute their polydipsia to a nearly constant thirst. Dipsogenic DI is usually idiopathic, but it can also be caused by organic structural lesions in the hypothalamus. Finally, primary polydipsia is sometimes caused by physicians, nurses, lay practitioners, or health writers who recommend a high fluid intake for valid (e.g., recurrent nephrolithiasis) or unsubstantiated reasons of health. Occasionally fluid intake rises to such extraordinary levels that the excretory capacity of the kidneys is exceeded and dilutional hyponatremia develops (>20 L/day). Intense drinking binges can transiently achieve symptomatic levels of hyponatremia with total daily volumes of water intake of less than 20 L if it is ingested sufficiently rapidly.

Clinical Disturbances of Calcium, Magnesium, and Phosphate Metabolism

8

DISORDERS OF CALCIUM HOMEOSTASIS

The extracellular calcium concentration is tightly maintained and reflects the actions of multiple hormones (parathyroid hormone [PTH], calcitonin, and vitamin D) on bone, intestine, kidney, and parathyroid tissue. This homeostatic system is modulated by dietary and environmental factors (including vitamins, hormones, medications, and mobility). The normal total extracellular calcium concentration is 9 to 10.5 mg/dL (2.25 to 2.65 mcmol/L), of which 50% is bound to serum proteins and the remainder exists as free ionized calcium. The ionized calcium concentration is pathophysiologically relevant. Although in most instances an alteration in ionized calcium is reflected by altered total calcium, such may not be the case when an abnormality in serum protein concentration is present. A useful rule is to add 0.8 mg/dL for every 1-mg depression in serum albumin below 4 mg/dL to "correct" for hypoalbuminemia.

Hypercalcemia

Signs and Symptoms
The clinical manifestations of hypercalcemia reflect both the degree of hypercalcemia and the rate of increase. Neuromuscular sequelae include mental status, depression, fatigue, and muscle weakness. Gastrointestinal complications include constipation, nausea, vomiting and rarely pancreatitis. Hypercalcemia causes polyuria and polydipsia, and significant hypercalcemia can lead to severe dehydration. Nephrolithiasis and nephrocalcinosis are

seen in 15% to 20% of patients with primary hyperparathyroidism (HPT). Hypercalcemia causes a shortened QT interval on electrocardiograms as a result of an increased rate of cardiac repolarization. Heart block and other arrhythmias also may be observed.

Diagnosis

Primary HPT and malignancy-associated hypercalcemia are responsible for most cases of hypercalcemia. In primary HPT, the serum PTH level is usually frankly elevated; in malignancy-associated hypercalcemia and in hypercalcemia from most other causes, PTH levels are low. An elevated parathyroid hormone-related protein level indicates humoral hypercalcemia of malignancy (although some forms of malignancy-associated hypercalcemia are not mediated by this circulating hormone). Approximately 10% of cases of hypercalcemia are due to other causes. Of particular importance in the evaluation of a hypercalcemic patient are the family history (because of familial syndromes), medication history (because of the several medication-induced forms of hypercalcemia), and the presence of other disease (such as granulomatous or malignant disease).

Causes of Hypercalcemia

Causes of hypercalcemia are listed in Table 8–1.

Primary Hyperparathyroidism

Primary HPT is caused by excess PTH secretion and accounts for 50% of cases of hypercalcemia. An incidental finding of hypercalcemia is the usual presentation, and the degree of hypercalcemia may be mild and intermittent. A single adenoma is the cause in 80% to 90% of patients. Carcinoma is rare. The disease is about three times more common in women than in men. Primary HPT rarely causes life-threatening hypercalcemia. The standard therapy for primary HPT remains parathyroidectomy. Indications include serum calcium levels greater than 1 mg/dL above normal, a history of life-threatening hypercalcemia, renal insufficiency, kidney stones, and hypercalciuria (>400 mg of calcium/24 hr). Medical surveillance is considered to be a reasonable alternative for individuals older than 50 years with no obvious symptoms and normal bone density. Such patients should receive close follow-up, including periodic measurements of bone density, renal function, and serum calcium. Although excision of a single enlarged parathyroid gland is curative, the finding of more than one enlarged gland raises the possibility of diffuse parathyroid hyperplasia and the syndrome of multiple endocrine neoplasia (MEN). When all

Table 8–1: Causes of Hypercalcemia

Common	Less Common
Primary hyperparathyroidism	Inherited disease
Adenoma	Multiple endocrine
Carcinoma	neoplasia type I or II
Hyperplasia	Familial hypocalciuric
Malignancy	hypercalcemia
Humoral hypercalcemia	Other
Lytic bone disease	Granulomatous disease
Ectopic 1,25-dihydroxyvitamin D	Drug induced
production	Lithium
	Vitamin D
	Thiazides
	Aminophylline
	Estrogens
	Vitamin A
	Milk-alkali syndrome
	Nonparathyroid
	endocrinopathies
	Immobilization
	Renal failure

glands are enlarged, removal of $3\frac{1}{2}$ glands or all 4 glands with forearm autotransplantation of a portion of the gland is advocated.

Parathyroid Carcinoma
Parathyroid carcinoma accounts for less than 1% of primary HPT. The diagnosis of parathyroid carcinoma may be difficult to make in the absence of metastases because the histologic appearance may be similar to that of atypical adenomas. In general, parathyroid carcinoma is not aggressive, and survival is common if the entire gland can be removed.

Malignancy
Humoral hypercalcemia of malignancy generally refers to the syndrome of malignancy-associated hypercalcemia caused by secretion of parathyroid hormone-related protein (80% of malignancy-associated hypercalcemia). Malignancies associated with humoral hypercalcemia of malignancy include lymphomas and squamous, renal cell, breast, and ovarian carcinomas. Patients are hypercalcemic and hypophosphatemic and hypercalciuric. Malignant lymphomas have been reported to produce 1,25-hydroxyvitamin D_2 in sufficient quantity to lead to elevated levels and hypercalcemia caused by bone resorption and increased

intestinal calcium absorption. Osteolytic metastases may produce severe pain, pathologic fractures, and hypercalcemia.

Inherited Disease

MULTIPLE ENDOCRINE NEOPLASIAS   MEN-I, an autosomal dominant disorder characterized by tumors of the parathyroid gland, pituitary, and pancreas, is the most common form of familial HPT. Primary HPT is caused by diffuse hyperplasia of all four glands in most patients. The gene defect in MEN-I is found in the *menin* gene, a possible tumor suppressor gene found on chromosome 11q13. MEN-IIA is also characterized by parathyroid hyperplasia and autosomal dominant inheritance. Associated findings are medullary thyroid carcinoma and pheochromocytoma. The MEN-IIA gene is on chromosome 10 and encodes the *RET* proto-oncogene. Treatment of the HPT is surgical: subtotal parathyroidectomy or total parathyroidectomy with autotransplantation of a portion of the excised parathyroid gland in the forearm.

FAMILIAL HYPOCALCIURIC HYPERCALCEMIA AND NEONATAL SEVERE HYPERPARATHYROIDISM   Familial hypocalciuric hypercalcemia (FHH), or familial benign hypercalcemia, is a rare autosomal dominant condition due to inactivating defects in the extracellular calcium receptor (CaR) located on chromosome 3q. The hypercalcemia is typically of mild to moderate severity (10.5 to 12 mg/dL) and asymptomatic. The PTH level is generally "inappropriately normal" in the presence of hypercalcemia. Urinary calcium excretion is not elevated, as would be expected in hypercalcemia of other causes. The fact that relative hypocalciuria persists even after parathyroidectomy in patients with FHH suggests a role of the CaR in regulating renal calcium handling. Differentiating primary HPT from FHH is critically important because the hypercalcemia in FHH is benign and does not respond to subtotal parathyroidectomy.

Two copies of CaR alleles bearing inactivating mutations cause neonatal severe hyperparathyroidism (NSHPT). This rare disorder, most often reported in the offspring of consanguineous parents with FHH, is characterized by severe hyperparathyroid hyperplasia, PTH elevation, and elevated extracellular calcium. Treatment is total parathyroidectomy followed by vitamin D and calcium supplementation. This disease is usually lethal without surgical intervention.

Medications

Hypercalcemia, often with elevated PTH levels, affects 5% to 10% of patients treated with lithium. The hypercalcemia is typically reversible, although lithium-independent HPT may develop after prolonged treatment. Vitamin A intoxication (ingestion of 100,000 units/day) may cause hypercalcemia, presumably from increased osteoclast-mediated bone resorption. Hypercalcemia is a well-recognized complication of thiazide diuretics. Because thiazides may exacerbate borderline hypercalcemia from other causes, severe hypercalcemia in a thiazide-treated patient should prompt further investigation.

Milk-Alkali Syndrome

The syndrome of hypercalcemia, alkalosis, and renal insufficiency caused by the ingestion of large amounts of calcium and antacids is known as the milk-alkali syndrome. With a decline in the use of antacids, the incidence of this syndrome had been declining, but the popularity of calcium supplementation has resulted in a recent upsurge in cases.

Vitamin D Intoxication

Hypercalcemia may develop in individuals ingesting vitamin D or vitamin D analogs, including 1,25-hydroxyvitamin D_2. The diagnosis is made by the history and detection of elevated 25-hydroxyvitamin D levels.

Immobilization

Immobilization can produce increased rates of bone resorption, decreased rates of bone formation, and hypercalcemia days to weeks after the start of complete bed rest. The hypercalcemia is reversible with resumption of activity.

Granulomatous Disease

Hypercalcemia is observed in 10% of patients with sarcoidosis. The cause of hypercalcemia is 1-hydroxylation of 25-hydroxyvitamin D to produce calcitriol by macrophages in sarcoid granulomata. Other granulomatous disorders have rarely been associated with altered hypercalcemia.

Management of Hypercalcemia

The treatment of mild chronic hypercalcemia should be focused on the underlying cause. However, immediate therapy is required for patients with acute severe hypercalcemia (>14 mg/dL [3.5 mmol/L]). Volume depletion is almost universal in severe hypercalcemia. Volume repletion and induction of saline diuresis prompt a caliuresis and are central to successful therapy. Patients should be initially given 200 to 300 mL/hr of 0.9% NaCl; this dose can then be lowered to 100 to 200 mL/hr, based on the clinical discretion of the treating physician. Once volume repletion is accomplished, loop diuretics, which block renal calcium absorption can be administered to augment the urinary calcium losses. Care should be taken not to use loop diuretics before volume expansion because this may trigger prerenal acute renal failure. Care must be taken to monitor the patient's volume status closely during the administration of large amounts of saline and diuretics, particularly in hospitalized patients with cardiac or pulmonary disease.

Bisphosphonates such as pamidronate (30 to 90 mg intravenously over 2 hours) and zoledronate (4 mg intravenously over 15 minutes) are highly effective in lowering the serum calcium concentration and can control it for several weeks. These drugs appear to be particularly efficacious in patients with malignancy. Calcitonin, an effective inhibitor of osteoclast bone resorption, has a rapid onset of action, but its effect is transient. Given as 4 to 8 units of salmon calcitonin/kg subcutaneously, this drug has minimal toxicity but is of limited use as the sole therapy for hypercalcemia. Plicamycin, previously called mithramycin, is a highly effective intravenous hypocalcemic agent that reduces the serum calcium concentration within hours of administration. Side effects include bone marrow, hepatic, and renal toxicity.

Glucocorticoids are the most effective drugs in the hematologic malignancies (e.g., multiple myeloma and Hodgkin disease) and disorders of vitamin D metabolism (e.g., granulomatous disease and vitamin D toxicity). In severely hypercalcemic patients (>18 mg/dL [4.5 mmol/L]), hemodialysis with a low- or no-calcium dialysate is an effective treatment.

Hypocalcemia

The clinical manifestations of hypocalcemia vary greatly among individual patients. The most common symptoms are muscle cramps and numbness in the digits. Bedside signs of hypocalcemia include ipsilateral facial muscle twitching in response to tapping of the facial nerve (Chvostek sign) and carpal spasm induced by brachial artery occlusion (Trousseau sign). Electrocardiographic changes include prolongation of the QT interval. Long-standing hypocalcemia may result in dry skin, coarse hair, and alopecia, and calcification of the basal ganglia and cerebral cortex may be detected by computed tomography in chronic hypocalcemia. The most common causes of hypocalcemia in the nonacute setting are hypoparathyroidism, hypomagnesemia, renal failure, and vitamin D deficiencies.

Acquired Hypoparathyroidism

Surgical hypoparathyroidism is the most common cause of acquired hypoparathyroidism. It is observed after total thyroidectomy for cancer or thyrotoxicosis, radical neck dissection, and repeated operations for parathyroid adenoma. Transient hypoparathyroidism and hypocalcemia are quite common after total thyroidectomy. Removal of a single hyperfunctioning parathyroid adenoma can result in transient hypercalcemia because of hypercalcemia-induced suppression of PTH secretion from the normal glands.

Magnesium-Related Disorders

Both hypomagnesemia and hypermagnesemia are associated with hypocalcemia. Mg^{2+} is an extracellular CaR agonist and infusion of magnesium or hypermagnesemia inhibits PTH secretion. Chronic severe hypomagnesemia results in hypocalcemia from intracellular Mg^{2+} depletion and its effect on parathyroid gland function. The appropriate therapy is Mg^{2+} repletion; in the absence of adequate Mg^{2+} repletion, the hypocalcemia is resistant to PTH or to vitamin D therapy.

Autoimmune Disease

Type I polyglandular autoimmune syndrome, also referred to as APECED (autoimmune polyendocrinopathy, candidiasis, ectodermal dystrophy syndrome), is a recessive disorder. Its cardinal features are childhood onset of hypoparathyroidism in association with adrenal insufficiency and mucocutaneous candidiasis. Autoantibodies against parathyroid tissue have been reported in a significant percentage of patients with hypoparathyroidism, but the causative role of these antibodies is unclear.

Vitamin D-Related Disorders

Because vitamin D_3 is normally produced by the skin from 7-dehydrocholesterol in the presence of sunlight, vitamin D deficiency requires both dietary deficiency and lack of exposure to the sun. Prolonged vitamin D deficiency causes rickets (a disorder of mineralization of growing bone) and osteomalacia (a disorder of mineralization of formed bone). Elevation of PTH levels is generally observed. The diagnosis is confirmed by measurement of serum 25-hydroxyvitamin D levels. Populations at risk include hospitalized patients, nursing home residents, and breast-feeding infants of mothers with diets low in vitamin D. Vitamin D deficiency may also be seen after gastrectomy, in Crohn disease and celiac sprue, and after intestinal resection due to malabsorption of vitamin D. Vitamin D deficiency with hypocalcemia is commonly seen in patients with renal insufficiency and is due in part to impaired 1α-hydroxylation of vitamin D. Disorders of altered vitamin D metabolism represent a second group of vitamin D–related hypocalcemias. They may be acquired or inherited. Medications, most notably phenytoin and phenobarbital, can increase the rate of hepatic metabolism of vitamin D.

Medications
Bisphosphonates, plicamycin, and calcitonin, all of which inhibit bone resorption, may depress serum calcium to subnormal levels. Administration of citrated blood during massive transfusion can cause hypocalcemia. Similarly, significant hypocalcemia may occur after plasmapheresis.

Foscarnet (trisodium phosphonoformate) can cause hypocalcemia through the chelation of extracellular calcium ions; normal total calcium measurements may not reflect ionized hypocalcemia.

Critical Illness
In critically ill patients, total calcium measurements may be poor indicators of the ionized calcium concentration (e.g., hypoproteinemia, acid-base disturbances, and dialysis therapy). Thus, it is particularly important to measure ionized calcium in this setting. Hypocalcemia has been reported to be present in 70% of patients in intensive care units.

Genetic Disorders of Parathyroid Hormone
Dysfunction or Altered Responsiveness
A variety of inherited or genetic disorders can cause hypocalcemia including DiGeorge syndrome and pseudohypoparathyroidism. For a more detailed discussion of these disorders, see Chapter 22, Clinical Disturbances of Calcium, Magnesium and Phosphate Metabolism, in *Brenner and Rector's The Kidney.*

Treatment of Hypocalcemia
Treatment of acute hypocalcemia depends on the severity of the depression in serum calcium and the presence of clinical manifestations. Oral calcium supplementation may be sufficient treatment for mild hypocalcemia; severe hypocalcemia with evidence of neuromuscular effects or tetany is treated with intravenous calcium. Typically, 1 to 3 g of calcium gluconate is given intravenously over a period of 10 to 20 minutes, followed by slow intravenous calcium infusion. Dialysis may be the appropriate treatment if severe hyperphosphatemia is also present. Correction of hypomagnesemia and hyperphosphatemia should also be undertaken

when present. Treatment of chronic hypocalcemia depends on the underlying cause, for instance, correction of hypomagnesemia or vitamin D deficiency. The principal therapy for primary disorders of parathyroid dysfunction or PTH resistance is dietary calcium supplementation and vitamin D therapy. Correction of serum calcium to the low-normal range is generally advised; correction to normal levels may lead to frank hypercalciuria.

DISORDERS OF MAGNESIUM HOMEOSTASIS

Hypomagnesemia and Magnesium Deficiency

Extracellular fluid Mg^{2+} accounts for only 1% of total body Mg^{2+}; therefore, serum Mg^{2+} concentrations correlate poorly with overall Mg^{2+} status. The incidence of hypomagnesemia ranges from 20% to 44% in patients admitted to intensive care units and is associated with a twofold increased mortality.

Etiology and Diagnosis

Mg^{2+} deficiency may be caused by decreased intake or intestinal absorption; increased losses via the gastrointestinal tract, kidneys, or skin; or rarely, sequestration in the bone compartment. The first step in determining the etiology is to distinguish between renal Mg^{2+} wasting and extrarenal causes of Mg^{2+} loss by measuring the urinary Mg^{2+}-to-creatinine ratio (>0.02 mg/mg = Mg^{2+} wasting state). If renal Mg^{2+} wasting has been excluded, the losses must be extrarenal in origin and the underlying cause can usually be identified from the case history.

Extrarenal Causes

NUTRITIONAL DEFICIENCY Approximately 20% to 25% of alcoholics have frank hypomagnesemia. Protein-calorie malnutrition in countries where the staple dietary food is cassava, which is particularly low in Mg^{2+} content, may be associated with hypomagnesemia. Patients receiving parenteral nutrition have a high incidence of hypomagnesemia due to associated medical conditions, a poorly understood increase in daily Mg^{2+} requirements and the refeeding syndrome, whereby overzealous parenteral feeding of severely malnourished patients causes hyperinsulinemia, and a rapid cellular uptake of Mg^{2+}.

INTESTINAL MALABSORPTION Generalized malabsorption syndromes caused by conditions such as celiac disease, Whipple disease, and inflammatory bowel disease are often associated with intestinal Mg^{2+} wasting and Mg^{2+} deficiency. Previous intestinal resection, particularly of the distal part of the small intestine, is also an important cause of Mg^{2+} malabsorption. Similarly, Mg^{2+} deficiency can be a late complication of jejunoileal bypass surgery performed for the treatment of obesity.

CUTANEOUS LOSSES Hypomagnesemia may be observed after prolonged intense exertion. About one fourth of the decrement in serum Mg^{2+} can be accounted for by losses in sweat, with the remainder most likely being due to transient redistribution into the intracellular space. Hypomagnesemia occurs in 40% of patients with severe burn injuries during the early period of recovery due to cutaneous losses, which can exceed 1 g/day.

REDISTRIBUTION TO BONE COMPARTMENT Hypomagnesemia may occasionally accompany the profound hypocalcemia of hungry bone syndrome observed in some patients with HPT and severe bone disease immediately after parathyroidectomy.

Renal Magnesium Wasting
POLYURIA Renal Mg^{2+} wasting occurs with osmotic diuresis, during recovery from ischemic injury in the transplanted kidney, and during postobstructive diuresis. In the latter, it is likely that residual tubule reabsorptive defects persisting from the primary renal injury play as important a role as polyuria itself in inducing renal Mg^{2+} wasting.

EXTRACELLULAR FLUID VOLUME EXPANSION Chronic therapy with Mg^{2+}-free parenteral fluids, either crystalloid or hyperalimentation, can cause renal Mg^{2+} wasting, in part because of expansion of the extracellular fluid volume. Renal Mg^{2+} wasting is also characteristic of hyperaldosteronism.

DEFECTIVE Na^+ REABSORPTION IN DISTAL NEPHRON Loop diuretics inhibit paracellular Mg^{2+} reabsorption. Hypomagnesemia is therefore a common finding in patients receiving chronic loop diuretic therapy. Thiazides also inhibit renal Mg^{2+} reabsorption by an incompletely understood mechanism.

HYPERCALCEMIA Elevated serum ionized Ca^{2+} levels directly induce renal Mg^{2+} wasting and hypomagnesemia. In HPT, the hypercalcemia-induced tendency for Mg^{2+} wasting is counteracted by the action of PTH, which stimulates Mg^{2+} reabsorption; therefore, Mg^{2+} deficiency is rare.

TUBULE NEPHROTOXINS Multiple tubulotoxins are associated with hypermagnesuria. The most commonly implicated drugs include cisplatin, the aminoglycosides, amphotericin B, pentamidine, and cyclosporine. The hypomagnesemia associated with cisplatin is dose-related and may persist for months, even, years, after cessation of therapy. Cyclosporine causes renal Mg^{2+} wasting and hypomagnesemia in patients after renal and bone marrow transplantation.

INHERITED RENAL Mg^{2+}-WASTING DISORDERS Other rare causes of Mg^{2+}-wasting include isolated familial hypomagnesemia, familial hypomagnesemia, and primary hypomagnesemia with hypocalcemia. Bartter and Gitelman syndromes are discussed further in Chapter 18, Inherited Disorders of the Renal Tubule.

Clinical Manifestations
Hypomagnesemia may cause symptoms and signs of disordered cardiac, neuromuscular, and central nervous system function. However, most patients with hypomagnesemia are completely asymptomatic. Thus, the clinical importance of hypomagnesemia remains controversial. Furthermore, many of the cardiac and neurologic manifestations attributed to Mg^{2+} deficiency may also be explained by the frequent coexistence of hypokalemia and hypocalcemia in the same patient.

Treatment
Given the clinical manifestations outlined earlier, it seems prudent to replete magnesium in all Mg^{2+}-deficient patients with a significant underlying cardiac or seizure disorder, in patients with concurrent severe hypocalcemia or hypokalemia, and in patients with isolated asymptomatic hypomagnesemia if it is severe (<1.4 mg/dL). Individuals who are being maintained by parenteral nutrition should receive Mg^{2+} supplementation. The recommended oral daily allowance of Mg^{2+} in adults is 350 mg (29 mEq) for men and 280 mg (23 mEq) for women.

INTRAVENOUS REPLACEMENT The initial rate of repletion depends on the urgency of the clinical situation. In a patient who is actively having seizures or who has a cardiac arrhythmia, 8 to 16 mEq (1 to 2 g of $MgSO_4$) may be administered intravenously over a 2- to 4-minute period. The magnitude of the Mg^{2+} deficit is difficult to gauge clinically and cannot be readily deduced from the serum Mg^{2+} concentration. In general, though, the average deficit can be assumed to be 1 to 2 mEq/kg body weight. A simple regimen for nonemergency Mg^{2+} repletion is to administer 64 mEq (8 g) of $MgSO_4$ over the first 24 hours and then 32 mEq (4 g) daily for the next 2 to 6 days. It is important to remember that serum Mg^{2+} levels rise early whereas intracellular stores take longer to replete, so Mg^{2+} repletion should continue for at least 1 to 2 days after the serum Mg^{2+} level normalizes. In patients with renal Mg^{2+} wasting, additional Mg^{2+} may be needed to replace ongoing losses. In patients with a reduced glomerular filtration rate, the rate of repletion should be reduced by 25% to 50%, and the serum Mg^{2+} level should be checked often.

The main adverse effects of Mg^{2+} repletion are due to hypermagnesemia and include facial flushing, loss of deep tendon reflexes, hypotension, and atrioventricular block. Monitoring of tendon reflexes is a useful bedside test to detect Mg^{2+} overdose. In addition, intravenous administration of large amounts of $MgSO_4$ results in an acute decrease in the serum ionized Ca^{2+} level and therefore can precipitate tetany.

ORAL REPLACEMENT A number of oral Mg^{2+} salts are available; however, they all cause diarrhea in high doses. Magnesium hydroxide and magnesium oxide are alkalinizing salts with the potential to cause systemic alkalosis, whereas the sulfate and gluconate salts may potentially exacerbate K^+ wasting. The appropriate dose of each salt can be estimated, if ongoing losses are known, by determining its content of elemental Mg^{2+} and assuming a bioavailability of approximately 33% for normal intestinal function. In patients with intestinal Mg^{2+} malabsorption, this dose may need to be increased two- to four-fold. In patients with inappropriate renal Mg^{2+} wasting, potassium-sparing diuretics such as amiloride and triamterene, may reduce renal Mg^{2+} losses. These drugs may be particularly useful in patients whose Mg^{2+} deficiency is refractory to oral repletion or requires such high doses of oral Mg^{2+} that diarrhea develops.

Hypermagnesemia

Etiology

RENAL INSUFFICIENCY Significant hypermagnesemia is rare even in advanced renal insufficiency, unless the patient has received exogenous Mg^{2+} in the form of antacids, cathartics, or enemas.

EXCESSIVE Mg^{2+} INTAKE Hypermagnesemia can occur in individuals with a normal glomerular filtration rate when the rate of Mg^{2+} intake exceeds the renal excretory capacity. It has been reported with excessive oral ingestion of Mg^{2+}-containing antacids and cathartics and with the use of rectal magnesium sulfate enemas and is observed with large parenteral doses of Mg^{2+}, such as those given for preeclampsia.

Clinical Manifestations

Initial manifestations are hypotension, nausea, vomiting, facial flushing, urinary retention, and ileus (serum Mg^{2+} > 4 to 6 mg/dL

[1.75 to 2.76 mmol/L]). If untreated, it may progress to flaccid skeletal muscular paralysis and hyporeflexia, bradycardia and bradyarrhythmias, respiratory depression, coma, and cardiac arrest. An abnormally low (or even negative) serum anion gap may be a clue to hypermagnesemia, but it is not consistently observed and probably depends on the nature of the anion that accompanies the excess body Mg^{2+}.

CARDIOVASCULAR SYSTEM   Manifestations include hypotension, cutaneous flushing, sinus or junctional bradycardia, and sinoatrial, atrioventricular, and His bundle conduction block. Cardiac arrest as a result of asystole is often the terminal event.

NERVOUS SYSTEM   Flaccid skeletal muscle paralysis and hyporeflexia are observed when the serum Mg^{2+} concentration exceeds 8 to 12 mg/dL. Respiratory depression is a serious complication of advanced Mg^{2+} toxicity. Smooth muscle paralysis also occurs and is manifested as urinary retention, intestinal ileus, and pupillary dilatation. Signs of central nervous system depression, including lethargy, drowsiness, and eventually coma, are seen.

Treatment
Mild cases of Mg^{2+} toxicity in individuals with good renal function may require no treatment other than cessation of Mg^{2+} ingestion. For serious toxicity, temporary antagonism of the effect of Mg^{2+} may be achieved by the administration of intravenous Ca^{2+} (1 g of calcium gluconate, repeated after 5 minutes if necessary). Renal excretion of Mg^{2+} can be enhanced by saline diuresis and by the administration of furosemide. In patients with renal failure hemodialysis efficiently removes Mg^{2+}.

DISORDERS OF PHOSPHATE HOMEOSTASIS

Hyperphosphatemia

Hyperphosphatemia is generally defined as a serum phosphate level greater than 5 mg/dL (1.6 mmol/L). The serum phosphorus level usually exhibits diurnal variation with levels being lowest in the late morning and peaking in the first morning hours.

Causes
The clinical causes of hyperphosphatemia can be broadly classified into one of three groups: reduced phosphate excretion, excess intake of phosphorus, and redistribution of cellular phosphorus.

DECREASED RENAL PHOSPHATE EXCRETION Chronic renal failure is by far the most common cause of hyperphosphatemia. Increased fractional excretion of PO_4 is a compensatory mechanism until the glomerular filtration rate falls to less than 24 mL/min. Hyperphosphatemia caused by decreased renal function is reviewed extensively in Chapter 30 in the context of renal osteodystrophies.

INCREASED PHOSPHORUS INTAKE Exogenous intake of phosphorus sufficient to cause hyperphosphatemia is rare in the absence of renal insufficiency. Great caution in administration of phosphate, particularly in the form of phosphate-containing enemas, must be taken in individuals with renal insufficiency and in children.

REDISTRIBUTION OF PHOSPHORUS The causes of hyperphosphatemia due to cellular redistribution include:

- **Respiratory Acidosis.** Chronic respiratory acidosis can lead to hyperphosphatemia, renal PTH resistance, and hypocalcemia. The effect is more pronounced in acute respiratory acidosis. Efflux of phosphate from cells into the extracellular space is responsible.
- **Tumor Lysis.** Tumor lysis syndrome is a well-described complication of the treatment of hematologic malignancies associated with hyperphosphatemia. Lymphoblasts are particularly high in phosphorus and hyperphosphatemia after induction chemotherapy for leukomatous and lymphomatous disorders may be observed.
- **Pseudohyperphosphatemia.** Incorrect laboratory readings of hyperphosphatemia from patient samples may occur in certain settings as a result of interference with the analysis. This problem is most common in the case of paraproteinemia (as in multiple myeloma or Waldenström macroglobulinemia). Hyperlipidemia, hyperbilirubinemia, and sample dilution problems are rare causes.

Clinical Manifestations and Treatment
Most of major clinical manifestations of hyperphosphatemia stem from hypocalcemia, discussed earlier this chapter. Treatment of chronic hyperphosphatemia is generally accomplished through dietary phosphate restriction and administration of oral phosphate binders. Acute hyperphosphatemia in association with hypocalcemia requires rapid attention. Severe hyperphosphatemia in patients with reduced renal function or acute renal failure, particularly in those with tumor lysis

syndrome, may require hemodialysis or a continuous form of renal replacement therapy. Volume expansion may increase urinary phosphate excretion, as can administration of acetazolamide.

Hypophosphatemia

Only a small percentage (about 1%) of total body phosphorus is extracellular. Thus, although hypophosphatemia may reflect total body phosphorus depletion, such need not be the case. Hypophosphatemia is relatively common in hospitalized patients and is present in a significant proportion of chronic alcoholics.

Clinical Manifestations

Mild hypophosphatemia does not typically cause symptoms. Patients with symptoms usually have serum phosphate levels less than 1 mg/dL. Severe hypophosphatemia impairs muscle function as a result of adenosine triphosphate depletion. Overt heart failure and respiratory failure as a result of decreased muscle performance may be observed. Rhabdomyolysis is a well-recognized complication of severe hypophosphatemia. Because cell breakdown may lead to the release of intracellular phosphate, normophosphatemia or hyperphosphatemia in this setting may mask the existence of true phosphate depletion. Chronic phosphate depletion leads to increased bone resorption and, if prolonged, rickets and osteomalacia may result. Hypophosphatemia leads to decreased proximal tubule reabsorptive function, and frank hypercalciuria can result. This hypercalciuria is not solely the result of renal calcium handling but also reflects increased calcium release from bone and increased intestinal calcium absorption.

Diagnosis

The probable cause of hypophosphatemia may be immediately apparent from the clinical findings (e.g., in a malnourished patient with alcoholism or anorexia). Shifts of phosphorus from the extracellular to the intracellular space generally occur in the acute setting (e.g., respiratory alkalosis or treatment of diabetic ketoacidosis). In hospitalized patients, hypophosphatemia caused by shifts of phosphorus into the intracellular compartment are much more common than hypophosphatemia caused by renal losses. If the underlying diagnosis is not immediately apparent, it can be clinically useful to determine the rate of urine phosphorus excretion. High urine phosphorus in the setting of hypophosphatemia suggests HPT, a renal tubule defect, or a form of rickets.

Causes of Hypophosphatemia

INCREASED RENAL EXCRETION Hypophosphatemia caused by increased urinary phosphate excretion is generally the result of either excess PTH or an inherited disorder of renal phosphate handling in the proximal tubule. Excess PTH directly decreases renal phosphate reabsorption, thereby leading to increased renal phosphate excretion and hypophosphatemia.

ACUTE RENAL FAILURE AND RECOVERY FROM ACUTE TUBULAR NECROSIS Hyperphosphatemia is the typical derangement observed in patients with acute renal failure. However, confounding factors in the setting of critical illness may contribute to the development of hypophosphatemia in some instances: administration of phosphate-binding antacids, refeeding syndrome, and mechanically induced respiratory alkalosis. In addition, during the diuretic phase of recovery from acute tubular necrosis, significant urinary losses of phosphate may lead to hypophosphatemia.

RENAL TRANSPLANTATION Hypophosphatemia is well described in patients after renal transplantation; however, severe hypophosphatemia is rare. Persistent HPT is not the sole mechanism of hypophosphatemia. Renal tubule dysfunction and diuretic and immunosuppressive medications are all contributory factors.

FANCONI SYNDROME Increased urine phosphorus excretion is a typical feature of the defect in proximal tubule transport known as Fanconi syndrome.

DECREASED INTESTINAL ABSORPTION The causes of hypophosphatemia due to decreased intestinal absorption include:

- **Malnutrition.** Malnutrition is an uncommon cause of hypophosphatemia. Increased renal reabsorption of phosphorus can compensate for all but the most severe decreases in oral phosphate intake.
- **Malabsorption.** Phosphorus absorption occurs primarily in the duodenum and jejunum, and small intestinal malabsorption may lead to hypophosphatemia. Heavy use of phosphate-binding antacids may also result in hypophosphatemia.
- **Vitamin D–Mediated Disorders.** Deficiency of vitamin D leads to decreased intestinal absorption of phosphorus. In addition, vitamin D deficiency leads to HPT and a consequent PTH-mediated increase in renal phosphorus.

REDISTRIBUTION The causes of hypophosphatemia due to cellular redistribution include:

- **Respiratory Alkalosis.** Respiratory alkalosis, as may occur during mechanical ventilation, decreases serum phosphorus levels. It has been suggested that in the hypophosphatemia seen in respiratory alkalosis, carbon dioxide diffusion from the intracellular space increases intracellular pH, stimulates glycolysis, and increases the formation of phosphorylated carbohydrates, thereby leading to a fall in extracellular phosphorus levels.
- **Refeeding.** In chronically malnourished individuals, including patients with anorexia nervosa, rapid refeeding can result in significant hypophosphatemia. The mechanism is related to increased cellular phosphate uptake and utilization. The incidence of refeeding-related hypophosphatemia is quite high in hospitalized patients receiving parenteral nutrition and may occur after even very short periods of starvation. The use of a parenteral nutrition formula containing 13.6 mEq of phosphorus/L appears to prevent this complication. Higher amounts may be required in patients with diabetes or chronic alcoholism.
- **Special Situations: Alcoholism and Diabetes.** Hypophosphatemia is a particularly common and often severe problem in alcoholic patients with poor nutritional intake, vitamin D deficiency, and heavy use of phosphate-binding antacids. Refeeding or administration of intravenous glucose (or both) in this patient population stimulates shifts of phosphorus into cells, thereby leading to the development of severe hypophosphatemia and on occasion rhabdomyolysis. Hypophosphatemia is an extremely common complication of the treatment of diabetic ketoacidosis because insulin administration stimulates the cellular uptake of phosphorus. However, routine administration of phosphate in this setting before the development of frank hypophosphatemia is discouraged because it may lead to significant hypocalcemia.

INHERITED DISORDERS Hypophosphatemia is observed in a variety of inherited disorders including X-linked hypophosphatemia, autosomal dominant hypophosphatemic rickets, and hereditary hypophosphatemic rickets with hypercalciuria. For a more detailed discussion of these disorders see Chapter 22, Clinical Disturbances of Calcium, Magnesium and Phosphate Metabolism, in *Brenner and Rector's The Kidney.*

Treatment
Because serum levels of phosphorus are a good reflection of total body stores, it is difficult to predict the amount of phosphorus

necessary to correct phosphorus deficiency. In mild or moderate hypophosphatemia (>2 mg/dL), oral repletion with low-fat milk (containing 0.9 mg of phosphorus/mL) is effective. In individuals intolerant of milk, potassium phosphate or sodium phosphate preparations can be used (up to 3.5 g/day in divided doses). Intravenous phosphorus repletion is generally reserved for individuals with severe (<1 mg/dL) hypophosphatemia. One standard regimen is to administer 2.5 mg/kg body mass of elemental phosphorus over a 6-hour period for severe asymptomatic hypophosphatemia and 5 mg/kg body mass of elemental phosphorus over a 6-hour period for severe symptomatic hypophosphatemia.

III

Pathogenesis of Renal Disease

Acute Renal Failure

9

DEFINITIONS, INCIDENCE, AND CLASSIFICATION

Acute renal failure (ARF) is a syndrome characterized by a rapid decline in the glomerular filtration rate (GFR) with retention of waste products such as blood urea nitrogen (BUN) and creatinine. ARF is an independent risk factor for mortality and is associated with a significant prolongation in length of hospital stay. ARF may complicate a host of diseases that for purposes of diagnosis and management are conveniently divided into three categories:

- Prerenal ARF (55% to 60%)
- Intrinsic ARF (35% to 40%)
- Postrenal ARF (<5%)

The diagnosis of ARF usually hinges on serial analysis of BUN and serum creatinine levels; however, these are relatively insensitive indices of the GFR which may fall by up to 50% before the serum creatinine levels rise above the normal range, because the initial decrement in creatinine filtration by glomeruli is matched by enhanced creatinine secretion by proximal tubule cells. The GFR may also fall without a marked elevation in serum creatinine levels in patients with reduced muscle mass (e.g., elderly patients); the same is true for BUN levels in patients with conditions causing urea generation (e.g., malnutrition or liver disease). Furthermore, BUN or serum creatinine values may rise without an acute decline in GFR in patients with preexisting chronic kidney disease in the setting of enhanced urea or creatinine production.

ETIOLOGY OF ACUTE RENAL FAILURE

Prerenal Azotemia

Prerenal azotemia is the most common cause of ARF. By definition, the integrity of renal parenchymal tissue is maintained and GFR is corrected rapidly with restoration of renal perfusion. Untreated, severe renal hypoperfusion may contribute to the development of ischemic acute tubule necrosis (ATN) and the two syndromes often coexist. Prerenal azotemia can complicate any disease characterized by hypovolemia, low cardiac output, systemic vasodilatation, or intrarenal vasoconstriction (Table 9–1). Glomerular filtration is preserved during mild hypoperfusion (mean systemic blood pressure > 80 mm Hg) through several compensatory mechanisms (see Chapter 4, Control of Extracellular Volume and the Pathophysiology of Edema Formation). These compensatory renal responses are blunted by a variety of drugs including angiotensin-converting enzyme inhibitors, angiotensin receptor antagonists and nonsteroidal anti-inflammatory drugs (NSAIDs). The use of these agents can trigger prerenal ARF in the setting of relatively modest decreases in renal perfusion pressure if

Table 9–1: Major Causes of Prerenal Azotemia

Intravascular volume depletion
    Hemorrhage
    Gastrointestinal losses
    Renal losses (overzealous diuresis, osmotic diuresis, diabetes
        insipidus)
    Increased insensible losses
    "Third-space" losses (pancreatitis, crush syndrome)
Decreased cardiac output
    Cardiac failure
    Systemic vasodilatation
    Drugs: antihypertensives, afterload reduction, anesthetics,
        drug overdoses
    Sepsis, liver failure, anaphylaxis
Renal vasoconstriction
    Norepinephrine, ergotamine, liver disease, sepsis,
        hypercalcemia
Pharmacologic agents that acutely impair autoregulation and
    glomerular filtration rate in specific settings
    Angiotensin-converting enzyme inhibitors in renal artery
        stenosis or severe renal hypoperfusion
    Nonsteroidal anti-inflammatory drugs during renal hypoperfusion

they are administered to high-risk individuals including those with preexisting renal disease and elderly patients. Occasionally prerenal ARF can be triggered by direct renal vasoconstriction without overt systemic hypotension as occurs in the setting of hypercalcemia or vasoconstrictor administration or with the use of a calcineurin inhibitor (cyclosporine or tacrolimus).

Intrinsic Renal Azotemia

From a clinicopathologic viewpoint, it is helpful to categorize intrinsic renal failure as follows:

- Diseases involving large renal vessels
- Diseases of the renal microvasculature and glomeruli
- Ischemic and nephrotoxic ATN
- Tubulointerstitial diseases

Diseases of Large Renal Vessels, Microvasculature, and Tubulointerstitium

Bilateral occlusion of the large renal vessels or unilateral occlusion in a single functioning kidney is a rare cause of ARF. Acute renal artery occlusion is usually caused by atheroemboli that are dislodged from an atheromatous aorta during arteriography, angioplasty, or aortic surgery. Outside of the immediate posttransplantation period, renal vein thrombosis is an exceedingly rare cause of ARF and is usually only encountered as a complication of the nephrotic syndrome in adults or of severe dehydration in children.

Virtually any disease that compromises blood flow within the renal microvasculature may induce ARF. These disorders include inflammatory (e.g., glomerulonephritis and vasculitis) and noninflammatory (e.g., malignant hypertension) diseases of the vessel wall, thrombotic microangiopathies, and hyperviscosity syndromes. Disorders of the tubulointerstitium that induce ARF, other than ischemia or tubule cell toxins, include allergic interstitial nephritis, bilateral pyelonephritis, allograft rejection, and, rarely, infiltrative disorders such as sarcoid, lymphoma, or leukemia.

Acute Tubule Necrosis

The pathologic term ATN and the clinical term ARF are often used interchangeably to refer to ischemic and nephrotoxic renal injury. The clinical course of ATN can be divided into three phases: the initiation phase, the maintenance phase, and the recovery phase. The initiation phase is the period during which patients are exposed to the ischemia or toxin and parenchymal renal injury is evolving but not yet established. ATN is potentially preventable during this period, which may last hours to days. This is followed by a maintenance phase, during which parenchymal injury is established and GFR stabilizes at a value of 5 to 10 mL/min. The maintenance phase typically lasts 1 to 2 weeks but may be prolonged for 1 to 12 months before the recovery phase, which is the period during which patients recover renal function through repair and regeneration of renal tissue. Its onset is typically heralded by a gradual increase in urine output and a fall in serum creatinine level, although the latter may lag behind the onset of diuresis by several days. This "post-ATN" diuresis may reflect appropriate excretion of salt and water accumulated during the maintenance phase, osmotic diuresis induced by filtered urea and other retained solutes, and/or the actions of diuretics administered to hasten salt and water excretion. Occasionally, diuresis may be inappropriate and excessive if recovery of tubule reabsorptive processes lags behind glomerular filtration, although this phenomenon is more common after relief of urinary tract obstruction.

Ischemic ATN and prerenal azotemia are part of a spectrum of manifestations of renal hypoperfusion with prerenal azotemia being a response to mild or moderate hypoperfusion and ischemic ATN being the result of more severe or prolonged hypoperfusion usually coexistent with other renal insults (from vasoactive drugs or nephrotoxins). In its more extreme form, renal hypoperfusion may result in bilateral renal cortical necrosis and irreversible renal failure (<5%). Ischemic ATN is observed most commonly in patients who have had major surgery trauma or have severe hypovolemia, overwhelming sepsis, or burns. ATN in these settings is often multifactorial in origin and results from the combined effects of hypovolemia, sepsis-induced vasodilation, toxins released by damaged tissue (myoglobin), and the administration of nephrotoxic antibiotics. Table 9–2 lists the toxins that are most commonly associated with ATN. The nephrotoxicity of most agents is dramatically increased in the presence of borderline or overt renal ischemia, sepsis, or other renal insults.

Nonoliguric ATN complicates 10% to 30% of courses of aminoglycoside antibiotics, even when blood levels are in the therapeutic range. Important risk factors for aminoglycoside nephrotoxicity include the use of high or repeated doses or prolonged therapy, preexisting renal insufficiency, advanced age, volume depletion, and the coexistence of renal ischemia, sepsis, or other nephrotoxins. ARF is usually detected during the

Table 9–2: Exogenous Nephrotoxins Associated with the Development of Acute Tubule Necrosis

Antibiotics
  Aminoglycosides
  Acyclovir
  Indinavir
Amphotericin B
Chemotherapeutic agents
  Cisplatin
  Ifosfamide
Anti-inflammatory and immunosuppressive agents
  Nonsteroidal antiinflammatory drugs (including
    cyclooxygenase-2 inhibitors)
  Cyclosporine/tacrolimus
Radiocontrast agents
Organic solvents
  Ethylene glycol
  Toluene
Poisons
  Paraquat

second week of therapy, but it may manifest earlier in the presence of ischemia or other nephrotoxins. ARF is common in patients who receive prolonged courses of amphotericin B. Amphotericin B infusion occasionally triggers an immediate fall in GFR by inducing direct renal vasoconstriction; however, more commonly ATN develops as the cumulative dose reaches 1 g and is often associated with biochemical signs of tubule dysfunction including hypomagnesemia, relative hypokalemia, and a non-anion gap acidosis. High-dose intravenous acyclovir can cause ARF in the volume depleted patient as a result of intratubule precipitation of crystals, and the presentation is characterized by colic, nausea, and vomiting. A similar syndrome is now recognized in patients receiving the oral antiretroviral drug indinavir. A Fanconi-like syndrome is seen in up to 40% of patients receiving the novel antiviral agents adefovir and cidofovir. ATN complicates up to 70% of courses of cisplatin and ifosfamide, two commonly used chemotherapeutic agents. Cisplatin causes direct injury to the proximal tubule and may cause severe hypomagnesemia, even in the absence of ARF, which may persist long after therapy has been stopped. Ifosfamide-induced ATN is being recognized increasingly and is often associated with Fanconi syndrome.

ATN complicates up to 30% of cases of rhabdomyolysis. Intratubular obstruction has been implicated as a central event in the pathophysiology of ATN induced by some other endogenous (e.g., myeloma light chains and uric acid) and exogenous (e.g., ethylene glycol) nephrotoxins. Casts, composed of filtered immunoglobulin light chains and other urinary proteins such as Tamm-Horsfall protein, induce ARF in patients with multiple myeloma (myeloma-cast nephropathy). Acute uric acid nephropathy typically complicates treatment of lymphoproliferative or myeloproliferative disorders and is usually associated with other biochemical evidence of tumor lysis such as hyperkalemia, hyperphosphatemia, and hypocalcemia. Acute uric acid nephropathy is rare when plasma concentrations are less than 15 to 20 mg/dL (885 to 1180 mmol/L) but may be precipitated at relatively low levels by volume depletion or low urine pH.

Postrenal Azotemia

Urinary tract obstruction accounts for fewer than 5% of occurrences of ARF. Because one kidney has sufficient clearance capacity to excrete the nitrogenous waste products generated daily, ARF resulting from obstruction requires either obstruction of urine flow between the external urethral meatus and the bladder neck, bilateral ureteric obstruction, or unilateral ureteric obstruction in a patient with only one functioning kidney or with underlying chronic renal insufficiency. Obstruction of the bladder neck, the most common cause of postrenal azotemia, may complicate prostatic disease (e.g., hypertrophy, neoplasia, and infection), neurogenic bladder, or therapy with anticholinergic drugs. Less common causes of acute lower urinary tract obstruction include blood clots, calculi, and urethritis with spasm. Ureteric obstruction may result from intraluminal obstruction (e.g., calculi, blood clots, or sloughed renal papillae), infiltration of the ureteric wall (e.g., neoplasia), or external compression (e.g., retroperitoneal fibrosis, neoplasia or abscess, or inadvertent surgical ligature). During the early stages of obstruction (hours to days), continued glomerular filtration leads to increased intraluminal pressure upstream of the site of obstruction. This results in gradual distention of the proximal ureter, renal pelvis, and calyces and a fall in GFR.

Clinical Features, Urinary Findings, and Confirmatory Tests

See Chapter 1, Clinical Assessment of the Patient with Kidney Disease.

Renal Failure Indices for Differentiation of Prerenal Azotemia and Ischemic Acute Tubule Necrosis

Differential Diagnosis of Acute Renal Failure in Specific Clinical Settings

ACUTE RENAL FAILURE AFTER AN INTRAVENOUS CONTRAST STUDY   The differential diagnosis of ARF after angiography includes the following:

- Contrast nephropathy
- Atheroembolic renal disease
- Renal infarction (e.g., aortic dissection)

Risk factors for the development of contrast nephropathy include chronic renal insufficiency (serum creatinine level > 2 mg/dL [176 mcmol/L]), diabetic nephropathy, cardiac failure, jaundice, volume depletion, large volumes of contrast material, and the coincident use of angiotensin-converting enzyme-inhibitors or NSAIDs. Creatinine levels usually peak after 3 to 5 days in contrast nephropathy and return to the normal range within 5 to 7 days. In atheroembolic renal disease, the initial rise occurs over a similar time frame; however, the renal failure is typically irreversible. Patients with contrast nephropathy usually present with benign urine sediment, concentrated urine, and low fractional excretion of Na^+.

ACUTE RENAL FAILURE IN A PATIENT WITH CANCER   Most ARF in patients with cancer is caused either by prerenal azotemia induced by vomiting, often in the presence of NSAIDs, or by intrinsic renal azotemia triggered by chemotherapeutic drugs or the products of tumor lysis. Rarer causes include hypercalcemia of malignancy, tumor-associated glomerulonephritis, hemolytic uremic syndrome or thrombotic thrombocytopenic purpura induced by drugs or irradiation, or infiltration of the renal vessels or urinary collecting system by tumor. The leukemias have long been associated with the development of ARF, usually as a result of tumor lysis syndrome or acute urate nephropathy, which can sometimes develop before the administration of chemotherapeutic agents. The differential diagnosis of ARF in association with multiple myeloma is wide and includes hypovolemic prerenal ARF, hypercalcemia, cryoglobulinemia, hyperviscosity syndrome, contrast nephropathy, myeloma cast nephropathy, light-chain deposition disease, plasma cell infiltration, vascular amyloidosis, sepsis caused by immunocompromise, and ATN induced by drugs or tumor lysis syndrome.

ACUTE RENAL FAILURE IN PREGNANCY   Ischemic ATN may be provoked by postpartum hemorrhage or abruptio placentae and less commonly by amniotic fluid embolism or sepsis. Glomerular filtration is usually normal in mild or moderate preeclampsia; however, ARF may complicate severe disease. In this setting, ARF is typically transient and is found in association with intrarenal vasospasm, marked hypertension, neurologic abnormalities, and laboratory evidence of abnormal liver function, thrombocytopenia, and coagulation abnormalities. A distinct variant of preeclampsia, the HELLP syndrome (*h*emolysis, *el*evated *l*iver enzymes, and *l*ow *p*latelet count), is characterized by an initial benign course that can rapidly deteriorate with marked hemolysis and derangement of coagulation and hepatic and renal function. This presentation contrasts with that of postpartum hemolytic uremic syndrome or thrombocytopenic thrombolytic purpura, which typically occurs with normal pregnancy; is characterized by thrombocytopenia, microangiopathic anemia, and normal prothrombin and partial thromboplastin times; and often causes long-term impairment of renal function.

ACUTE RENAL FAILURE AFTER CARDIOVASCULAR SURGERY ARF requiring dialytic support is seen in 1% to 5% of patients undergoing coronary bypass grafting procedures. ARF in this setting can usually be attributed to prerenal azotemia, ischemic ATN, atheroembolic disease, or the effects of radiocontrast material administered perioperatively. The pattern of rise in the serum creatinine level may be extremely helpful in the differential diagnosis of ARF in this setting. As noted earlier, prerenal azotemia is typified by rapid fluctuations in serum creatinine values that usually precede surgery and mirror changes in systemic hemodynamics and renal perfusion. In ischemic ATN the rise in serum creatinine postoperatively is sustained and returns to baseline over days to weeks. Independent preoperative risk factors for the development of ATN after cardiovascular surgery include advanced age, creatinine clearance less than 60 mL/min, peripheral vascular disease, cardiomegaly, and a left ventricular ejection fraction of less than 35%. Intraoperative risk factors include emergency surgery, bypass time longer than 100 minutes, intra-aortic balloon pump insertion, and combined valvular and coronary revascularization procedures.

ACUTE RENAL FAILURE IN ASSOCIATION WITH PULMONARY DISEASE The coexistence of ARF and pulmonary disease (pulmonary renal syndrome) classically suggests a diagnosis of Goodpasture syndrome, Wegener granulomatosis, or another vasculitis. The detection of circulating antineutrophil cytoplasmic antibodies, antiglomerular basement membrane antibodies, or hypocomplementemia can be useful in the differentiation of these diseases although the urgent need for definitive diagnosis and treatment may mandate a lung or renal biopsy. More commonly ARF and pulmonary disease coexist owing to volume overload or pulmonary infection in the critically ill patient.

ACUTE RENAL FAILURE IN ASSOCIATION WITH LIVER DISEASE
The term *hepatorenal syndrome* (HRS) is widely misused. It should be reserved for a syndrome of irreversible ARF that complicates advanced liver disease, hepatic failure, or portal hypertension. The syndrome is characterized hemodynamically by intense intrarenal vasoconstriction with concomitant peripheral vasodilation. Most patients have evidence of advanced cirrhosis and the syndrome is uncommon outside of this setting or that of fulminant viral or alcoholic hepatitis. HRS almost certainly represents the terminal stage of a hypoperfusion state that begins early in the course of chronic liver disease. The diagnosis of HRS is one of exclusion. Other diagnoses that must be entertained in the patient with ARF and liver disease are prerenal ARF due to gastrointestinal losses, drug toxicity, combined hepatitis and tubulointerstitial nephritis induced by drugs or infectious agents, and multiorgan involvement in vasculitides (e.g., hepatitis C–induced cryoglobulinemia). The BUN and serum creatinine values are characteristically deceptively low, despite marked impairment of GFR, because of impaired urea generation and coexisting muscle wasting. The urinary findings include a benign sediment and a low FENa value. The most common precipitant of the HRS in patients with compensated cirrhosis is spontaneous bacterial peritonitis. Other trigger factors include vigorous diuresis, paracentesis, gastrointestinal bleeding, infections, minor surgery, or the use of NSAIDs and other drugs. Death is almost invariable in true HRS and is usually caused by hepatic failure, infection, hemorrhage, or circulatory failure.

COMPLICATIONS OF ACUTE RENAL FAILURE

Intravascular Volume Disturbance

Intravascular volume overload is a common consequence of ARF and manifests clinically as mild hypertension, increased jugular venous pressure, bibasilar lung crackles, pleural effusions or ascites, peripheral edema, increased body weight, and life-threatening pulmonary edema. Hypervolemia may be particularly troublesome in patients receiving multiple intravenous medications, sodium bicarbonate for correction of acidosis, or enteral or parenteral nutrition. Moderate to severe hypertension is unusual in ATN and should suggest other diagnoses, such as malignant hypertension, scleroderma renal crisis, or a primary glomerular pathologic condition. A vigorous osmotic diuresis may complicate the recovery phase of ARF and precipitate intravascular volume depletion and a delay in recovery of renal function.

Electrolyte Disturbances

Hyponatremia due to a combination of impaired free-water clearance and the ingestion of water or administration of hypotonic intravenous solutions can cause hyponatremia, which can be severe. Hyperkalemia is a common and potentially life-threatening complication. The serum potassium level typically rises by 0.5 to 1 mEq/L/day in oligoanuric patients, but the rate of rise may be higher in rhabdomyolysis or the tumor lysis syndrome. Mild hyperkalemia (< 6 mEq/L) is usually asymptomatic. Higher levels are often associated with electrocardiographic (ECG) abnormalities, typically peaked T waves, prolongation of the PR interval, flattening of P waves, widening of the QRS complex, and left axis deviation. These changes may precede the onset of life-threatening cardiac arrhythmias such as bradycardia, heart block, ventricular tachycardia or fibrillation, and asystole. Hypokalemia is unusual in ARF but may complicate nonoliguric ATN caused by aminoglycosides, cisplatin, or amphotericin B.

Mild hyperphosphatemia (5 to 10 mg/dL [1.6 to 3.2 mmol/L]) is a common consequence of ARF, and hyperphosphatemia may be severe (10 to 20 mg/dL [3.2 to 6.4 mmol/L]) in highly catabolic patients or when ARF is associated with rapid cell death, as in rhabdomyolysis or tumor lysis. Hypocalcemia is usually asymptomatic, possibly because of the counterbalancing effects of acidosis on neuromuscular excitability. However, symptomatic hypocalcemia can occur in patients with rhabdomyolysis or acute pancreatitis or after treatment of acidosis with bicarbonate. Clinical manifestations of hypocalcemia include perioral paresthesias, muscle cramps, seizures, hallucinations and confusion, and, on the ECG, prolongation of the QT interval and nonspecific T-wave changes. Mild asymptomatic hypermagnesemia is usual in oliguric ARF and reflects impaired excretion of ingested magnesium (dietary magnesium, magnesium-containing laxatives, or antacids). Hypomagnesemia occasionally complicates nonoliguric ATN associated with cisplatin or amphotericin B and, as with hypokalemia, probably reflects injury to the thick ascending limb, the principal site for Mg^{2+} reabsorption. Hypomagnesemia is usually asymptomatic but may occasionally manifest as neuromuscular instability, cramps, seizures, cardiac arrhythmias, or resistant hypokalemia or hypocalcemia.

Acid-Base Disturbance

ARF is commonly complicated by metabolic acidosis, typically with a widening of the serum anion gap. The acidosis may be severe (daily fall in plasma $HCO_3^- > 2$ mEq/L) if the generation of H^+ is increased by additional mechanisms (e.g., diabetic or fasting ketoacidosis; lactic acidosis complicating generalized tissue hypoperfusion, liver disease, or sepsis; metabolism of ethylene glycol). Metabolic alkalosis is an uncommon finding but may complicate overzealous correction of acidosis with bicarbonate or prerenal ARF triggered by loss of gastric secretions by vomiting or nasogastric aspiration.

Uremic Syndrome

Protracted periods of severe ARF or short periods of catabolic, anuric azotemia often lead to the development of the uremic syndrome. Clinical manifestations of the uremic syndrome include pericarditis, pericardial effusion, and cardiac tamponade; gastrointestinal complications such as anorexia, nausea, vomiting, and ileus; and neuropsychiatric disturbances including lethargy, confusion, stupor, coma, agitation, psychosis, asterixis, myoclonus, hyperreflexia, restless leg syndrome, focal neurologic deficits, and seizures.

MANAGEMENT OF ACUTE RENAL FAILURE

Prerenal Azotemia

By definition, prerenal azotemia is rapidly reversible on restoration of renal perfusion. Hypovolemia caused by hemorrhage is ideally corrected with packed red blood cells if the patient's condition is hemodynamically unstable or if the hematocrit is dangerously low. In the absence of active bleeding or hemodynamic instability, isotonic saline may suffice. Isotonic saline is the appropriate replacement fluid for plasma losses (e.g., burns or pancreatitis). The composition of urinary or gastrointestinal fluids vary greatly, but they are usually hypotonic and, accordingly, initial replacement is best achieved with hypotonic solutions (e.g., 0.45% saline). Colloid solutions should be used sparingly in prerenal ARF, and renal function should be monitored regularly. The risk of hyperoncotic renal failure is minimized by concomitant use of appropriate crystalloid solutions. Cardiac failure may require aggressive management with loop diuretics, antiarrhythmic drugs, positive inotropes, and/or preload- or afterload-reducing agents.

Fluid management may be particularly challenging in patients with prerenal ARF and cirrhosis. These subjects typically have intense intrarenal vasoconstriction and expanded total plasma volume because of pooling of blood in the splanchnic circulation, effective hypovolemia may be present. Therefore, the relative contribution of hypovolemia to ARF in this type of hepatic failure can be determined only by administration of a fluid challenge. Fluids should be administered slowly, because nonresponders may have an increase in ascites formation or pulmonary edema or both. Spontaneous bacterial peritonitis is a common trigger factor for HRS in patients with advanced cirrhosis and ascites. The administration of albumin (1.5 g/kg on diagnosis and 1 g/kg on day 3) in combination with standard antibiotic therapy in this setting has been demonstrated to reduce the incidence of HRS and improve patient survival. Paracentesis can be used to remove large volumes of ascitic fluid. Although it is controversial, simultaneous administration of albumin intravenously is thought by some investigators to minimize the risk of prerenal ARF and full-blown HRS during large-volume paracentesis. Indeed, large-volume paracentesis may occasionally improve GFR, possibly by lowering intra-abdominal pressure and promoting blood flow in renal veins. Vasopressin (V_1) receptor agonists, either alone or in combination with the α-agonist midodrine, have shown promise in the reversal of established HRS. In one small, prospective study, a combination of octreotide (100 to 200 mcg subcutaneously three times daily) and midodrine (7.5 to 12.5 mg three times daily), titrated to achieve a rise in mean arterial pressure of at least 15 mm Hg, in combination with daily intravenous albumin, resulted in a striking improvement in renal function and prolonged survival.

Intrinsic Renal Azotemia

Prevention
Optimization of cardiovascular function and intravascular volume is the single most important maneuver in the management of acute intrinsic azotemia. There is compelling evidence that aggressive restoration of intravascular volume dramatically reduces the incidence of ATN after major surgery, trauma, and burns. The importance of maintaining euvolemia in high-risk clinical situations has been demonstrated most convincingly with contrast nephropathy. Prophylactic infusion of saline

(0.45% N. Saline; 1 mL/kg for 12 hours before and after procedure) appears to be more effective in preventing ARF than administration of other commonly used agents such as mannitol and furosemide. Prophylactic administration of oral acetylcysteine (600 mg twice daily, 24 hours before and 24 hours after the procedure), in combination with hydration, reduced the incidence of contrast nephropathy in patients with moderate renal insufficiency in several, but not all, clinical trials.

Diuretics, NSAIDs (including cyclooxygenase-2 inhibitors), angiotensin-converting enzyme inhibitors, and other vasodilators should be avoided in patients with suspected true or effective hypovolemia, because they may convert prerenal azotemia to ischemic ATN. Careful monitoring of circulating drug levels appears to reduce the incidence of ARF associated with aminoglycoside antibiotics. There is convincing evidence that once-daily dosing with these agents affords equal antimicrobial activity and less nephrotoxicity than do conventional regimens. The use of lipid-encapsulated formulations of amphotericin B may offer some protection against renal injury. Several other agents are commonly used to prevent ARF in specific clinical settings. Allopurinol is useful for limiting uric acid generation in patients at high risk for acute urate nephropathy. Amifostine, an organic thiophosphate, has been demonstrated to ameliorate cisplatin nephrotoxicity in patients with solid organ or hematologic malignancies. Forced diuresis and alkalinization of urine may attenuate renal injury caused by uric acid or methotrexate. *N*-Acetylcysteine limits acetaminophen-induced renal injury if given within 24 hours of ingestion, and dimercaprol, a chelating agent, may prevent heavy metal nephrotoxicity. Both ethanol and fomepizole inhibit ethylene glycol metabolism to oxalic acid and other toxic metabolites and can prevent the development of ATN after toxic ingestion. (See Chapter 39, Extracorporeal Management of Poisoning.)

Specific Therapies
Despite intensive investigation, no specific therapy exists to accelerate recovery from ATN. Judicious volume management, treatment of complications, and avoidance of further injury are the mainstays of therapy. "Renal dose dopamine" (1 to 3 mg/kg/min) has been widely advocated for the management of oliguric ARF; however, it has *not* been demonstrated to prevent or alter the course of ischemic or nephrotoxic ATN in prospective, controlled clinical trials. The administration of high-dose intravenous diuretics to individuals with oliguric ARF is a common practice. Although this strategy may minimize fluid

overload, there is no evidence that it alters the mortality rate or the dialysis-free survival rate. Similarly, no adequate data exist to support the routine administration of mannitol to oliguric patients. Moreover, when it is administered to severely oliguric or anuric patients, it can trigger expansion of intravascular volume, pulmonary edema, and severe hyponatremia due to an osmotic shift of water from the intracellular to the intravascular space and its use is to be discouraged. ARF caused by other intrinsic renal diseases, such as acute glomerulonephritis or vasculitis, may respond to corticosteroids, alkylating agents, and/or plasmapheresis, depending on the primary disease.

Management of Complications

Metabolic complications such as intravascular volume overload, hyperkalemia, hyperphosphatemia, and metabolic acidosis are almost invariable in oliguric ARF, and preventive measures should be taken from the time of diagnosis. Prescription of nutrition should be designed to meet caloric requirements and minimize catabolism. In addition, doses of drugs excreted via the kidney must be adjusted for the degree of renal impairment.

INTRAVASCULAR VOLUME MANAGEMENT After correction of intravascular volume deficits, salt and water intake should be adjusted to match losses (e.g., urinary, gastrointestinal, drainage site, and insensible losses). Intravascular volume overload can usually be managed by restriction of salt and water intake and the use of diuretics. In the volume-overloaded patient, high doses of loop diuretics such as furosemide (bolus doses of up to 200 mg or up to 20 mg/hr as an intravenous infusion) or sequential thiazide and loop diuretic administration may be required if there is no response to conventional doses. Diuretic therapy should be discontinued in resistant patients to avoid complications such as ototoxicity. Ultrafiltration or dialysis may be required for removal of volume if conservative measures fail. Hyponatremia associated with a fall in effective serum osmolality can usually be corrected by restriction of water intake.

ELECTROLYTE DISTURBANCES Mild hyperkalemia (<5.5 mEq/L) should be managed initially by restriction of dietary potassium intake and elimination of potassium supplements and potassium-sparing diuretics. Moderate hyperkalemia (5.5 to 6.5 mEq/L) in patients without clinical or ECG evidence of hyperkalemia can usually be controlled by administration of K^+-binding ion-exchange resins such as sodium polystyrene sulfonate (15 to 30 g every 3 or 4 hours) with sorbitol (50 to 100 mL of 20% solution) by mouth or as a retention enema. Loop diuretics also increase K^+ excretion in diuretic-responsive patients. Emergency measures should be used for patients with serum K^+ values greater than 6.5 mEq/L and for all patients with ECG abnormalities or clinical features of hyperkalemia. Infusion of intravenous insulin (10 units of regular insulin) and glucose (50 mL of 50% dextrose) promotes K^+ shift into cells within 30 to 60 minutes, a benefit that lasts for several hours. Use of intravenous albuterol (0.5 mg in 100 mL of 5% dextrose over 5 minutes) or nebulized albuterol (10 to 20 mg) also promotes an intracellular shift of K^+. Calcium solutions such as calcium gluconate (10 mL of 10% solution intravenously over 5 minutes) antagonize the cardiac and neuromuscular effects of hyperkalemia and provide a valuable emergency temporizing measure, whereas other agents reduce the serum K^+ concentration. Dialysis is indicated if hyperkalemia is resistant to these measures. Hyperphosphatemia can usually be controlled by restriction of dietary phosphate intake and oral administration of agents (e.g., aluminum hydroxide, calcium carbonate, or sevelamer) that reduce absorption of PO_4^{3-} from the gastrointestinal tract. Hypocalcemia does not usually require treatment unless it is severe, as may occur in patients with rhabdomyolysis or pancreatitis or after administration of bicarbonate.

ACID-BASE BALANCE   Metabolic acidosis does not require treatment unless the serum bicarbonate concentration falls to less than 15 mEq/L. More severe acidosis can be corrected by either oral or intravenous bicarbonate administration. Initial rates of replacement should be based on estimates of bicarbonate deficit and adjusted thereafter according to serum levels. Patients should be monitored for complications of bicarbonate administration, including volume overload, hypernatremia, and metabolic alkalosis.

NUTRITIONAL MANAGEMENT   If the duration of renal insufficiency is likely to be short and the patient is not catabolic, then dietary protein should be restricted to less 0.8 g/kg of body weight/day. Catabolic patients, including those receiving continuous renal replacement therapy, may receive up to 1.4 mg/kg/day. Total caloric intake should not exceed 35 kcal/kg/day and will typically range from 25 to 30 kcal/kg/day. The enteral route of nutrition is preferred, because it avoids the morbidity associated with parenteral nutrition while providing support to intestinal function.

GENERAL MANAGEMENT ISSUES   Anemia may necessitate blood transfusion or the administration of recombinant human erythropoietin if it is severe or if recovery is delayed. Uremic bleeding usually responds to desmopressin, correction of anemia, estrogens, or dialysis. Febrile patients must be investigated aggressively for infection and may require treatment with broad-spectrum antibiotics while the clinician awaits identification of specific organisms. Meticulous care of intravenous cannulas, Foley catheters, and other invasive devices is mandatory. There is no indication for the prophylactic administration of antibiotic therapy.

Indications for and Modalities of Dialysis

When approaching the patient with ARF who requires renal replacement therapy (RRT), one should ask the following questions:

- When is it best to initiate RRT?
- What access is best?
- Which RRT modality should be used?
- What degree of solute clearance is required?

Indications
Absolute indications for RRT in ARF include the following:

- Symptomatic uremia (e.g., asterixis, pericardial rub, or encephalopathy)
- Metabolic acidosis/hyperkalemia/volume overload refractory to medical management

Relative indications include rapidly rising BUN and creatinine levels without evidence of imminent renal recovery when the development of uremic or other complications can reasonably be expected to supervene without intervention. "Renal support" indications involve the use of RRT to facilitate administration of total parenteral nutrition, fluid removal in congestive heart failure, and total fluid management in the patient with multiorgan failure. Knowing when to initiate RRT for patients in the intensive care unit (ICU) is a complex decision. Traditionally, the occurrence of a life-threatening indication for renal replacement has dictated timing. However, when one considers renal support requirements and the extremely high mortality in these patients, earlier intervention may be appropriate in selected patients.

Vascular Access
Vascular access for patients in the ICU is an important and often overlooked aspect of extracorporeal therapy. Poor access can lead to significant recirculation and inadequate blood flows, resulting in less efficient solute clearance. Factors determining catheter function include location of catheter placement and

catheter design. Temporary catheters range in length from 15 to 24 cm. The 15-cm catheters are designed for placement via the right internal jugular vein, although in most men and larger women, catheters of 19 to 20 cm may be required to reach the superior vena cava–right atrial junction. Catheters 20 cm and longer are designed for left internal jugular and femoral approaches. Dialysis catheters in the ICU should be placed in the internal jugular or the femoral position; the right internal jugular vein is usually preferred and femoral catheter length should exceed 19 cm to minimize recirculation. Subclavian access should be avoided whenever possible because it is associated with an unacceptable rate of central vein thrombosis and stenosis.

Catheter care is designed to prevent malfunction and infection. Malfunction is usually related to thrombus or fibrin sheath formation. Prevention of malfunction with any particular type of locking solution is not proved. Most institutions continue to use heparin or 4% citrate. When catheter dysfunction is present, line reversal may be successful and recirculation characteristics are acceptable. Infection is prevented by use of excellent local care and observation. In addition, studies have demonstrated reduced infection rates in acute catheters with the use of local antibiotic ointment on a dry gauze pad at the exit site. Importantly the risk of bloodstream infection rises dramatically after 1 week in patients with femoral catheters and 3 weeks in patients with internal jugular catheters. It is reasonable to try to limit catheter duration to within these periods. If a catheter exit site infection is recognized, the catheter should be removed immediately.

Modalities of Renal Replacement

No dialytic modality has been demonstrated to offer a definitive survival benefit in ARF. Continuous renal replacement therapy (CRRT) offers recognized advantages in continuous fluid and solute control but has never been convincingly shown to reduce mortality. Intermittent hemodialysis (IHD) can be performed, and recently attention has shifted to increasing its frequency to more than the traditional three times weekly. Slow low-efficiency daily dialysis (SLEDD) increases volume control and solute clearance compared with IHD and approaches that achieved with CRRT. Peritoneal dialysis is also used in the ICU but requires an intact peritoneal cavity. A decision on which modality to select depends on local preference, cost, and availability of therapies. Regardless of the RRT utilized, the goals should always be to improve the patient's fluid and electrolyte and acid-base balances, allowing for an optimal chance of renal and patient recovery.

CONTINUOUS RENAL REPLACEMENT THERAPIES   With the advent of safe placement of double-lumen venous catheters, CRRT options in general have developed into continuous venovenous modalities. A roller pump ensures constant blood flow and generates hydraulic pressure for ultrafiltration. Standard solutions are isotonic and use lactate as their bicarbonate equivalent; however, tailored solutions may use bicarbonate or citrate as the base. Anticoagulation options include systemic heparinization, prostacyclin infusion, or regional citrate anticoagulation. The latter approach offers several advantages including the provision of highly effective local anticoagulation with prolonged filter half-life without the need for systemic anticoagulation. This approach is particularly useful in patients with heparin-induced thrombocytopenia and in those with a high risk of bleeding in whom systemic anticoagulation is contraindicated. In slow continuous ultrafiltration (SCUF), the extracorporeal system is simplified to include a blood system hooked inline with a high-efficiency or high-flux membrane. As blood passes through the membrane, plasma water and solutes also pass through the membrane to allow formation of an ultrafiltrate, which is discarded. No replacement fluids or dialysate fluids are required. Although SCUF is a purely convective modality, the ultrafiltrate volume is limited to inputs plus desired losses and hence not enough volume is generated to control azotemia or significant metabolic disorders. This therapy is reserved for patients with residual renal function, but high volumes of input or significant fluid overload with a "relative" oliguria.

CRRT modalities designed for fluid and metabolic control require higher volumes of ultrafiltrate and hence require replacement fluid, dialysate fluid, or a combination of both. *Continuous venovenous hemofiltration* (CVVH) is an extracorporeal circuit with a double-lumen venous catheter hooked to an extracorporeal system with a blood pump, high-efficiency or high-flux dialysis membrane, and replacement fluid. As with SCUF, pure convection produces the ultrafiltrate, but much greater volumes are generated. Volume status and metabolic improvements are maintained by the addition of replacement fluid in the circuit. Replacement fluid can be added pre or postfilter. Prefilter replacement offers the benefit of less hemoconcentration within the dialysis membrane but decreases clearances up to 15%. Postfilter replacement maintains efficiency of the circuit but may be associated with an increase in thrombosis of the extracorporeal circuit.

Continuous venovenous hemodialysis (CVVHD) is an extracorporeal circuit with a double-lumen venous catheter hooked to an extracorporeal system with a blood pump, high-efficiency or high-flux dialysis membrane, and dialysate fluid. As with IHD, the dialysate runs countercurrent to the blood pathway, and as with other forms of CRRT, low efficiency is maintained by limiting the dialysate volume to 1 to 3 L/hr. Although considered a diffusive therapy, certainly convection occurs due to significant back-filtration.

Continuous venovenous hemodiafiltration (CVVHDF) consists of an extracorporeal circuit with a double-lumen venous catheter hooked to an extracorporeal system with a blood pump, high-efficiency or high-flux dialysis membrane, and both replacement and dialysate fluid. In general, this combination is used to increase clearance; however, CVVHDF can be used to simplify citrate delivery for anticoagulation. Clearly, both diffusive and convective forces determine solute clearances.

INTERMITTENT THERAPIES *Conventional hemodialysis* is typically delivered in the ICU setting three to four times a week with a standard clearance goal prescribed, similar to that for end-stage renal disease; however, recent evidence suggests that daily dialysis reduces mortality and aids renal recovery. The major complications of acute intermittent hemodialysis are associated with rapid shifts in plasma volume and solute composition, the angioaccess procedure, and the necessity for anticoagulation. Intradialytic hypotension is common in patients undergoing acute intermittent hemodialysis and usually occurs in the following circumstances:

- Overestimation of the extent of intravascular volume overload
- Rapid removal of fluid that is not matched by a flux of fluid into the intravascular space from the interstitial and cellular compartments
- Impairment of the patient's compensatory responses as a result of microvascular disease, sepsis, or vasodilatory medications (e.g., nitrates or antihypertensive medication)

Hypotension may be particularly problematic in critically ill patients with ATN and concurrent sepsis, hypoalbuminemia, malnutrition, or large third-space losses. Management of intradialytic hypotension requires careful assessment of intravascular volume by invasive hemodynamic monitoring if necessary; prescription of realistic ultrafiltration targets; and close observation for tachycardia or hypotension during dialysis. The immediate management of hypotension involves the discontinuation of hemofiltration, placement of the patient in the Trendelenburg position, and rapid infusion of 250 to 500 mL of normal saline. Other complications including the dialysis disequilibrium syndrome are discussed in Chapter 36, Hemodialysis. SLEDD has been developed to be a hybrid therapy between continuous and intermittent therapy. Blood flows and dialysate flows are slowed to 100 to 200 and 200 to 300 mL/min, respectively, and the therapy is prolonged to 8 to 12 hours/day. This slower form of dialysis theoretically allows for more hemodynamic stability with increased clearances compared with conventional hemodialysis. SLEDD also allows for time off the extracorporeal circuit, allowing the patient to travel to diagnostic studies.

Peritoneal dialysis can also be utilized in the ICU. It offers the advantages of lack of anticoagulation and vascular problems, hemodynamic stability, and is performed with relatively inexpensive and simple systems. The disadvantages include the need for an intact peritoneum, hyperglycemia, potential respiratory embarrassment due to increased abdominal pressure, the risk of peritonitis, and less clearance than can be obtained with SLEDD or CRRT.

Postrenal Azotemia

Management of postrenal azotemia usually involves a multidisciplinary approach and requires close collaboration among the nephrologist, urologist, and radiologist. This topic is reviewed extensively in Chapter 22. Urethral or bladder neck obstruction is usually relieved temporarily by transurethral or suprapubic placement of a bladder catheter, which provides a window for identification and treatment of the obstructing lesion. Similarly, ureteric obstruction may be treated initially by percutaneous catheterization of the dilated ureteric pelvis or ureter. Indeed, obstructing lesions can often be removed percutaneously (e.g., calculus or sloughed papilla) or bypassed by insertion of a ureteric stent (e.g., carcinoma). Most patients experience an appropriate diuresis for several days after relief of obstruction; however, approximately 5% develop a transient salt-wasting syndrome, because of delayed recovery of tubule function relative to GFR that may require intravenous fluid replacement for maintenance of blood pressure.

OUTCOME

The mortality rate among patients with acute intrinsic renal azotemia varies from less than 10% in obstetric-related ARF to more than 70% in cases associated with multiple organ failure. Factors associated with a poor prognosis include male sex, advanced age, oliguria (< 400 mL/day), and a rise in the serum creatinine value of more than 3 mg/dL (265 mcmol/L). Most patients who survive an episode of ARF recover sufficient renal function to live normal lives. However, ARF is irreversible in approximately 5% of patients, usually as a consequence of complete cortical necrosis, and necessitates long-term renal replacement therapy with dialysis or transplantation. An additional 5% of patients show progressive deterioration in renal function after an initial recovery phase, probably because of hyperfiltration and subsequent sclerosis of remnant glomeruli.

Primary Glomerular Disease

10

GENERAL DESCRIPTION OF GLOMERULAR SYNDROMES

Proteinuria

Proteinuria can be caused by systemic overproduction (e.g., multiple myeloma with Bence Jones proteinuria), tubular dysfunction (e.g., Fanconi syndrome), or glomerular dysfunction. It is important to identify patients in whom the proteinuria is a manifestation of substantial glomerular disease as opposed to those patients who have benign transient or postural (orthostatic) proteinuria.

Isolated proteinuria is a mild transient proteinuria that typically accompanies physiologically stressful conditions, including fever, exercise, and congestive heart failure.

Orthostatic proteinuria is defined by the absence of proteinuria while the patient is in a recumbent posture and its appearance during upright posture, especially during exercise. It is most common in adolescents. The total amount of protein excretion in a 24-hour period is generally less than 1 g. The diagnosis is made by comparing the protein excretion in two 12-hour urine collections, one recumbent and one during ambulation. Importantly, patients should be recumbent for at least 2 hours before their ambulatory collection is completed to avoid the possibility of contamination of the "recumbent" collection by urine formed during ambulation. The diagnosis of orthostatic proteinuria requires that protein excretion during recumbency be less than 50 mg during those 8 hours. Patients should be followed on an annual basis until the proteinuria resolves and the long-term prognosis is typically excellent.

Fixed proteinuria is present whether the patient is upright or recumbent. The proteinuria disappears in some patients, whereas others have a more ominous glomerular lesion that portends an

175

adverse long-term outcome. The prognosis depends on the persistence and severity of the proteinuria. If proteinuria disappears, it is less likely that the patient will develop hypertension or a reduced glomerular filtration rate (GFR). These patients must be evaluated periodically for as long as the proteinuria persists.

Plasma cell dyscrasias can produce monoclonal proteins, immunoglobulin, free light chains, and combinations of these. Light chains are filtered at the glomerulus and may appear in the urine as Bence Jones protein. The detection of urine immunoglobulin light chains can be the first clue to a number of important clinical syndromes associated with plasma cell dyscrasias that involve the kidney. Unfortunately, urine immunoglobulin light chains may not be detected by reagent strip tests for protein. However, plasma cell dyscrasias may also manifest as proteinuria or albuminuria when the glomerular deposition of light chains causes disruption of the normally impermeable glomerular capillary wall. The diagnosis of a plasma cell dyscrasia can be considered when a tall, narrow band on electrophoresis suggests the presence of a monoclonal γ-globulin or immunoglobulin light chain either in the urine or plasma.

Nephrotic Syndrome

The nephrotic syndrome is characterized by proteinuria of more than 3.5 g/day associated with edema, hyperlipidemia, and hypoalbuminemia. In addition to the primary glomerular diseases discussed below, the nephrotic syndrome may be caused by a large number of identifiable disease states (Table 10–1).

Hematuria

Hematuria is the presence of an excessive number of red blood cells in the urine and is categorized as either microscopic (visible only with the aid of a microscope) or macroscopic (urine that is tea-colored or cola-colored, pink, or even red). An acceptable definition of microscopic hematuria is more than two red blood cells per high-power field in centrifuged urine. The urinary dipstick method detects one to two red blood cells per high-power field and a negative dipstick examination virtually excludes hematuria.

Dysmorphic red cells on urine microscopy provide strong evidence for glomerular bleeding, known as *glomerular hematuria*. The findings of proteinuria (especially >2 g/day) and/or red blood cell casts enhance the possibility that hematuria is of

Table 10–1: Causes of the Nephrotic Syndrome

- Idiopathic nephrotic syndrome due to primary glomerular disease
- Nephrotic syndrome associated with specific etiologic events or in which glomerular disease arises as a complication of other diseases:

1. Medications
   - Organic, inorganic, elemental mercury
   - Organic gold
   - Penicillamine, bucillamine
   - "Street" heroin
   - Probenecid
   - Captopril
   - Nonsteroidal anti-inflammatory drugs
   - Lithium
   - Interferon alfa
2. Allergens, venoms, immunizations
   - Bee sting
   - Pollens
3. Infections
   a. Bacterial—poststreptococcal granulonephritis, infective endocarditis, "shunt nephritis," leprosy, syphilis (congenital and secondary), *Mycoplasma* infection, tuberculosis, chronic bacterial pyelonephritis with vesicoureteral reflux
   b. Viral—hepatitis B, hepatitis C, cytomegalovirus, infectious mononucleosis (Epstein-Barr virus), herpes zoster, vaccinia, human immunodeficiency virus type I
   c. Protozoal—malaria (especially quartan malaria), toxoplasmosis
   d. Helminthic—schistosomiasis, trypanosomiasis, filariasis
4. Neoplastic
   a. Solid tumors (carcinoma and sarcoma): lung, colon, stomach, breast
   b. Leukemia and lymphoma: Hodgkin disease
   c. Graft-versus-host disease after bone marrow transplantation
5. Multisystem disease
   - Systemic lupus erythematosus
   - Henoch-Schönlein purpura/IgA nephropathy
   - Amyloidosis (primary and secondary)
6. Heredofamilial and metabolic disease
   - Diabetes mellitus
   - Hypothyroidism (myxedema)
   - Graves diseases
   - Amyloidosis (familial Mediterranean fever and other hereditary forms, Muckle-Wells syndrome)
   - Podocyte mutations
   - Congenital nephrotic syndrome (Finnish type)
7. Miscellaneous
   - Pregnancy-associated (preeclampsia, recurrent, transient)
   - Chronic renal allograft failure

glomerular origin. The differential pathologic diagnosis of glomerular hematuria without proteinuria, renal insufficiency, or red blood cell casts is IgA nephropathy, thin basement membrane nephropathy, hereditary nephritis, or histologically normal glomeruli. When hematuria is accompanied by 1 to 3 g/day proteinuria but no significant renal insufficiency, IgA nephropathy is the most likely specific cause. Patients with hematuria and subacute renal failure usually have an aggressive glomerulonephritis with crescents. However, a definitive diagnosis requires a renal biopsy. The potential benefits of renal biopsy in patients with hematuria and no proteinuria or renal insufficiency ("isolated hematuria") include a reduction of patient and physician uncertainty and the accompanying anxiety by establishment of a specific diagnosis. However, isolated glomerular hematuria may not warrant a renal biopsy for many patients because the findings often do not affect management. Nonglomerular causes of isolated hematuria are discussed in Chapter 2, Laboratory Assessment of Kidney Disease; Clearance, Urinalysis and Kidney Biopsy.

Nephritic Syndrome

The nephritic syndrome is characterized by inflammatory injury to the glomerular capillary wall. It presents clinically as abrupt onset renal dysfunction with oliguria, hematuria with red cell casts, hypertension, and subnephrotic proteinuria. The distinction between the nephritic and nephrotic syndrome is generally easily made on the basis of clinical and laboratory features. Common diseases that present as the nephritic syndrome include poststreptococcal glomerulonephritis, IgA nephropathy, lupus nephritis, and immune complex glomerulonephritis associated with infection.

Rapidly Progressive Glomerulonephritis/Crescentic Glomerulonephritis

The term "rapidly progressive glomerulonephritis" (RPGN) refers to a clinical syndrome characterized by a rapid loss of renal function (days to weeks), often accompanied by oliguria or anuria and features of glomerulonephritis (red cell casts/proteinuria). These aggressive glomerulonephritides usually are associated with extensive crescent formation and, hence, the clinical term RPGN is sometimes used interchangeably with the pathologic term "crescentic glomerulonephritis." Renal diseases other than crescentic glomerulonephritis that can cause the signs and symptoms of RPGN include thrombotic microangiopathy and atheroembolic renal disease.

The three major immunopathologic categories of crescentic glomerulonephritis are as follows:

- Immune complex
- Pauci-immune (antineutrophil cytoplasmic antibody [ANCA] associated)
- Anti–glomerular basement membrane (GBM) disease

In a patient who has RPGN clinically and crescentic glomerulonephritis identified by light microscopy of a renal biopsy specimen, the precise diagnostic categorization of the disease requires integration of clinical, serologic, immunohistologic, and electron microscopic data (Fig. 10–1).

GLOMERULAR DISEASES THAT CAUSE NEPHROTIC SYNDROME

Minimal Change Glomerulopathy

Minimal change glomerulopathy is most common in children, accounting for 70% to 90% of cases of nephrotic syndrome in children younger than 10 years of age and 50% of cases in older children. Minimal change glomerulopathy also causes 10% to 15% of cases of primary nephrotic syndrome in adults. The disease may also affect elderly patients in whom there is a higher propensity for the clinical syndrome of minimal change glomerulopathy and acute renal failure.

Pathology
Minimal change glomerulopathy has no glomerular lesions by light microscopy or only minimal focal segmental mesangial prominence. Immunofluorescence staining in minimal change disease is negative for immunoglobulins and complement components. The pathologic sine qua non of minimal change glomerulopathy is effacement of visceral epithelial cell foot processes observed by electron microscopy.

Clinical Features and Natural History
The cardinal clinical feature of minimal change glomerulopathy in children is the relatively abrupt onset of proteinuria and development of the nephrotic syndrome with heavy proteinuria, hypoalbuminemia, and hyperlipidemia. Minimal change glomerulopathy in adults is frequently associated with hypertension and

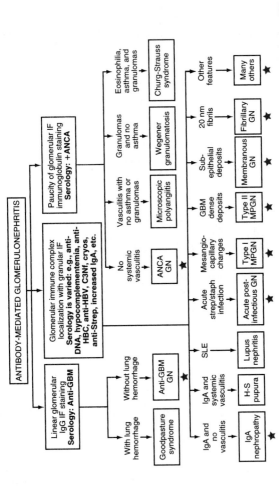

Figure 10–1. Algorithm for categorizing glomerulonephritis that is known or suspected of being mediated by antibodies. This categorization applies to glomerulonephritis with crescents as well as to glomerulonephritis without crescents. The diseases with stars beneath them can be considered primary glomerular diseases, whereas those without stars are secondary to (components of) systemic diseases.

acute renal failure, the latter especially in the older than 60 age-group. Minimal change glomerulopathy has been associated with several other conditions, including viral infections, pharmaceutical agents, malignancy, and allergy. There may be a history of a drug reaction before the onset of minimal change glomerulopathy. In this setting most patients also manifest pyuria and renal insufficiency as a consequence of the simultaneous development of acute tubulointerstitial nephritis. This process has been described most commonly with nonsteroidal anti-inflammatory drugs. A history of food allergy should be elicited because there is an association in some patients. Minimal change glomerulopathy is associated with malignancies (usually Hodgkin disease), but it may also occur with solid tumors.

Laboratory Findings

The ubiquitous laboratory feature of minimal change glomerulopathy is severe proteinuria. Microscopic hematuria is seen in fewer than 15% of patients. Volume contraction may lead to a rise in both hematocrit and hemoglobin. The erythrocyte sedimentation rate is increased as a consequence of hyperfibrinogenemia as well as hypoalbuminemia. The serum albumin concentration is generally less than 2 g/dL and, in more severe cases, less than 1 g/dL. Total cholesterol, low-density lipoprotein, and triglyceride levels are increased. Pseudohyponatremia has been observed in the setting of marked hyperlipidemia. Renal function is usually normal, although a minority of patients have substantial acute renal failure, as discussed earlier. Immunoglobulin (Ig) G levels may be profoundly decreased—a factor that may result in susceptibility to infections. Complement levels are typically normal in patients with minimal change glomerulopathy.

Treatment

CHILDREN Prednisone 60 mg/m^2/day will induce a remission in more than 90% of patients within 4 to 6 weeks of therapy. Once remission has been obtained, an alternate-day schedule should begin within at least 4 weeks of the response to decrease the incidence of steroid-induced side effects. In children who have received empirical treatment, a renal biopsy is indicated when there is failure to respond to a 4- to 6-week course of prednisone.

ADULTS For an adult, the dose of prednisone is 1 mg/kg body weight, not to exceed 80 mg/day. In adult patients response rates are typically lower and a full response to corticosteroid treatment may take up to 15 weeks.

MANAGEMENT OF RELAPSE   As few as 25% of patients have a long-term remission, 25% to 30% have infrequent relapses (no more than one a year), and the remainder have frequent relapses, a dependency on steroid treatment, or resistance to steroid treatment. Patients with relapses or steroid-dependent nephrotic patients typically require cytotoxic therapy with either cyclophosphamide or chlorambucil. Both cyclophosphamide and chlorambucil have profound side effects that include life-threatening infection, gonadal dysfunction, hemorrhagic cystitis, bone marrow suppression, and mutagenic events. In patients unresponsive to alkylating therapy, the question is whether other forms of therapy are indicated. End-stage renal failure is rare in minimal change glomerulopathy, and, in light of this fact, additional forms of therapy must be considered carefully with respect to the cumulative toxicity of immunosuppressive and cytotoxic drugs.

STEROID-RESISTANT MINIMAL CHANGE GLOMERULOPATHY   In approximately 5% of children minimal change glomerulopathy appears to be steroid-resistant. Reasons for steroid resistance include inaccurate diagnosis (e.g., focal segmental glomerulonephritis), noncompliance with therapy, and occasionally malabsorption in very edematous patients. Therapeutic options in true steroid resistance include cyclosporine, which induces remissions in up to 90% of patients, albeit with a high relapse rate upon withdrawal.

Focal Segmental Glomerulosclerosis

Focal segmental glomerulosclerosis (FSGS) should not be considered a single disease but rather a diagnostic term for a clinicopathologic syndrome that has multiple causes and pathogenic mechanisms. The ubiquitous clinical feature of the syndrome is proteinuria, and the ubiquitous pathologic feature is focal segmental glomerular consolidation and scarring. As shown in Table 10–2, FSGS may appear to be a primary renal disease or may be associated with a variety of other conditions. The yearly incidence of primary FSGS has risen from less than 10% to approximately 25% of adult nephropathies over the last two decades. A substantial portion of this increase may be attributable to an increase in the collapsing variant of FSGS and FSGS caused by obesity. Notably, the relative incidence of FSGS is higher for blacks than for whites.

Pathology
FSGS is by definition a focal process, i.e., not all glomeruli are involved, and the glomeruli are segmentally sclerotic, i.e.,

Table 10–2: Focal Segmental Glomerulonephritis (FSGS)

Primary (idiopathic) FSGS
  Typical (not otherwise specified) FSGS
  Glomerular tip lesion variant of FSGS
  Collapsing glomerulopathy variant of FSGS
  Perihilar variant of FSGS
  Familial FSGS
Secondary FSGS
  With HIV disease (typically collapsing variant)
  With intravenous drug abuse
  With glomerulomegaly (usually peripheral vascular)
    Morbid obesity
    Sickle cell disease
    Cyanotic congenital heart disease
    Hypoxic pulmonary disease
  Reduced nephron numbers (usually perihilar variant)
    Unilateral renal agenesis
    Oligomeganephronia
    Reflux interstitial nephritis
    Postfocal cortical necrosis
    Postnephrectomy
  Drug toxicity
    Pamidronate (collapsing FSGS)
    Lithium
  Familial FSGS
    α-Actinin 4 mutations (autosomal recessive)
    Podocin mutations (autosomal recessive)
    Nephrin mutations (autosomal recessive)

portions of the involved glomeruli may appear normal by light microscopy. Nonsclerotic glomeruli and segments usually have no staining for immunoglobulins or complement. The ultrastructural features of FSGS on electron microscopy include focal foot process effacement.

Clinical Features and Natural History
Proteinuria is the hallmark of primary FSGS. The degree of proteinuria varies from non-nephrotic (1 to 2 g/day) to massive proteinuria (>10 g/day). Hematuria, which can be gross, occurs in more than one half of patients, and approximately one third of patients present with some degree of renal insufficiency. Hypertension is found as a presenting feature in one third of patients. Patients with a variant of FSGS known as "collapsing FSGS" typically have more severe proteinuria and renal insufficiency. The rapidity of onset of FSGS is similar to the clinical

presentation of minimal change glomerulopathy. Predictors of a poor outcome in primary FSGS include nephrotic range proteinuria, renal insufficiency, and failure to respond to corticosteroid therapy. Neither the degree of scarring within the glomerulus nor the number of glomeruli that are totally obsolescent is predictive of long-term renal outcome; however, significant interstitial fibrosis and tubular atrophy correlate with poor prognosis.

Laboratory Findings

Hypoproteinemia is common in patients with FSGS, and the serum albumin concentration may fall to less than 2 g/dL, especially in patients with the collapsing variant. Hypogammaglobulinemia and hyperlipidemia are typical. Serum complement components are generally in the normal range in FSGS. Serologic testing for human immunodeficiency virus infection should be obtained for patients with FSGS, especially those with the collapsing pattern.

Treatment

Angiotensin-converting enzyme (ACE) inhibitors decrease proteinuria and the rate of progression to end-stage renal disease in proteinuric renal disease including FSGS. Indeed, ACE inhibition may provide a substantial reduction in proteinuria and a long-term renoprotective effect that may be equal to or greater than that of immunosuppressive therapy. Indeed, in patients who have less than 3 g/day proteinuria, a trial of ACE inhibition without recourse to immunosuppression may be warranted as first-line therapy. Response rates to immunosuppressive therapy in primary FSGS are approximately 45% for complete remission, 10% for partial remission, and 45% for no response. In children, the initial treatment of FSGS is similar to that of minimal change glomerulopathy. In adults with nephrotic range proteinuria, recommended doses of prednisone include 1 mg/kg, up to 80 mg/day for up to 16 weeks. The prolonged course in adults is based on the finding that in adults the median time for complete remission is 3 to 4 months. Among adult patients who have a relapse after a prolonged remission (>6 months), a repeat course of corticosteroid therapy may again induce a remission. In steroid-dependent patients who have frequent relapses, alternative strategies include the introduction of cyclosporine (5 mg/kg/day). The practice of using higher doses of corticosteroids to reach remission has resulted in alternative therapeutic approaches, including the administration of methylprednisolone boluses of 30 mg/kg/day to a maximum of 1 g given every other day for 6 doses, followed by this same dose on a weekly basis for 10 weeks; subsequently, similar doses are given on a tapering schedule.

These very high doses of corticosteroids may have significant short- and long-term side effects.

Alternatives to Corticosteroid Therapy

FSGS-resistant prednisone may be induced into remission with cyclosporine. In steroid-resistant FSGS, patients treated with cyclosporine, complete remission rates are approximately 20% with partial remission rates in the 40% to 70% range. However, as with minimal change disease, the withdrawal of treatment results in relapse in more than 75% of patients. Relapse rates may be minimized by maintenance of therapy for 12 months after induction of remission followed by a slow taper. However, long-term treatment with cyclosporine is associated with the development of tubular atrophy, tubulointerstitial fibrosis, and renal insufficiency. Clinical studies have failed to convincingly demonstrate the effectiveness of cytotoxic drugs, including cyclophosphamide, or plasmapheresis in the treatment of FSGS in both adults and children.

C1q Nephropathy

C1q nephropathy is a relatively rare cause of proteinuria and nephrotic syndrome that can mimic FSGS clinically and histologically. The diagnosis is based on the presence of mesangial immune complex deposits that have conspicuous staining for C1q accompanied by staining for IgG, IgM, and C3. Patients with C1q nephropathy are predominantly black, male, and aged between 15 and 30 years. Many are asymptomatic, but 50% present with edema, 40% with hypertension, and 30% with hematuria. Renal survival at 3 years is 84%, and treatment with corticosteroids does not provide any improvement in proteinuria or preservation of renal function.

Membranous Glomerulopathy

Idiopathic membranous glomerulopathy is the most common cause of nephrotic syndrome in adults (25%) and can occur as an idiopathic (primary) or secondary disease. Secondary membranous glomerulopathy is caused by autoimmune diseases (e.g., lupus erythematosus or autoimmune thyroiditis), infection (e.g., hepatitis B or hepatitis C), drugs (e.g., penicillamine or gold), and malignancies (e.g., colon cancer or lung cancer). In 20% to 30% of patients older than age 60, membranous glomerulopathy is ass~~~~ a malignancy. The peak incidence of membranou~ is in the fourth or fifth decade of life. Altho~

with membranous glomerulopathy present with the nephrotic syndrome, 10% to 20% of patients have less than 2 g/day.

Pathology

The characteristic histologic abnormality in membranous glomerulopathy is diffuse global capillary wall thickening and the presence of subepithelial immune complex deposits.

Clinical Features and Natural History

Patients with membranous glomerulopathy usually present with the nephrotic syndrome.

The onset is usually not associated with any prodromal disease process or other antecedent infections. Hypertension early in the disease process is variable. Most patients present with normal or slightly decreased renal function and if progressive renal insufficiency develops, its course is usually relatively indolent. Causes of an abrupt decline in renal function include overzealous diuresis, crescentic transformation (ANCA/anti-GBM associated), or acute bilateral renal vein thrombosis. Patients with membranous nephropathy are hypercoagulable to a greater extent than other nephrotic patients. Consequently, venous thrombosis, including renal vein thrombosis, is reported more often in patients with membranous glomerulopathy than in those with other nephrotic glomerulopathies. The high prevalence of deep vein thrombosis in patients with membranous glomerulopathy (up to 45%) has led to the use of prophylactic anticoagulation for patients with proteinuria greater than 10 g/day.

Approximately 35% of patients develop end-stage renal disease by 10 years, and 25% can expect a complete spontaneous remission of proteinuria within 5 years. Spontaneous remission may take 36 to 48 months to develop. Risk factors for progression include renal insufficiency at presentation, persistent proteinuria, male sex, advanced age (older than 50 years) and poorly controlled hypertension. In addition to the clinical prognostic features, the presence of advanced membranous glomerulopathy on renal biopsy, tubular atrophy, and interstitial fibrosis are also associated with a poor outcome.

Laboratory Findings

Proteinuria is usually more than 3 g of protein per 24 hours and may exceed 10 g/day in 30% of patients, whereas microscopic hematuria is present in 30% to 50% of patients. Macroscopic hematuria is distinctly uncommon. Renal function is typically preserved at presentation. Hypoalbuminemia is observed if proteinuria is severe. Complement levels are normal; however, the complex of terminal complement components known as C5b-9 is found in the urine in some patients. Tests for hepatitis B, hepatitis C, and syphilis for immunologic disorders such as lupus, mixed connective tissue disease, and cryoglobulinemia should be performed to exclude secondary causes.

Treatment

The management of primary membranous glomerulopathy is controversial. Common therapeutic approaches include the following:

- Supportive care including ACE inhibition, lipid-lowering therapy, and anticoagulation therapy if required
- Corticosteroids (usually prednisone or methylprednisolone)
- Alkylating agents, such as chlorambucil or cyclophosphamide, with or without concurrent corticosteroid treatment
- Cyclosporine

All patients should receive supportive care, including the use of ACE inhibitors or adrenergic receptor blockers and lipid-lowering agents and consideration for use of prophylactic anticoagulation therapy.

CORTICOSTEROIDS Three large, prospective, randomized trials have been conducted in adult patients to examine the efficacy of oral corticosteroid therapy, and the outcomes have differed. A pooled analysis of randomized trials and prospective studies suggested a lack of benefit for corticosteroid therapy in inducing a remission of the nephrotic syndrome. It has been argued that higher dosages (60 to 200 mg every other day) of prednisone and a longer course of therapy (up to 1 year) are required to effect a response. However, the side effects of extended high-dose corticosteroid therapy are substantial and the risk-benefit ratio may not favor corticosteroid therapy in most, if not all, patients.

CYCLOPHOSPHAMIDE Cytotoxic drugs have been used in the treatment of idiopathic membranous glomerulopathy including cyclophosphamide and chlorambucil. A regimen of chlorambucil (0.2 mg/kg/day) alternating monthly with daily prednisone (0.5 mg/kg/day) in combination with intravenous pulse methylprednisolone (1 g/day) for the first 3 days of each month has been demonstrated to lead to a higher and more rapid rate of remission in addition to stabilization of renal function. Cyclophosphamide may be at least as effective as chlorambucil when used in a similar dosing protocol. The risk-to-benefit ratio of these aggressive treatment protocols must be acceptable to the patient who must be informed of the heightened long-term risk of transitional cell carcinoma of the bladder and of lymphoma. Thus, these more aggressive strategies for membranous glomerulopathy should probably only be considered for patients with evidence of progressive deterioration of renal function and/or adverse prognostic features.

OTHER FORMS OF IMMUNOSUPPRESSIVE THERAPY The use of cyclosporine given in dosages of 4 to 5 mg/kg/day has resulted in improvement in proteinuria and stability of renal function in many patients with membranous glomerulopathy. However, worsening of proteinuria occurs in most patients soon after the cessation of cyclosporine therapy, and biopsy studies have documented persistent deposition of immunoglobulin and complement in cyclosporine-treated patients. The role of mycophenolate mofetil in the therapy of membranous nephropathy remains to be elucidated.

Membranoproliferative Glomerulonephritis (Mesangial Capillary Glomerulonephritis)

Membranoproliferative glomerulonephritis (MPGN) is characterized by diffuse global capillary wall that often has a double-contoured appearance and either subendothelial deposits (type I MPGN) or deposits within the mesangium and basement membrane (type II MPGN). Most patients with idiopathic MPGN are children, with an equal proportion of males to females for both type I and type II diseases. Although the pathologic findings indicate that type I MPGN is an immune complex disease, the identity of the nephritogenic antigen is unknown in most patients. In type II MPGN an autoantibody, C3 nephritic factor, that triggers persistent activation of the complement cascade occurs in more than 60% of patients and may be responsible for disease in these patients.

Clinical Features and Natural History
The clinical presentations of MPGN are as follows:

- Nephrotic syndrome (50%)
- Combination of asymptomatic hematuria and proteinuria (25%)
- Acute nephritic syndrome (25%)

Hypertension is typically mild, and renal dysfunction occurs in at least one half of patients. When present at the outset of disease, renal dysfunction portends a poor prognosis. Membranoproliferative glomerular diseases are also associated with a number of other disease processes (Table 10–3). A wide variety of infectious and autoimmune conditions are associated with

MPGN, suggesting that, in addition to the known association with hepatitis, infections by themselves may present with MPGN. A small number of patients have an X-linked deficiency of C2 or C3 with or without partial lipodystrophy. In addition to partial lipodystrophy, congenital complement deficiency states and deficiency of α_1-antitrypsin also predispose to MPGN type I.

In general, one third of patients with type I MPGN will have a spontaneous remission, one third will have progressive disease, and one third will have a disease process that waxes and wanes but never completely disappears. The 10-year renal survival is 40% to 60%; however, non-nephrotic patients have a 10-year

Table 10–3: Classification of Membranoproliferative Glomerulonephritis

Idiopathic
    Type I
    Type II
    Type III
Secondary
    Infections
        Hepatitis C and B
        Visceral abscesses
        Infective endocarditis
        Shunt nephritis
        Quartan malaria
        Schistosoma nephropathy
        Mycoplasma infection
    Rheumatologic diseases
        Systemic lupus erythematosus
        Scleroderma
        Sjögren syndrome
        Sarcoidosis
        Mixed essential cryoglobulinemia with or without hepatitis C infection
        Anti–smooth muscle syndrome
Malignancy
    Carcinoma
    Lymphoma
    Leukemia
Inherited
    $\alpha 1$-Antitrypsin deficiency
    Complement deficiency (C2 or C3), with or without partial lipodystrophy

survival of more than 80%. The parameters suggestive of poor prognosis in idiopathic MPGN type I include hypertension, renal insufficiency, nephritic syndrome, and cellular crescents on biopsy. The prognosis for patients with type II disease is worse than that for those with type I disease because it is associated with a higher rate of crescentic glomerulonephritis and chronic tubulointerstitial nephritis at the time of biopsy. Clinical remissions of type II MPGN are rare, and recurrence in transplanted kidneys occurs much more regularly than for type I MPGN. Type III MPGN occurs in a very small number of children and young adults. These patients may have clinical features and outcomes quite similar to those of MPGN type I.

Laboratory Findings
Hematuria is the hallmark of the patients presenting with MGPN and may be microscopic or macroscopic. The degree of proteinuria varies widely. Renal insufficiency occurs in a variable number of patients, but it is the most ominous feature of the acute nephritic syndrome. Serologic and clinical evidence of cryoglobulinemia, hepatitis C, hepatitis B, osteomyelitis, subacute bacterial endocarditis, or infected ventriculoatrial shunt should be sought in type I MGPN. C3 is persistently depressed in approximately 75% to 90% of patients with MPGN. C3 nephritic factor is found in 60% of patients with type II MPGN.

Treatment
The treatment of type I MPGN is based on the underlying cause of the disease process. Thus, the therapy for MPGN associated with cryoglobulinemia and hepatitis C should be focused on treating hepatitis C virus infection (interferon/ribavirin), whereas the treatment of MPGN associated with lupus or with scleroderma should be based on the principles of care for those rheumatologic conditions. Most recommendations for the treatment of idiopathic type I MPGN are limited to studies in children in whom low-dose prednisone therapy improves renal survival. Whether similar effects are achieved in adults has never been subjected to a prospective randomized trial. In addition to glucocorticoids, a host of other forms of immunosuppressive and anticoagulant treatments have been used in the treatment of type I MPGN including dipyridamole, aspirin, and warfarin with and without cyclophosphamide. However, definitive prospective data are lacking. Unfortunately, there is no good form of therapy for MPGN type II. This problem in clinical decision making is compounded by the fact that MPGN type II recurs almost invariably in renal transplant patients, especially if crescentic disease was present in the native renal biopsy.

GLOMERULONEPHRITIS

The syndrome of glomerulonephritis is characterized by the following:

- Hematuria with or without red blood cell casts
- Proteinuria
- Hypertension
- Renal insufficiency

The spectrum of clinical presentation ranges from asymptomatic hematuria to the acute nephritic syndrome. A diagnostic algorithm is shown in Figure 10–1.

Acute Poststreptococcal Glomerulonephritis

Acute poststreptococcal glomerulonephritis (PSGN) is a disease that affects primarily children, with the peak incidence between the ages of 2 and 6 years. It may occur as part of an epidemic or as a sporadic disease, and rarely PSGN and rheumatic fever occur concomitantly. The incidence of acute PSGN is on the decline in developed countries, but it remains static in developing countries. Epidemic PSGN is often associated with skin infections as opposed to pharyngitides in developed countries. Overt glomerulonephritis is found in about 10% of children at risk, but when one includes subclinical disease as evidenced by microscopic hematuria, about 25% of children at risk are affected. In some developing countries, acute PSGN remains the most common form of acute nephritic syndrome among children.

Clinical Features and Natural History

The syndrome of acute PSGN can present with a spectrum of severity ranging from asymptomatic to oliguric acute renal failure. A latent period is present (7 to 21 days) from the onset of pharyngitis to that of nephritis. The hematuria is microscopic in more than two thirds of patients. Hypertension occurs in more than 75% of patients and is usually mild to moderate in severity. It is most evident at the onset of nephritis and typically subsides promptly after diuresis. Antihypertensive treatment is necessary in only about one half of patients. Signs and symptoms of congestive heart failure may occur in as many of 40% of elderly patients with PSGN. Edema may be the presenting symptom in two thirds of patients, and is present in up to 90% of patients. Ascites and anasarca may occur in children. Encephalopathy is not common and affects children more often than adults. This encephalopathy is not always attributable to severe hypertension, but may be the result of central nervous system vasculitis.

The clinical manifestations of acute PSGN typically resolve in 1 to 2 weeks as edema and hypertension disappear after diuresis. Both the hematuria and proteinuria may persist for several months, but usually resolve within a year. The long-term persistence of proteinuria and especially albuminuria may indicate the persistence of a proliferative glomerulonephritis. The differential diagnosis of acute PSGN includes IgA nephropathy/Henoch-Schönlein purpura, MPGN, or acute crescentic glomerulonephritis. The occurrence of an acute nephritis in the setting of persistent fever should raise the suspicion of a peri-infectious glomerulonephritis, such as that occurring with an occult abscess or infective endocarditis.

Laboratory Findings

Hematuria, microscopic or gross, is nearly always present in acute PSGN. Microscopic examination of urine typically reveals the presence of dysmorphic red blood cells or red blood cell casts. Proteinuria is nearly always present but is typically in the subnephrotic range. Proteinuria in the nephrotic-range may occur in as many as 20% of patients and is more common in adults than in children. A pronounced decline in the glomerular filtration rate is unusual in children and is more common in the elderly population. Throat or skin cultures may reveal group A streptococci; however, serologic studies are superior for evaluating the presence of recent streptococcal infection. The antibodies most commonly studied for the detection of a recent streptococcal infection are antistreptolysin-O (ASO), antistreptokinase, antihyaluronidase, antideoxyribonuclease-B, and antinicotinyladenine dinucleotidase. An elevated ASO titer greater than 200 units may be found in 90% of patients; however, a rise in titer is more specific than the absolute level of an individual titer. Serial ASO titer measurements with a twofold or greater rise are highly indicative of a recent infection. The serial estimation of complement components is important in the diagnosis of PSGN. Early in the acute phase, the levels of hemolytic complement activity (CH-50 and C3) are reduced. These levels return to normal, usually within 8 weeks, and the presence of persistently depressed C3 levels suggests an alternative diagnosis.

Treatment

Treatment of acute PSGN is largely supportive care. Children almost invariably recover from the initial episode. Indeed, even the presence of acute renal failure in adults is not necessarily associated with a poor prognosis. Thus, there is little evidence to suggest the need for any form of immunosuppressive therapy.

Supportive therapy may require the use of loop diuretics such as furosemide to ameliorate volume expansion and hypertension. In patients with substantial volume expansion and marked pulmonary congestion whose condition does not respond to diuretic therapy, dialysis support may be appropriate. Importantly, potassium-sparing agents, including triamterene, spironolactone, and amiloride, should not be used in this disease state because patients can develop substantial hyperkalemia. Usually patients undergo a spontaneous diuresis within 7 to 10 days after the onset of their illness and no longer require supportive care. There is no evidence to date that the early treatment of streptococcal disease, either pharyngitic or cellulitic, alters the risk of development of PSGN. The long-term prognosis of patients with PSGN is not as benign as was previously considered. Widespread crescentic glomerulonephritis results in an increased number of obsolescent glomeruli associated with tubulointerstitial disease and may herald a progressive loss of functional renal mass over time.

IgA Nephropathy

IgA nephropathy is one of if not the most common form of glomerulonephritis. The disease process was initially considered to be a benign form of hematuria but is now recognized as a significant cause of ESRD. It is most common in the second and third decades of life, and it is much more common in males than in females. IgA nephropathy can only be definitively diagnosed by the immunohistologic demonstration of mesangial immune deposits that stain dominantly or codominantly for IgA. The mechanisms responsible for the glomerular injury in IgA nephropathy are poorly understood but may involve the synthesis of structurally abnormal IgA molecules.

Clinical Features and Natural History
The typical presenting features of IgA nephropathy are as follows:

- Macroscopic hematuria (40% to 50%)
- Microscopic hematuria (40%)
- Nephritic syndrome (10%)
- Malignant hypertension (<5%)

Episodes of macroscopic hematuria tend to occur in close temporal relationship to upper respiratory infection, including tonsillitis or pharyngitis. This timing differs from that for PSGN, which has an interval period of 7 to 14 days between the onset of infection and overt hematuria. Macroscopic hematuria may be entirely asymptomatic, but more often is associated with dysuria that may prompt the treating physician to consider bacterial cystitis. Systemic symptoms are often found, including nonspecific symptoms such as malaise, fatigue, muscle aches and pains, and fever. Microscopic hematuria and proteinuria persist between episodes of macroscopic hematuria. Associated hypertension is common. Patients presenting with the nephrotic syndrome may have a widespread proliferative glomerulonephritis or coexistence of IgA nephropathy and minimal change glomerulopathy.

IgA nephropathy may be the glomerular expression of a systemic disease—Henoch-Schönlein purpura—and many authorities consider them part of one spectrum of disease. Although IgA nephropathy was previously thought to have a relatively benign prognosis, it is estimated that renal insufficiency may occur in 20% to 30% of patients within 2 decades of the original presentation. Renal failure typically follows a slowly progressive course, but a minority of patients with IgA manifest a fulminant course resulting in a rapid progression to end-stage renal disease. Clinical features that predict a poor prognosis include sustained hypertension, persistent proteinuria greater than 1 g, impaired renal function, and the nephrotic syndrome. In general, persistent microscopic hematuria is associated with a poor prognosis. It is important to note that acute renal failure associated with macroscopic hematuria does not affect the long-term prognosis and may reflect acute tubular injury rather than crescentic disease. Histologic features associated with progression to end-stage renal disease include interstitial fibrosis, tubular atrophy, and glomerular scarring. Whether crescents found on renal biopsy constitute a poor prognostic factor is controversial.

Laboratory Findings
Typical findings include microscopic hematuria on urinalysis and dysmorphic erythrocytes on urine microscopy. Proteinuria is found in many patients with IgA nephropathy, although most subjects have less than 1 g of protein/day. There are no specific serologic or laboratory tests to diagnose IgA nephropathy or Henoch-Schönlein purpura. Although serum IgA levels are elevated in up to 50% of patients, the presence of elevated IgA levels in the circulation is not specific for IgA nephropathy. Levels of complement such as C3 and C4 are typically normal.

Treatment
As in any form of chronic renal insufficiency, antihypertensive therapy is essential in preventing progressive glomerular injury.

ACE inhibition is specifically indicated in proteinuric patients. Recent studies suggest that corticosteroid treatment may have important beneficial effects. A prospective, randomized trial has demonstrated that in patients with urine protein excretion of 1 to 3.5 g daily, and plasma creatinine concentrations of 1.5 mg/dL (133 mcmol/L) or less, intravenous methylprednisolone for 3 consecutive days in months 1, 3, and 5 combined with oral prednisone given at a dosage of 0.5 mg/kg every other day for months 1 through 6 results protected against loss of renal function. Patients with IgA nephropathy who have concurrent minimal change glomerulopathy also benefit from corticosteroid therapy. More aggressive treatment may be appropriate in patients with rapidly progressive IgA nephropathy. Treatment options in this setting include low-dose oral prednisone and cyclophosphamide for 3 months followed by 2 years of azathioprine, which has been demonstrated to improve renal survival in patients with baseline creatinine greater than 1.5 mg/dL (133 mcmol/L). It is reasonable to treat crescentic disease in IgA nephropathy in a manner similar to that for other forms of crescentic glomerulonephritis using pulse methylprednisolone, oral prednisone, or cyclophosphamide, individually or in combination.

The advent of treatment of IgA nephropathy with fish oil is based on a study demonstrating a marked improvement in renal outcome in patients treated with 12 g of fish oil containing ω-3 fatty acids daily for 2 years. The enthusiasm for this approach has been tempered by two other, much smaller, trials that showed absolutely no benefit of fish oil, and a recent meta-analysis of the available trials suggested that there was no significant benefit of fish oil therapy in most patients. If any effect is to be observed with fish oil therapy, it is probably seen in those individuals who have heavy proteinuria.

Other Glomerular Diseases That Cause Hematuria

The clinical designation of benign familial hematuria often refers to thin basement membrane nephropathy. The prevalence of thin basement membrane nephropathy in the general population has been estimated to be approximately 5% to 10%. Males and females are equally affected and are typically found to have microscopic hematuria when they are adolescents or young adults. Macroscopic hematuria and proteinuria are uncommon. The pattern of hematuria is sometimes familial, and results from assessing the urine of family members can further complement a diagnosis. Persistent isolated hematuria is also present in hereditary nephritis associated with Alport syndrome, which is usually associated with an X-linked dominant form of inheritance and is associated with hearing loss and ocular abnormalities. The syndrome of loin pain hematuria is another condition associated with hematuria. This uncommon syndrome occurs primarily in young women. The clinical picture is reminiscent of IgA nephropathy. There are recurrent episodes of gross hematuria, usually with flank pain that is typically described as dull or aching. Patients sometimes have fever, malaise, and anorexia. Hypertension and proteinuria are uncommon. The treatment of loin pain hematuria usually begins with cessation of oral contraceptives, which have been associated with disease development, or treatment with anticoagulant drugs.

Fibrillary Glomerulonephritis and Immunotactoid Glomerulopathy

Nomenclature

Fibrillary glomerulonephritis and immunotactoid glomerulopathy are glomerular diseases that are characterized by patterned deposits seen by electron microscopy. There is controversy over how to categorize these diseases. Most renal pathologists distinguish fibrillary glomerulonephritis from immunotactoid glomerulopathy based on the presence of fibrils of approximately 20-nm diameter in the former and larger 30- to 40-nm diameter microtubular structures in the latter. The etiology and pathogenesis of fibrillary glomerulonephritis and immunotactoid glomerulopathy are not known, but both conditions have been associated with lymphoproliferative diseases.

Epidemiology and Clinical Features

Fibrillary glomerulonephritis is relatively uncommon. It is observed in less than 1% of native renal biopsies. Patients typically present with a mixture of features of both nephrotic and nephritic syndromes. Proteinuria is typically in the nephrotic range. Renal insufficiency, hematuria, and hypertension are common at the time of presentation. There appears to be a racial predilection, with a higher incidence in white patients. Immunotactoid glomerulopathy is less commonly observed, and some controversy exists as to whether it is truly a glomerular disease separate from fibrillary glomerulopathy. It appears to be more commonly associated with lymphoproliferative disease. The prognosis in patients with either of these diseases is dismal; 40% to 50% of patients develop end-stage renal disease within 6 years of presentation. Predictors of a poor outcome in both conditions include the degree of proteinuria and the severity of the associated hypertension.

Treatment

At this time, there is no convincingly effective form of treatment for patients with either fibrillary glomerulonephritis or immunotactoid glomerulopathy. Treatment efforts with either glucocorticoids or alkylating agents such as cyclophosphamide have proven unsuccessful. Nonetheless, it is possible that the treatment of the underlying malignancy, if one is detected, may improve the renal outcome. Fibrillary glomerulonephritis recurs in most renal allografts although the rate of deterioration in the allograft appears to be slower.

RAPIDLY PROGRESSIVE GLOMERULONEPHRITIS AND CRESCENTIC GLOMERULONEPHRITIS

Immune Complex–Mediated Crescentic Glomerulonephritis

Most patients with immune complex crescentic glomerulonephritis have clinical or pathologic evidence of a specific category of primary glomerulonephritis. However, a minority of patients with immune complex crescentic glomerulonephritis do not have patterns of immune complex localization that readily fit into the specific categories, and this category is sometimes called idiopathic crescentic immune complex glomerulonephritis. The light microscopic appearance of crescentic immune complex glomerulonephritis reflects the underlying category of glomerulonephritis in the most aggressive expressions (e.g., MPGN, PSGN, or IgA).

Treatment

Therapy for crescentic immune complex glomerulonephritis is influenced by the nature of the underlying category of immune complex glomerulonephritis. For example, acute PSGN with 50% crescents might not prompt the same therapy as IgA nephropathy with 50% crescents. However, there are inadequate data from controlled prospective trials to guide therapy for most forms of crescentic immune complex glomerulonephritis. Some nephrologists extrapolate from experience with lupus nephritis and choose to use immunosuppressive drugs in patients with crescentic immune complex disease, which they would not use if the glomerular lesions appeared less aggressive. For the minority of patients who have idiopathic immune complex crescentic glomerulonephritis, the most common treatment is immunosuppressive therapy with pulse methylprednisolone followed by prednisone at a dosage of 1 mg/kg/day, which is then tapered over the second to third month to an alternate-day regimen until it is completely discontinued. In patients with a rapid decline in renal function, cytotoxic agents in addition to corticosteroids may be considered. There is evidence that immune complex crescentic glomerulonephritis is less responsive to immunosuppressive therapy than is either anti-GBM or ANCA crescentic glomerulonephritis.

Anti–Glomerular Basement Membrane Glomerulonephritis

Anti-GBM disease accounts for about 10% to 20% of crescentic glomerulonephritides. This disease is characterized by circulating antibodies to the GBM and deposition of IgG or rarely IgA along the GBM. Anti-GBM disease occurs as a renal-limited disease (anti-GBM glomerulonephritis) and as a pulmonary-renal vasculitic syndrome (Goodpasture syndrome). The incidence of anti-GBM disease has two peaks with respect to age. The first peak is in the second and third decades of life and the second peak is in the sixth and seventh decade. The first peak has a male preponderance and higher frequency of pulmonary hemorrhage (Goodpasture syndrome), whereas the second peak has a predominance of women who more often have renal-limited disease. Genetic susceptibility to anti-GBM disease is associated with HLA-DR2 specificity.

Clinical Features and Natural History

The onset of renal anti-GBM disease is typically characterized by an abrupt, acute glomerulonephritis with severe oliguria or anuria. There is a high risk of progression to end-stage renal disease if appropriate therapy is not instituted promptly. Prompt treatment with plasmapheresis, corticosteroids, and cyclophosphamide results in patient survival of approximately 85% and renal survival of approximately 60%. The onset of disease may be associated with arthralgias, fever, and myalgias; however, gastrointestinal complaints or neurologic disturbances are rare. Goodpasture syndrome is characterized by the presence of pulmonary hemorrhage concurrent with glomerulonephritis. The pulmonary manifestation is usually severe, and pulmonary hemorrhage may be life-threatening. The occurrence of pulmonary hemorrhage is far more common in smokers than in nonsmokers and may also be associated with environmental exposure to hydrocarbons or exposure to other agents, such as cocaine or upper respiratory tract infections.

Laboratory Findings

Renal involvement in anti-GBM disease typically causes an acute nephritic syndrome with hematuria, including dysmorphic erythrocyturia and red blood cell casts. The diagnostic laboratory finding in anti-GBM disease is detection of circulating antibodies to GBM, specifically to the α-3 chain of type IV collagen. These antibodies are detected by radioimmunoassay or enzyme immunoassay in approximately 90% of patients. Up to 30% of patients also have circulating ANCAs.

Treatment

The standard treatment for anti-GBM disease includes intensive plasmapheresis combined with corticosteroids and cyclophosphamide or azathioprine. Plasmapheresis consists of removal of 2 to 4 L of plasma and replacement with a 5% albumin solution continued on a daily basis until circulating antibody levels become undetectable. In patients with pulmonary hemorrhage, clotting factors should be replaced by administration of fresh-frozen plasma at the end of each treatment. Prednisone should be administered at a dose of 1 mg/kg body weight for at least the first month and then tapered to alternate-day therapy during the second and third months of treatment. Cyclophosphamide is administered either orally (at a dosage of 2 mg/kg/day) or intravenously at a starting dose of 0.5 g/m^2 body surface area. The dose of cyclophosphamide must be adjusted with consideration for the degree of impairment of renal function and the white blood cell count. Cytotoxic therapy is usually continued for about 6 to 12 months. Aggressive plasmapheresis, even in patients with severe renal insufficiency, may have an ameliorative effect and provide improved long-term patient and renal survival. The major prognostic marker for the progression to end-stage renal disease is the serum creatinine level at the time of initiation of treatment. Patients with a serum creatinine level greater than 7 mg/dL (620 mcmol/L) are unlikely to recover sufficient renal function to discontinue renal replacement therapy. Aggressive immunosuppression should probably be withheld in patients with disease limited to the kidney who present with widespread glomerular and interstitial scarring on renal biopsy and a serum creatinine level greater than 7 mg/dL (620 mcmol/L). Once remission of anti-GBM disease is achieved with immunosuppressive therapy, recurrent disease is rare. Similarly, the recurrence of anti-GBM disease after renal transplantation is also rare. However, transplantation should be delayed until after the disappearance or substantial diminution of anti-GBM antibody in the circulation.

Pauci-Immune Crescentic Glomerulonephritis

The characteristic feature of pauci-immune crescentic glomerulonephritis is a focal necrotizing and crescentic glomerulonephritis in association with circulating ANCAs. Pauci-immune crescentic glomerulonephritis usually is a component of a systemic small vessel vasculitis, but some patients have renal-limited (primary) pauci-immune crescentic glomerulonephritis. The presence of arteritis in a biopsy specimen from a patient with pauci-immune crescentic glomerulonephritis indicates that the glomerulonephritis is a component of a more widespread vasculitis, such as microscopic polyangiitis, Wegener granulomatosis, or the Churg-Strauss syndrome. The pathogenesis of pauci-immune crescentic glomerulonephritis is currently not fully understood. Although many patients have circulating ANCAs, it has not been conclusively proven that ANCAs are involved in the pathogenesis of pauci-immune small vessel vasculitis or glomerulonephritis.

Clinical Features and Natural History

Most patients with pauci-immune necrotizing crescentic glomerulonephritis and ANCAs have glomerular disease as part of a systemic small vessel vasculitis. However, the disease is clinically limited to the kidney in about one third of patients. When it is part of a systemic vasculitis, patients may present with a pulmonary-renal, dermal-renal, or multisystem disease. Common sites of involvement include the lungs, upper airways, sinuses, ears, eyes, gastrointestinal tract, skin, peripheral nerves, joints, and central nervous system. The three major ANCA-associated syndromes are microscopic polyangiitis, Wegener granulomatosis, and Churg-Strauss syndrome. Even when patients have no clinical evidence or extrarenal manifestation of active vasculitis, systemic symptoms consisting of fever, fatigue, myalgias, and arthralgias are common.

In some patients the disease follows an indolent course of slow decline in function and less active urine sediment in which episodes of focal necrosis and hematuria resolve with focal glomerular scarring. Subsequent relapses result in cumulative damage to glomeruli.

The presence of pulmonary hemorrhage is the most important determinant of patient survival in patients with ANCA small vessel vasculitis. With regard to the risk of end-stage renal disease, the most important predictor of outcome is the entry serum creatinine level at the time of initiation of treatment. The presence of advanced interstitial fibrosis is an independent risk factor for outcome only in patients with entry serum creatinine levels of less than 3 mg/dL (265 mcmol/L).

Laboratory Findings

Approximately 80% to 90% of patients with pauci-immune necrotizing and crescentic glomerulonephritis will have circulating ANCA. With indirect fluorescence microscopy on alcohol-fixed neutrophils, ANCAs show two patterns of staining: perinuclear (P-ANCA) and cytoplasmic (C-ANCA). The two major antigen specificities for ANCA are myeloperoxidase (MPO) and proteinase 3 (PR3). With rare exceptions, anti-MPO antibodies produce a P-ANCA pattern of staining on indirect immunofluorescence microscopy, whereas anti-PR3 antibodies cause a C-ANCA pattern of staining. About two thirds of patients with pauci-immune necrotizing crescentic glomerulonephritis without clinical evidence of systemic vasculitis will have MPO-ANCA or P-ANCA, and approximately 30% will have PR3-ANCA or C-ANCA. The frequency of MPO-ANCA relative to PR3-ANCA is higher in patients with renal-limited disease than in patients with microscopic polyangiitis or Wegener granulomatosis. Maximal sensitivity and specificity with ANCA testing is best performed when both immunofluorescence and antigen-specific assays are performed. Antigen-specific assays may be either enzyme-linked immunosorbent assays or radioimmune assays. The positive predictive value of a positive ANCA result depends on the signs and symptoms of disease in the patient who is tested. The positive predictive value of a positive ANCA result in a patient with classic features of RPGN is 95%. Although the positive predictive value is not good in patients with hematuria and normal renal function, the negative predictive value is greater than 95%.

Urinalysis findings in pauci-immune crescentic glomerulonephritis include hematuria with dysmorphic red blood cells, with or without red blood cell casts, and proteinuria. The degree of proteinuria ranges widely. The serum creatinine level usually is elevated at the time of diagnosis and is rising, although a minority of patients will have relatively indolent disease. Serum complement component levels are typically within normal limits.

Treatment

The treatment of pauci-immune crescentic glomerulonephritis involves varying regimens of corticosteroids and cyclophosphamide. In view of the potentially explosive and fulminant nature of this disease, induction therapy should be instituted using pulse methylprednisolone at a dosage of 7 mg/kg/day for 3 consecutive days followed by daily oral prednisone, as well as cyclophosphamide, either orally or intravenously. Prednisone is usually started at a dosage of 1 mg/kg/day for the first month, then tapered to an alternate-day regimen, and then discontinued by the end of third to fourth month of treatment. When a regimen of monthly intravenous doses of cyclophosphamide is used, the starting dose should be about 0.5 g/m^2 and adjusted upward to 1 g/m^2 based on the 2-week leukocyte count nadir. A regimen based on daily oral cyclophosphamide should begin at a dosage of 2 mg/kg/day and adjusted downward as needed to keep a nadir leukocyte count greater than 3000 m^3. The usual length of therapy with cyclophosphamide is 6 to 12 months. For patients in whom remission is not achieved by that time, continuing treatment for a longer duration is a reasonable approach. In some patients, the monthly intravenous regimen is not sufficiently immunosuppressive, necessitating daily oral cyclophosphamide treatment (which results in a higher cumulative dosage). An alternative proposed regimen is based on the use of cyclophosphamide for the first 3 months of treatment followed by azathioprine 2 mg/kg/day for an additional 6 to 12 months. Plasmapheresis does not provide any added benefit over immunosuppressive treatment alone in patients with renal-limited disease or in patients with mild to moderate renal dysfunction. However, the use of plasmapheresis in addition to immunosuppressive therapy may be beneficial in the subset of patients who require dialysis at the time of presentation. Trimethoprim-sulfamethoxazole has been suggested to be of benefit in the treatment of patients with Wegener granulomatosis. The beneficial effect, if any, seems to be limited to the upper respiratory tract, and this antibiotic combination is unlikely to have a role in the treatment of pauci-immune crescentic glomerulonephritis alone.

The chance of recovery of renal function in patients presenting with advanced renal failure requiring renal replacement therapy is diminished compared with that of patients who do not require dialysis at presentation (50% versus 70%). It appears that in this patient group the adjunctive use of plasmapheresis in addition to an immunosuppressive regimen is of benefit in improving the renal outcome. Continuing immunosuppressive therapy beyond 12 weeks in a patient who is still receiving dialysis is unlikely to be of added benefit. Because of the clinically observed increased risk of severe bone marrow suppression with the use of cyclophosphamide in patients receiving dialysis, such treatment should be pursued with extreme caution. The rate of recurrence for ANCA small vessel vasculitis in general, including pauci-immune necrotizing glomerulonephritis alone, is about 20%. A positive ANCA test result at the time of transplantation does not seem to be associated with an increased risk of recurrent disease.

Whether a renal biopsy is essential to the management of ANCA-associated pauci-immune glomerulonephritis depends on a number of factors, including the diagnostic accuracy of ANCA testing, the pretest probability of finding pauci-immune glomerulonephritis, the value of knowing the activity and chronicity of the renal lesions, and the risk associated with immunotherapy of ANCA pauci-immune necrotizing glomerulonephritis. Based on a study of 1000 patients with proliferative or necrotizing glomerulonephritis or both and a positive test for either PR3-ANCA or MPO-ANCA, the positive predictive value of ANCA testing was found to be 86% with a false-positive rate of 14% and a false-negative rate of 16%. Considering the serious risks inherent to treatment with high-dose corticosteroids and cytotoxic agents, it is prudent to confirm the diagnosis and characterize the activity and chronicity of ANCA-associated pauci-immune crescentic glomerulonephritis by renal biopsy unless the patient is too ill to tolerate the procedure.

Secondary Glomerular Disease | *11*

LUPUS NEPHRITIS

Lupus nephritis (LN) is a frequent and potentially serious complication of systemic lupus erythematosus (SLE). Renal involvement worsens morbidity and mortality rates in lupus, and patient outcomes are also adversely affected through complications of therapy. Approximately 25% to 50% of unselected patients with lupus have clinical renal disease at disease onset, and up to 60% of adults with SLE develop renal disease during their lifetime. Renal involvement in SLE is defined for diagnostic purposes as persistent proteinuria exceeding 500 mg daily or the presence of cellular casts. The deposition of circulating immune complexes plays a major role in the development of LN. Glomerular and vascular damage may also be potentiated by hypertension and a thrombotic microangiopathy triggered by the presence of antiphospholipid (APL) antibodies.

Pathology of Lupus Nephritis

The renal biopsy in LN may show a number of different histopathologic patterns. In addition, overlapping patterns may occur, and histologic progression from one lesion to another may occur spontaneously or with therapy. The World Health Organization (WHO) has developed a uniform classification system that is both accurate and precise. In the most recent 2003 WHO classification, biopsy results of patients with lupus are classified into one of six categories according to glomerular changes by light microscopy, immunofluorescence, and electron microscopy (Table 11–1). The WHO classification system is useful as a prognostic and therapeutic guide, with grade IV disease having the worst outcome. Biopsy specimens are also graded for features of activity (potentially reversible lesions) and chronicity (irreversible lesions).

Table 11–1: World Health Organization Classification of Lupus Nephritis

Class Description
I. Normal glomeruli (by LM, IF, EM)
II. Mesangial glomerulonephritis
    Normocellular mesangium by LM but mesangial deposits by IF or EM
    Mesangial hypercellularity with mesangial deposits by IF or EM
III. Focal segmental proliferative glomerulonephritis
IV. Diffuse proliferative glomerulonephritis
V. Membranous glomerulonephritis

EM, electron microscopy; IF, immunofluorescence; LM, light microscopy.

Clinical Manifestations

The clinical manifestations of kidney involvement in SLE are varied. Renal involvement often develops concurrently or shortly after the onset of SLE and may follow a protracted course with periods of remissions and exacerbations. Patients with WHO class I disease often have no or at most mild evidence of clinical renal disease. Likewise, most patients with disease confined to the mesangial regions of the glomeruli (WHO class II) have minimal clinical renal findings, including an inactive urinary sediment, proteinuria of less than 1 g daily, and a normal serum creatinine level. WHO class III, focal proliferative LN, is often associated with active lupus serology, although the degree of serologic activity does not correlate with the severity or extent of the histologic damage. Hypertension and an active urinary sediment are commonly present and proteinuria is usually greater than 1 g daily. Up to 25% of these patients will have an elevated serum creatinine level at presentation. Patients with class IV disease typically have high anti-DNA antibody titers, renal dysfunction, hypertension, low serum complement levels, and a very active urinary sediment, with erythrocytes and red blood cell casts on urinalysis. Virtually all patients have proteinuria, and up to 50% present with the nephrotic syndrome. Patients with lupus membranous nephropathy, WHO class V, typically present with proteinuria, edema, and other manifestations of the nephrotic syndrome. Although serologic activity is often mild, up to 60% of patients with membranous neuropathy have a low serum complement level and an elevated anti-DNA antibody titer. End-stage LN, WHO class VI, is usually the result of "burned out" LN of long duration. It is often the end result of years of lupus flares alternating with periods of inactivity.

Serologic Tests

Abnormal autoantibody production is the hallmark of SLE. The presence of antibodies directed against nuclear antigens (ANAs) and especially against DNA (anti-DNA) are included in the American Rheumatism Association's diagnostic criteria for SLE and are commonly used to monitor the course of patients with SLE. However, the ANA titer does not correlate well with the severity of renal involvement in SLE. Autoantibodies directed against double-stranded DNA (anti-dsDNA) are a more specific but less sensitive marker of SLE. A variety of other autoantibodies are commonly present in patients with lupus, including anti-Sm, anti-nuclear riboprotein, anti-Ro/serum amyloid A (SSA), and anti-La/serum amyloid B (SSB), but these do not predict renal involvement. Levels of total hemolytic complement (CH50) and complement components are usually decreased during active renal disease, and this decrease may precede a clinical flare. Other immunologic abnormalities commonly detected in patients with lupus include elevated levels of circulating immune complexes, a positive lupus band test, and the presence of cryoglobulins. Mixed immunoglobulin (Ig) G-IgM cryoglobulins may be found in patients with SLE and active renal disease. A false-positive result for a Venereal Disease Research Laboratory (VDRL) test due to the presence of APL antibodies is also common.

Monitoring Clinical Disease

LN is typically a chronic disease with relapses and remissions. It is important in the management of patients with lupus to be able to predict clinical and renal relapses and prevent their occurrence through the judicious use of immunosuppressive agents. Serial measurement of serologic tests of clinical activity has been used to predict flares of lupus activity. Circulating serum levels of anti-dsDNA typically rise as the clinical activity of SLE increases and usually before there is a clinical renal deterioration. Likewise, serum total hemolytic complement levels typically decline preceding or concurrent with the onset of active clinical disease. An increase in proteinuria from levels of less than 1 g daily to greater than this amount and certainly from low levels to nephrotic levels is a clear indication of either increased activity or a change in renal histologic class.

Drug-Induced Lupus

A variety of medications may induce a lupus-like syndrome or exacerbate an underlying predisposition to development of SLE.

Although a number of drugs have produced this entity, those metabolized by acetylation such as procainamide and hydralazine are common causes. Drug-induced lupus occurs more commonly in patients with a genetic decrease in hepatic N-acyltransferase activity, called *slow actylators*. Clinical manifestations of drug-induced lupus include fever, rash, myalgias, arthralgias and arthritis, and serositis. Renal involvement is relatively uncommon in drug-induced disease.

Pregnancy and Systemic Lupus Erythematosus

Pregnancy in patients with LN has also been associated with worsening of renal function. Risk factors for loss of renal function include active disease within the previous 6 months and coexistent hypertension, proteinuria, and renal impairment at baseline. Patients with elevated serum creatinine levels are most likely to have worsening of renal function and also have the highest risk for fetal loss (which may exceed 50%). Both high-dose corticosteroids and azathioprine have been used in pregnant patients with lupus, but mycophenolate and cyclophosphamide are contraindicated. Other risk factors for fetal loss include the presence of anticardiolipin antibodies, hypertension, or heavy proteinuria.

Dialysis and Transplantation

The percentage of patients with LN who develop end-stage renal disease (ESRD) ranges from 10% to 30%. Most patients who develop ESRD have resolution of their extrarenal manifestations of disease and serologic activity. In general, most renal transplant programs allow patients with active SLE to undergo a period of dialysis for 3 to 12 months to allow clinical and serologic disease activity to become quiescent. Allograft survival rates in patients with ESRD due to LN are comparable to those for the rest of the ESRD population. The rate of recurrent SLE in the allograft is less than 5%.

Course and Prognosis of Lupus Nephritis

The prognosis is defined in part by the initial pattern and severity of renal involvement. However, ultimately the outcome is modified by therapy, exacerbations of the disease, and complications of treatment. Patients with lesions limited to the renal mesangium generally have an excellent course and prognosis. Patients with mild WHO class III disease typically respond well to therapy, and fewer than 5% develop renal failure during 5-year follow-up. Patients with diffuse proliferative disease have the least favorable prognosis. Nevertheless, the prognosis for this group has markedly improved in recent years and the 5-year renal survival is higher than 90% in some series of patients treated with modern immunosuppressive therapy. Clinical risk factors for a poor outcome in diffuse proliferative disease include age older than 30, male sex and African-American race, nephrotic-range proteinuria, disease relapse, and elevated creatinine levels. Patients with combined severe activity and chronicity (Activity Index >7 plus Chronicity Index >3) as well as those with the combination of cellular crescents and interstitial fibrosis appear to have a worse prognosis.

Treatment of Lupus Nephritis

Class I and II Lupus Nephritis
WHO class I and II LN do not merit renal-specific therapy, and patients should be treated only for extrarenal manifestations of SLE.

Class III Lupus Nephritis
There is no general consensus on the treatment of patients with focal proliferative LN. Patients who have moderate proliferative lesions involving only a few glomeruli, with no necrotizing features and no crescent formation, have a good prognosis, and LN often resolves with a short course of high-dose corticosteroid therapy. Patients, in whom larger amounts of the glomerular surface area are involved, with necrotizing features and crescent formation, require more vigorous therapy similar to that for patients with WHO class IV lesions.

Class IV Lupus Nephritis
The most appropriate form of treatment regimen for patients with diffuse proliferative LN is still widely debated. Currently, widely used agents include high-dose daily or alternate-day corticosteroids, azathioprine, intravenous pulse methylprednisolone, oral or intravenous cyclophosphamide, cyclosporine, and mycophenolate mofetil (MMF). All of the current regimens of immunosuppressive therapy have the potential for major side effects, and no agent is universally effective.

Higher doses of corticosteroids during the early treatment period appear to be more effective compared with low-dose therapy (<30 mg prednisone daily) and are the standard of care. A typical steroid regimen is 1 mg/kg/day of prednisone, which is converted to 2 mg/kg/day on alternate days after 4 to 6 weeks of treatment and slowly tapered thereafter. If a second immunosuppressive agent is added, it is usually cyclophosphamide, azathioprine, or MMF.

CYCLOPHOSPHAMIDE   A series of controlled trials have established intravenous cyclophosphamide as an effective agent in the prevention of renal failure in patients with severe class III and class IV LN. A typical regimen is 6 monthly intravenous boluses beginning with 0.75 g/m^2 of body surface area and increasing to a maximum of 1 g/m^2 given in a saline solution over 30 to 60 minutes, assuming that the white blood cell count remains greater than 3000/mm^3. This may then be followed by 3 monthly pulses for up to 24 months. The dose of intravenous cyclophosphamide must be reduced in patients with significant renal impairment. Complications include hemorrhagic cystitis, alopecia, menstrual abnormalities, and premature menopause, which is most common in women older than 25 years of age who have received intravenous cyclophosphamide treatment for more than 6 months.

PULSE METHYLPREDNISOLONE   Pulse methylprednisolone may be considered in patients with severe active disease who develop acute renal failure. A typical regimen is three consecutive daily doses of 1-g pulses. In recent trials at the National Institutes of Health, pulse corticosteroids have been found to be less effective than intravenous cyclophosphamide for preventing progressive renal failure. Combination therapy with intravenous cyclophosphamide may offer improved remission rates, albeit at the cost of a higher incidence of short-term side effects.

MYCOPHENOLATE MOFETIL   Emerging evidence suggests that MMF may offer efficacy equivalent to that of cyclophosphamide with a lower incidence of side effects, particularly infectious complications. Although the results of recent trials are very promising in terms of a therapy with fewer side effects (especially with no bladder problems, amenorrhea, alopecia, and so forth), it has been appropriately stressed that these results are only of short duration compared with results for many of the cyclophosphamide studies.

AZATHIOPRINE   Prospective trial data in patients with proliferative LN who received induction therapy with intravenous cyclophosphamide for 6 months suggested that oral azathioprine is as efficacious as 3 monthly intravenous boluses of cyclophosphamide as a maintenance therapy.

Class V Lupus Nephritis

For patients with membranous lupus nephropathy, conflicting data about the course, prognosis, and response to treatment have been reported. The degree, if any, of a superimposed proliferative lesion can greatly influence the course of the disease in an individual patient. Some patients with pure membranous lupus nephropathy have a prolonged course of asymptomatic proteinuria or the nephrotic syndrome yet little progression to renal failure over time. Others with active serologic activity, severe nephrotic syndrome, and a progressive course may benefit from intervention. In the past this has often been achieved with short-term high-dose daily or alternate-day corticosteroids. However, evidence of associated class III or IV disease may mandate the concomitant administration of a second agent such as cyclophosphamide or MMF.

ANTIPHOSPHOLIPID ANTIBODY SYNDROME

The presence of APL antibodies may be associated with glomerular disease, large-vessel renal involvement, and coagulation problems in dialysis and renal transplant patients. A variety of APL antibodies including anticardiolipin antibodies, antibodies causing a false-positive VDRL test result, the lupus anticoagulant, and antibodies directed against plasma proteins that may be bound to phospholipids (antibodies to β_2-glycoprotein-1) have been identified in patients with renal disorders. Of patients with APL antibodies, 30% to 50% have the primary APL syndrome in which there is no associated autoimmune disease. APL antibodies have also been found in 25% to 45% of patients with SLE, although most of these patients never manifest the clinical features of the APL syndrome. APL antibodies are also found with a variety of infections (e.g., hepatitis C and human immunodeficiency virus [HIV]) and drug reactions, but these are not usually associated with the clinical spectrum of the APL syndrome.

The clinical features of the APL syndrome relate to thrombotic events and consequent ischemia. Systemic features include superficial and deep venous thromboses, arterial thromboses, fetal miscarriages (due to placental thrombosis), pulmonary hypertension, cerebral infarcts with transient ischemic attacks, strokes, memory impairment, and other neurologic manifestations. Renal involvement occurs in as many as 25% of patients with primary APL syndrome. The most common clinical renal features are proteinuria, at times in the nephrotic range, an active urinary sediment, hypertension, and progressive renal dysfunction. With major renal arterial involvement, evidence of renal infarction may be present, and renal vein thrombosis may be silent or present with sudden flank pain and a decrease in renal function. Renal pathologic characteristics include thrombosis of blood vessels ranging from the glomerular capillaries to the main renal artery and vein.

Treatment

The optimal treatment of patients with APL antibodies or APL syndrome or both is unclear. Some practitioners treat patients without evidence of the APL syndrome and no thrombotic events with only daily aspirin therapy. For patients with the full APL syndrome, either primary or secondary to SLE, high-dose anticoagulation therapy (international normalized ratio > 3) has proven to be more effective than no therapy, aspirin alone, or low-dose anticoagulation therapy for preventing recurrent thromboses. The role of immunosuppressive agents has yet to be defined. Rarely, in patients who cannot tolerate anticoagulation therapy because of recent bleeding episodes, who have thromboembolic events despite adequate anticoagulation therapy, or who are pregnant, plasmapheresis with corticosteroids and other immunosuppressives have been used with some success.

MIXED CONNECTIVE TISSUE DISEASE

Many features of mixed connective tissue disease overlap with those of SLE, scleroderma, and polymyositis. Patients typically have a distinct serologic profile characterized by a very high ANA titer, often with a speckled pattern, and antibodies directed against a specific ribonuclease-sensitive extractable nuclear antigen, U1RNP. The incidence of renal disease has been reported to vary from 10% to 26% in adults and from 33% to 50% in children with mixed connective tissue disease. Most patients with renal involvement have mild or minimal clinical manifestations with only microhematuria and proteinuria of less than 500 mg daily. However, heavy proteinuria and the nephrotic syndrome occur in up to one third of patients. Other patients have severe hypertension and acute renal failure resembling "scleroderma renal crisis" (see later). In general, glomerular lesions resemble the spectrum found in SLE, whereas vascular lesions, when present, resemble those found in scleroderma. Corticosteroid therapy in mixed connective tissue disease is effective for treating the inflammatory features of joint disease and serositis. Glomerular involvement can vary as in SLE, and treatment is generally directed to the glomerular lesion in a fashion similar to that for treating active LN.

POLYARTERITIS NODOSA

Polyarteritis nodosa (PAN) is seen in two patterns:

- *Classic* PAN is a systemic necrotizing vasculitis primarily affecting muscular arteries, often at branch points, producing lesions of varying ages with focal aneurysm formation.
- *Microscopic* polyangiitis is a necrotizing vasculitis affecting small arteries, veins, and capillaries, involving multiple viscera, including the lung and dermis, and producing lesions of similar age, usually without aneurysms.

In many patients features of both patterns overlap. Moreover, both presentations of polyarteritis may be associated with circulating antineutrophil cytoplasmic antibodies (ANCAs) and histologic evidence of a pauci-immune segmental necrotizing and crescentic glomerulonephritis similar to those seen in patients with isolated pauci-immune idiopathic rapidly progressive glomerulonephritis. Polyarteritis is more common in males than in females and occurs most often in the fifth and sixth decades of life. Although a number of diseases have been associated with glomerular disease and a systemic and/or renal vasculitis, true idiopathic polyarteritis is a primary vasculitis. A *secondary* vasculitis that is associated with hepatitis B or C infection, cryoglobulinemia, SLE, and Schönlein-Henoch purpura is usually readily distinguished.

Pathogenesis

The vasculitis of polyarteritis may be mediated by a number of diverse pathogenetic factors including humoral vascular immune deposits, cellular immunity, endothelial cytopathic factors, and antineutrophilic cytoplasmic antibodies. ANCAs may play a pathogenetic role in a manner similar to that seen in Wegener granulomatosis.

Renal Features

In the microscopic form of the disease, features of vasculitis and glomerulonephritis are seen, whereas in the classic pattern features of renal ischemia and infarction predominate because of larger vessel disease. Hypertension is common in polyarteritis (50%), and most patients have laboratory evidence of their renal involvement at presentation. Most patients have urinary sediment changes with microscopic hematuria and often red blood cell casts. Proteinuria is found in most patients, but the nephrotic syndrome is rarely present. In microscopic polyarteritis the severity of the clinical renal findings correlates with the degree of glomerular involvement. Patients with normal creatinine clearance are likely to have normal glomeruli on biopsy or only ischemic glomerular changes. Presenting symptoms related to kidney disease are uncommon in classic polyarteritis with the exception of hypertension but may include hemorrhage from a renal artery aneurysm, flank pain, and gross hematuria. Angiographic examination reveals multiple rounded, saccular aneurysms of medium-sized vessels in about 70% of patients with classic PAN.

Laboratory Tests

The erythrocyte sedimentation rate (ESR) is elevated in almost all patients and is usually associated with anemia, leukocytosis, eosinophilia, and thrombocytosis. Most patients are ANA negative and have normal serum complement levels. Results of tests for circulating immune complexes and rheumatoid factor are often positive. Cryoglobulins may reflect associated hepatitis B infection (<10% of patients). Patients with classic PAN are ANCA negative and a positive test result suggests either microscopic polyarteritis or Wegener granulomatosis.

Prognosis and Treatment

Left untreated, the overall prognosis for patients with polyarteritis is dismal, with 5-year survival rates of less than 15%. Indicators for poor prognosis include older age, delayed diagnosis, gastrointestinal tract involvement, and severe renal involvement. Aggressive early therapy to stop the disease process is believed to be crucial in preventing residual organ damage. Initial therapy of polyarteritis usually consists of high-dose cyclophosphamide (e.g., 1 to 2 mg/kg/day), adjusted to avoid leukopenia, commonly given along with high-dose corticosteroid therapy (e.g., 60 mg of prednisone daily). The steroid dose is then tapered over time. Monthly intravenous boluses of cyclophosphamide (0.5 to 1 g/m^2) appear to have efficacy equivalent to oral regimens and a better side effect profile. Plasmapheresis may benefit a subset of patients with severe glomerulonephritis requiring dialysis. For patients with ESRD, immunosuppressive therapy should be continued for 6 months to 1 year after the disease appears to be inactive to manage extrarenal complications. The risk of recurrence after transplantation ranges from 15% to 20%.

CHURG-STRAUSS SYNDROME (ALLERGIC GRANULOMATOSIS)

Churg-Strauss syndrome, or allergic granulomatosis, is a rare systemic disease characterized by vasculitis, asthma, organ infiltration by eosinophils, and peripheral eosinophilia. There is no gender predominance, and the mean age of diagnosis is 50 years.

Pathology

The spectrum of glomerular involvement in Churg-Straus syndrome is wide. It extends from normal renal tissue through focal segmental necrotizing glomerulonephritis into diffuse and global glomerulonephritis with severe necrotizing features and crescents. Vasculitis of the renal vessels may be noted also.

Pathogenesis

Although the pathogenesis of Churg-Strauss syndrome is unclear, an allergic or hypersensitive mechanism is suggested by the presence of asthma, hypereosinophilia, and elevated plasma levels of IgE. It is likely that ANCAs may play a role akin to that in Wegener granulomatosis and microscopic polyarteritis.

Clinical and Laboratory Features

Patients may have initial constitutional symptoms such as weight loss, fatigue, malaise, and fever. Characteristic extrarenal features include asthma (present in >95% of patients), an allergic diathesis, allergic rhinitis, and peripheral eosinophilia. Asthmatic disease typically precedes the onset of the vasculitis by years, but it may occur simultaneously, and the severity of the asthma does not necessarily parallel the severity of the vasculitis. A chest radiograph may show patchy infiltrates, nodules, diffuse interstitial disease, and even pleural effusion. This multisystem disease can affect the heart with pericarditis, heart failure, and/or ischemic disease; the gastrointestinal tract with abdominal pain, ulceration, diarrhea, or bowel; and the skin with subcutaneous nodules, petechiae, and purpuric lesions. Mononeuritis multiplex is common, but migrating polyarthralgias and arthritis occur less often. Laboratory evaluation typically reveals anemia, leukocytosis, and an elevated ESR. Eosinophilia is universally present and may reach 50% of the total peripheral count. The degree of eosinophilia and the ESR may correlate with disease activity. Rheumatoid factor is often positive and C-reactive protein levels are increased, whereas serum complement, hepatitis markers, circulating immune complexes, ANAs, and cryoglobulins are usually negative. ANCA levels have been elevated in a large percentage of patients with Churg-Strauss syndrome. Usually patients are perinuclear ANCA positive, but some are positive for cytoplasmic ANCA. The clinical renal findings in Churg-Strauss syndrome are also quite diverse; however, renal involvement rarely predominates. Microscopic hematuria and mild proteinuria are common, but nephrotic-range proteinuria is rare. In pure Churg-Strauss syndrome, renal failure is uncommon although it occurs in patients with overlap syndromes.

Prognosis, Course, and Treatment

Patients may have several phases of the syndrome over many months or years. There may be a prodromal phase of asthma or allergic rhinitis followed by a phase of peripheral blood and tissue eosinophilia remitting and relapsing over months to years before development of systemic vasculitis. A shorter duration of asthma before the onset of vasculitis has been associated with a worse prognosis. Survival rates in treated patients are approximately 90% at 1 year and 70% at 5 years. Patients with significant cardiac and/or gastrointestinal involvement have a worse prognosis. Corticosteroid therapy is successful in most patents with Churg-Strauss syndrome. The disease responds rapidly to high daily oral prednisone therapy and even relapses respond to retreatment. Patients with resistant disease may benefit from concomitant treatment with other immunosuppressive agents, such as azathioprine and cyclophosphamide.

GLOMERULAR INVOLVEMENT IN OTHER VASCULITIDES (TEMPORAL ARTERITIS, TAKAYASU DISEASE, AND LYMPHOMATOID ARTERITIS)

Temporal Arteritis

Temporal arteritis, or giant cell arteritis, is a systemic vasculitis with a characteristic giant cell vasculitis of medium-sized and large arteries. The disease is the most common form of arteritis in Western countries. It is primarily a disease of the elderly, with an average age of onset of symptoms of 72 years. Extracranial vascular involvement occurs in 10% to 15% of patients. Renal manifestations are rare and generally mild, consisting of mild hematuria and proteinuria, without renal functional impairment.

Abnormal urinary sediment changes disappear with standard corticosteroid therapy.

Takayasu Arteritis

Takayasu arteritis is a rare vasculitic disease of unknown pathogenesis characterized by inflammation and stenosis of medium-sized and large arteries, with a predilection for the aortic arch and its branches. The disease most commonly affects young women between 10 and 40 years of age, and Asians are much more commonly affected. Renal involvement is characterized by an obliterative arteritis of the main renal artery or narrowing of the renal ostia by abdominal aortitis, leading to renovascular hypertension. Arteriography is usually used to make the diagnosis of Takayasu arteritis, although computed tomography and magnetic resonance imaging have been used as well. Laboratory abnormalities reveal mild anemia, elevated ESR, increased levels of C-reactive protein, and elevated gamma globulin levels, but results of other serologic tests are normal. Hypertension may be severe and occurs in 40% to 60% of patients; however, renal failure is uncommon.

Treatment
In most patients, corticosteroids are effective therapy for the vasculitis and systemic symptoms, and further vascular deterioration is suppressed. Other immunosuppressive agents including methotrexate, cyclophosphamide, and mycophenolate have also been used successfully.

HENOCH-SCHÖNLEIN PURPURA

Henoch-Schönlein purpura (HSP) is a systemic vasculitis syndrome with involvement of the skin and gastrointestinal tract and joints in association with a glomerulonephritis characterized by prominent IgA deposition. IgA immune complexes deposit in the skin, kidney, and other organs in association with an inflammatory reaction of the vessels. Children are far more commonly affected than adults, although the disease can occur at any age. More severe renal disease occurs in older children and adults.

Clinical Findings

The classic tetrad in HSP includes dermal involvement, gastrointestinal disease, joint involvement, and glomerulonephritis.

Constitutional symptoms such as fever, malaise, and fatigue and weakness may be associated with active isolated dermal involvement or full-blown systemic disease. Skin lesions commonly found on the lower and upper extremities may also be seen on the buttocks or elsewhere. They are characterized by urticarial macular and papular reddish-violaceous lesions and may be discrete or may coalesce into palpable purpuric lesions. On skin biopsy there is a leukocytoclastic angiitis with evidence of IgA-containing immune complexes along with IgG, C3, and properdin but not C4 or C1q. Gastrointestinal manifestations are present in 25% to 90% of patients and may include colicky pain, nausea and vomiting, melena, hematochezia, and intussusception. Rheumatologic involvement is most common in the ankles and knees and less common in the elbows and wrists and may consist of arthralgias or frank arthritis with painful, tender effusions. Renal involvement ranges from 40% to 60% of patients and is characterized by a proliferative nephritis with prominent IgA deposition. The onset of the renal disease usually follows the onset of the systemic manifestations by days to weeks. Patients commonly have microscopic hematuria, an active urinary sediment, and proteinuria. Up to one half of patients with clinical renal involvement develop the nephrotic syndrome, and some have a nephritic picture.

Course, Prognosis, and Treatment

In most patients HSP is a self-limited disease with a good long-term outcome. In general, there is a good correlation between the clinical renal presentation and the ultimate prognosis. Patients with focal mesangial involvement and only hematuria and mild proteinuria tend to have an excellent prognosis. A poor renal prognosis is predicted by an acute nephritic presentation, persistent nephrotic syndrome, older age, IgA deposits extending from the mesangium out along the peripheral capillary walls, and especially the presence of a greater percentage of crescents on renal biopsy. There is no proven therapy for HSP. Although steroids have been associated with decreased abdominal and rheumatologic symptoms, they have not been proven to ameliorate the renal lesions in any controlled fashion. Patients with severe clinical features and especially those with more crescents on biopsy may benefit from more aggressive intervention with pulse methylprednisolone followed by oral corticosteroid therapy. Other regimens used in this setting have included varying combinations of corticosteroids, azathioprine, cyclophosphamide, chlorambucil, plasmapheresis, and intravenous immune gamma globulin.

SJÖGREN SYNDROME

Sjögren syndrome is characterized by a chronic inflammatory cell infiltration of the exocrine salivary and lacrimal glands and is associated with the "sicca complex" of xerostomia and xerophthalmia. Although this disease may present as an isolated exocrine gland disorder, patients may have a systemic inflammatory disease with renal involvement. Serologic abnormalities include hypergammaglobulinemia, circulating rheumatoid factor, cryoglobulins, autoantibodies such as homogeneous or speckled-pattern ANA, anti-Ro/SSA, and anti-La/SSB, but serum complement levels are generally normal unless the patient has associated SLE. The major clinical renal manifestations reflect tubulointerstitial involvement, distal renal tubular acidosis, impaired concentrating ability, hypercalciuria, and less commonly proximal tubule defects. Most patients have relatively normal urinalysis results with only mild elevations of the serum creatinine level. In patients with glomerular lesions, hematuria, proteinuria, and renal insufficiency are found. Some patients develop the full nephrotic syndrome, whereas others may develop renal vasculitis with prominent hypertension and renal insufficiency. Patients with immune complex glomerulonephritis and Sjögren syndrome are generally treated in a fashion similar to that for those with SLE, and patients with vasculitis generally receive cytotoxic therapy similar to that for other necrotizing vasculitides.

SARCOIDOSIS

The most common renal manifestations of sarcoidosis are interstitial nephritis (typically granulomatous), nephrolithiasis, and functional abnormalities of the tubule. Glomerular disease is uncommon and may be the coincidental expression of two unrelated disease processes in one individual rather than a result of the sarcoidosis itself. A variety of glomerular lesions have been described in patients with sarcoidosis including minimal-change disease, focal segmental glomerulosclerosis, membranous nephropathy, IgA nephropathy, membranoproliferative glomerulonephritis (MPGN), and proliferative and crescentic glomerulonephritis. Some patients have granulomatous renal interstitial nephritis in addition to the glomerular lesions, whereas others have only extrarenal histologic documentation of the sarcoidosis. The clinical presentation of glomerular disease in sarcoidosis is usually proteinuria, an active urinary sediment at times, and most commonly the nephrotic syndrome. Patients have been treated with various forms of immunosuppression including steroids, depending on their glomerular lesions.

AMYLOIDOSIS

Amyloidosis comprises a diverse group of systemic and local diseases characterized by the deposition of fibrils in various organs. Amyloid fibrils bind Congo red (leading to characteristic apple green birefringence under polarized light), have a characteristic ultrastructural appearance, and contain a 25-kD glycoprotein, serum amyloid P component. In primary (AL) amyloidosis, the deposited fibrils are derived from the variable portion of immunoglobulin light chains produced by a clonal population of plasma cells. Secondary (AA) amyloidosis is due most often to the deposition of serum amyloid A protein in chronic inflammatory states. Forms of hereditary amyloid involving the kidney include mutations in transthyretin, fibrinogen A chain, apolipoprotein A_1, lysozyme, apolipoprotein AII, cyclostatin C, and gelosin.

Primary and Secondary Amyloidosis

In primary amyloidosis, fibrils are composed of the N-terminal amino acid residues of the variable region of an immunoglobulin light chain. The kidneys are the most common major organ to be involved by AL amyloid, and the absence of other organ involvement does not exclude amyloidosis as a cause of major renal disease. Multiple myeloma occurs in up to 20% of patients with primary amyloidosis. Amyloidosis should be suspected in all patients with circulating serum monoclonal M proteins and approximately 90% of patients with primary amyloidosis will have a paraprotein spike in the serum or urine by immunofixation. The median age at presentation is approximately 60 years and fewer than 1% of patients are younger than 40 years. Men are affected twice as often as women. Presenting symptoms include weight loss, fatigue, lightheadedness, shortness of breath, peripheral edema, pain due to peripheral neuropathy, and purpura. Patients may have hepatosplenomegaly, macroglossia, and, rarely, enlarged lymph nodes.

Secondary amyloidosis is due to the deposition of amyloid A (AA) protein in patients with chronic inflammatory diseases. Secondary amyloidosis is observed in rheumatoid arthritis, inflammatory bowel disease, familial Mediterranean fever, and bronchiectasis and occasionally in poorly treated osteomyelitis. The diagnosis of amyloidosis must be established by tissue biopsy of an affected organ. Liver and kidney biopsy results are positive in as many as 90% of clinically affected patients. A diagnosis may be made with less invasive techniques such as fat pad aspirate or rectal biopsy. Serum amyloid P whole-body scintigraphy, after injection of radiolabeled serum amyloid P, may allow the noninvasive diagnosis of amyloidosis as well as allow quantification of the extent of organ system involvement. Results of this test may be positive even when tissue biopsy results have been negative and are more accurate in secondary than in primary amyloidosis.

Clinical manifestations of renal disease depend on the location and extent of amyloid deposition. Renal involvement predominates as the primary organ system involved in AL amyloidosis. Most patients have proteinuria, approximately 25% of patients have nephrotic syndrome at diagnosis, and others present with varying degrees of azotemia. Proteinuria is almost universal, but the urinalysis results are typically otherwise normal. More than 90% of patients with proteinuria greater than 1 g/day have a monoclonal protein in the urine. The amount of glomerular amyloid deposition does not correlate well with the degree of proteinuria. Despite the literature suggestion of enlarged kidneys in AL amyloidosis, by ultrasonography most patients have normalsized kidneys. Hypertension is found in 20% to 50% of patients, but many have orthostatic hypotension due to autonomic neuropathy. Occasionally patients have predominantly tubule deposition of amyloid with tubule defects such as distal renal tubular acidosis and nephrogenic diabetes insipidus.

Course, Prognosis, and Treatment

The prognosis of patients with AL amyloidosis is poor, with some series having a median survival of less than 2 years. The baseline serum creatinine level at diagnosis and the degree of proteinuria are predictive of the progression to ESRD. The median time from diagnosis to onset of dialysis is 14 months and from dialysis to death is only 8 months. Factors associated with decreased patient survival include evidence of cardiac involvement, λ versus κ proteinuria, and an elevated serum creatinine level. The optimal treatment for AL amyloidosis is unclear. Most treatments focus on methods to decrease the production of monoclonal light chains akin to myeloma therapy using chemotherapeutic drugs such as melphalan and prednisone, high-dose dexamethasone, chlorambucil, and cyclophosphamide. Recent reports using high-dose melphalan followed by an allogeneic bone marrow or stem cell transplant have given promising results. Thus, for younger patients with predominantly renal involvement, stem cell transplantation is a reasonable alternative therapy for AL amyloidosis. Regardless of whether chemotherapy or marrow transplant is used, the treatment of patients with amyloidosis and nephrotic syndrome involves supportive care measures. These may include judicious use of diuretics and salt restriction in those with nephrotic edema, treatment of orthostatic hypotension (autonomic neuropathy) with compression stockings, fludrocortisone, and midodrine, an oral α-adrenergic agonist.

The treatment of AA amyloidosis focuses on the treatment of the underlying inflammatory disease process. Alkylating agents have been used to control AA amyloidosis due to rheumatologic diseases in a number of studies, and responses including decreased proteinuria and prolonged renal survival have been noted. In patients with familial Mediterranean fever colchicine has long been used successfully to prevent febrile attacks. However, in patients with nephrotic syndrome at presentation or an elevated serum creatinine level, colchicine does not appear to prevent progression to ESRD.

MONOCLONAL IMMUNOGLOBULIN DEPOSITION DISEASE

Monoclonal immunoglobulin deposition disease, which includes light chain deposition disease (LCDD), light and heavy chain deposition disease (LCDD/HCDD), and heavy chain deposition disease (HCDD), is a systemic disease caused by the overproduction and extracellular deposition of a monoclonal immunoglobulin protein. In LCDD the constant region of the immunoglobulin light chain is typically deposited. Patients with LCDD are generally older than 45 years of age, and many patients have or subsequently develop frank myeloma or lymphoplasmacytic B cell disease such as lymphoma or Waldenström macroglobulinemia. Patients with renal involvement usually have significant glomerular involvement and thus present with heavy proteinuria accompanied by hypertension and renal insufficiency. The prognosis for patients with LCDD is uncertain and appears to be better than that for AL amyloidosis. As in amyloidosis, death is often attributed to cardiac disease or infectious complications. Treatment with melphalan and prednisone has led to stabilization or improvement in renal function in some patients. However, therapy is not successful in patients with a plasma creatinine level higher than 4 mg/dL (350 mcmol/L). Patient survival is about

90% at 1 year and 70% at 5 years, with renal survival of 67% and 37% at 1 and 5 years, respectively. Bone marrow or stem cell transplantation may be the optimal treatment for many patients with LCDD in the future.

GLOMERULAR DISEASE IN MYELOMA

Renal impairment is a common complication of multiple myeloma, occurring in 50% of patients. Renal involvement includes myeloma cast nephropathy, LCDD, AL amyloidosis, plasma cell infiltration, and glomerulonephritis. Other factors, such as hypercalcemia, hyperuricemia, infection, hyperviscosity, and nephrotoxic drugs, can precipitate or exacerbate acute and chronic renal failure. Glomerular and vascular lesions are usually restricted to those patients with associated AL amyloidosis or monoclonal LCDD or HCDD or both (see previous section). The glomeruli are usually spared and appear normal by light microscopy or have only mild glomerular basement membrane (GBM) thickening or minor amounts of mesangial matrix deposition without mesangial hypercellularity. In rare patients, glomerular crystals with an associated granulomatous reaction or exudates of proteinaceous material in the urinary space have been reported. Crescentic glomerulonephritis and MPGN have also been reported rarely, mostly in patients with associated cryoglobulinemia.

Myeloma Kidney

Myeloma cast nephropathy, also referred to as *myeloma kidney,* is an important cause of acute renal failure in myeloma. The underlying pathogenesis involves the precipitation of filtered light chains within the tubule lumen and the subsequent obstruction of urine flow. Light chains may also be directly toxic to the proximal tubule cells and can trigger the development of Fanconi syndrome. Patients are equally susceptible to cast nephropathy whether the filtered light chain is of the κ or λ variety, and an inherent ability to bind with Tamm-Horsfall protein is an important determinant of whether or not the light chain precipitates. Other factors favoring the development of cast nephropathy include a low urine flow rate as may occur during volume depletion, hypercalcemia, and diuretic or nonsteroidal anti-inflammatory drug use. Clinical findings include features of myeloma including a serum and urine paraprotein and occasionally evidence of Fanconi syndrome (proximal renal tubular acidosis and glycosuria). Of note, a routine urine dipstick test may not detect the positively charged light chains and hence quantitative determination of urine protein should be performed if cast nephropathy is suspected. The definitive diagnosis requires a renal biopsy. The pathologic findings include preservation of the normal glomerular architecture and tubular casts that stain positive for either κ or λ light chains on immunofluorescence. Management involves treatment of exacerbating factors including removal of offending agents (diuretics, nonsteroidal anti-inflammatory drugs, or angiotensin-converting enzyme inhibitors [ACEs]), volume expansion, treatment of hypercalcemia, and possibly the induction of an alkaline diuresis, although this last point remains controversial. Ultimately clearance of the paraprotein is required, and this is effected by chemotherapy aimed at the underlying plasma cell dyscrasia. Anecdotal and small retrospective studies suggest a role for plasmapheresis in the management of patients with a high paraprotein burden and acute renal injury in whom conservative measures have failed to improve renal function. Plasmapheresis may also have a role in patients with hyperviscosity syndrome leading to a failure of filtration within the glomerular capillary bed (plasma oncotic pressure > capillary hydraulic pressure within the glomerular capillary).

WALDENSTRÖM MACROGLOBULINEMIA

Waldenström macroglobulinemia is a syndrome characterized by a circulating monoclonal IgM protein in association with a B-cell lymphoproliferative disorder. This slowly progressive disorder occurs in older patients who present with fatigue, weight loss, bleeding, visual disturbances, peripheral neuropathy, hepatosplenomegaly, lymphadenopathy, anemia, and often a hyperviscosity syndrome. Renal involvement is uncommon but may manifest as microscopic hematuria and proteinuria, which may be nephrotic. Patients may have enlarged kidneys. The pathologic changes seen in Waldenström macroglobulinemia are varied. Some patients have invasion of the renal parenchyma by neoplastic lymphoplasmacytic cells. Acute renal failure associated with intraglomerular occlusive thrombi of the IgM paraprotein has also been reported. By immunofluorescence these glomerular "thrombi" stain for IgM and a single light chain, consistent with monoclonal IgM deposits. By electron microscopy the deposits contain nonamyloid fibrillar or amorphous electron-dense material. Other potential presentations include MPGN with an associated type I or II cryoglobulinemia, LCDD, and intratubule cast deposition similar to that seen in myeloma cast nephropathy and amyloidosis. Treatment of Waldenström macroglobulinemia consists of therapy directed against the lymphoproliferative disease with alkylating agents and at times plasmapheresis for hyperviscosity signs and symptoms. Newer therapies include fludarabine, cladribine, interferon (IFN)-α, rituximab, and marrow transplantation.

MIXED CRYOGLOBULINEMIA

Cryoglobulinemia refers to a pathologic condition caused by the production of circulating immunoglobulins that precipitate on cooling and resolubilize on warming. It is associated with a variety of infections as well as collagen-vascular disease and lymphoproliferative diseases. Cryoglobulins have been divided into three major groups based on the nature of the circulating immunoglobulin:

- Type I: The cryoglobulin is a single monoclonal immunoglobulin often found associated with Waldenström macroglobulinemia or myeloma.
- Type II: The cryoglobulin is a monoclonal immunoglobulin (IgM fl in >90%) directed against polyclonal IgG and has rheumatoid factor activity.
- Type III: The cryoglobulin contains polyclonal IgG and IgM directed against polyclonal IgG. Most patients with types II and III mixed cryoglobulins have been shown to have hepatitis C virus (HCV) infection.

Clinical and Laboratory Findings

Most patients with cryoglobulinemia are asymptomatic. Type I disease typically presents with symptoms related to peripheral hyperviscosity including livido reticularis, Raynaud phenomenon, or digital ischemia. Systemic manifestations of type II disease are more nonspecific and include weakness, malaise, Raynaud phenomenon, arthralgias and arthritis, hepatosplenomegaly, peripheral neuropathy, and purpuric skin lesions. Renal disease occurs at presentation in less than one fourth of patients but develops in as many as 50% over time. Renal disease due to cryoglobulin deposition within the kidney in most patients has a slow, indolent course characterized by proteinuria, hypertension hematuria, and renal insufficiency. However, in up to one third of patients an acute nephritic picture develops. A rapidly progressive glomerulonephritis presentation is rare. About 20% of patients present with the nephrotic syndrome. Some studies of type II cryoglobulinemia have shown evidence of hepatitis B infection. However, recent studies have clearly documented

HCV as a major cause of cryoglobulin production in most patients previously believed to have essential mixed cryoglobulinemia (types II and III). Antibodies to HCV antigens have been documented in the serum, and HCV RNA and anti-HCV antibodies are enriched in the circulating cryoglobulins. HCV antigens have also been localized by immunohistochemical analysis in the glomerular deposits. Low levels of total complement and especially C4 are common. The diagnosis rests on the demonstration of a circulating cryoglobulin.

Course and Treatment

The treatment of cryoglobulinemia is based both on the severity of symptoms and the underlying etiology. Mild disease in the absence of end-organ injury should be managed conservatively (analgesics and avoidance of cold). In patients with type I disease who have evidence of end-organ injury, therapy is directed against the underlying lymphoproliferative disease with steroids and cyclophosphamide in idiopathic cases. Most cases of type II and III disease are associated with HCV infection and are managed with a combination of interferon-alfa and ribavirin. In severe disease with fulminant renal involvement therapy may be initiated with plasmapheresis to remove the circulating cryoglobulin, corticosteroids to control the inflammatory response, and oral cyclophosphamide to prevent new cryoglobulin generation. Although this regimen typically eliminates the acute inflammatory injury, activation of hepatitis C replication is a real concern, and antiviral therapy should proceed in parallel with immunosuppressive therapy. Most patients have episodic exacerbations of their systemic and renal disease. Mean patient survival is 70% at 5 years after diagnosis, with death typically resulting from infection and cardiovascular disease. Renal survival is more than 80% at 10 years.

HEREDITARY NEPHRITIS, INCLUDING ALPORT SYNDROME

Alport syndrome is an inherited (usually X-linked) disorder associated with progressive renal failure, hearing loss, and ocular abnormalities. Renal failure develops due to structural abnormalities in the GBM consequent to abnormalities in the *COL4A5* gene encoding the α5 subunit of collagen type IV. Alport syndrome accounts for 2.5% of children and 0.3% of adults with ESRD in the United States.

Clinical Features

The disease usually manifests in children or young adults as microscopic hematuria, with episodic gross hematuria that may be exacerbated by respiratory infections or exercise. Proteinuria is usually mild at first and increases progressively with age. Hypertension is a late manifestation. Slowly progressive renal failure is common, and ESRD usually occurs in males between the ages of 16 and 35. Because this is usually an X-linked disorder, most females have only mild disease. More severe disease in females suggests an autosomal pattern of inheritance. High-frequency sensorineural deafness occurs in 30% to 50% of patients and is always accompanied by renal involvement. Ocular abnormalities occur in 15% to 30% of patients. Anterior lenticonus is virtually pathognomonic of Alport syndrome.

Course and Treatment

Recurrent hematuria and proteinuria may be present for many years, followed by the insidious onset of renal failure. Virtually all affected males develop ESRD, but there is considerable interkindred variability in the rate of progression. The rate of progression within male members of an affected family is usually, but not always, relatively constant. There is no proven therapy for Alport syndrome. Because weakening of the GBM appears important, it has been proposed that reduction of intraglomerular pressures with aggressive control of hypertension and use of ACE inhibitors might slow the rate of progression in patients with hereditary nephritis. Renal transplantation may be performed in patients with hereditary nephritis. Allograft survival is comparable to that in other patients with ESRD. In approximately 2% to 4% of patients receiving a renal transplant, anti-GBM antibody disease may develop, particularly after a second transplant. The GBM antibodies are directed against the Goodpasture antigen in the $\alpha 5$ chain, which presumably does not exist in the kidneys of patients with hereditary nephritis and is thus recognized as being a non-self antigen.

THIN GLOMERULAR BASEMENT MEMBRANE DISEASE

Benign familial hematuria describes a condition that differs from Alport disease in its benign course and lack of progression. The true incidence of thin GBM disease is unknown; reports evaluating patients with isolated hematuria suggest that 20% to 25% of such patients have thin GBM disease.

Clinical Features

The disease usually presents in childhood with microhematuria. Hematuria is usually persistent but may be intermittent in some patients. Episodic gross hematuria may occur, particularly with upper respiratory infections. Patients do not typically have overt proteinuria, but when present, this may suggest progression of disease.

Pathogenesis

In most kindreds with benign familial hematuria, the disorder appears to be transmitted in an autosomal dominant pattern. Thin GBM disease has been linked to the *COL4A3* and *COL4A4* genes, suggesting that type IV collagen defects can cause both benign hematuria and Alport syndrome.

INHERITED MUTATIONS OF PODOCYTE PROTEINS

Two novel proteins have been associated with the steroid-resistant nephrotic syndrome in childhood: nephrin and podocin.

Nephrin: Congenital Nephrotic Syndrome of the Finnish Type

Congenital nephrotic syndrome of the Finnish type (CNF) was originally described in Finland, but has been reported in other countries. The gene responsible for this form of nephrotic syndrome has been called *NPHS1*, and the gene product is a podocyte protein named nephrin.

Clinical Features

The disease manifests in utero with heavy proteinuria, and the affected infants are small for gestational age. Infants exhibit massive proteinuria, ascites, anasarca, and polycythemia associated with a failure to thrive and recurrent infectious complications. Associated abnormalities include pyloric stenosis and severe gastroesophageal reflux, resulting in aspiration pneumonia. The glomerular filtration rate progressively declines, and most infants develop renal failure within the first few years of life.

Pathogenesis

CNF is inherited in an autosomal recessive pattern. The gene affected in this disorder has been localized to chromosome 19 (19q13.1) and has been termed *NPHS1;* the gene product is known as nephrin. In the kidney, nephrin expression is restricted to the podocyte and localizes to the slit diaphragm and its precise function is unknown. Prenatal diagnosis is possible.

Treatment

Treatment strategies to support infants include intravenous albumin substitution, optimizing nutrition, administration of thyroxin, and anticoagulation, until bilateral nephrectomy can be performed (at around 1 year of life). Patients are maintained on dialysis until renal transplantation (at around 2 years of age). Other authors have reported success in reducing proteinuria, thus avoiding nephrectomy, with ACE inhibition in combination with indomethacin.

Podocin: Autosomal Recessive Nephrotic Syndrome

Podocin mutations have also been reported in patients with familial steroid-resistant nephrotic syndrome. The clinical course is characterized by early-childhood onset of proteinuria, rapid progression to ESRD, and focal segmental glomerulosclerosis on the kidney biopsy. The podocin (*NPHS2*) gene is located on chromosome 1q25-1q31. Podocin has been localized to the slit diaphragm and colocalizes with nephrin. Podocin and nephrin interact at the level of the slit diaphragm, possibly to maintaining podocyte ultrastructural integrity.

α-Actinin-4: Autosomal Dominant Nephrotic Syndrome

Mutations in α-actinin-4 have been associated with an autosomal dominant form of focal and segmental glomerulonephritis. The phenotype in these families is characterized by subnephrotic proteinuria and progressive renal insufficiency. The penetrance is high, but a small number of persons do not have clinical disease. *NPHS2* mutations have also been identified in adult-onset focal segmental glomerulosclerosis.

FABRY DISEASE (ANGIOKERATOMA CORPORIS DIFFUSUM UNIVERSALE)

Fabry disease is an X-linked inborn error of glycosphingolipid metabolism involving a lysosomal enzyme, α-galactosidase A.

It is characterized by an accumulation of globotriaosylceramide and related neutral glycosphingolipids, leading to multiorgan dysfunction.

Clinical Features

The estimated incidence in males is 1 in 40,000 to 60,000. The initial clinical presentation begins in childhood with episodic pain in the extremities and acroparesthesias. Renal involvement presents with hematuria and proteinuria, which often progress to nephrotic levels with progressive renal failure by the fifth decade. The skin is commonly involved with reddish-purple macules (angiokeratomas) typically found on the abdomen, buttocks, hips, genitalia, and upper thighs. The nervous system is involved, with peripheral and autonomic neuropathy. Premature arterial disease of coronary vessels leads to myocardial ischemia and arrhythmias at a young age. Corneal opacities are seen in virtually all homozygotes and most heterozygotes. Posterior capsular cataracts, edema of the retina and eyelids, and tortuous retinal and conjunctival vessels may also be seen in the eye. Up to one third of female carriers have been reported to have significant disease manifestations.

Pathogenesis

Deficiency of α-galactosidase leads to accumulation of globotriaosylceramide, especially in the vascular endothelium, with subsequent ischemic organ dysfunction. Accumulation in podocytes leads to proteinuria.

Diagnosis

The diagnosis in affected males may be established by measuring levels of α-galactosidase-A in plasma or peripheral blood leukocytes. Female carriers may have enzyme levels in the low to normal range; to diagnose female carriers, the specific mutation in the family must be demonstrated. Prenatal diagnosis can be made in amniotic fluid by measuring amniocyte enzyme levels.

Treatment

Two randomized, controlled trials have shown that recombinant human α-galactosidase-A replacement therapy is safe and can improve clinical parameters including neuropathic pain and creatinine clearance. Treatment has also been shown to decrease microvascular endothelial deposits of globotriaosylceramide in the kidney. Enzyme replacement therapy should be administered as early as possible in all males with Fabry disease (including those with ESRD) and in female carriers with substantial disease manifestations.

SICKLE CELL NEPHROPATHY

See Chapter 15, Microvascular Diseases of the Kidney.

LECITHIN-CHOLESTEROL ACYLTRANSFERASE DEFICIENCY

This a familial disorder characterized by proteinuria, anemia, hyperlipidemia, and corneal opacity. In initial reports, most patients were of Scandinavian origin; however, subsequent reports have been from other countries.

Clinical Features

The triad of anemia, nephrotic syndrome, and corneal opacities suggests lecithin-cholesterol acyltransferase (LCAT) deficiency. Renal disease is a universal finding, with albuminuria noted early in life. Proteinuria increases in severity during the fourth and fifth decades, often with development of the nephrotic syndrome and progressive renal failure. Most patients are mildly anemic with target cells and poikilocytes on the peripheral smear. There is evidence of low-grade hemolysis. Corneal opacities, which appear as grayish spots over the cornea accompanied by a lipoid arcus, are noted during childhood.

Diagnosis

Patients have little or no LCAT activity in their blood circulation because of mutations in the *LCAT* gene. In patients suspected of having LCAT deficiency, measurements of the plasma enzyme should be performed. Other abnormalities of lipids often accompany LCAT deficiency. The plasma is turbid, the total cholesterol level varies, triglyceride levels are increased, the high-density lipoprotein level is reduced, and all fractions contain higher amounts of cholesterol.

Treatment

A low-lipid diet or use of lipid-lowering drugs has not been shown to be of benefit. Plasma infusions may provide reversal of erythrocytic abnormalities, but long-term benefits have yet to be demonstrated. The lesions may recur in the allograft, but renal function is adequately preserved.

GLOMERULAR INVOLVEMENT WITH BACTERIAL INFECTIONS

Infectious Endocarditis

In the preantibiotic era, *Streptococcus viridans* was the most common causative organism in endocarditis-related glomerulonephritis. However, with the use of prophylactic antibiotics in patients with valvular heart disease and an increase in intravenous drug use, *Staphylococcus aureus* has replaced *S viridans* as the primary pathogen. The incidence of glomerulonephritis with endocarditis with *S aureus* ranges from 22% to 78%, being higher in those series consisting predominantly of intravenous drug users.

Clinical Features
Renal complications of infectious endocarditis include infarcts, abscesses, and glomerulonephritis (all of which may coexist). The spectrum of glomerulonephritis ranges from mild asymptomatic urinary abnormalities including hematuria, pyuria, and albuminuria to rapidly progressive renal failure with crescents. Although hypocomplementemia is common, it is not seen invariably. Most patients demonstrate activation of the classic pathway, and the degree of complement activation correlates with the severity of renal impairment. Circulating immune complexes have been found in the serum in up to 90% of patients. Mixed cryoglobulins and rheumatoid factor may also be present.

Pathogenesis
Endocarditis-related glomerulonephritis is an immune complex–mediated disease. The demonstration of hypocomplementemia, antibody deposition in the glomeruli, and the detection of bacterial antigen in the deposits supports this hypothesis.

Treatment
With the initiation of antibiotic therapy, the manifestations of glomerulonephritis begin to subside. Plasmapheresis and

corticosteroids has been reported to promote renal recovery in some patients with renal failure. However, the risk from worsening of the infectious aspects of the disease while ameliorating the immunologic manifestations should be kept in mind when this approach is used.

Shunt Nephritis

Ventriculovascular (ventriculoatrial or ventriculojugular) and ventriculoperitoneal shunts used for the treatment of hydrocephalus may become colonized with microorganisms, most commonly *Staphylococcus albus* (75%). Patients commonly present with fever, arthralgia, and malaise. Anemia, hepatosplenomegaly, and lymphadenopathy are found on examination. Renal manifestations include hematuria (microscopic or gross), proteinuria (nephrotic syndrome in 30% of patients), azotemia, and hypertension. Laboratory abnormalities include the presence of rheumatoid factor, cryoglobulins, elevated ESR and C-reactive protein levels, hypocomplementemia, and the presence of circulating immune complexes.

Treatment

Antibiotic therapy and prompt removal of the infected catheter lead to remission of the glomerulonephritis.

Other Bacterial Infections and Fungal Infections

Congenital, secondary, and latent forms of syphilis may rarely be complicated by glomerular involvement. Patients are usually nephrotic, and proteinuria usually responds to penicillin therapy. Membranous nephropathy with varying degrees of proliferation and with granular IgG and C3 deposits is the most common finding on biopsies. Renal involvement including azotemia, proteinuria, nephrotic syndrome, renal tubule defects, and hematuria is not uncommon in leprosy, especially with the lepra reaction.

Rarely, presentation with rapidly progressive glomerulonephritis and ESRD can occur. Mesangial proliferation, diffuse proliferative glomerulonephritis, crescentic glomerulonephritis, membranous nephropathy, MPGN, microscopic angiitis, and amyloidosis all may be seen in kidney biopsies. Membranous nephropathy, MPGN, crescentic glomerulonephritis, and amyloidosis have been associated with *Mycobacterium tuberculosis*. *Mycoplasma* has been reported to be associated with the nephrotic syndrome and rapidly progressive glomerulonephritis. Antibiotics do not seem to alter the course of the disease. Acute glomerulonephritis with hypocomplementemia has been reported with pneumococcal infections. Proliferative glomerulonephritis with deposition of IgG, IgM, complements C1q, C3, and C4, and pneumococcal antigens have been observed in renal biopsies. Patients with *Brucella* infections may present with hematuria and proteinuria (usually nephrotic) and varying degrees of renal functional impairment. Improvement is usually seen after antibiotic treatment, but histologic abnormalities, proteinuria, and hypertension may persist. Mesangial proliferation, focal and segmental proliferation, diffuse proliferation, and crescents may be found in renal biopsies. Immunofluorescence may show no deposits, IgG, or occasionally IgA deposition. Asymptomatic urinary abnormalities may be seen in as many as 80% of patients infected with *Leptospira*. Patients usual present with acute renal failure due to tubulointerstitial nephritis. Rarely, mesangial or diffuse proliferative glomerulonephritis may be seen.

GLOMERULAR INVOLVEMENT WITH PARASITIC DISEASES

Malaria

Clinically overt glomerular disease is uncommon in falciparum malaria (*Plasmodium falciparum*). However, severe falciparum malaria may manifest with hemoglobinuric acute renal failure. In quartan malaria (*Plasmodium malariae*) with renal involvement, proteinuria is the cardinal manifestation and significant hematuria is unusual. Serum complement levels may be depressed in early stages of the disease. Progression to end-stage renal failure occurs within 3 to 5 years. Spontaneous remissions may occur but are rare. Antimalarial treatment fails to improve the renal outcome, and the response to steroids is disappointing.

Schistosomiasis

Schistosomiasis is a visceral parasitic disease caused by the blood flukes of the genus *Schistosoma*. *Schistosoma mansoni* and *Schistosoma japonicum* cause cirrhosis of the liver and *Schistosoma hematobium* causes cystitis. Glomerular involvement in *mansoni* infection includes mesangial proliferation, focal sclerosis, membranoproliferative lesions, crescentic changes, membranous nephropathy, amyloidosis, and eventually ESRD.

Schistosomal antigens have been demonstrated in renal biopsies in such patients. Treatment with antiparasitic agents does not appear to influence progression of renal disease. *Schistosoma hematobium* is occasionally associated with the nephrotic syndrome, which may respond to antiparasitic treatment.

Leishmaniasis

Leishmaniasis, also known as kala-azar, is caused by *Leishmania donovani*. Renal involvement in kala-azar appears to be mild and reverts with antileishmanial treatment. Renal biopsies show mesangial proliferation or focal proliferation. IgG, IgM, and C3 may be observed in areas of proliferation. Amyloidosis may also complicate kala-azar.

Trypanosomiasis and Filariasis

Trypanosoma brucei, Trypanosoma gambiense, and *Trypanosoma rhodesiense* cause African sleeping sickness and have rarely been associated with proteinuria. Filariasis is caused by organisms in the genera *Onchocerca, Brugia, Loa,* and *Wuchereria.* Hematuria and proteinuria (including nephrotic syndrome) have been described. Renal manifestations may appear with treatment of infection. Renal biopsy findings have included mesangial proliferative glomerulonephritis with C3 deposition, diffuse proliferative glomerulonephritis, and collapsing glomerulopathy.

GLOMERULAR INVOLVEMENT WITH VIRAL INFECTIONS

Human Immunodeficiency Virus–Associated Nephropathy

Clinical Features

HIV-associated nephropathy (HIVAN) was first reported in 1984 and is characterized by a collapsing form of focal glomerulosclerosis. There is a strong predilection for HIVAN among black HIV-infected patients with a black-to-white ratio of 12:1. Although intravenous drug use has been the most common risk factor for HIVAN, the disease has been seen in all groups at risk for acquired immunodeficiency syndrome (AIDS). HIVAN usually occurs in patients with a low CD4 count, but full-blown AIDS is certainly not a prerequisite for the disease. The prevalence of HIVAN in patients who test positive for HIV is reported to be 3.5%. The clinical features of HIVAN include proteinuria, typically in the nephrotic range (and often massive), and renal insufficiency. Some patients, however, present with subnephrotic-range proteinuria and urinary sediment findings of microhematuria and sterile pyuria. Renal ultrasound studies in HIVAN show echogenic kidneys with preserved or enlarged size (average of more than 12 cm) despite the severe renal insufficiency.

Pathogenesis

HIV appears to be able to infect glomerular endothelial cells and to a lesser degree mesangial cells in vitro. HIV-1 RNA is detectable in renal tubule epithelial cells and glomerular epithelial cells (visceral and parietal) by in situ hybridization in human subjects. Based on animal models, it appears likely that a viral gene product or indirect effects on host cytokine production mediate glomerular injury.

Course and Treatment

The natural history of HIVAN during the early part of the AIDS epidemic was characterized by rapid progression to ESRD. However, early institution of zidovudine antiviral therapy in HIVAN is associated with an improvement in outcome. The role of combined antiviral therapies and the use of newer agents in the treatment of HIVAN have been investigated in small numbers of patients with apparent beneficial effect. Indeed, the incidence of HIVAN-related ESRD has decreased substantially with the introduction of highly active antiretroviral therapy. At present the therapy for HIVAN should include use of multiple antiviral agents as for HIV-infected patients without nephropathy. Use of ACE inhibitors or angiotensin II receptor blockers is likely to be beneficial and should be considered in all patients.

GLOMERULAR MANIFESTATIONS OF LIVER DISEASE

Hepatitis B

Hepatitis B antigenemia is associated with membranous nephropathy, MPGN, and PAN. In countries where the virus is endemic (sub-Saharan Africa, Southeast Asia, and Eastern Europe) hepatitis B–associated nephropathy occurs predominantly in children with a 4:1 male preponderance. In the industrialized world where hepatitis B is acquired by parenteral routes or sexually, the nephropathy affects mainly adults and has a clinical course different from that of the endemic form.

Clinical Features

Most patients present with proteinuria or the nephrotic syndrome and have normal renal function at the time of presentation. Urinary erythrocytes may be present, but most patients have a bland sediment. Liver disease may be absent (carrier state) or chronic and clinically mild. Serum aminotransferase levels may be normal or modestly elevated. Liver biopsies in these patients often show chronic active hepatitis. Some patients ultimately develop cirrhosis as seen in their biopsies. Spontaneous resolution of the carrier state often occurs with resolution of renal abnormalities.

Treatment

In children with a mild endemic form of hepatitis B–associated nephropathy, no treatment other than supportive care is advocated and spontaneous recovery is common. In patients with progressive renal dysfunction, IFN-alfa has been used with mixed results. Steroid treatment does not significantly improve proteinuria and may potentially enhance viral replication. Nucleoside analogs including lamivudine, adefovir, and lobucavir also have clinical utility in treating hepatitis B infection; their role in treating the nephropathy remains to be established. Use of preemptive lamivudine therapy in renal transplant recipients has improved survival compared with that for historical control subjects.

Hepatitis C

Renal diseases associated with HCV infection include MPGN with or without associated mixed cryoglobulinemia and membranous glomerulopathy (see Chapter 10, Primary Glomerular Disease, and earlier). The MPGN is most often type I, with fewer instances of type III. Rare occurrences of diffuse proliferative and exudative glomerulonephritis, polyarteritis, and fibrillary and immunotactoid glomerulopathy have also been described in association with HCV. Most patients have evidence of liver disease as reflected by elevated plasma transaminase levels. However, transaminase levels are normal in some patients, and a history of acute hepatitis is often absent.

Pathogenesis

The pathogenesis of HCV-related nephropathies is immune complex mediated. HCV-specific proteins have been isolated from glomerular lesions. The disappearance of viremia in response to IFN (see later) is associated with a diminution of proteinuria; a relapse of viremia is accompanied by rising proteinuria.

Treatment

A number of reports have demonstrated a beneficial response to IFN-α therapy in patients with HCV-induced renal disease. Vasculitic symptoms, viral titers, proteinuria, and, in some studies, the plasma creatinine level improve in 50% to 60% of patients receiving IFN-α for periods up to 1 year. Cessation of IFN therapy, however, is associated with recurrence of viremia and cryoglobulinemia in most patients in these studies. IFN therapy may paradoxically exacerbate proteinuria and hematuria that appears to be unrelated to viral antigenic effects. Combination therapy with ribavirin and IFN may offer benefits over therapy with IFN-α alone. However, the combination therapy may not be well tolerated in the presence of significant renal dysfunction. IFN-α treatment of renal transplant patients with HCV has been associated with acute renal failure and acute humoral rejection. Cyclophosphamide treatment has been used successfully in HCV glomerulonephritis, even if the condition is IFN-α resistant. Cyclophosphamide treatment may be associated with a temporary, reversible increase in viral load.

Cirrhosis

Cirrhotic glomerulonephritis is usually a clinically silent disease; however, the diagnosis can be suspected by finding proteinuria or abnormalities of the urine sediment. Glomerular morphologic abnormalities with IgA deposition have been noted in more than 50% of patients with cirrhosis at both necropsy and biopsy, although this has also been found in some autopsies of noncirrhotic kidneys. Clinically, there may be mild proteinuria or hematuria, or both. Rarely, HSP with rapidly progressive glomerulonephritis has been described in association with cirrhosis.

GLOMERULAR LESIONS ASSOCIATED WITH NEOPLASIA

The occurrence of glomerular syndromes, both nephrotic and nephritic, may be associated with malignancy, but this is rare (<1%). Glomerular disease may be seen with a wide variety of malignancies. Carcinomas of the lung, stomach, breast, and colon are most often associated with glomerular lesions. Membranous nephropathy is the most common lesion associated with carcinoma. Patients older than 50 years of age presenting with nephrotic syndrome should be examined for the presence of a malignancy.

Clinical and Pathologic Features

Clinically, the glomerulopathy of neoplasia may be manifested by proteinuria or nephrotic syndrome, an active urine sediment, and diminished glomerular filtration. Significant renal impairment is uncommon and is usually associated with the proliferative forms of glomerulonephritis. In evaluating an ESR in patients with nephrotic syndrome, one should note that most such patients have an ESR higher than 60 mm/hr, with roughly 20% having ESRs higher than 100 mm/hr. As a result, an elevated ESR alone in a patient with the nephrotic syndrome (or with ESRD) is not an indication to evaluate the patient for an occult malignancy or underlying inflammatory disease.

Membranous Nephropathy

Lesions of membranous nephropathy may be associated with malignancies in 10% to 40% of patients. Malignancies include carcinoma of the bronchus, breast, colon, and stomach and Hodgkin disease, among others. In some instances successful treatment of the neoplasm has induced a partial or complete remission of the associated glomerulopathy.

Minimal-Change Disease or Focal Glomerulosclerosis

Minimal-change disease or focal glomerulosclerosis may occur in association with Hodgkin disease and less often with other lymphoproliferative disorders or solid tumors.

Proliferative Glomerulonephritides and Vasculitides

Both MPGN and rapidly progressive glomerulonephritis have been described in patients with solid tumors and lymphomas, although the etiologic relationship between these conditions is not proven. The association is probably strongest for MPGN and chronic lymphocytic leukemia and may be related to circulating cryoglobulins.

Thrombotic Microangiopathy

Hemolytic-uremic syndrome–thrombotic thrombocytopenic purpura can occur in patients with malignancy. An underlying carcinoma of the stomach, pancreas, or prostate may be associated with hemolytic-uremic syndrome. More commonly, however, antitumor therapy is implicated: mitomycin, the combination of bleomycin and cisplatin, and radiation plus high-dose cyclophosphamide before bone marrow transplantation all can lead to hemolytic-uremic syndrome, which may first become apparent months after therapy has been discontinued.

Tubulointerstitial Diseases

12

Progressive inflammation or injury to the tubulointerstitial region typically destroys extensive amounts of kidney tissue and, as a result, usually produces irreversible chronic kidney disease. Interstitial inflammation can begin either from within the interstitial compartment or as a secondary event after glomerular or vascular injury, and if left unchecked, can evolve into irreversible tubulointerstitial fibrosis. Although some forms of injury to the tubulointerstitial compartment are the result of toxic insult or exposure to infection and drugs, much of the inflammatory process is immunologically mediated. Many studies have pointed to the degree of tubulointerstitial fibrosis as an accurate prognostic marker of severe interstitial disease in a variety of glomerular diseases.

ACUTE INTERSTITIAL NEPHRITIS

Primary acute interstitial nephritis is now recognized as a common renal disease, accounting for approximately 1% to 15% of all renal biopsies. This estimate is consistent with chart review data indicating that chronic interstitial nephritis accounts for approximately 25% of instances of permanent renal failure.

Pathology

The hallmark of acute primary interstitial nephritis is the infiltration of inflammatory cells into the interstitial compartment with sparing of glomeruli. An associated minimal change–like lesion is often observed with use of nonsteroidal anti-inflammatory drugs (NSAIDs). In chronic interstitial nephritis, the cellular infiltrate is largely replaced by interstitial fibrosis, which accounts for the irregular and contracted gross appearance of the kidney. *Chronic* is a relative term, because fibrotic changes can be seen

241

within 7 to 10 days of initiation of an inflammatory process. A third pathologic category can be seen in either the acute or chronic setting, namely, granuloma formation. In acute granulomatous interstitial nephritis, the granulomas are sparse and non-necrotic, giant cells are rare, and an accompanying interstitial nephritis is common. The granulomas of the chronic lesion contain more giant cells, and if due to tuberculosis, they may become necrotic. Drugs are a common cause of this lesion in the acute setting. Sarcoidosis or tuberculosis should be considered when granulomas are seen in chronic disease.

Clinical Features

The typical presentation of acute interstitial nephritis (AIN) is acute renal failure, most commonly in an asymptomatic patient who has experienced an intervening illness or who was given a new medication. Occasionally, the nephritis is severe enough to result in the need for renal replacement therapy. The classic signs of drug-associated AIN include the following:

- Fever (75%)
- Skin rash (50%)
- Eosinophilia (80%)

The entire triad is, however, observed in fewer than one third of patients. Immunoglobulin E levels are occasionally increased. Other symptoms include lumbar pain due to distention of the renal capsule from diffuse swelling of the kidney. The onset of drug-induced nephritis ranges from days to weeks after initiation of therapy. The onset of renal failure can be precipitous (days), especially in those patients who are reexposed to a nephropathic agent; conversely, it can be protracted, with a steadily declining glomerular filtration rate over months. A history of a previous allergic reaction is only rarely obtained.

Dipstick evaluation typically reveals mild to moderate proteinuria and hematuria in most patients. Gross hematuria is uncommon. The sediment typically shows red and white blood cells. White blood cell casts are occasionally observed. The finding of eosinophils in the urine suggests allergic interstitial nephritis. The absence of eosinophiluria should never discourage the diagnostic pursuit of AIN.

Serum creatinine levels are usually elevated. The magnitude of proteinuria in acute tubulointerstitial disease is usually modest and nearly always less than 3 g/24 hr. Nephrotic-range proteinuria is not usually seen in AIN unless there is a coexisting glomerular lesion after exposure to NSAIDs. The fractional excretion of

Na^+ is usually greater than 1. Affected patients are often oliguric, but nonoliguric renal failure also occurs. Oliguria may be related to interstitial inflammation severe enough to cause tubular obstruction and impede urine flow. Tubular defects and tubular syndromes such as Fanconi syndrome and renal tubular acidosis are rarely observed in AIN and are more common with chronic tubulointerstitial diseases. The kidney in AIN is usually normal or slightly increased in size by echographic criteria. Many features of the patient's history, presentation, urinalysis, and laboratory evaluation may suggest the diagnosis of AIN. Unfortunately, none of these findings are pathognomonic, and ultimately the diagnosis can only be established with certainty by renal biopsy. Therefore, a biopsy should be performed in patients with acute renal failure who present with signs or symptoms suggestive of an interstitial process and in whom obstructive nephropathy and prerenal azotemia have been excluded.

Etiology

The causative factors leading to AIN are usually limited to a few broad categories. In our experience drugs are the predominant etiologic agents today, followed by infection, and then by autoimmune idiopathic lesions.

Drugs

A list of potentially offending pharmacologic agents is presented in Table 12–1. Although a multitude of agents have been reported to cause AIN, most cases result from a relatively restricted number

Table 12–1: Common Causes of Acute Interstitial Nephritis

Drugs
    Antibiotics, especially β-lactams, rifampin, and sulfa drugs
    Nonsteroidal anti-inflammatory drugs, including selective
      cyclooxygenase-2 inhibitors
    Diuretics
    H_2 antagonists and proton pump inhibitors
Infection
    Bacteria, including streptococci, staphylococci, *Legionella,*
      Brucella, and *Salmonella*
    Viruses including Epstein-Barr virus, cytomegalovirus, human
      immunodeficiency virus, and polyomavirus
Idiopathic
    Anti–tubular basement membrane disease
    Tubulointerstitial nephritis and uveitis syndrome

of agents of which the β-lactam antibiotics are the best-studied group. Methicillin was widely implicated in the development of AIN but is no longer in widespread use. Generic penicillin and ampicillin are commonly implicated in acute tubulointerstitial disease, whereas nafcillin has only rarely been observed to produce AIN. It should be remembered that recurrent AIN, after an initial insult with one penicillin derivative, has occurred with the use of a different penicillin or even with a cephalosporin. Prominent among the other antimicrobials associated with AIN are sulfonamides, quinolones, and rifampin. Rifampin appears to be most often associated with acute tubulointerstitial disease in conjunction with intermittent or discontinuous dosing. NSAID-associated AIN appears in two forms. The first is an occasional pure lesion, with or without papillary necrosis, but without any glomerular disease. The second is a combined lesion of minimal-change glomerulonephritis and AIN. This combined lesion has also recently been described with selective cyclooxygenase-2 inhibitors. Patients with the combined lesion can present with nephrotic-range proteinuria, nephrotic syndrome, and renal failure. The interstitial lesion can appear as early as 1 week after medication is begun, but more commonly is seen after several months to 1 year of use. Lesions in most patients respond to removal of the offending NSAID; however, if renal function does not improve within 1 to 2 weeks or if there is an associated minimal-change lesion then steroid therapy should be considered. Finally, alternative medicines, particularly some Chinese herb preparations, idiosyncratically produce renal failure. Sometimes this has been rapidly progressive (or subacute) interstitial nephritis, but occasional patients appear with acute renal failure.

Infection
AIN and renal failure can be seen in the setting of systemic infection. Whereas drugs are clearly the most common etiologic agents for AIN in adults, studies from the pediatric literature suggest that infections, particularly streptococcal, are the most common etiologic factor. The interstitial lesion seems to be a response to disseminated infection and not simply a matter of hematogenous seeding of the kidney with bacteria. Renal failure from infection-related AIN generally resolves with treatment of the underlying infection, and steroid therapy, although sometimes advocated, is often not needed. Human immunodeficiency virus has not been shown to directly cause an isolated interstitial nephritis; however, it has been emphasized recently that tubulointerstitial lesions are common with this infection for a variety of factors. These include opportunistic infections with

cytomegalovirus, cryptococcus, or histoplasmosis, nephrocalcinosis, and use of sulfa drug derivatives. Similarly, renal allograft recipients may be susceptible to Epstein-Barr virus and cytomegalovirus infections. Polyomavirus is increasingly recognized as a cause of renal insufficiency in immunosuppressed patients with renal allografts. Renal biopsies typically demonstrate viral intranuclear inclusions within the tubular epithelium. Current clinical approaches to this entity include diminution of immunosuppression and antiviral therapy.

Idiopathic Acute Interstitial Nephritis

Idiopathic interstitial nephritis may account for up to 30% of cases of AIN. The predominance of mononuclear cells in the interstitial infiltrate, the presence of constitutional symptoms, and the spontaneous nature of the lesion all suggest an immunologic basis. In humans, anti-3M-1 antibodies have been observed in several different clinical settings. As discussed before, linear deposition of anti–tubular basement membrane antibodies have been observed in 70% of patients with anti–glomerular basement membrane disease. Anti–tubular basement membrane staining occurs without anti–glomerular basement membrane antibodies occasionally and in this case the target antigen appears to be 3M-1. Most commonly, however, anti–tubular basement membrane antibodies appear in the setting of renal transplantation. Most of these antibodies probably result from 3M-1 polymorphisms in which a 3M-1$^+$ transplanted kidney is placed in a 3M-1$^-$ recipient. Unlike drug-induced lesions, the idiopathic forms of interstitial nephritis are rarely associated with rash or eosinophilia, although fever is common. The absence of obvious predisposing factors for AIN should not bias one against consideration of this diagnosis in an otherwise appropriate clinical setting. The potentially subtle nature of AIN forms the basis for many diagnostic renal biopsies. One particular category of patients with idiopathic AIN has received special attention: those with tubulointerstitial nephritis and uveitis (the so-called TINU syndrome). These patients are usually adolescent girls, or occasionally adults, who present with constitutional symptoms, reduced renal function and tubule dysfunction, bone marrow or lymphoid granulomas, and uveitis during some point in the course of disease. On renal biopsy, evidence of AIN is seen, sometimes with fibrosis. The prognosis in children seems to be excellent with or without treatment with steroids, whereas the prognosis is more guarded in adults. Adult patients are generally treated with corticosteroids, and partial recovery of renal function may occur over several weeks.

Course and Treatment

The primary therapeutic approach to AIN is to identify the inciting factor and remove or treat it as appropriate. Withdrawal of the offending agent, usually a drug, often results in an improvement in renal function within several days in many patients. The likelihood of complete recovery, however, appears to be inversely proportional to the duration of renal failure. Prolonged and active tubulointerstitial injury and a subsequent lack of total resolution have their pathologic correlates in irreversible interstitial fibrosis. Unless an offending agent can be identified and removed, progression to end-stage renal disease is likely. In idiopathic AIN, although spontaneous resolution may occur, more than 50% of patients are left with residual renal dysfunction. In the absence of a prompt response to withdrawal of an inciting insult, early institution of corticosteroid therapy appears appropriate. Although no prospective data are available, steroid therapy is commonly used in acute interstitial disease. This trial of corticosteroids consists of a dosage equivalent to 1 mg/kg/day of prednisone in patients with no contraindications to prednisone therapy. Improvement in renal function should begin within 1 to 2 weeks of initiation of treatment, in which case the drug can be discontinued after 4 to 6 weeks. If no improvement is seen within the first 2 weeks, the addition of a second agent such as cyclophosphamide (2 mg/kg/day) may be considered; if successful, this treatment should be continued for up to 1 year with appropriate monitoring of the white blood cell count. Lack of any evidence of improvement after 6 weeks of combined therapy should lead to discontinuation of both agents. The presence of marked interstitial fibrosis on renal biopsy specimens suggests a more appropriate diagnosis of chronic interstitial nephritis and militates against the use of immunosuppressive therapy.

CHRONIC INTERSTITIAL NEPHRITIS

Clinical Features

Unless a patient is found to have an abnormal urinalysis or elevated serum creatinine level from a screening test, patients with chronic interstitial disease present either because of systemic symptoms of a primary disease or because of nonspecific symptoms of renal failure. These nonspecific symptoms depend on the severity of the renal failure but may include lassitude, weakness, nausea, nocturia, and sleep disturbances. Typical laboratory findings in these patients include non–nephrotic-range proteinuria, microscopic hematuria and pyuria, glycosuria, and positive urine culture results in up to

30% of patients. Acidifying and concentrating defects are common. Chronic interstitial disease from some causes displays characteristic patterns of tubular dysfunction (proximal or distal renal tubular acidosis) or marked early concentrating defects (primary medullary dysfunction). Anemia occurs relatively early in the course of certain forms of chronic interstitial disease, presumably because of early destruction of erythropoietin-producing interstitial cells.

Etiology

Chronic interstitial nephritis can occur in association with a number of diseases of diverse etiology. Table 12–2 provides

Table 12–2: Common Causes of Chronic Interstitial Nephritis

Metabolic disturbances
    Hypercalcemia/nephrocalcinosis
    Hyperoxaluria
    Hypokalemia
    Hyperuricemia
Drugs and toxins
    Analgesics
    Cadmium
    Lead
    Nitrosoureas
    Herbs
    Lithium
    Cyclosporine
Immune mediated
    Renal allograft rejection
    Sjögren syndrome
    Sarcoidosis
Infection
    Direct infection
    Malacoplakia
    Xanthogranulomatous pyelonephritis
Obstructive and mechanical disorders
    Tumors
    Stones
    Outlet obstruction
    Vesicoureteral reflux
Miscellaneous
    Endemic nephropathy
    Radiation nephritis
    Progressive glomerular disease
    Extracorporeal shock wave lithotripsy

a more exhaustive list of common and rare cause of chronic interstitial disease.

Endemic Nephropathy

Balkan nephropathy is a form of chronic interstitial disease endemic to areas of Bulgaria, the former Yugoslavia, and Romania. Its cause remains unknown, although it has been attributed over the years to long-term exposure to lead, infection, environmental agents (including fungus-contaminated foodstuffs), and genetic factors, alone or in combination. The disease typically manifests clinically in the fourth or fifth decade of life, and the consensus is that this is a slowly progressive disease. There is no specific diagnostic test for Balkan nephropathy, which makes early diagnosis difficult. Asymptomatic patients typically have elevated excretion of "tubule" proteins (lysozyme, light chains, β_2-microglobulin, and retinal binding protein), increased enzymuria (N-acetyl-β-D-glucosaminidase), and submaximal urinary concentrating ability. The kidneys are normal in size in the latent stages of the disease and become small with progressive disease. Various series have reported that anywhere from 2% to 47% of patients with Balkan nephropathy develop uroepithelial tumors.

Sarcoidosis

Sarcoidosis most commonly affects the kidney through disordered Ca^{2+} metabolism. Many patients with sarcoidosis have either hypercalcemia or normocalcemic hypercalciuria, which can lead to concentrating defects, depress glomerular filtration, or result in nephrocalcinosis or nephrolithiasis. Although autopsy series have demonstrated that noncaseating granulomas are present within the renal interstitium in 15% to 30% of patients with sarcoidosis, it is unusual for these pathologic abnormalities to result in clinically apparent renal dysfunction. However, a small subset of patients with sarcoidosis develop granulomatous interstitial nephritis that leads to renal insufficiency. The renal dysfunction is associated with tubular defects including glycosuria, concentrating defects, and renal tubular acidosis. It is unusual to see renal sarcoidosis without other apparent organ involvement. The pathologic findings in renal sarcoidosis consist of interstitial non-caseating granulomas, composed of giant cells, histiocytes, and lymphocytes that may virtually replace most of the cortical volume, severely distorting the tubular architecture. These patients often have an impressive therapeutic response to corticosteroid therapy, with improvement in glomerular filtration and improvement in histologic findings. Cyclophosphamide is occasionally used in patients with sarcoidosis that is refractory to corticosteroids or in those who are intolerant of corticosteroids.

Radiation Nephritis
Radiation nephritis is uncommon today because protocols for the administration of therapeutic radiation have been altered to take into account the risk of renal injury. An acute form of radiation nephritis is seen within 1 year after radiation and presents with hypertension, anemia, and edema. A more insidious chronic form presents primarily with diminished glomerular filtration, hypertension, and occasionally proteinuria. A small number of patients can develop malignant hypertension with accelerated loss of renal function. Another pattern of less severe renal injury after radiation is that of isolated proteinuria, which can occur more than a decade after radiation and may be persistent or intermittent. The common pathologic finding in patients with chronic radiation nephritis is interstitial fibrosis. Because hypertension commonly accompanies radiation nephritis, it is difficult to separate the effects of the radiation and hypertension on the fibrotic process. Radiation nephritis is dose-dependent, affecting most of those exposed to more than 2300 rads. It can be prevented by shielding of the kidney, or, alternatively, by fractionating doses, which increases renal tolerance to the damaging effects of radiation. However, even with fractionated schedules, patients exposed to other nephrotoxins (e.g., chemotherapeutic agents, antibiotics, or radiocontrast agents) have an increased risk for toxicity.

Analgesic Nephropathy
See Chapter 16, Toxic Nephropathy.

Uric Acid Nephropathy
Chronic hyperuricemia has been proposed as an independent risk factor for chronic interstitial nephritis and progressive renal failure. Historically, chronic hyperuricemia associated with chronic interstitial disease was called *gouty nephropathy*. However, this association has been challenged by some authorities who suggested that most cases reflect the effects of hypertension, vascular disease, stones, or aging rather than hyperuricemia per se. This is an important question, especially because many patients with chronic renal failure have serum uric acid levels greater than 10 mg/dL (550 mcmol/L), attributable to diminished glomerular filtration and the effects of diuretics. The existence of gouty nephropathy received another challenge by the finding that infusion of ethylenediamine tetraacetic acid into patients with gout and interstitial disease elicits an abnormal increase in lead excretion, which suggests that heavy metal intoxication may be the primary event resulting in hypertension, interstitial disease, and hyperuricemia. Despite the clear associations between lead

intoxication and hyperuricemia, it is still controversial whether chronic hyperuricemia alone can lead to interstitial disease. Although underexcretion of uric acid is often clinically assumed to not be harmful to the kidney, this assumption may not be true. If hyperuricemia in chronic renal failure can accelerate disease progression, then it is an important metabolic abnormality to specifically treat.

Hypokalemic Nephropathy

Long-standing hypokalemia can cause chronic interstitial nephritis. There are both inherited and acquired forms of hypokalemic nephropathy. The inherited form is human leukocyte antigen linked and is characterized by primary renal wasting of K^+ and normal blood pressure, but elevated renin, aldosterone, and urinary prostaglandin E excretion. These patients have an interstitial nephritis with progressive renal failure. A pathologic characteristic of both the acquired and inherited forms of nephropathy is the finding of vacuoles in the proximal convoluted tubules, the composition of which is unknown. The cause of this condition may be hypokalemia that stimulates ammoniagenesis (because of the associated intracellular acidosis), which then elicits complement activation, initiating the influx of immune cells into the interstitium.

Oxaloses

Hyperoxaluria occurs in the setting of inborn errors of metabolism, increased bowel absorption or oxalate, or acute massive oxalate loads. Primary hyperoxaluria is due to a defect in either the 2-oxoglutarate: glyoxylate carboligase (type I) or the 2-glyceric dehydrogenase (type II). These patients develop chronic renal failure typically before reaching adulthood. Patients with inflammatory bowel disease or ileal-jejunal bypass surgery have increased bowel absorption of oxalate and can develop chronic renal insufficiency, which can be progressive. Ethylene glycol ingestion or ascorbic acid overdoses result in acute massive oxalate loads and acute renal failure associated with intrarenal obstruction by intratubular precipitation of oxalic acid crystals. In each setting the pathogenesis appears to be intraluminal obstruction by oxalate crystals, followed by progressive tubule atrophy and fibrosis.

Lead and Cadmium Nephropathy

See Chapter 16, Toxic Nephropathy.

Chinese Herb Nephropathy

See Chapter 16, Toxic Nephropathy.

Course and Therapy

Most forms of chronic interstitial nephritis cause slowly progressive renal functional deterioration. General therapeutic principles include treating the primary diseases and identifying and eliminating any exogenous agents (drugs or heavy metals) or conditions (obstruction or infection) associated with the chronic interstitial lesion. Other prudent maneuvers include good control of blood pressure (particularly angiotensin-converting enzyme inhibition) and treatment of electrolyte disturbances (particularly metabolic acidosis, hyperuricemia, and hyperphosphatemia). More specific therapies, such as chelation in lead nephropathy and corticosteroids in sarcoidosis, were discussed earlier. Many of the entities discussed in this chapter present with moderate to advanced renal failure and have no specific therapy.

Urinary Tract Infection, Pyelonephritis, and Reflux Nephropathy

13

BACTERIOLOGY OF URINARY TRACT INFECTION

General Considerations: The Urine Culture and Urinalysis

There is incomplete correlation between the clinical symptoms of urinary tract inflammation and the presence of true urinary tract infection (UTI), so objective evidence of the presence and the type of infection is of great importance.

Urine cultures with at least 10^5 colony-forming units (CFU)/mL of a bacterial species (often termed *significant bacteriuria*) have a high probability of indicating true infection; those with lesser numbers of CFUs (*insignificant bacteriuria*) probably reflect contamination. However, women who present with symptoms of acute, uncomplicated UTI are thought to have true infection when at least 10^3 CFU/mL of a single species of uropathogen are found on quantitative culture. In patients with symptoms of acute pyelonephritis (fever, rigors, and flank pain, with or without dysuria or frequency), the cutoff is at least 10^4 CFU/mL. Circumstances associated with lower densities of bacteria in the urine when the patient has true infection include acute urethral syndrome, infection with *Staphylococcus saprophyticus* and *Candida* species, prior administration of antimicrobial therapy, rapid diuresis, extreme acidification of the urine, obstruction of the urinary tract, and extraluminal infection. Polymicrobial UTI is uncommon and is observed in only a few clinical situations: long-term urinary catheterization or inadequate emptying of the bladder, particularly when repeated instrumentation is necessary or when there is a fistulous communication between the urinary tract and the gastrointestinal or female genital tracts.

Outside of these clinical scenarios, the isolation of two or more bacterial species on urine culture usually signifies a contaminated specimen.

Examination of the urine for leukocytes is another validation test that can be applied in the evaluation of patients with possible UTI. When a randomly collected urine sample is examined in a hemocytometer and at least 10 leukocytes/mm^3 are found, there is a high probability of clinical infection. Most symptomatic women with pyuria without significant bacteriuria have a UTI with either bacterial uropathogens present in colony counts of less than 10^5 CFU/mL (which will respond to appropriate antimicrobial therapy) or associated with some other condition. Possibilities include *Chlamydia trachomatis* infection, interstitial cystitis, genitourinary tuberculosis, and contiguous infection resting on the ureter or bladder and inducing "sympathetic inflammation" in the urine. In patients with indwelling urinary catheters, the finding of pyuria does not necessarily indicate infection.

Etiologic Agents

Bacterial Pathogens

- Enterobacteriaceae (including *Escherichia coli* and *Escherichia faecalis*) account for more than 95% of UTIs.
- Previous antimicrobial therapy, instrumentation, and urinary obstruction favor other organisms including *Serratia marcescens* and *Pseudomonas aeruginosa*.
- *S saprophyticus* is an important cause of symptomatic UTI in young, sexually active women.
- In contrast, the organisms that commonly colonize the distal urethra and skin of both men and women and the vagina of women rarely cause UTI (*Staphylococcus epidermidis*, corynebacteria, lactobacilli, and *Gardnerella vaginalis*).
- The kidney is the most common extrapulmonary site of tuberculosis; the tubercle bacilli reach the kidney from the lung by the hematogenous route.

Fungal Pathogens

- *Candida* species are the most common cause of fungal infection of the urinary tract. Most such infections occur in patients with indwelling Foley catheters who have been receiving broad-spectrum antibacterial therapy, particularly if diabetes mellitus is also present or corticosteroids are being administered.

Other Pathogens

- *C trachomatis* has been clearly shown to be an important cause of the acute urethral syndrome.

- *Ureaplasma urealyticum* also causes a significant number of cases of urethritis (albeit fewer than *C trachomatis*).

Pathogenesis

Two potential main routes of infection occur:

- *Ascending infection.* Most infections of the kidney result from the inoculation of bacteria derived from the gastrointestinal tract into the urethra, from there to the bladder, and finally to the kidney. The most common mechanism for introducing bacteria into the bladder in women is through sexual intercourse, particularly if intercourse is coupled with the presence of virulent bacteria in the vagina. The normal bladder is capable of clearing itself of organisms within 2 to 3 days by simple voiding. Clinically, clearing of bacteriuria does not occur in the presence of inadequate bladder emptying, foreign bodies or stones in the bladder, increased vesical pressure, or previous inflammation of the bladder mucosa.
- *Hematogenous seeding of the kidney as a consequence of bloodstream infection (<3% of patients).* The spectrum of organisms responsible differs from that seen in ascending infection and includes *Staphylococcus aureus*, *Salmonella species*, *P aeruginosa*, and *Candida*.

Host Factors Influencing Infection

Risk factors for development of a UTI include the following:

- Urinary tract obstruction
- Vesicoureteric reflux (VUR)
- Instrumentation of the urinary tract (including catheterization)
- Pregnancy
- Diabetes mellitus
- Nephrolithiasis
- Neurologic disorders with bladder involvement

Vesicoureteral Reflux
An important host defense against ascending infection from the bladder to the kidneys is the competency of the vesicoureteral valve. Indeed, the combination of VUR and infected urine is the most common factor predisposing to chronic pyelonephritic scarring, particularly in infants and children. Failure of this vesicoureteric valve mechanism is most commonly due to shortening of the intravesical portion of the ureter caused by abnormal lateral localization of the ureteral orifices (primary VUR).

In children, VUR may also be secondary, occurring in association with other anomalies including meningomyelocele, paraurethral diverticulum, posterior urethral valves, ureteral duplications, hypospadias, and ureteroceles. VUR occurs in 18% of adults who have spinal cord injuries and in a variable percentage of adults with bladder tumors, prostatic hypertrophy, and urinary tract stones.

The severity of VUR, which can be unilateral or bilateral, may vary considerably. The severity of reflux is graded as follows:

- Grade I: Reflux partly up the ureter
- Grade II: Reflux up to the pelvis and calices without dilation; normal caliceal fornices
- Grade III: Same as grade II, but with mild or moderate dilation and tortuosity of the ureter and no blunting of the fornices
- Grade IV: Moderate dilation and tortuosity of the ureters, pelvis, and calices; complete blunting of fornices
- Grade V: Gross dilation and tortuosity of the ureter, pelvis, and calices; absent papillary impressions in the calices

The clinical significance of VUR is emphasized by the fact that 30% to 50% of children with recurrent infection and 85% to 100% of children and 50% of adults with chronic pyelonephritic scarring demonstrate VUR on cystography. Progressive renal scarring typically appears in the more severe forms of reflux and almost always in the presence of infected urine. It must be stressed, however, that in many infants and children with VUR, pyelonephritic scarring never develops, and VUR may disappear either spontaneously or with antibacterial therapy in up to 80% of ureters after long-term follow-up. Even severe reflux associated with scarring may disappear, although reflux is more likely to cease if it is mild or moderate and if the kidneys are unscarred.

Intrarenal Reflux
Whereas VUR is responsible for the ascent of bacteria into the renal pelvis, considerable evidence now suggests that the spread of infection from the pelvis into the cortex occurs because of a phenomenon known as *intrarenal reflux*. In this setting contrast medium instilled into the bladder during voiding cystourethrography permeates the renal parenchyma as far as the renal capsule. VUR and intrarenal reflux, in combination, are almost certainly the major mechanisms responsible for the renal inflammation and scarring characteristic of chronic pyelonephritis. Scarring appears to occur early in life, possibly even in utero. Indeed, the development of new scars in children is unusual beyond the age of 5 years (and possibly the age of 2 years), regardless of proven episodes of UTI, suggesting that the early detection of

UTI and the gross forms of VUR is essential if renal scarring is to be prevented.

NATURAL HISTORY OF BACTERIURIA AND PYELONEPHRITIS

Frequency and Epidemiology of Urinary Tract Infection

UTI is predominantly a female disease. Among adult women, the incidence and prevalence of bacteriuria are related to age, degree of sexual activity, and form of contraception used. There is an incomplete correlation between the presence of bacteriuria and the occurrence of clinical symptoms. Dysuria occurs each year in approximately 20% of women between the ages of 24 and 64 years. Of those seeking medical care, one third have the acute urethral syndrome, and two thirds have a UTI. As the aging process progresses and prostatic disease becomes more common, the frequency of UTI in men rises dramatically. By age 70, the frequency of bacteriuria reaches a level of 3.5% in otherwise healthy men and a level of greater than 15% in hospitalized men. Other populations at high risk of UTI include pregnant women and renal transplant recipients (see Chapter 17, The Kidney and Hypertension in Pregnancy and Chapter 40, Clinical Aspects of Renal Transplantation).

Clinical Impact of Urinary Tract Infection

Urinary Tract Infection, Renal Failure, and Hypertension
There is little evidence that uncomplicated UTI beginning in adult life, by itself, leads to progressive chronic renal injury. In contrast to the experience in adults, bacteriuria may have a significant impact in children. As discussed in detail earlier, the combination of VUR and UTI in children younger than 5 years of age can have potentially disastrous consequences and may be resolved by early recognition and prolonged therapy with prophylactic antibiotic regimens.

CLINICAL PRESENTATIONS

In dealing with the patient who presents with possible UTI, the tasks of the clinician are the following:

1. To define the microbial etiologic agent causing the symptoms and the ideal form of antimicrobial management.

2. To make a judgment as to the anatomic site of infection within the urinary tract.
3. To ascertain the risk of complicating structural or functional disease of the urinary tract that might alter clinical management and, when indicated, carry out diagnostic tests such as cystoscopy, voiding cystourethrography, ultrasonography, radioscintigraphy, or excretory urography.

Acute Urinary Tract Infection

Acute Uncomplicated Cystitis

By far the most common clinical symptoms associated with UTI that cause patients to seek medical attention are those referable to the lower urinary tract: dysuria, frequency, nocturia, and suprapubic discomfort. Approximately 10% to 20% of women of reproductive age seek medical attention each year for these symptoms. Of these, two thirds have significant bacteriuria, whereas one third (those with the acute urethral syndrome) do not. Of the patients with significant bacteriuria, 50% to 70% have infection restricted to the bladder, but the remainder have covert infection of the upper urinary tract as well. Women with the acute urethral syndrome can be divided into two groups. Approximately 70% have pyuria on urinalysis and have true infection. For the most part these patients have infection with *C trachomatis* or with the usual bacterial uropathogens (e.g., *E coli* or *S saprophyticus*) but in less than significant numbers (10^2 to 10^4/mL). The remaining 30% of patients with the acute urethral syndrome, but no pyuria, have no known microbial etiologic agent for their symptoms. Presumably, these symptoms result from trauma related to intercourse, local irritation, or allergy.

Recurrent Cystitis

Recurrent symptoms of lower urinary tract inflammation may be due to either relapsing infection or reinfection. Relapse is caused by reappearance of the same organism from a sequestered focus, usually within the kidney in women or the prostate in men, shortly after completion of therapy. In reinfection, the course of therapy has successfully eradicated the original infection, and there is no sequestered focus, but organisms are reintroduced from the fecal reservoir. More than 80% of all recurrences are due to reinfection. The most important cause of recurrent symptoms of lower urinary tract inflammation in adult men is prostatitis. Acute bacterial prostatitis is a febrile illness associated with chills; perineal, back, or pelvic pain; dysuria; and urinary frequency and urgency. Bladder outlet obstruction may be present; on physical examination, the prostate is enlarged, tender, and indurated. Chronic prostatitis, in contrast, may be more occult; asymptomatic infection is manifested as recurrent bacteriuria or variable low-grade fever with back or pelvic discomfort. Urinary symptoms are usually due to reintroduction of infection into the bladder from a chronic prostatic focus that has been inadequately treated and only temporarily suppressed by a previous course of antimicrobial therapy.

Acute Pyelonephritis
The clinical findings associated with full-blown acute pyelonephritis are familiar: rigors, fever, back and loin pain (with exquisite tenderness or percussion of the costovertebral angle), often with colicky abdominal pain, nausea and vomiting, dysuria, frequency, and nocturia. Although bacteremia may complicate the course of symptomatic pyelonephritis in any patient, it is seldom associated with septic shock. When shock or disseminated intravascular coagulation occurs in the setting of pyelonephritis, the possibility of complicating obstruction must be ruled out. In one particularly important form of obstructive uropathy, which is associated with acute papillary necrosis, the sloughed papilla may obstruct the ureter. This form of obstruction should be particularly suspected in diabetic patients with severe pyelonephritis and high-grade bacteremia, especially if the response to therapy is delayed. In children younger than 2 years of age, fever, vomiting, nonspecific abdominal complaints, or failure to thrive may be the only manifestation of acute pyelonephritis. In older children, clinical manifestations resemble more closely those seen in adults, although the reappearance of enuresis may be a marker for the decreased urinary concentrating ability that is sometimes associated with renal infection.

Complicated Urinary Tract Infection
The term *complicated UTI* encompasses a wide range of clinical syndromes. The common element is the presence of bacterial infection of the urinary tract in patients with structurally or functionally abnormal urinary tracts, intrinsic renal disease, or a systemic process that renders the patient particularly susceptible to bacterial invasion. The range of organisms causing such infections is far broader than that noted for uncomplicated infection, and the level of antibiotic resistance of these bacteria is also greater than that seen in isolates from the general population. Because the therapeutic requirements and management strategies for complicated UTI are different from those for uncomplicated infection (discussed later), this differentiation is clinically important.

Chronic Pyelonephritis and Reflux Nephropathy

Unlike the dramatic clinical presentation of many patients with acute pyelonephritis, chronic disease typically has a more insidious course. Clinical signs and symptoms may be divided into two categories: (1) those related directly to infection and (2) those related to the degree and the location of injury within the kidney. Surprisingly, the infectious aspects of the disease may be minor. Although intermittent episodes of full-blown pyelonephritis may occur, these are the exception. More common is asymptomatic bacteriuria, symptoms referable to the lower urinary tract (dysuria and frequency), vague complaints of flank or abdominal discomfort, and intermittent low-grade fevers. Much more striking than the infectious or inflammatory symptoms are the physiologic derangements that result from the long-standing tubulointerstitial injury. These derangements include hypertension, an inability to conserve Na^+, decreased concentrating ability, and a tendency to develop hyperkalemia and acidosis. Although all of these are seen to some extent in all forms of renal disease, in patients with tubulointerstitial nephropathy such as this, the degree of physiologic derangement is out of proportion to the degree of renal failure (or serum creatinine level elevation).

The diagnosis of chronic pyelonephritis is based either on pathologic findings or on specific radiologic findings seen with excretory urography. Radiologic features include focal, coarse cortical scarring with underlying retraction of the papillae and blunting and dilation of the calices. Scars are most commonly observed in the upper and lower poles. The laboratory findings are as nonspecific as the clinical findings. Although pyuria is usually present, it may be absent, particularly if no active infection is present. Less common is the presence of white blood cell casts on urinalysis. Bacteriuria may or may not be demonstrable. Proteinuria is typically less than 1 g/day of protein.

DIAGNOSTIC EVALUATION

History and Physical Examination

When a patient with a single acute episode of symptomatic UTI is examined, the first consideration is whether there are signs or symptoms suggesting the presence or imminent development of systemic sepsis: spiking fevers, rigors, tachypnea, colicky abdominal pain, and exquisite loin pain. Such patients require immediate attention and parenteral therapy in a hospital setting. If the patient does not exhibit acute sepsis, attention turns to concerns such as a previous history of UTIs, renal disease, and conditions such as diabetes mellitus, neurologic conditions, a history of renal stones, and previous genitourinary tract manipulation—conditions that could predispose to UTI and could affect the efficacy of therapy. A careful neurologic examination can be particularly important in suggesting the possibility of a neurogenic bladder.

The patient with a history of recurrent UTIs merits special attention in terms of obtaining a clear history of sexual activity, response to therapy, and temporal relationships of recurrences to the cessation of therapy. Thus, women with recurrent bacterial UTIs temporally related to intercourse could benefit from the administration of antibiotics after each sexual exposure. In the woman with the acute urethral syndrome due to *C trachomatis* infection, UTI may respond only temporarily to antichlamydial therapy, because of reinfection from the untreated sexual partner; cure occurs when both individuals are treated simultaneously.

Women with recurrent UTIs who have relapsing infection usually present within 4 to 7 days of completing a course of therapy of 14 days or less, whereas those with recurrent reinfection usually have a longer interval between episodes unless bladder dysfunction or some other disturbance of urinary tract function is present. Similarly, men with persistent prostatic foci of infection often have a relapse promptly after a similar conventional course of therapy. When the patient with possible chronic pyelonephritis and reflux nephropathy is examined, two types of information should be sought: the history of UTI in childhood and during pregnancy, and the possible presence of pathophysiologic consequences such as hypertension, proteinuria, polyuria, nocturia, and frequency.

Urine Tests

Dipstick Tests

The most commonly used dipstick test is the Griess nitrate reduction test, which depends on the bacterial reduction of nitrate in the urine to nitrite. This test is most accurate on first-morning urine specimens and is reasonably effective in identifying infection due to Enterobacteriaceae but fails to detect infection due to gram-positive organisms and *Pseudomonas*. False-negative results may also be caused by diuresis, because bladder incubation is necessary for bacteria to reduce nitrates. Because of its simplicity, this test is best used as part of a home or epidemiologic screening program, particularly if multiple specimens can be evaluated from a single individual. The combination of the nitrate test with a test for leukocyte esterase on a single, inexpensive dipstick that can be read in less than 2 minutes has greatly increased the utility of this approach. False-negative test results can be caused by proteinuria and the presence of gentamicin or cephalexin in the urine.

Dip-Slide Methods

A variety of dip-slide methods in which plastic paddles with agar on their surfaces are immersed in the urine, drained, and incubated are available. An agar medium selective for gram-negative organisms (e.g., MacConkey agar) is usually present on one side of the paddle or slide, and a nonselective medium that supports the growth of most bacterial species, including gram-positive organisms, is present on the other side. After overnight incubation, the numbers of colonies on both agar surfaces are then compared with standardized pictures of inoculated dip-slides to achieve a semiquantitative estimation of the number of organisms present. Positive slides can then be sent to a reference laboratory for species identification and antibiotic susceptibility testing. The technique is useful for office or home screening.

Radiologic and Urologic Evaluations

The primary objective of radiologic and urologic evaluations in UTI is to delineate abnormalities that would lead to changes in the medical or surgical management of the patient.

1. An ultrasound study is indicated to rule out obstruction in patients requiring hospital admission for bacteremic pyelonephritis. Patients with septic shock require such procedures on an emergency basis because these patients often cannot be effectively resuscitated unless their "pus under pressure" is relieved by some form of drainage procedure that bypasses the obstruction.
2. Children with first or second UTIs, particularly those younger than 5 years of age, should undergo both excretory urography and voiding cystourethrography for detection of obstruction, VUR, and renal scarring. Dimercaptosuccinic acid scanning is a sensitive technique for detecting scars, and serial studies can be useful in assessing the course of scarring and the success of preventive regimens. However, this approach does not delineate anomalies in the pyelocaliceal system or the ureters. The aim of this imaging effort in children is to identify those who might benefit from intensive medical evaluation, particularly prolonged antimicrobial prophylaxis. Because active infection by itself can produce VUR, it is usually recommended that the

radiologic procedures be delayed until 4 to 8 weeks after the eradication of infection, although some groups perform these studies as early as 1 week after infection.

3. Most men with bacterial UTI have some anatomic abnormality of the urinary tract, most commonly bladder neck obstruction resulting from prostatic enlargement. Therefore, anatomic investigation, starting with a good prostatic examination and then proceeding to excretory urography or urinary tract ultrasound studies with postvoiding views, should be performed in all male patients with UTI.

4. Routine anatomic evaluation of all women with recurrent UTIs is not recommended. Characteristics of women who might benefit from anatomic studies include patients whose UTI fails to respond to appropriate antimicrobial therapy or those who have a rapid relapse after such therapy; patients with continuing hematuria; patients with infection with urea-splitting bacteria; patients with symptoms of continuing inflammation, such as night sweats; and patients with symptoms of possible obstruction, such as back or pelvic pain that persists despite adequate antimicrobial therapy.

TREATMENT

Acute Uncomplicated Cystitis in Young Women

The treatment of choice is short-course therapy with trimethoprim-sulfamethoxazole or a fluoroquinolone, both of which are superior to β-lactam drugs in the treatment of UTI. The antibacterial spectrum of activity of these drugs is such that the normal anaerobic and microaerophilic vaginal flora, which provide colonization resistance against the major uropathogens, are left intact. In contrast, β-lactam drugs, such as amoxicillin, appear to promote vaginal colonization with uropathogenic *E coli*. Unfortunately, antimicrobial resistance has increased significantly since the early 1990s, particularly to trimethoprim-sulfamethoxazole. There is wide variation in different geographic areas in terms of the incidence of bacterial resistance to trimethoprim-sulfamethoxazole, and the prescribing physician is obligated to obtain such information for his or her community of practice. If the incidence is higher than 20%, then it is recommended that a fluoroquinolone be prescribed as the drug of choice.

A 3-day course of therapy is superior to a single dose with either trimethoprim-sulfamethoxazole or a fluoroquinolone. Early recurrence is significantly more common with single-dose therapy.

Short-course therapy should therefore never be given to women who fall into the following categories: patients with overt pyelonephritis; patients with symptoms of longer than 7 days' duration; patients with underlying structural or functional defects of the urinary system; immunosuppressed individuals; patients with indwelling catheters; and patients with a high probability of infection with antibiotic-resistant organisms. Because acute uncomplicated UTI in otherwise healthy women is so common, the range of organisms causing the infection is so well defined, their antimicrobial susceptibility is so uniform, and the efficacy and lack of side effects of short-course therapy are now so well established, a cost-effective approach that minimizes both laboratory studies and the need for visits to the physician is widely used (Fig. 13–1).

Recurrent Urinary Tract Infection in Young Women

Before the physician embarks on an antimicrobial approach to prevent reinfection, simple interventions for the woman such as voiding immediately after sexual intercourse and switching from a diaphragm and spermicide-based contraceptive strategy to some other approach should be implemented. If these measures are not effective, then other preventive regimens can be considered. The most popular prophylactic regimen currently used in women susceptible to recurrent UTI is low-dose trimethoprim-sulfamethoxazole; as little as half a tablet (trimethoprim, 40 mg; sulfamethoxazole, 200 mg) three times weekly at bedtime is associated with an infection frequency of less than 0.2 per patient-year. Another option is the use of a fluoroquinolone. A variation of these efficacious continuous prophylaxis programs is to use a fluoroquinolone or trimethoprim-sulfamethoxazole as postcoital prophylaxis. An important unanswered question is the duration of prophylactic therapy against recurrent UTI: One option is to continue therapy for 6 months and then to discontinue it. If infection then recurs, prophylaxis can be reinstituted for periods of 1 to 2 years or longer. Because of concerns about adverse effects, compliance, and cost in the long-term prophylaxis of recurrent UTI, another approach is to provide women having histories of recurrent infections with a supply of trimethoprim-sulfamethoxazole and a fluoroquinolone. The patient is then instructed to initiate single-dose therapy with the onset of symptoms; further medical attention is sought only when the symptoms do not abate or the number of treated episodes exceeds four in a 6-month period.

The approach to the minority of patients with relapsing infection is different. Two factors may contribute to the pathogenesis of

WOMEN WHO PRESENT WITH COMPLAINTS
OF DYSURIA AND FREQUENCY

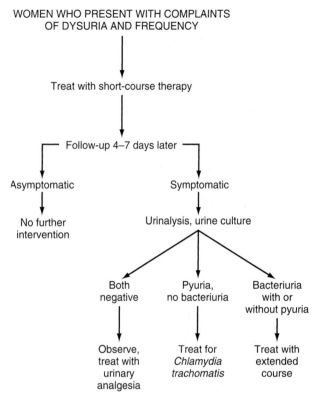

Figure 13–1. Clinical approach to the woman with dysuria and frequency. (Modified from Tolkoff-Rubin NE, Wilson ME, Zuromskis P, et al: Single-dose amoxicillin therapy of acute uncomplicated urinary tract infections in women. *Antimicrob Agents Chemother* 25:626, 1984.)

relapsing infection in women: (1) deep tissue infection of the kidney that is suppressed but not eradicated by a 14-day course of antibiotics; and (2) a structural abnormality of the urinary tract (e.g., calculi). UTIs in at least some of these patients respond to a 6-week course of therapy. Most true relapses occur within 1 week of the cessation of antimicrobial therapy, and virtually all occur within 1 month, so information concerning the timing of the recurrences can be helpful in establishing the diagnosis. Knowledge of the bacterial species isolated and the antibiotic susceptibility pattern of the species can help in deciding whether it is the same organism or one different from the original pathogen. The response to short-course therapy in such women is helpful in making the management decision: if the UTI responds to short-course therapy, it is likely that the patient has been having recurrent reinfection and is thus a candidate for long-term prophylaxis; if the UTI does not respond to short-course therapy, it is probable that the patient has been having relapsing infection and is thus a candidate for imaging of the renal tract and an intensive course of prolonged therapy.

Acute Uncomplicated Cystitis in Older Women

Whereas symptoms referable to the lower urinary tract in younger women are almost invariably due to uropathogens and *C trachomatis* (see earlier), other possibilities exist in older women. In particular, in symptomatic women with pyuria and negative culture results, the possibility of genitourinary tuberculosis and diverticulitis or a diverticular abscess impinging on the bladder or ureters should be considered, rather than chlamydial infection, which represents a major cause of such infections in younger women. The antimicrobial strategies discussed before for the management of acute cystitis in younger women are applicable in postmenopausal women as well. In addition, however, other interventions have an important role in this population. Several studies have now shown that estrogen replacement therapy, either locally by use of a vaginal cream or systemically with oral therapy, restores the atrophic genitourinary tract mucosa of the postmenopausal woman and is associated with a reappearance of lactobacilli in the vaginal flora, a fall in vaginal pH, and decreases in vaginal colonization by Enterobacteriaceae. In addition, regular intake of cranberry juice significantly reduces the occurrence of both bacteriuria and pyuria in elderly women.

Acute Uncomplicated Pyelonephritis in Women

There are three goals in the antimicrobial therapy of symptomatic pyelonephritis: control or prevention of the development of urosepsis, eradication of the invading organism, and prevention of recurrences. Use of ampicillin, amoxicillin, or first-generation cephalosporins as the initial therapy for pyelonephritis is not recommended when the nature and the susceptibility of the infecting organism are unknown because 20% to 30% of isolates are now resistant to these drugs. If possible, a Gram stain of the urine should be performed to establish whether gram-positive cocci are present or if that information is not available, the initial therapy should include intravenous ampicillin (or vancomycin) plus gentamicin to provide adequate coverage for both enterococci and the more common gram-negative uropathogens. If only gram-negative bacilli are present, there are a large number of choices, ranging from parenteral trimethoprim-sulfamethoxazole and fluoroquinolones to gentamicin; broad-spectrum cephalosporins such as ceftriaxone, aztreonam, and the β-lactam–β-lactamase inhibitor combinations; and imipenem-cilastatin. In general, the last agents on the list are reserved for patients with more complicated histories, previous episodes of pyelonephritis, and recent urinary tract manipulations. Initial control with any effective parenteral regimen, followed by oral trimethoprim-sulfamethoxazole or fluoroquinolone for eradication, is the cornerstone of the therapeutic strategy. In patients with milder disease, who are free of nausea and vomiting, advantage can be taken of the excellent antimicrobial spectrum and bioavailability of drugs such as trimethoprim-sulfamethoxazole and the fluoroquinolones to prescribe oral therapy for the entire therapeutic course. Once the patient has been afebrile for 24 hours (usually within 72 hours of initiation of therapy), there is no inherent benefit to maintaining parenteral therapy.

Urinary Tract Infection in Pregnancy

See Chapter 17, The Kidney and Hypertension in Pregnancy.

Urinary Tract Infections in Men

UTI is uncommon in men younger than 50 years of age, although UTI without associated urologic abnormalities can occur under the following circumstances: in homosexual men, in men having intercourse with women colonized with uropathogens, and in men with the acquired immunodeficiency syndrome. Such individuals should never be treated with short-course therapy; rather, 10- to 14-day regimens of trimethoprim-sulfamethoxazole or a fluoroquinolone should be regarded as standard therapy unless antimicrobial intolerance or an unusual pathogen requires an alternative approach. In men older than 50 years of age with UTIs, tissue invasion of the prostate, the kidneys, or both should be assumed, even in the absence of overt signs of infection at these sites. Because of the inflammation usually present, acute bacterial prostatitis initially responds well to the same array of antimicrobial agents used to treat UTIs in other populations. However, after a conventional course of therapy of 10 to 14 days, relapse is common. It is now recognized that intensive therapy for at least 4 to 6 weeks and as many as 12 weeks is required to sterilize the urinary tract in many of these men. The drugs of choice for this purpose, assuming that the invading organisms are susceptible, are trimethoprim-sulfamethoxazole, trimethoprim (in the individual allergic to sulfonamides), and the fluoroquinolones. Prolonged treatment with each of these has a greater than 60% chance of eradicating infection. When relapse occurs, a choice then has to be made among three therapeutic approaches: (1) long-term antimicrobial suppression, (2) repeated treatment courses for each relapse, and (3) surgical removal of the infected prostate gland under coverage of systemic antimicrobial therapy. The choice from among these approaches depends on the age, sexual activity, and general condition of the patient; the degree of bladder outlet obstruction present; and the level of suspicion that prostate cancer could be present. In addition to the usual uropathogens that cause a UTI in men, one additional entity merits attention. After instrumentation of the urinary tract, most commonly after repeated insertion of a Foley catheter, infection with *S aureus* may occur; the use of antistaphylococcal therapy and the removal of the foreign body are required for cure.

Treatment of Childhood Urinary Tract Infection

The treatment of full-blown pyelonephritis in the child is similar to that in the adult: broad-spectrum parenteral therapy until the antimicrobial susceptibility pattern of the infecting organism is known, followed by narrow-spectrum, least-toxic therapy parenterally until the patient is afebrile for 24 to 48 hours. A prolonged 1- to 3-month course of oral therapy is then instituted. Follow-up urine cultures within a week of completion of therapy and at frequent intervals for the next year are indicated. In children with acute, uncomplicated UTI, conventional 7- to 14-day regimens are appropriate, although many UTIs respond to short-course therapy. The one major difference in the approach to children as opposed to that in adults is that fluoroquinolones are not used in children because of possible adverse effects on developing cartilage. Recurrent UTIs in children, particularly in those with renal scarring or demonstrable VUR, is dealt with by long-term prophylaxis with agents such as trimethoprim-sulfamethoxazole (2 mg/kg per dose once or twice per day of the trimethoprim component, which gives 10 mg/kg per dose of the sulfamethoxazole component), nitrofurantoin (2 mg/kg/day as single dose), or methenamine mandelate (50 mg/kg/day in three divided doses). Sulfonamides are less effective because of the emergence of resistance. An auxiliary intervention that can be effective in some children with recurrent UTI is the aggressive treatment of constipation, particularly if this is present in conjunction with urinary incontinence. Results of trials comparing medical therapy with surgical correction of VUR in children have failed to show significant benefit from the surgical approach in terms of renal function, progressive scarring, or renal growth, despite the fact that the technical aspects of the surgical repair could be accomplished satisfactorily. As a result, current views are to aggressively prevent scarring with prolonged antimicrobial therapy and close monitoring as primary therapy. Surgical correction is reserved for the child who, in a 2- to 4-year period, appears to not be showing a response to medical therapy.

Complicated Urinary Tract Infection

The term *complicated UTI,* by its nature, encompasses infections in a heterogeneous group of patients with a wide variety of structural and functional abnormalities of the urinary tract and kidney. Therapy should be targeted primarily to symptomatic UTIs because there is little evidence to show that treatment of asymptomatic bacteriuria in this population of patients either alters the clinical condition of the patient or is likely to be successful. The one exception to this rule is if the asymptomatic patient is scheduled for instrumentation of the urinary tract. In this instance, sterilization of the urine before manipulation and continuation of antimicrobial therapy for 3 to 7 days after manipulation can prevent serious morbidity and even mortality from urosepsis. Because of the broad range of infecting pathogens and their varying sensitivity patterns, culture data are essential in prescribing therapy for symptomatic patients. If therapy is needed before such information is available, the initial therapy must encompass a far broader spectrum than that for other groups of patients. Thus, in a patient with apparent pyelonephritis or urosepsis in a complicated setting, initial therapy with regimens such as ampicillin plus gentamicin, imipenem-cilastatin, and piperacillin-tazobactam is indicated. In the patient who is more subacutely ill, trimethoprim-sulfamethoxazole or a fluoroquinolone appears to be a reasonable first choice.

Every effort should be made to correct the underlying complicating factor, whenever possible, in conjunction with the antimicrobial therapy. If this is possible, a prolonged 4- to 6-week "curative" course of therapy in conjunction with the surgical manipulation is appropriate. If such correction is not possible, shorter courses of therapy (7 to 14 days), targeted to control symptoms, appear to be more appropriate. For patients with frequent symptomatic relapses, long-term suppressive therapy should be considered. A particular subgroup of patients susceptible to complicated UTI are those with neurogenic bladders resulting from spinal cord injury. In these patients, intermittent self-catheterization with clean catheters and methenamine prophylaxis have been shown to decrease the morbidity associated with UTI.

Catheter-Associated Urinary Tract Infection

Infections of the urinary tract are by far the most common cause of hospital-acquired infection. Approximately 2% to 4% of these patients develop gram-negative sepsis, and such events can contribute to the mortality of patients. Although bacteriuria is inevitable with long-term catheterization, certain guidelines can be used to delay the onset of such infections and to minimize the rate of acquisition of antibiotic-resistant pathogens. Critically important in this regard are sterile insertion and care of the catheter, use of a closed drainage system, and prompt removal. Isolation of patients with catheter-associated bacteriuria from other patients with indwelling bladder catheters will also decrease the spread of infection. Whether techniques such as the use of silver ion–coated catheters, the use of disinfectants in collecting bags, and other local strategies offer additional benefit is still unclear, although topical meatal care with povidone-iodine may be especially useful. Systemic antimicrobial therapy can delay the onset of bacteriuria and can be useful in clinical situations in which the time of catheterization is clearly limited (e.g., in association with gynecologic or vascular surgery and kidney transplantation). Treatment of catheter-associated UTI requires good clinical judgment. In any patient who is symptomatic from the infection, immediate therapy with effective antibiotics is indicated, with the use of the same antimicrobial strategies described before for other forms of complicated UTI. In an asymptomatic patient, no therapy is indicated. Patients with long-term indwelling catheters rarely become symptomatic unless the catheter is obstructed or is eroding through the bladder mucosa. In patients who do become symptomatic, antibiotics should be given, and close attention should be focused on changing the catheter or changing the type of urinary drainage.

Candidal Infection of the Urinary Tract

Clear-cut guidelines for the treatment of candidal infection of the urinary tract are not available. The following approaches are ones we currently advocate:

1. In patients with catheter-associated candidal UTI, we remove the preceding catheter, insert a three-way catheter, and infuse an amphotericin rinse for a period of 3 to 5 days These measures appear to eradicate the infection with a greater than 75% success rate. Success is increased if contributing factors such as hyperglycemia, corticosteroid use, and antibacterial therapy can be eliminated.
2. In patients with candiduria without an indwelling catheter, our preference is to use fluconazole, 200 to 400 mg/day for 10 to 14 days.
3. Any patient with candiduria who is to undergo instrumentation of the urinary tract, we administer systemic therapy with amphotericin or fluconazole to prevent the consequences of transient candidemia.

SPECIAL FORMS OF PYELONEPHRITIS

Xanthogranulomatous Pyelonephritis

Xanthogranulomatous pyelonephritis is an uncommon form of chronic bacterial pyelonephritis characterized by the destruction of renal parenchyma and the presence of granulomas, abscesses, and collections of lipid-filled macrophages. Women are affected more often than men (2:1), and the lesions typically affect only one kidney. Most patients present with renal pain, recurrent UTI, fever (of undetermined nature), malaise, anorexia, weight loss, and constipation. Most patients have a history of previous calculous disease, obstructive uropathy, or diabetes mellitus, and 38% have undergone urologic procedures. The diagnosis of xanthogranulomatous pyelonephritis should be considered in patients with a history of chronic infection and certain radiologic features including unilateral renal enlargement, a nonfunctioning kidney as seen on an intravenous urogram, the presence of renal calculi, angiographic demonstration of an avascular mass or masses with stretched attenuated intrarenal vessels, and an irregular impaired nephrogram with prominent avascular areas. Bacterial cultures of the urine are almost invariably positive, and *Proteus mirabilis* and *E coli* are the organisms most commonly cultured. The pathogenesis of xanthogranulomatous pyelonephritis is unclear, although it seems certain that the condition is caused by bacterial infection and accentuated by urinary obstruction. Most kidneys with xan-thogranulomatous pyelonephritis are removed surgically, largely because a correct preoperative diagnosis is rarely made, but studies suggest that diagnosis by a combination of clinical and radiologic features is possible in 40% of patients.

Malakoplakia

Malakoplakia is a rare, histologically distinct inflammatory reaction usually caused by enteric bacteria and affecting many organs but most commonly the urinary tract. In most patients, the condition is confined to the urinary bladder mucosa, where it appears as soft, yellow, slightly raised, often confluent plaques 3 to 4 cm in diameter. It is most common in middle-aged women with chronic UTI. Renal malakoplakia occurs in the same clinical setting as xanthogranulomatous pyelonephritis—chronic infection and obstruction—and there is considerable overlap in the gross histologic features of both conditions. *E coli* is the most common organism cultured from urine. Clinical findings usually include flank pain and signs of active renal infection. Bilateral involvement has been reported, as has a clinical presentation simulating acute renal failure. The pathogenesis of malakoplakia is unclear, but about one half of cases are associated with immunodeficiency or autoimmune disorders, including hypogammaglobulinemia.

Disorders of the Renal Arteries and Veins

14

This chapter focuses on (1) acute thrombosis of the renal artery, (2) thromboembolism of the renal arteries, (3) renal artery aneurysms, (4) dissecting aneurysms of the renal artery, and (5) acute and chronic renal vein thrombosis. Other conditions, such as atheroembolic renal disease and causes of renovascular hypertension are considered in Chapter 15, Microvascular Diseases of the Kidney, and Chapter 25, Renovascular Hypertension and Ischemic Nephropathy, respectively.

ACUTE OCCLUSION OF THE RENAL ARTERY

Traumatic Renal Artery Thrombosis

Blunt abdominal trauma is a major cause of acute renal artery thrombosis. The main renal artery, renal vein, or branch vessels may be injured in trauma, resulting in lacerations, contusions, or thrombosis. Thrombosis, the most common injury, is usually unilateral and more commonly left-sided, but it may be bilateral and occurs in 1% to 3% of patients with severe blunt abdominal trauma. The major concern with acute thrombosis is severe renal ischemia and the rapid progression to renal infarction. Common clinical signs and symptoms associated with renal artery thrombosis include flank and abdominal pain, nausea, vomiting, and fever. The finding of anuria should raise the suspicion of bilateral thrombosis or thrombosis of a solitary functioning kidney. Gross or microscopic hematuria is common but may be absent in one fourth of patients, and mild proteinuria is often present. Marked elevations of lactate dehydrogenase may be noted. Serum aspartate aminotransferase and alanine aminotransferase levels may be increased, but not to the same extent as the lactate dehydrogenase level.

A rapid diagnosis is critical, and spiral computed tomography (CT) with contrast is the preferred diagnostic study. The key findings of main renal artery thrombosis are the absence of renal parenchymal enhancement with contrast material (CT nephrogram) and the lack of contrast material excretion (CT pyelogram). In some patients, enhancement of the peripheral renal cortex ("cortical rim sign") may be seen, which is presumably the result of capsular or collateral perfusion to the cortex. If the diagnosis is uncertain, renal angiography can provide the definitive diagnosis.

Nontraumatic Renal Artery Thrombosis

Nontraumatic renal artery thrombosis occurs rarely. Thrombosis of preexisting atherosclerotic plaques is the most common setting for arterial thrombosis. Inherited disorders of the anticoagulant pathways (e.g., factor V Leiden mutation) do not appear to play a major role in the formation of arterial thrombosis. However, renal artery thrombosis has been described in the acquired hypercoagulable states such as the antiphospholipid syndrome and in heparin-induced thrombocytopenia. Acute renal artery occlusion in renal allografts due to technical failure of the anastomosis usually occurs within several weeks after surgery, with consequent graft loss.

Thromboembolism of the Renal Artery

Thromboemboli to the renal arteries usually originate from the heart. Various cardiac diseases and arrhythmias, in particular atrial fibrillation, are associated with thromboemboli. The risk of renal artery thromboembolism is relatively low with only approximately 2% of peripheral thromboemboli involving the renal arteries.

Clinical Features of Renal Artery Thrombosis and Thromboembolism

The clinical features of renal artery occlusion are varied and depend on the size and extent of the thrombosis or emboli. Bilateral artery occlusion or occlusion in a solitary functioning kidney would be more likely to produce acute renal failure and anuria than would a unilateral embolism with a normal contralateral kidney. Patients commonly experience some degree of abdominal or flank pain, often with nausea and vomiting. The pain is often dull and unrelenting, but it may be absent, particularly with small infarcts. Gross hematuria may be present. Some patients may have had prior embolic events in one or both kidneys or in other organs. Abdominal or flank tenderness is usually present on physical examination, and signs of peritoneal irritation may be noted. Fever is common, and chills may occur. Hypertension can be severe, and it is the prominent clinical problem in some patients. Other organs, especially the brain or extremities, should be evaluated for signs of arterial embolization. Cardiac arrhythmias, particularly atrial fibrillation, the presence of valvular disease, or a recent myocardial infarction, should alert the clinician to the possibility of a cardiac source for the emboli.

Early diagnosis of acute arterial occlusion is often difficult, because the initial diagnostic considerations are usually focused on other, more common, diseases such as nephrolithiasis, pyelonephritis, acute myocardial infarction, acute cholecystitis, and acute tubular necrosis. A common laboratory abnormality is an elevated lactate dehydrogenase concentration, which may rise to 2000 international units/L with large infarctions. Most patients have microscopic hematuria and mild proteinuria. Leukocytosis may develop.

A rapid diagnosis is critical if acute intervention with thrombolysis or surgery is contemplated in the hope of preserving renal function. Spiral CT with contrast can furnish a rapid and accurate diagnosis and is considered the best initial test. Ultrasound of the renal vessels using doppler techniques is of limited value because it is technically difficult to visualize the entire renal arteries. Magnetic resonance angiography can show sharp images of the renal arteries and renal perfusion abnormalities, and has the added benefit of avoiding the risk of contrast nephropathy. Renal arteriography, the gold standard study, is the definitive method for diagnosis of renal artery occlusion and has the added advantage that thrombolysis can be administered right away if a thrombosis or embolus is found.

Therapy for Acute Occlusive Renal Arterial Disease

The duration of warm ischemic time, the degree of occlusion (complete or partial), and the size of the occluded artery or arteries (main, branch, or interlobar) are all factors determining whether renal function can be preserved through an intervention. The ischemic time is a crucial factor; most successful outcomes have occurred with a presumed renal ischemic time of less than 12 hours. In patients with a unilateral thrombosis and a functional contralateral kidney, the outcomes with surgery may not be better than those with observation and medical management, so the indication for surgery in this setting is uncertain. Surgical outcomes for preserving renal function in acute nontraumatic obstructions are mixed, and if intervention is considered necessary intra-arterial thrombolysis is preferable because of lower patient mortality rates. Either therapy is probably futile if complete occlusion of the renal artery has been present for a prolonged period.

RENAL ARTERY ANEURYSMS

Renal artery aneurysms (RAAs) are uncommon in the general population ($\approx 0.01\%$). In patients undergoing renal arteriography for the evaluation of renovascular hypertension, the incidence is as high as 1%. Many RAAs remain asymptomatic. However, the clinical concerns with RAAs are their potential to rupture, thrombose, cause distal embolization, or lead to renovascular hypertension. They may be located anywhere along the vascular tree, but most of them are found at the bifurcation of the renal artery or in the first-order branch arteries. Concomitant aortic, splenic, or mesenteric aneurysms are observed in 5% to 10% of patients. The primary cause may be a congenital weakness in the internal elastic lamina of the artery, although this is uncertain. Fusiform aneurysms are often seen in medial fibromuscular dysplasia. RAAs have also been described in polyarteritis nodosa, Takayasu arteritis, Ehlers-Danlos syndrome, and mycotic aneurysms.

Clinical Manifestations of Renal Artery Aneurysms

Most RAAs are asymptomatic; they are typically diagnosed as part of a workup for renovascular hypertension. Occasionally, such patients have flank pain. Acute onset or worsening flank pain should raise the concern of an expanding aneurysm, rupture and hemorrhage, thrombosis or thromboemboli with impending renal infarction, or dissection. A patient with rupture of an RAA, a potentially catastrophic event, may present with vascular collapse and hemorrhagic shock. Pregnant women make up a disproportionate number of those with RAA rupture. Emergency nephrectomy is usually required in this setting to control the hemorrhage.

Aneurysms larger than 4 cm in diameter should be electively resected, whereas those less than 2 cm in diameter can be safely followed with periodic imaging studies. There is uncertainty about mid-sized aneurysms, those between 2.1 and 4 cm. Indications for resection of aneurysms of less than 4 cm include significant expansion seen in any aneurysm during follow-up imaging studies, abdominal or flank pain, aneurysms of any size in young women of child-bearing age, an aneurysm to a solitary kidney, and renovascular hypertension, particularly with lateralization of renal renin levels. Given the technically demanding nature of RAA surgery, this intervention should be performed by surgeons with demonstrated expertise in renal artery reconstructive procedures. Catheter-based interventions of stent grafts and embolization techniques using microcoils and Gelfoam have been used to treat saccular or distal branch RAAs as an alternative to surgery.

Dissecting Aneurysms of the Renal Artery

Dissecting aneurysms of the renal artery are uncommon. Acute dissections may manifest in an explosive manner, with malignant hypertension, flank pain, and renal infarction. Chronic dissection most commonly manifests as renovascular hypertension. Acute dissection can occur spontaneously, and it can be precipitated by strenuous physical activity or trauma. Fibromuscular dysplasia and atherosclerosis are common predisposing factors that lead to intimal tears, medial necrosis of the artery wall, and dissection. Iatrogenic dissection due to angiographic procedures may occur from trauma induced by guide wires, catheters, or angioplasty balloons.

Symptoms include new-onset, accelerated, or worsening hypertension. Flank pain is common, and headache may occur, perhaps as a result of hypertension. In some cases, especially with lesions that develop from an angiographic procedure, the patient may be asymptomatic. Selective angiography is necessary for the diagnosis. Dissection on arteriography appears as an abrupt narrowing of the arterial lumen which is caused by the unfilled false lumen. The clinical outcome is varied. Some patients have persistent severe renovascular hypertension that may be resistant to medical therapy. These patients may benefit from revascularization (surgical/endovascular) or nephrectomy.

RENAL VEIN THROMBOSIS

Renal vein thrombosis (RVT) may be caused by trauma or tumor; however, it occurs most commonly in nephrotic patients, in whom the incidence has been reported to be as high as 40%. The most common underlying nephropathy associated with RVT is membranous nephropathy. An important factor in the causation of RVT in patients with the nephrotic syndrome is the presence of a hypercoagulable state. The use of oral contraceptives has also been implicated as an occasional cause of RVT. Dehydration has been clearly associated with RVT in infants. Most of these infants do not have the nephrotic syndrome or even significant proteinuria. This syndrome develops initially in the clinical setting of diarrhea, vomiting, and shock. Oliguria and hematuria rapidly ensue. Acute RVT may also occur in a newly transplanted kidney because of technical problems with the anastomosis. Patients with chronic thrombosis are usually asymptomatic, but patients with acute thrombosis may present with signs of renal infarction including costovertebral pain, fever, and gross hematuria. On occasion, acute RVT is bilateral, resulting in marked oliguric acute renal failure and flank pain.

Diagnosis

Inferior venacavography with selective catheterization of the renal vein establishes the diagnosis of RVT. Other diagnostic approaches include helical CT scanning, magnetic resonance venography, or duplex ultrasonography. A high incidence of false-negative findings in the diagnosis of RVT is seen with Doppler ultrasonography. Magnetic resonance venography is the procedure of choice for the noninvasive evaluation of acute RVT and offers the advantage of not requiring the use of intravenous contrast material.

Clinical Course and Treatment

The experience to date on the course, prognosis, and treatment of RVT in nephrotic patients is limited. However, small retrospective studies have suggested a high mortality with many patients succumbing to thromboembolic complications. Convincing evidence suggests that anticoagulant therapy reduces the incidence of new thromboembolic episodes and often reverses the deterioration of renal function that occurs with acute RVT. Heparin is the initial therapy of choice. In patients with a large renal vein thrombus and pulmonary embolism, the clearance of heparin is increased; and such patients may need higher doses of heparin in the early stages of therapy. Warfarin therapy is instituted after the patient has received satisfactorily anticoagulation therapy and is continued for as long as the patient remains nephrotic. The safety and efficacy of thrombolytic therapy have not been established.

Microvascular Diseases of the Kidney

15

HEMOLYTIC-UREMIC SYNDROME AND THROMBOTIC THROMBOCYTOPENIC PURPURA

The hemolytic-uremic syndrome (HUS) and thrombotic thrombocytopenic purpura (TTP) are closely related diseases characterized by microangiopathic hemolytic anemia with multiorgan dysfunction. A thrombotic microangiopathy is the underlying pathologic lesion in both syndromes. The diagnosis of HUS is made when renal failure is a predominant feature of the syndrome, as is common in children. When neurologic impairment predominates, the syndrome is then often referred to as TTP. Recent studies suggest that TTP and HUS may now be distinguished by measuring the plasma von Willebrand factor (VWF)–cleaving metalloproteinase activity, which has been shown to be deficient in most patients with TTP but not in those with HUS. However, in clinical terms many cases of TTP and HUS are still not easily distinguished; therefore, the broader term HUS/TTP remains in use.

Clinical Features

The diagnosis of HUS/TTP should be considered if the following clinical findings are present:

- Microangiopathic hemolytic anemia
- Thrombocytopenic purpura
- Acute renal failure
- Fever
- Neurologic symptoms

TTP is usually a sporadic disease, with an incidence of approximately 1 per 1 million persons per annum. It is more common in women (female-to-male ratio, 3:2 to 5:2) and although the peak incidence is in the third and fourth decade of life, TTP can affect any age-group. It is often accompanied by nonspecific constitutional symptoms, such as malaise, nausea, and vomiting. Neurologic symptoms are common at presentation (>85%) and include headache, altered mental status, paresis, aphasia, dysphasia, paresthesias, visual problems, seizures, and coma. Fever is an almost universal symptom. Renal involvement in TTP (>80%) is usually mild but can range from abnormal urinalysis to severe renal insufficiency that requires dialysis therapy. In HUS, hemolytic anemia and renal involvement are uniformly present. Acute renal failure is detected in 90% of patients, and neurologic symptoms occur less commonly than in TTP. Gastrointestinal prodromes (vomiting, diarrhea, and abdominal pain) typically occur a few days to weeks before disease onset. This is characteristically a disease of young children, and both sporadic and epidemic forms of HUS occur. The epidemic form is the typical presentation and is characteristically preceded by a diarrheal illness. Additional clinical findings in either TTP or HUS result from microvascular thromboses in the intestines, pancreas, skeletal muscle, and heart (intestinal perforation, pancreatitis, rhabdomyolysis, and congestive heart failure).

Laboratory Findings

The hallmark laboratory finding, essential for the diagnosis of HUS/TTP, is a microangiopathic hemolytic anemia. The laboratory findings include the following:

- Schistocytes on the peripheral smear (burr cells, helmet cells, and other fragments)
- Anemia (hemoglobin levels are < 6.5 mg/dL in 40% of patients)
- Reticulocytosis
- Elevated lactate dehydrogenase/low haptoglobin level
- Negative Coombs test results
- Thrombocytopenia (usually <60,000/mm^3)

Moderate leukocytosis may accompany the hemolytic anemia, but white cell counts rarely exceed 20,000/mm^3. In contrast to disseminated intravascular coagulation, the prothrombin time, partial thromboplastin time, fibrinogen level, and coagulation factors are normal.

Renal Involvement

Evidence of renal involvement is present in most patients with HUS/TTP. Microscopic hematuria and subnephrotic proteinuria are the most consistent findings. Male sex, hypertension, prolonged anuria, and hemoglobin levels greater than 10 g/L at onset are associated with a higher risk of renal sequelae in children. More than 90% of patients with HUS have significant renal failure at presentation, and one third of these are anuric. Dialysis is required for a large percentage of these patients. The mean duration of renal failure is 2 weeks. Severe acute renal failure or anuria occurs in fewer than 10% of patients with classic TTP.

Etiology

Although the etiologic mechanisms in HUS/TTP are not completely defined, the available data suggest that environmental factors (e.g., infection, drugs, and toxins), combined with a genetic predisposition in some patients, are responsible for initiation of thrombotic microangiopathy. The link between bacterial toxins and HUS offers the strongest etiologic evidence. Epidemiologic and laboratory data suggest that bacterial cytotoxins may be causative agents in HUS. Outbreaks of hemorrhagic colitis in children have led to the identification of a verotoxin-producing strain of *Escherichia coli* (serotype O157:H7) as a pathogenetic factor. Strong epidemiologic evidence links this strain to sporadic cases and outbreaks of HUS. Transmission of *E coli* O157:H7 appears to be caused by contaminated food, such as ground beef and other cattle products. Less commonly, HUS is associated with gastrointestinal and respiratory infections caused by other cytotoxin-producing bacteria, such as *Shigella dysenteriae* type I, *Salmonella typhi*, *Campylobacter jejuni*, and *Streptococcus pneumoniae*.

Drug-induced HUS/TTP is also well recognized. It is most commonly diagnosed in patients receiving chemotherapeutic agents (Table 15–1). Thrombotic microangiopathy, unrelated to chemotherapy, has been described in conjunction with acute promyelocytic leukemia and prostatic, gastric, and pancreatic carcinomas. The antiplatelet agents ticlopidine and clopidogrel have also been associated with the disease. In renal allograft recipients, calcineurin-induced HUS may occur during the first weeks after transplantation and reverses with the cessation of the calcineurin inhibitor (cyclosporine and FK506). HUS/TTP may occur after bone marrow transplantation independent of prior radiation or cyclosporine therapy. Other drugs and toxins less commonly associated with HUS/TTP are listed in Table 15–1. The association between HUS/TTP and pregnancy is also well recognized. Neurologic involvement predominates in the prepartum form, whereas severe renal failure is more typical in postpartum HUS/TTP. This condition differs from preeclampsia

Table 15–1: Hemolytic-Uremic Syndrome Thrombotic Thrombocytopenic Purpura: Causes and Associations

Infectious agents

Bacteria
   Escherichia coli O157:H7 (verotoxin-producing)
   Shigella dysenteriae type
   Salmonella typhi
   Streptococcus pneumoniae
   Campylobacter jejuni
   Yersinia pseudotuberculosis
   Pseudomonas species
   Bacteroides
   Mycobacterium tuberculosis

Viruses
   Togavirus (rubella)
   Coxsackievirus
   Echoviruses
   Influenza virus
   Epstein-Barr virus
   Rotaviruses
   Cytomegalovirus
   Human immunodeficiency virus

Drugs

Immunosuppressants
   Cyclosporine and FK-506
   OKT3

Chemotherapeutic agents
   Mitomycin C
   Cisplatin
   Daunorubicin
   Cytosine arabinoside
   Gemcitabine

Others
   Oral contraceptives
   Ticlopidine
   Clopidogrel

Pregnancy
   Prepartum or postpartum

Others
   Malignant neoplasm
   Transplantation
   Systemic lupus erythematosus
   Polyarteritis nodosa
   Primary glomerulopathies

in that consumptive coagulopathy is present in severe preeclampsia but is characteristically absent in HUS/TTP. A hereditary form of recurrent HUS/TTP related to a genetic deficiency of factor H, a regulatory protein of the alternative complement pathway, leading to low levels of complement C3, has been described.

Patients with TTP have very large circulating polymers of VWF in both the serum and fibrin deposits. A protease (ADAMTS13) responsible for cleavage of VWF multimers has been found to be deficient in patients with chronic relapsing TTP. Linkage studies have identified multiple mutations in the gene encoding ADAMTS13 located on chromosome 9 in patients with recurrent or familial TTP. Other investigators have demonstrated that patients with sporadic acute TTP have an acquired deficiency of VWF-cleaving protease activity related to the presence of immunoglobulin G autoantibodies directed against components of the enzyme that result in its functional inactivation. The VWF-cleaving protease deficiency and the presence of circulating autoantibodies have also reported in patients who developed TTP after treatment with the antiplatelet drugs ticlopidine or clopidogrel. Inefficient clearance of VWF polymers due to either a congenital or acquired loss of activity may lead to platelet aggregation and subsequent microvascular thrombosis. The polymers are consumed during TTP relapse, so their levels decrease. In contrast, children with diarrhea-associated HUS typically demonstrate no abnormalities in VWF-cleaving protease activity.

Prognosis and Treatment

With appropriate supportive care the mortality rate of HUS/TTP is approximately 6% and 10% in children and adults, respectively. Clinical features predictive of a poor outcome include older age, high polymorphonuclear neutrophil count at presentation, oliguria, and renal dysfunction. Younger children who present with the "typical" diarrheal prodrome have a better prognosis than older children with HUS that is not heralded by diarrhea. Supportive therapy, including dialysis, antihypertensive medications, blood transfusions, and management of neurologic complications, contributes to the improved survival of patients with HUS/TTP. Adequate fluid balance and bowel rest are important in treating typical HUS associated with diarrhea. Antibiotics given to treat infection caused by *E coli* O157:H7 increase the risk of overt HUS by 17-fold, probably by favoring the acute release of large amounts of preformed toxin after the injury to the bacterial cell membrane or by giving a selective advantage to

E coli O157:H7. On the other hand, in developing countries where hemorrhagic colitis is precipitated by *S dysenteriae* type I, early and empiric antibiotic therapy has been shown to shorten the duration of diarrhea and decrease the incidence of complications and therefore should be started early, even before the involved pathogen is identified. Platelet transfusions are avoided because of the risk of precipitous worsening of the patient's clinical status. It is postulated that transfused platelets, in combination with high circulating levels of von Willebrand multimers, induce further organ damage.

Among the therapeutic modalities used to treat patients with TTP, plasma exchange (plasmapheresis combined with fresh-frozen plasma replacement) is currently the treatment of choice for sporadic TTP. The advantage of plasmapheresis is that it removes inhibitory autoantibodies against VWF protease from the circulation while simultaneously replacing the protease enzyme. A significant benefit is observed in adults with acute TTP with response rates of between 60% and 80%. Although some benefit has been observed with plasma infusion alone, plasma exchange is more effective than plasma infusion for treatment of TTP. Usually plasma exchange is performed once a day and replaces one plasma volume (40 mL/kg). For patients with a poor initial response to treatment, plasma exchange may be intensified by increasing the volume of plasma replaced or, preferably, by initiating twice-daily exchange to minimize recycling of infused plasma. Plasma exchange should be performed daily until remission is achieved, i.e., normalization of platelet count, resolution of neurologic symptoms, or both. Because 85% of children with HUS recover with supportive therapy alone, plasma exchange is generally reserved for patients with poor prognostic indicators, and even in these patients, any beneficial effect is open to question.

Patients with refractory TTP that does not respond to plasma exchange therapy may benefit from therapy with adjunctive immunosuppression. Treatment options in this setting include azathioprine and cyclophosphamide. Cyclosporine is generally avoided because of its association with HUS/TTP. Although platelet thrombi are invariably present in the thrombotic angiopathies, therapy with aspirin and dipyridamole has proven ineffective. Fibrinolytic therapy with either streptokinase or urokinase is ineffective and increases the risk of bleeding. The prognosis for patients with cancer- and/or chemotherapy-induced HUS/TTP is poor despite treatment, and the role of plasmapheresis remains undefined. With drug-induced HUS/TTP, removal of the individual agent is mandated. However, the role, if any, for plasma exchange remains unclear.

Severe renal insufficiency resulting from HUS/TTP often requires dialysis. Renal transplantation has also been performed, but HUS/TTP may recur in the renal allograft. Calcineurin-based immunosuppressive regimens after transplantation may increase the risk of recurrence of HUS after renal transplantation. With the advent of novel potent immunosuppressive agents such as antithymocyte globulin, mycophenolate mofetil, and rapamycin, calcineurin-independent regimens may offer a lower risk of disease recurrence.

SYSTEMIC SCLEROSIS

Clinical Features

Systemic sclerosis is a rare disease affecting predominantly women between 30 and 50 years of age. The overall annual incidence is unclear, and estimates range from 2 to 20 cases per 1 million. Involvement of the skin and subcutaneous tissue is the predominant feature of systemic sclerosis. In the diffuse cutaneous form of the disease, thickening of the skin is observed on the face, trunk, and distal and proximal extremities. This phase is followed by sclerosis, which leads to a taut, shiny appearance of the skin and tapering of the fingertips (sclerodactyly). Other extrarenal manifestations include the following:

- Raynaud phenomenon (>90%)
- Telangiectasias on the skin of the face and upper torso
- Arthralgias or arthritis in most patients
- Myopathy of the shoulder and pelvic girdle (20%)
- Esophageal hypomotility or diminished tone of the lower esophageal sphincter (75%)
- Diffuse pulmonary fibrosis (45%)
- Pericarditis (20%)
- Myocardial fibrosis leading to arrhythmia (40%)

Laboratory Findings

Of patients with systemic sclerosis, 70% have a positive antinuclear antibody titer (<1:16), typically in a speckled or nucleolar pattern. Antibodies to DNA topoisomerase I (anti-Scl-70) are more specific; however, they are found in only 30% of patients with diffuse cutaneous involvement and in only 15% of those with the limited form of the disease. Anticentromere antibodies are present in one half of patients, most of whom have limited systemic sclerosis. Approximately 30% of the patients have positive tests for rheumatoid factor. Antibodies to double-stranded DNA are rarely noted.

Renal Involvement

Kidney involvement in systemic sclerosis occurs in up to 80% of patients and manifests as one of two non-mutually exclusive presentations:

- Slowly progressive chronic renal disease
- Scleroderma renal crisis (SRC)

Clinical indicators of chronic renal involvement in systemic sclerosis include proteinuria (30%), hypertension (24%), and decreased glomerular filtration rate (25%). The proteinuria is usually subnephrotic and occurs in 15% to 36% of the patients. Renal manifestations rarely antedate the other features of systemic sclerosis. SRC is characterized by the sudden onset of accelerated or malignant arterial hypertension, followed by rapidly progressive oliguric renal failure and occurs in between 5% and 15% of patients. Patients with the diffuse cutaneous form have a much higher risk for development of SRC than those with limited cutaneous systemic sclerosis. The symptoms are malignant hypertension, severe headaches, blurring of vision, encephalopathy, convulsions, and acute left ventricular failure. Oliguric acute renal failure supervenes shortly thereafter. The urinalysis reveals microscopic hematuria, granular casts, and modest proteinuria. SRC usually progresses rapidly to severe renal failure that requires dialysis. Other clinical manifestations of SRC include microangiopathic hemolytic anemia resulting from malignant hypertension-induced endothelial injury. It is postulated that SRC is caused by severe vasospasm, leading to cortical ischemia and enhanced production of renin and angiotensin II, which in turn perpetuate renal vasoconstriction. The role of the renin-angiotensin system in perpetuating renal ischemia is underscored by the finding of markedly elevated plasma renin activity and the significant benefit produced by angiotensin-converting enzyme (ACE) inhibition (see later).

Pathogenesis

The pathogenesis of systemic sclerosis is poorly understood. Postulated mechanisms include abnormal vasomotor control, enhanced collagen production, immune-mediated injury, and primary endothelial abnormalities. Although several antinuclear autoantibodies have been detected in patients with systemic sclerosis, it is unclear whether these immunologic changes constitute primary events in systemic sclerosis or are epiphenomena.

Management of Renal Complications

ACE inhibition has revolutionized the management of SRC. One-year patient survival rates have improved from less than 20% to more than 70% with the advent of ACE inhibitor agents. Close monitoring of renal function is required, and administration of an additional antihypertensive agent may be required to effect adequate hypertensive control. Blood pressure should be lowered gradually (10 to 20 mm Hg/day) to avoid renal hypoperfusion and acute tubular necrosis. Diuretics should be avoided because of their ability to stimulate renin release. Both peritoneal dialysis and hemodialysis have been used in the management of end-stage renal disease (ESRD) in patients with systemic sclerosis. Occasionally recovery of renal function is observed even after prolonged renal replacement therapy. Evidence exists to suggest that aggressive use of ACE inhibitors improves the chances of a spontaneous recovery of renal function. Renal transplantation for SRC-induced ESRD has been successfully performed; however, graft survival rates may be lower than the normal. Recurrence of systemic sclerosis in the transplanted kidney has been documented.

ATHEROEMBOLIC RENAL DISEASE

Atheroembolic renal disease results from embolization of cholesterol crystals from atherosclerotic plaques present in large arteries to the smaller arteries of the renal vasculature. Atheroembolic renal disease is an increasingly common and often under diagnosed cause of renal insufficiency in elderly patients. Risk factors include a history of ischemic cardiovascular disease, older age, hypertension, and diabetes mellitus. Precipitating factors including vascular surgery, arteriography, angioplasty, anticoagulation with heparin, and thrombolytic therapy are identified in only 50% of patients.

Clinical Features

Clinical manifestations usually appear 1 to 14 days after an inciting event, but their onset can be delayed for weeks. Clinical manifestations include the following:

- Livedo reticularis, "purple" toes or toe gangrene (40% to 50%)
- Fever, myalgias, headaches, and weight loss (<50%)

- Abdominal pain (intestinal embolization)
- Transient cerebral ischemia
- Renal failure (50%)

Accelerated hypertension is the most common manifestation of renal involvement. Renal insufficiency is usually subacute and advances in a stepwise fashion over a period of several weeks, leading to dependence on dialysis in up to 40% of patients. Of these, a significant number regain independent renal function after variable periods of dialytic support. A high degree of suspicion is required to diagnose atheroembolic renal disease. The differential diagnosis includes radiocontrast nephropathy, systemic vasculitis, drug-induced interstitial nephritis, and renal artery thrombosis or thromboembolism. The time course of decline in renal function may aid in the diagnosis of atheroembolic renal disease. Renal failure due to procedure-induced atheroembolic renal disease is characterized by a decline in renal function over 3 to 8 weeks.

Radiocontrast material–induced nephropathy, conversely, usually manifests earlier and often resolves within 2 to 3 weeks after appropriate intervention. Histologic demonstration of cholesterol crystals in small arteries and arterioles of target organs is the most definitive method of diagnosing atheroembolic renal disease. Kidney, muscle, and skin biopsy specimens are the most likely to yield a positive diagnosis. The characteristic histologic finding is cholesterol "clefts" within the small arterioles.

Laboratory Features

Renal involvement in the cholesterol crystal embolization syndrome is manifested by the following:

- Increased serum creatinine and blood urea nitrogen levels
- FeNa$^+$ greater than 1%
- Increased ESR, leukocytosis, and anemia
- Transient eosinophilia (60% to 80%)
- Eosinophiluria (30%)
- Hypocomplementemia (40%)

Outcome

Atheroembolic renal disease is associated with high morbidity and mortality. The most significant morbidity associated with atheroembolic renal disease is severe renal insufficiency that requires dialysis. This occurs in approximately 40% of patients, only one half of whom recover sufficient renal function to regain independence from dialysis. Mortality is significantly higher in patients who develop ESRD (>50%).

Treatment

No effective therapy for atheroembolic renal disease has been reported. Use of anticoagulants should be avoided because of the risk of precipitating more atheroembolization. In fact, withdrawal of anticoagulation may be beneficial. Despite the high mortality and the absence of effective therapy, kidney function improves in a minority of patients even after prolonged periods of renal insufficiency. An aggressive therapeutic approach with patient-tailored supportive measures, including statin therapy, withdrawal of anticoagulants, postponement of aortic procedures, control of hypertension and heart failure, dialysis therapy, and adequate nutritional support may be associated with favorable clinical outcome.

RENAL INVOLVEMENT IN SICKLE CELL DISEASE

Clinical Manifestations

Sickle cell anemia and occasionally the heterozygous forms of sickle cell disease can lead to multiple renal abnormalities, which include tubular, medullary, and glomerular dysfunction or a combination thereof. Clinical manifestations include the following:

- Microscopic and/or gross hematuria (>50%)
- Renal papillary necrosis (15% to 36%)
- Proteinuria (26% to 40%)
- Nephrotic syndrome (3%)
- Polyuria
- Progressive renal failure (5%)

The onset of proteinuric progressive renal failure usually occurs after age 30. Progression to ESRD occurs within 2 years in 50% of these patients, and survival time is approximately 4 years, even with dialysis therapy. Acute or chronic deterioration in renal function may reflect concomitant infection, rhabdomyolysis, or less commonly renal vein thrombosis or intravascular hemolysis. Sickling in the medullary microcirculation causes chronic medullary ischemia, which is manifested as an inability to maximally concentrate the urine, and in an incomplete form of distal renal tubule acidosis. A highly aggressive form of renal cell carcinoma has been described in some patients with sickle cell disease.

Pathogenesis

Hb-SS polymer formation is promoted by higher degrees of deoxygenation, increased intracellular hemoglobin concentration, and the absence of hemoglobin F. The pathogenesis of medullary renal lesions in sickle cell disease is attributed largely to microvascular occlusion. Erythrocytes passing through the vessels of the inner renal medulla and the renal papillae are vulnerable to sickling because of relative hypoxia and the high osmolality of the blood, which leads to cell shrinkage and increased hemoglobin concentration. The pathogenesis of sickle cell glomerulopathy is generally attributed to secondary hyperfiltration.

Treatment

The management of patients with sickle cell disease is targeted to limiting sickle cell crises and end-organ damage. Factors that trigger sickling, such as infection and dehydration, should be treated aggressively. Exposure to hypoxia, cold, or medications that may induce sickle cell crisis should be avoided. Treatment options include transfusion therapy and, more recently, bone marrow transplantation. Hydroxyurea increases the hemoglobin F concentration, which results in a more than 40% reduction in the median annual rate of pain crises. However, it is not known whether a reduction in the frequency of sickle cell crises translates to a lower incidence of renal disease. ACE inhibitors should be used in the presence of proteinuric renal insufficiency to retard disease progression. Patients with sickle cell disease who develop ESRD have a 60% survival rate at 2 years after the initiation of renal replacement therapy. Dialysis is the most common form of renal replacement therapy used. Kidney transplantation has been performed in small numbers of patients. One-year survival rates are broadly comparable with those for other causes of ESRD, but there is a trend toward lower allograft survival thereafter. Nevertheless, patient survival appears better with renal transplantation compared with maintenance hemodialysis.

Toxic Nephropathy | *16*

The kidney is particularly vulnerable to nephrotoxic renal injury by virtue of its rich blood supply (25% of cardiac output) and its ability to concentrate toxins to high levels within the medullary interstitium and the renal epithelial cells.

ANTIBACTERIAL AGENTS

Aminoglycoside Antibiotics

Aminoglycosides are valuable agents for the treatment of serious gram-negative infections. Nephrotoxicity is the major side effect of this group of antibiotics. Nonoliguric acute tubular necrosis complicates 10% to 30% of treatment courses of aminoglycoside antibiotics, even when blood levels are maintained within the therapeutic range. This figure increases to almost 50% with 14 days or more of therapy.

Clinical Features
- Nonoliguric acute renal failure (ARF)
- Onset in the second week of therapy (earlier with concomitant nephrotoxic insults)
- Slow recovery of function (6 to 8 weeks for full recovery)
- Direct tubular injury resulting in glucosuria, low-grade proteinuria, hypomagnesemia, hypocalcemia, and hypokalemia
- Risk factors including volume depletion, sepsis, hypokalemia, advanced age, concomitant administration of other nephrotoxins, and a multiple versus a single daily dosing schedule

Prevention
It is appropriate to think of aminoglycosides as being nephrotoxic in all patients who receive them. In most patients the nephrotoxicity is subclinical and is not detected by routine monitoring of serum creatinine levels. When aminoglycoside therapy

is empirically begun for an infection in a patient with presumed sepsis or other serious infection, therapy should be changed to a less toxic agent when culture results are available. Indeed, a "clinical response" in the absence of positive cultures is not usually sufficient justification for prolonged treatment with an empirically started aminoglycoside. In the attempt to minimize clinical nephrotoxicity, several points should be emphasized:

- Aminoglycoside nephrotoxicity is more common when large doses of aminoglycosides are given over prolonged periods.
- Peak and trough aminoglycoside blood levels are not reliable predictors of aminoglycoside nephrotoxicity.
- Aminoglycoside nephrotoxicity is more common when usual doses are given to individuals with renal impairment. Nomograms and formulas designed to estimate the aminoglycoside dosage in patients with renal failure reduce the number of treatment failures, but their use *does not* reduce the incidence of nephrotoxicity.
- In clinical practice once-daily aminoglycoside dosing schedules have clinical efficacy, and toxicity may be reduced.
- Concomitant administration of other nephrotoxins (radiographic contrast material, amphotericin, cisplatin, and diuretics) should be avoided.
- Extracellular fluid volume should be optimized during aminoglycoside therapy.

Penicillins and Cephalosporins

True nephrotoxic reactions with penicillins and cephalosporins are rare. More often, acute interstitial nephritis is the cause of altered renal function with these agents.

Vancomycin

Vancomycin is valuable for the treatment of gram-positive infections, particularly methicillin-resistant staphylococcal infections, *Staphylococcus epidermidis* infections, and *Clostridium difficile* diarrhea. The early formulations of this drug had a substantial nephrotoxic potential, but with current preparations, the incidence of nephrotoxicity is reported to be as low as 5%. Vancomycin may have a synergistic nephrotoxic effect with aminoglycoside antibiotics.

Sulfonamides

Most cases of sulfonamide-induced renal disease represent acute interstitial nephritis. However, in the presence of an acid urine (pH < 5.5), several of these agents are capable of tubular precipitation, causing an acute obstructive nephropathy, particularly when used in high dosage. Renal failure can be prevented by increasing fluid intake during therapy and by maintaining an alkaline urine, which increases the solubility of these drugs in the urine.

Amphotericin

ARF is common in patients who receive prolonged courses of amphotericin B and is almost inevitable when the cumulative dose reaches 1 g. The mechanism by which renal injury occurs involves both direct tubular injury and renal vasoconstriction. The clinical presentation is nonoliguric ARF, which is often preceded or accompanied by biochemical evidence of distal tubular injury. This is characterized clinically by the following:

- Loss of urinary concentration ability (polyuria/hypernatremia)
- Distal hypokalemic renal tubule acidosis (normal anion gap metabolic acidosis)
- Wasting of potassium and magnesium (hypomagnesemia and relative hypokalemia)

Fortunately, azotemia is rarely severe and is usually reversible with discontinuation of therapy. Risk factors for nephrotoxicity include volume depletion, renal impairment, and concomitant nephrotoxin administration. The role of salt depletion had led to the common practice of saline loading before and during drug administration. Newer preparations, including liposome-encapsulated amphotericin B and lipid complex formulations of the drug may have less nephrotoxic potential.

ANTIVIRAL AND ANTIPROTOZOAL AGENTS

Acyclovir

Acyclovir is excreted by the kidney and has a low solubility in urine. Given by the intravenous route in high doses (500 mg/m^2), it may cause nonoliguric ARF as a result of intratubular precipitation, leading to tubular obstruction. Clinical signs of nephrotoxicity include nausea, flank pain, and hematuria. Urinalysis may show needle-shaped crystals under polarizing light. Management requires volume expansion, withdrawal of therapy, and occasionally hemodialysis. Nephrotoxicity may be prevented by vigorous hydration before and during infusion.

Pentamidine

Intravenous pentamidine, commonly used to treat *Pneumocystis carinii* pneumonia, is associated with nephrotoxicity in 25% to 65% of patients. Analogous to that seen with aminoglycoside antibiotics, renal accumulation of pentamidine occurs after multiple dose administration. Hypocalcemia, hypomagnesemia, and hyperkalemia occur with prolonged therapy. Nephrotoxicity is enhanced by concomitant amphotericin B administration.

Foscarnet

Foscarnet is a pyrophosphate analog, which is used intravenously in the management of cytomegalovirus infections in immunocompromised patients. The kidney is the primary route of elimination, and nephrotoxicity occurs in up to two thirds of patients. The rise in plasma creatinine concentration is usually delayed until the second week of therapy. Polyuria and polydipsia are common due to interference with the action of antidiuretic hormone, and isolated nephrogenic diabetes insipidus has been reported. As with most tubular toxins the risk of renal injury is increased by concomitant administration of other nephrotoxins. The risk of nephrotoxicity can be reduced by concomitant administration of saline.

Antiretroviral Therapy

Indinavir
Indinavir can trigger crystalluria and nephrolithiasis due to the precipitation of indinavir monohydrate in the tubules. Asymptomatic crystalluria occurs in approximately 4% to 10% of treated patients. Fewer than 5% of patients develop symptoms of loin pain and hematuria.

Adefovir
Adefovir is a nucleoside reverse transcriptase inhibitor that is excreted unchanged in the urine. It mediates proximal tubular injury characterized by phosphaturia, low-grade proteinuria, and ARF. Discontinuation of therapy usually results in recovery of renal function.

RADIOCONTRAST AGENTS

Radiocontrast agent–induced nephrotoxicity is a common cause of hospital-acquired ARF. The incidence of nephrotoxicity varies, depending on the underlying risk factors and ranges from approximately 2% in normal individuals up to 40% in patients with established diabetic nephropathy. Risk factors for the development of contrast nephropathy are as follows:

- Renal insufficiency
- Volume depletion
- Congestive heart failure
- High-dose contrast studies (>125 mL)
- Diabetes mellitus/liver disease/multiple myeloma
- Coadministration of other nephrotoxins

Clinical Features

Renal failure may be oliguric or nonoliguric, the latter being common in patients with near-normal prior renal function. Most episodes of contrast nephrotoxicity are mild, and creatinine levels usually peak after 3 to 5 days and return to the normal range within 5 to 7 days. Patients usually present with a benign urine sediment, concentrated urine, and low fractional excretion of Na^+ and thus have many features of prerenal azotemia; however, in severe cases there may be evidence of tubule cell injury. The differential diagnosis includes atheroembolic renal disease and renal infarction (e.g., aortic dissection).

Prevention

Approaches to the prevention of radiocontrast nephropathy include the following:

- Volume expansion (1 mL/kg of 0.45% N-saline for 12 hours before and after procedures)
- Minimization of contrast material load and avoidance of early repeat studies
- Low or isosmolal agents in "high-risk" patients
- N-Acetylcysteine (400 mg orally twice a day) in "high-risk" patients

Of all of these interventions, the avoidance of volume depletion is the most critical. There is no compelling evidence suggesting a role for prophylactic hemofiltration or hemodialysis at this time.

DRUGS USED IN TRANSPLANTATION

Cyclosporine and FK-506

See Chapter 40, Clinical Aspects of Renal Transplantation.

ANTINEOPLASTIC DRUGS

Many chemotherapeutic drugs, effective in the management of solid organ and hematopoietic malignancies, are associated with a substantial risk of nephrotoxicity (Table 16–1).

Table 16–1: Chemotherapy-Related Nephrotoxicity

Agent	Reported Toxicity
Alkylating agents	
Cisplatin	Tubulointerstitial nephritis (TIN) occasionally irreversible; often acute renal failure (ATN)
Carboplatin	Less nephrotoxic than cisplatin; can cause acute renal failure secondary to TIN
Cyclophosphamide	Associated with hyponatremia; also causes hemorrhagic cystitis
Streptozocin	Nitrosourea compound; renal dysfunction in 65% of patients; acute renal failure secondary to TIN
Semustine, carmustine	Nitrosourea compounds that can lead to chronic deterioration in renal function 3 years after therapy; semustine is more nephrotoxic than carmustine
Ifosfamide	Nephrogenic diabetes insipidus and direct toxic injury to proximal and distal tubule
Antibiotics	
Mitomycin C	Hemolytic-uremic syndrome
Plicamycin	Nephrotoxic injury in as many as 40% of patients with long-term treatment; causes proximal and distal tubule damage
Antimetabolites	
Methotrexate	Volume expansion reduces nephrotoxic risk; intratubule deposition of 7-hydroxymethotrexate, a factor in toxicity; also causes direct tubule damage; associated with nonoliguric acute renal failure
Cytarabine	Associated with TIN
6-Thioguanine	Parenteral administration and high doses associated with azotemia and acute renal failure syndrome
5-Fluorouracil	Associated with acute renal failure, often in combination with other drugs; less nephrotoxic than methotrexate
Interleukin-2	High doses cause acute renal failure in $\approx 90\%$; avoid use with nonsteroidal anti-inflammatory drugs

Cisplatin

Cisplatin (*cis*-diamminedichloroplatinum) is a highly effective antineoplastic agent in testicular, ovarian, small cell of the lung, head, neck, and bladder cancers. Nephrotoxicity is a major complication of cisplatin therapy, occurring in up to 25% of patients receiving first courses of cisplatin. The incidence rises thereafter with repeated courses of the drug. An unusual feature of cisplatin nephrotoxicity compared with that for most pharmacologic nephrotoxic agents is that in many patients, the renal damage is irreversible.

Clinical Features

The usual pattern of cisplatin nephrotoxicity is a dose-related and cumulative form of renal failure noted after one or more doses of the drug. The clinical features of cisplatin nephrotoxicity include the following:

- Nonoliguric ARF
- Isosthenuria
- Hypophosphatemia
- Hypomagnesemia and relative hypokalemia
- Modest proteinuria (<1 g/day)

The renal magnesium wasting state associated with cisplatin may be severe and may be accompanied by hypocalcemia and tetany. The peak incidence of hypomagnesemia occurs after 3 weeks of therapy and is exacerbated by the concomitant use of other drugs, particularly aminoglycoside antibiotics.

The following points are important in the prevention of cisplatin nephrotoxicity:

- Concomitant use of other nephrotoxins should be avoided.
- Doses of cisplatin exceeding 25 to 33 mg/m^2/wk predispose to nephrotoxicity.
- A urine output of at least 100 mL/hr for several hours before and after a dose of cisplatin reduces the incidence of nephrotoxicity. The administration of cisplatin in hypertonic saline may also lower the risk of nephrotoxicity.
- Amifostine, an organic thiophosphate, has been demonstrated to ameliorate cisplatin nephrotoxicity in patients with solid organ or hematologic malignancies.
- New platinum compounds, including carboplatin, may have less significantly nephrotoxicity.

Cyclophosphamide

The primary renal side effect of cyclophosphamide therapy is hyponatremia, which has been observed with doses greater than 50 mg/kg. This effect is dissipated approximately 24 hours after the drug has been discontinued and is caused via a direct antidiuretic effect in the distal nephron and not through increased levels of vasopressin.

Semustine

Semustine is lipid soluble and therefore has been used as a chemotherapeutic agent in the treatment of malignant brain tumors because it crosses the blood-brain barrier easily. High-dose therapy (1500 mg/m^2) in children with brain tumors resulted in a pattern of insidious renal failure, leading to renal insufficiency some 3 to 5 years after the onset of therapy. Doses greater than 1400 mg/m^2 for therapy of malignant melanoma in adults have resulted in chronic interstitial nephritis.

Ifosfamide

The incidence of clinical nephrotoxicity is believed to be less than 10%, but some instances of irreversible renal failure have been noted. Ifosfamide mediates proximal tubular injury that is associated with the development of Fanconi syndrome. Patients with preexisting renal dysfunction may be more vulnerable to the nephrotoxic effects of ifosfamide. Nephrogenic diabetes insipidus has also been linked to therapy with ifosfamide.

Mitomycin C

Administration of mitomycin C is associated with the development of a microangiopathic hemolytic anemia. The pathogenesis probably involves direct endothelial injury, and this complication has also been associated with other chemotherapeutic agents, including bleomycin, 5-fluorouracil, and gemcitabine. Management of this complication is largely supportive and involves removal of the offending agent.

Methotrexate

ARF is usually observed in the setting of high-dose intravenous methotrexate administration used in autologous bone marrow transplantation protocols. High-dose therapy given without concomitant volume expansion or urinary alkalinization is associated with nephrotoxicity in at least 10% of treated patients. The clinical course of methotrexate toxicity is usually nonoliguric renal failure. It is important to recognize this early because any reduction in glomerular filtration rate may result in very high levels of methotrexate, thereby incurring a risk for other toxicities of the drug. Forced diuresis and alkalinization of urine may attenuate the renal injury caused by methotrexate. High doses of folinic acid may be helpful in this setting.

6-Thioguanine

Intravenous doses of 6-thioguanine exceeding 800 mg/m^2 have been associated with reversible ARF. The use of oral 6-thioguanine has not been shown to be nephrotoxic.

Interleukin-2

High-dose parenteral interleukin-2 infusions can trigger a severe capillary leak syndrome, leading to edema, hypotension, and a reversible fall in glomerular filtration rate. Patients with preexisting renal failure may have a prolonged course of ARF. Management of ARF in this setting is largely supportive and involves maintenance of intravascular volume and blood pressure, as well as avoidance of other nephrotoxic insults. Older patients and those with chronic renal insufficiency have a high risk for the development of the capillary leak syndrome, and alternative treatment approaches may need to be considered.

TUMOR CELL LYSIS

See Chapter 9, Acute Renal Failure.

IMMUNOGLOBULIN THERAPY

Intravenous infusion of immunoglobulin preparations that contain sugar additives such as glucose, maltose, or sucrose can result in ARF accompanied by vacuolization and swelling of renal proximal tubular cells. The nephrotoxicity is related to osmotic-induced renal tubular injury. Risk factors for this lesion include advancing age, underlying diabetes mellitus, and preexisting chronic renal failure.

HEAVY METALS

Lead Nephropathy

The proximal tubule is the major site of injury, and acute intoxication is associated with development of Fanconi syndrome.

This syndrome appears to be rapidly reversible with chelation therapy. Chronic lead intoxication has been associated with the development of hypertension and chronic renal failure in some, but not all, studies.

Clinical Features

The classic clinical presentation of chronic lead nephropathy is a benign urinary sediment, modest proteinuria (<2 g), hyperuricemia, and hypertension. Gouty arthritis affects about one half of patients with lead nephropathy.

Diagnosis

The blood lead concentration is relatively insensitive for assessing cumulative body stores of lead. The best available method of screening for lead toxicity is the use of two 1-g doses of sodium calcium edetate. After the injections, a 24-hour urine sample is collected. Normal adults excrete up to 650 mg of lead chelate in the urine; patients with a serum creatinine level greater than 1.5 mg/dL (132 mcmol/L) should have urine collected for 48 or 72 hours because the excretion of lead may be delayed in these individuals.

Management

The therapy for lead nephropathy consists of three weekly 1-g treatments of sodium calcium edetate intramuscularly. The end point of therapy is a lead chelate product that is normal. Chelation therapy is effective in reversing acute lead nephropathy, but there is no convincing evidence that it reverses the established interstitial disease.

Cadmium Nephrotoxicity

Cadmium is a metal with a wide variety of industrial uses, including the manufacture of glass, metal alloys, and electrical equipment. Exposure to cadmium principally results from occupational exposure, consuming cadmium-tainted food, and smoking cigarettes.

Clinical Features

Clinical nephrotoxicity is manifested by aminoaciduria, glycosuria, renal tubular acidosis, and the excretion of metallothionein and β_2-microglobin. Given the deposition of cadmium in bone as well as kidney, it is not surprising that many patients have a combination of renal failure and severe osteopenia that may lead to fractures. Hypercalciuria may lead to recurrent nephrolithiasis. Chronic renal insufficiency is linked to heavy cadmium exposure and can lead to end-stage renal failure.

Diagnosis

The relationship between urinary excretion of cadmium and urinary creatinine concentration is a reliable indicator of the total body cadmium burden. The recommendation of the American Conference of Governmental Industrial Hygienists is that a value of 5 mg of cadmium/g of creatinine in the urine is the occupational exposure limit for cadmium.

Treatment

Minimization of cadmium exposure is the key therapeutic approach. If cadmium exposure is eliminated, the usual trend is for renal function to stabilize, but continued deterioration is not usual. The general consensus is that in most instances cadmium-induced tubular interstitial disease is not reversible, and the use of sodium calcium edetate has not improved renal function dramatically.

Mercury

Mercury can cause both acute and chronic renal injury. The former usually occurs as a result of accidental exposure to mercury vapor and presents as acute tubule necrosis due to a direct toxic effect on the proximal tubule cells. In patients with acute mercury intoxication, the administration of 2,3-dimercaprol leads to some improvement in the natural history of the disease. A blood mercury level greater than 3 mg/dL or a urine level greater than 50 mg/g creatinine is considered abnormal, but the relationship of these values to overt disease is not always clear. The renal consequences of endemic methyl mercury poisoning are surprisingly benign, consisting only of tubular proteinuria with typically no changes in serum creatinine levels or significant albuminuria. The evidence for a progressive decline in renal function with chronic ingestion is not impressive.

ALTERNATIVE MEDICINE

Aristolochic Acid Nephropathy

Aristolochic acid nephropathy, also referred to as Chinese herb nephropathy, is a subacute form of renal failure (Table 16–2). The disorder is linked to the nephrotoxin *Aristolochia fangchi*. The typical clinical syndrome occurs in young women with severe anemia, proteinuria, and renal failure progressing to end-stage renal failure over several months. There is also an increased incidence of uroepithelial tumors in patients who

Table 16–2: Nephrotoxicity of Alternative Medicine Preparations

Preparation	Reported Toxicity
Aristolochic acid	Chronic tubulointerstitial nephritis (TIN) with rapid course of end-stage renal disease, Fanconi syndrome, increased risk of uroepithelial cancer
Ephedra (ma huang)	Hypertension, increased risk of nephrolithiasis consisting of ephedra and its metabolites
St. John's wort	Induces liver microsomal enzymes with increased degradation of drugs such as cyclosporine
Star fruit juice (carambola juice)	Acute oxalate nephropathy
Vitamin C	Oxalate nephropathy
Creatine	Acute TIN
Non juice (*Morinda citrifolia*)	High potassium content leading to hyperkalemia in patients with chronic renal failure
Rohu or Indian carp (*Labeo rohita*)	Acute renal failure
Cat's claw (Uno'de gato)	Acute TIN

develop end-stage renal disease due to aristolochic acid nephropathy.

Ephedra (Ma Huang)

Ephedra is commonly used for a variety of reasons: asthma, flu symptoms, weight reduction, euphoria, and sexual enhancement, among others. Ephedra stimulates α-adrenergic receptors and has been reported to cause hypertension, palpitations, seizures, and strokes. Use of this supplement is associated with an increased risk of kidney stones that contain ephedrine and its metabolites.

Star Fruit Juice

Star fruit is used to produce carambola juice, which is a popular beverage in Asia. Pure fresh juice ingested for traditional remedies contains high quantities of oxalate and has been reported to cause acute oxalate nephropathy.

Vitamin C

Vitamin C is normally metabolized to oxalic acid and is not associated with renal toxicity when ingested at therapeutic doses.

There have been several reports of patients with ARF due to acute oxalate nephropathy related to ingestion of large doses of vitamin C used as a nonprescription vitamin supplement.

ANTIRHEUMATIC AGENTS

Penicillamine

Up to 7% of treated patients treated with penicillamine develop the nephrotic syndrome (membranous pattern of injury) within the first 6 to 8 months of therapy, but the onset of proteinuria may be delayed up to 6 years. Proteinuria typically disappears when the drug is stopped. A more serious but less common complication of penicillamine is the development of ARF due to a crescentic, rapidly progressive glomerulonephritis. Pulse prednisone, cyclophosphamide, and plasmapheresis have all been used to treat this disorder with some success.

Gold

The prevalence of proteinuria (usually subnephrotic) in therapeutic gold administration is approximately 30%. Membranous and minimal-change pathologic changes are the most commonly observed. A decline in the glomerular filtration rate is unusual in gold-treated patients, but both severe renal failure and nephrotic syndrome have been reported.

Nonsteroidal Anti-Inflammatory Drugs

The incidence of nephrotoxicity caused by nonsteroidal anti-inflammatory drugs (NSAIDs) is low. However, the widespread use of these agents means that even with a relatively low incidence rate, nephrotoxicity will be commonly seen. There are several forms of NSAID nephrotoxicity, including the following:

- Vasomotor acute renal failure (see Chapter 9, Acute Renal Failure)
- Acute tubulointerstitial nephritis often associated with nephrotic-range proteinuria (see Chapter 12, Tubulointerstitial Diseases)
- Sodium retention, hyperkalemia, and hyponatremia
- Chronic renal failure

Several of the effects of NSAIDs on the kidney are linked to the inhibition of renal prostaglandin synthesis. Clinical studies examining the specific cyclooxygenase-2 inhibitors celecoxib and rofecoxib suggest that these drugs are associated with a renal toxicity profile similar to that associated with use of traditional NSAIDs.

Nonsteroidal Anti-Inflammatory Drug–Induced Chronic Renal Failure and Analgesic Nephropathy

Analgesic nephropathy is a chronic renal disease characterized by renal papillary necrosis and chronic interstitial nephritis. The early reports of analgesic nephropathy were from patients who consumed combination products containing phenacetin. However, the removal of phenacetin from clinical use has not been followed by the expected reduction in the incidence of the syndrome, suggesting that the use of combination products per se is an important etiologic factor. The disease is more common in women by a factor of two to six and has a peak incidence in middle age. Patients typically have consumed compound analgesics on a daily basis for many years. Patients with analgesic nephropathy have predominantly tubulomedullary dysfunction characterized by impaired concentrating ability, acidification defects, and occasionally a salt-losing state. Proteinuria tends to be low to moderate in quantity. Pyuria is common, and the urine is often sterile. Occasionally hematuria is noted, but persistent hematuria should raise the possibility of a uroepithelial tumor because these tumors occur with greater frequency in patients with a history of analgesic nephropathy.

The diagnosis of analgesic nephropathy is often difficult to establish with certainty because the disease is slowly progressive and the symptoms and signs are nonspecific. Patients are often reluctant to admit to heavy usage of analgesics and, therefore the condition is either misdiagnosed or not diagnosed at all until the renal failure is far advanced. Noncontrast computed tomography scanning may reveal papillary calcifications, papillary necrosis with sloughing, decreased renal size, and irregular renal contours. Management of the condition involves withdrawal of the offending agent; however, if the degree of renal injury is advanced, then progression to end-stage renal failure may be inevitable.

A number of reports have suggested that chronic use of NSAIDs alone may also lead to chronic renal insufficiency. Reports have documented a twofold increase in the risk for chronic renal failure associated with the previous daily use of NSAIDs. Given the possible linkage of chronic NSAID use with the development of chronic renal failure, it has become common clinical practice to recommend the use of acetaminophen whenever possible for analgesia. However, heavy use of acetaminophen (more than one pill per day) and medium to high cumulative intake (1000 or more pills in a lifetime) both appear to double the odds of end-stage renal disease, suggesting that long-term daily use of acetaminophen should be discouraged. A recent organized review by a consensus panel of the National Kidney Foundation suggested that ingestion of aspirin and NSAID combinations should not be encouraged because of an increased risk of renal failure, that habitual consumption of analgesics should be discouraged and monitoring is recommended when such use is mandatory, that combination analgesics should be available by prescription only with an explicit warning to physicians that the habitual consumption of these combination products could lead to the insidious development of chronic renal failure, and that there should be an explicit warning to consumers regarding NSAID ingestion.

DRUGS USED IN INFLAMMATORY BOWEL DISEASE

Mesalazine and Olsalazine

Sulfasalazine is used in the treatment of inflammatory bowel disease. New formulations of this drug such as mesalazine and olsalazine are free of sulfapyridine and improve the delivery of 5-aminosalicylic acid to the small bowel. 5-Aminosalicylic acid is converted to acetyl-5-aminosalicylic acid in the bowel epithelium. Early tubular injury in humans is characterized by increased excretion of tubular proteins such as β_2-microglobulin. Renal function in patients who receive these agents on a chronic basis should be monitored closely.

ANGIOTENSIN-CONVERTING ENZYME INHIBITORS

Angiotensin-converting enzyme (ACE) inhibitors have been observed to cause reversible ARF in the setting of hypotension and/or congestive heart failure. The reason for this phenomenon appears to be related to the role that angiotensin II plays in sustaining the glomerular filtration rate under conditions of hypoperfusion. In this setting an increase in efferent arteriole resistance may be required to maintain the intracapillary glomerular pressure at a level sufficiently high to sustain glomerular filtration. The increase in efferent vascular tone is in large part due to the vasoconstrictive effect of angiotensin II. Under these conditions ACE inhibitors blunt the vasoconstrictive effect of angiotensin II at the efferent arteriole, which therefore leads to a decline in efferent arteriolar resistance. This decline in efferent arteriole resistance leads to a fall in glomerular capillary pressure and then to a fall in glomerular filtration rate.

The clinical settings in which these physiologic changes become important are as follows:

- Decreased absolute circulating volume (hemorrhage or volume depletion).
- Bilateral renal artery stenosis (>70%) or renal artery stenosis in a single functioning kidney.
- Decreased effective circulating volume (severe congestive heart failure). This is more pronounced if cardiac filling pressures decline during the course of therapy (overzealous diuresis).
- Small-vessel disease of the kidney (severe nephrosclerosis). Even though the main renal arteries are patent, the obstruction to renal perfusion occurs more distally in arcuate and interlobular vessels, leading to another type of functional renal ischemia.

The result of all these interrelationships is that if a decline in renal function follows the use of an ACE inhibitor, in the absence of an obvious alternative etiology, underlying obstructive renal artery disease should be suspected. The diagnosis of this condition is considered at length in Chapter 25, Renovascular Hypertension and Ischemic Nephropathy. If the decline in renal function occurs upon exposure to an ACE inhibitor in the context of congestive heart failure, then a reduction in the dose of the drug, liberalization of salt in the diet of the patient, or a decrease in diuretic therapy may improve renal function without obviating the beneficial effect of the drug on afterload reduction. Rarely ACE inhibitors have been associated with allergic interstitial nephritis.

HYDROCARBONS

Chronic hydrocarbon exposure may predispose individuals to the development of several different types of renal disease. Acute tubular necrosis, chronic interstitial nephritis, and glomerulonephritis have all been described. The pathogenesis of hydrocarbon-induced renal disease is not known with certainty, but the possibility that solvents cause renal damage and thereby release a tubular antigen that results in an autoimmune reaction is a theory that is held in some regard. Another hypothesis is that potentially toxic immune factors arise independently of hydrocarbon exposure and that hydrocarbons facilitate the deposit of these mediators in renal tissue.

The Kidney and Hypertension in Pregnancy

17

RENAL ANATOMY AND FUNCTION DURING PREGNANCY

The kidney increases 1 cm in length, and kidney volume increases by 30% in pregnancy. More striking is the development of the physiologic hydronephrosis of pregnancy, which may persist for up to 12 weeks postpartum.

CARDIOVASCULAR AND RENAL PHYSIOLOGY IN PREGNANCY

Blood Pressure

Blood pressure and peripheral vascular resistance fall soon after conception. Peripheral vasodilatation manifests as palmar erythema and spider telangiectasia. Although a rise in both systolic and diastolic pressures occurs after the 28th week of gestation, blood pressure at term remains below that of nonpregnant age-matched control subjects.

Blood Volume

Blood volume increases by approximately 50% in pregnancy. A greater increase in plasma than in red blood cell volume causes the "physiologic anemia" of pregnancy. The major stimulus for the development of edema is Na^+ retention, compression of the inferior vena cava by the enlarged uterus, and a reduction in colloid osmotic pressure. Limiting the time a pregnant woman spends standing and sleeping in a lateral recumbent position usually helps to minimize edema.

Renal Blood Flow and Glomerular Filtration Rate

Early in pregnancy a rise in renal blood flow triggers an increase in the glomerular filtration rate (GFR) (up to 45%), which remains elevated until term. The practical consequences of the changes in GFR are that in normal pregnancy the average blood urea nitrogen (8.7 ± 1.5 mg/dL [1.45 ± 0.5 mmol/L]) and serum creatinine levels (0.46 ± 0.13 mg/dL [40 ± 11.5 mmol/L]) are significantly lower than normal.

Renal Tubule Function

Despite normal renal water handling, pregnant women have a decrease in serum Na^+ of approximately 5 mEq/L and a decrease in plasma osmolality of approximately 10 mOsm/kg H_2O due to a decrease in the osmotic threshold for antidiuretic hormone secretion. In contrast, a small number of pregnant women develop transient diabetes insipidus due to placental vasopressinase activity during the latter stages of pregnancy. This can be treated with the synthetic antidiuretic hormone analog, desmopressin (DDAVP), which is not metabolized by vasopressinase.

The high serum progesterone level in pregnancy causes a compensated respiratory alkalosis. The arterial partial pressure of carbon dioxide (Pco_2) decreases by approximately 10 mm Hg, and arterial pH increases slightly to 7.44. Chronic respiratory alkalosis is accompanied by a decrease in plasma HCO_3^- to 18 to 20 mEq/L. This reduction in total buffering capacity predisposes pregnant women to more severe acidosis with the development of either ketoacidosis or lactic acidosis. The changes in renal hemodynamics during pregnancy also result in enhanced excretion of uric acid and glucose. The net effect of these changes is a decrease in serum uric acid level to between 2.5 and 4 mg/dL (150 to 216 mmol/L) early in pregnancy and the development of glucosuria during pregnancy in a significant minority of women.

HYPERTENSION AND PREECLAMPSIA

Hypertension is the most common medical complication of pregnancy. A rise in blood pressure in pregnancy virtually always indicates the presence of one of following conditions:

1. Preeclampsia (toxemia)
2. Preeclampsia superimposed on chronic hypertension or renal disease
3. Chronic essential hypertension
4. Gestational hypertension

The decrease in blood pressure observed in pregnancy makes the upper limit of normal blood pressure in nonpregnant women, 140/90 mm Hg, of little clinical significance. A blood pressure in excess of 125/75 mm Hg before the 32nd week of gestation and 125/85 mm Hg thereafter is associated with a significant increase in fetal risk and as such should be considered to be hypertension. Blood pressure measurement during early pregnancy has value in the detection of women in whom preeclampsia will ultimately develop during the later stages of pregnancy. The frequency of preeclampsia increases linearly with an increase in systolic pressure in the first trimester from 100 to 134 mm Hg, and preeclampsia develops in late pregnancy in one third of women with a mean arterial pressure higher than 90 mm Hg during the second trimester, compared with only 2% of those with a lower mean arterial pressure.

CLINICAL FEATURES AND EPIDEMIOLOGY OF PREECLAMPSIA

The clinical onset of preeclampsia may be insidious and not accompanied by overt symptoms. Headache, visual disturbances, epigastric pain, and feelings of apprehension may occur. The usual sequence is rapid weight gain with edema, particularly of the hands and face, accompanied by increased blood pressure and proteinuria. Rarely, proteinuria precedes the hypertension. Proteinuria in preeclampsia can range from minimal levels to the nephrotic range, but preeclampsia does not cause microscopic hematuria. Some patients with preeclampsia have severe proteinuria with minimal hypertension, and in others the hypertension is preeminent. Preeclampsia usually begins after the 32nd week of pregnancy, but it may begin earlier, particularly in women with preexisting renal disease or hypertension. When it occurs during the first trimester, it is pathognomonic of a hydatidiform mole. The disease may be seen postpartum, with hypertension and convulsions occurring within 24 to 48 hours after delivery. The condition usually resolves within 10 days after delivery.

The disease has a bimodal frequency, being more common in young primiparous and older multiparous women (>40 years of age). The presence of underlying essential hypertension, diabetes mellitus, or renal disease increases the risk of pre-eclampsia. Other risk factors for preeclampsia are twin pregnancies, the antiphospholipid syndrome, fetal hydrops, insulin resistance, a family history of preeclampsia, and hydatidiform mole. A paternal contribution to the pathogenesis of preeclampsia is suggested by the finding that men who were themselves the product of a preeclamptic pregnancy were 2.1 times more likely than control subjects to be the father in a pregnancy complicated by preeclampsia.

Physical examination reveals puffy edema of the face and hands. Diastolic hypertension is prominent, with the systolic pressure usually being lower than 160 mm Hg. Systolic blood pressure greater than 200 mm Hg points to preeclampsia superimposed on underlying chronic hypertension. Ophthalmoscopic examination shows segmental arteriolar narrowing with a wet, glistening appearance indicative of retinal edema; hemorrhages and exudates are rare. Pulmonary edema is a common complication of preeclampsia and is usually caused by left ventricular failure. Central nervous system excitability is reflected in hyperreflexia.

Because preeclampsia is a multisystem disease, its presentation often mimics that of other diseases. Thrombocytopenia may be prominent and may suggest idiopathic thrombocytopenic purpura; when accompanied by neurologic features, it resembles thrombotic thrombocytopenic purpura. A microangiopathic anemia with hemolysis is common. The HELLP syndrome comprises severe preeclampsia with *h*emolysis, *e*levated *l*iver enzymes, and *l*ow *p*latelet count. Jaundice, which may be severe, particularly when hemolysis occurs, and abnormalities of liver function tests suggest hepatitis.

In preeclampsia, the GFR falls by 60% to 80%. The plasma urate level rises, often before a measurable rise in the serum creatinine or urea nitrogen level is seen. Because there is no increase in urate production in preeclampsia, hyperuricemia indicates decreased renal clearance and is a valuable marker to differentiate preeclampsia from other causes of hypertension in pregnancy when a decrease in urate clearance does not occur. A serum urate level greater than 5.5 mg/100 mL is a strong indicator of the presence of preeclampsia, and when it exceeds 6 mg/100 mL, the disease is usually severe. Hyperuricemia correlates well with the clinical severity of preeclampsia and with fetal survival. Emerging novel biomarkers of preeclampsia include placental soluble fms-like tyrosine kinase 1 (sFlt1), an antagonist of vascular endothelial growth factor and placental growth factor. Circulating sFlt1 levels are elevated in established preeclampsia and in early pregnancy increased levels of sFlt-1 and reduced levels of placental growth factor predict the subsequent development of preeclampsia.

Treatment of Preeclampsia

The first objective is to prevent preeclampsia. Proper prenatal care with attention to adequate but not excessive weight gain and careful monitoring of blood pressure and urinary protein concentration reduce the frequency and severity of the disease. The physician must carefully evaluate all women who have a rise in blood pressure during late pregnancy for evidence of preeclampsia, because it is the most frequent cause of maternal mortality. Hypertension with clinical or laboratory evidence of systemic disease must be presumed to represent preeclampsia. Although all hypertension in pregnancy poses a risk to mother and child, preeclampsia poses the greatest risk. If the presumptive diagnosis is preeclampsia, hospitalization is indicated, whereas a rise in blood pressure without evidence of preeclampsia can be treated on an outpatient basis. The definitive treatment for preeclampsia is delivery of the fetus.

If the disease is mild (blood pressure < 140/90 mm Hg, proteinuria < 500 mg/24 hr, normal renal function, serum urate level < 4.5 mg/dL [265 mmol/L], normal platelet count, and no evidence of hemolysis or hepatic involvement), bed rest is usually sufficient therapy to lower the blood pressure and allow time for estimation of fetal size and maturity. If fetal size and maturation are thought to be adequate, delivery is indicated. If fetal size and maturation are of concern and there is no evidence of worsening of preeclampsia, the pregnancy can be continued under expert supervision in a tertiary center. Any sign of worsening of the disease should be an indication for delivery, particularly if the pregnancy is of 32 weeks' duration or longer.

If the blood pressure is greater than 140/95 mm Hg with decreased renal function, hyperuricemia, or proteinuria greater than 500 mg/24 hr, delivery is indicated in pregnancies thought to be more than 32 weeks' duration. Blood pressure should be lowered to 140/90 mm Hg before delivery. Antihypertensive therapy lessens the likelihood of a rise in blood pressure during delivery with potential complications of congestive heart failure or cerebral hemorrhage. Methyldopa or the α/β-adrenergic antagonist labetalol can be given orally. Diuretics are avoided because of the reduction in plasma volume that accompanies preeclampsia.

If the blood pressure is greater than 160/100 mm Hg, parenteral labetalol therapy may be needed. The rapid duration of action of intravenous hydralazine and the reflex tachycardia it induces make it less desirable than labetalol. Sodium nitroprusside is contraindicated because of the possibility of fetal cyanide toxicity. Whether treatment of hypertension in preeclampsia affects the underlying disease is less clear, but it is not unreasonable to assume that hypertension is a factor adversely affecting endothelial cell function. Antihypertensive therapy can prevent pulmonary edema and cerebral hemorrhage, two severe complications of preeclampsia. However, the presence of convulsions (eclampsia) or the HELLP syndrome is always an indication for delivery.

Obstetricians in the United States have relied on magnesium sulfate, a mild vasodilator, for the treatment of preeclampsia. However, at therapeutic serum Mg^{2+} levels, there is suppression of myoneuronal transmission, which can cause respiratory paralysis, leading to maternal death. Vital capacity and maximal inspiratory and expiratory pressures fall in pregnant women receiving magnesium sulfate. Nevertheless, two prospective studies comparing magnesium sulfate with phenytoin demonstrated that magnesium sulfate was superior in preventing seizures, and it remains the drug of choice.

If preeclampsia occurs during the second trimester, when delivery of the infant is not compatible with fetal survival, a difficult decision must be made by the mother and physician. In general, termination of pregnancy is indicated if the pregnancy is less than 24 weeks' duration because of the combination of high maternal morbidity (HELLP syndrome, eclampsia, and placental abruption) and poor fetal outcome (<5% survival). After 24 weeks fetal survival may be increased by prolonging the pregnancy with treatment of the hypertension.

ESSENTIAL HYPERTENSION IN PREGNANCY

Pregnant women with chronic essential hypertension have an increased risk of preeclampsia, abruptio placentae, intrauterine growth restriction, and second-trimester fetal death. Both the degree of fetomaternal risk and the benefit of blood pressure control appear to be directly linked to the severity of the hypertension and to the presence or absence of proteinuria. Because these women usually are taking antihypertensive medication before pregnancy, it is important to maintain whatever therapy has controlled their hypertension, with the exception of angiotensin-converting enzyme inhibitors and angiotensin receptor blockers. Angiotensin-converting enzyme inhibitors have been associated with increased fetal loss, renal tubular dysplasia, perinatal acute renal failure, and other congenital anomalies. Recent studies have not demonstrated adverse fetal outcomes resulting from the use of angiotensin-converting inhibitors in the first trimester only. Therefore, if unintended exposure is limited to the first trimester, termination of the pregnancy is not always indicated.

Baseline investigations in the pregnant patient with hypertension should include routine urinalysis and culture, measurement of serum creatinine, blood urea nitrogen, and glucose levels and electrolytes, and spot urine protein-to-creatinine ratio. There has been some reluctance to treat hypertension in pregnant women with essential hypertension. Although antihypertensive therapy may result in fewer exacerbations of hypertension, a lower incidence of proteinuria, and improved perinatal outcome, the overall benefit in women with mild to moderate hypertension may be small. Indeed, as in the nonpregnant population, the beneficial effect of antihypertensive therapy is demonstrated best at higher levels of blood pressure. Factors that would favor antihypertensive treatment include coexisting diabetes mellitus, chronic renal insufficiency, or left ventricular dysfunction.

The optimal management of mild to moderate hypertension in pregnancy (systolic blood pressure of 140 to 169 mm Hg and diastolic blood pressure of 90 to 109 mm Hg) is not well defined. Although the risk of development of severe hypertension decreases with treatment, other outcomes, such as perinatal mortality and the incidence of preeclampsia, do not appear to be reduced. The optimal degree of blood pressure control in the woman with mild to moderate hypertension is also a matter of conjecture. An excessive decrease in maternal mean arterial pressure may be associated with a higher proportion of small-for-gestational-age infants. The central α-adrenergic agonist, methyldopa, has been used extensively in pregnancy and has been shown to diminish second-trimester stillbirth. It is generally well tolerated, but somnolence is occasionally problematic. Other options include β-blockers and the Ca^{2+} channel blockers. Atenolol is widely used in pregnancy; however, some authorities favor labetalol as the agent of choice. The Ca^{2+} channel blockers merit mention from the standpoint of their common use for hypertension and because of interest in their potential to exert tocolytic effects on the uterus.

Nifedipine is the most widely studied agent and is recognized as an alternative agent to methyldopa or a β-blocker in the management of essential hypertension in pregnancy. No definitive data exist to recommend one agent over another in terms of either maternal or fetal outcome. The target blood pressure is controversial. Some authorities advocate a blood pressure less than 140/90 mm Hg in all patients, whereas others advocate blood pressure of 140 to 150/80 to 90 with lower goals only in patients with evidence of end-organ injury.

GESTATIONAL HYPERTENSION

Hypertension that appears during late pregnancy, is not associated with signs of preeclampsia and disappears after delivery is termed *gestational hypertension*. Women with gestational hypertension are usually multiparous and often overweight and have a family history positive for hypertension; essential hypertension ultimately develops in many of them. Management includes bed rest, and, if required, treatment with an antihypertensive agent such as atenolol, labetalol, methyldopa, or nifedipine.

PREECLAMPSIA SUPERIMPOSED ON CHRONIC HYPERTENSION

Chronic essential hypertension may be associated with underlying nephrosclerosis. Any increase in blood pressure during pregnancy is transmitted to the glomerulus because of impaired autoregulation of glomerular pressure, which may trigger or worsen proteinuria (see later discussion). When this occurs, the distinction between preeclampsia and increased proteinuria induced by glomerular hypertension is difficult. Hyperuricemia or a rise in the serum creatinine level suggests preeclampsia.

ACUTE FATTY LIVER OF PREGNANCY

Acute fatty liver of pregnancy occurs in 1 in 13,000 pregnancies. More than 90% of cases occur in the third trimester. Patients typically present with nonspecific symptoms related to hepatic insufficiency; abdominal pain is often severe but is not invariably present. Laboratory findings suggest hepatic failure (marked elevation of bilirubin and lesser elevation of hepatic enzyme levels). A microangiopathic hemolytic anemia with thrombocytopenia and prolonged clotting times may develop. Of women with acute fatty liver of pregnancy 60% develop acute renal failure. There is no specific treatment for this disease, and delivery is indicated as soon as the medical condition of the mother allows. The prognosis appears to depend on the quality of supportive obstetric care. Recently inherited defects in mitochondrial β-oxidation of fatty acids by long-chain 3-hydroxyacyl coenzyme A dehydrogenase (LCHAD) deficiency have been implicated in the development of this disorder. Therefore, the mother and child should be evaluated for LCHAD deficiency.

RENAL DISEASE COMPLICATING PREGNANCY

Bacteriuria

Urinary tract infections (UTIs) occur with the same frequency in pregnant as in nonpregnant women. However, they are important clinically because of their greater propensity to progress to pyelonephritis. Women with diabetes or sickle cell trait or disease, as well as those from lower socioeconomic groups, have a higher prevalence of UTI in pregnancy. The increased capacity of the urinary collecting system combined with slowed emptying and vesicoureteral reflux is a major factor accounting for the increased occurrence of serious UTI in pregnancy. Maternal risks associated with UTI include the development of bacteremia, septic shock, and decreases in renal function. Risks to the fetus include midtrimester abortion and a twofold increase in perinatal mortality when UTI occurs within 2 weeks of delivery. Only one half of pregnant women with bacteriuria are symptomatic, which is the rationale for obtaining a screening urine culture at the initial prenatal visit. On the other hand, many pregnant women with symptoms suggestive of bacteriuria do not have an infection, because nocturia, polyuria, and stress incontinence are common complaints during uncomplicated pregnancy.

Because of the potential for fetal and maternal morbidity as a consequence of bacteriuria, infection, even if asymptomatic, should be treated. Short courses of therapy for 3 to 5 days are effective. Sulfonamides, nitrofurantoin, ampicillin, and cephalexin have been considered to be relatively safe for use in early pregnancy; sulfonamides are avoided near term because of a possible role in the development of kernicterus. Trimethoprim is usually avoided because of evidence of toxic effects in the fetus at high doses in experimental animals, although it has been used successfully in humans during pregnancy without evidence of toxicity or teratogenicity. Fluoroquinolones are avoided because of possible adverse effects on fetal cartilage development. Our preference is the use of ampicillin or cephalosporins—the drugs that have been used most extensively in pregnancy. In pregnant women with overt pyelonephritis, admission to the hospital for parenteral therapy should be the standard of care; β-lactam drugs, aminoglycosides, or both are the cornerstone of therapy, followed by prolonged oral therapy (2 to 3 weeks) for eradication of the infection. If the UTI is difficult to eradicate or the history is suggestive of underlying disease, then evidence of structural abnormalities should be sought.

Asymptomatic Urinary Abnormalities: Proteinuria and Hematuria

The development of proteinuria during pregnancy may be an indicator of unmasked kidney disease, worsening of preexisting renal disease, de novo development of renal disease, or development of preeclampsia. In normal pregnancy, both because of the increase in GFR and because of an increase in glomerular capillary permeability to albumin, there is increased urinary excretion of albumin. When corrected for GFR, fractional albumin excretion increases by approximately 80%. Nevertheless, in otherwise healthy pregnant women, this should not result in a 24-hour urinary excretion of protein of greater than 200 to 250 mg. As is true for renal disease in general, urinary protein excretion of greater than 1 to 2 g/day suggests a glomerular process, whereas tubulointerstitial disease may produce less proteinuria.

The presence of red blood cells in the urine is almost always the result of an organic process. Although preeclampsia causes glomerular lesions and proteinuria, it does not cause hematuria. Therefore, the finding of hematuria, particularly with red blood cell casts, in a patient with preeclampsia suggests the presence of underlying renal disease (membranous nephropathy, focal glomerulosclerosis, and systemic lupus erythematosus). If a pregnancy becomes complicated by the apparent development of glomerulonephritis, a biopsy of the kidney is often contemplated. If a specific diagnosis is required immediately (e.g., rapidly progressive glomerulonephritis), then a renal biopsy can be safely performed in a pregnant patient. If the usual guidelines for renal biopsy are followed (i.e., control hypertension and avoid aspirin for 7 to 10 days before biopsy), complications occur no more often than in nongravid patients.

Acute Renal Failure

Acute renal failure during pregnancy usually presents as one of three forms:

- Acute tubule necrosis (ATN)
- Renal cortical necrosis
- Postpartum acute renal failure

Rarely, fatty liver of pregnancy or obstructive uropathy causes acute renal failure. The general diagnostic approach is the same as that in the nonpregnant patient. This approach requires careful physical examination of the patient to look for signs of volume depletion and evaluation of the urinary sediment for evidence of ATN or a glomerular/tubulointerstitial process. If urinary tract obstruction is suspected, abdominal ultrasonography can be performed to rule out hydronephrosis. However, because of the physiologic hydronephrosis of pregnancy, this diagnosis can be difficult to make with certainty.

Acute Tubule Necrosis

ATN occurs as a complication of many conditions, most commonly sepsis or hypotension. This condition has become rare in industrialized nations and now affects only about 1 in 20,000 pregnancies. In the first trimester, septic abortion accounts for most patients with ATN. Sepsis caused by any gram-negative organism results in hypotension, leading to acute renal failure. When *Clostridium perfringens* is the responsible bacterium, *Clostridium*-induced myonecrosis of the uterus may be a source of myoglobin, leading to pigment-induced ATN. In late pregnancy, acute renal failure is a complication of preeclampsia or placental abruption. ATN is a rare complication of preeclampsia, occurring in 1% to 2% of patients, probably due to diffuse endothelial cell swelling resulting in renal ischemia. The HELLP syndrome is a complication of preeclampsia, occurring in 2% to 12% of patients who have preeclampsia, with ATN developing in 5% to 10% of these. Abruptio placentae can cause ATN, but it is also the most common cause of renal cortical necrosis. Severe volume depletion due to hemorrhage, which results renal ischemia, is presumed to be the cause of ATN in this setting.

Renal Cortical Necrosis

Most cases of acute cortical necrosis are caused by abruptio placentae, but other causes include septic abortion, severe preeclampsia, amniotic fluid embolism, and a retained fetus. Renal cortical necrosis should also be suspected when oliguria or anuria persists for longer than 1 week. Definitive diagnosis may be made by renal biopsy or, preferably, by renal arteriogram. The renal arteriogram shows patchy blood flow or an absent nephrogram. Cortical necrosis is seen more often in older women and multigravidas, although age and multiple pregnancies may not be independent risk factors but merely factors associated with the development of obstetric complications. A large number of patients with cortical necrosis never recover renal function or recover renal function transiently with later development of end-stage renal disease.

Postpartum Hemolytic-Uremic Syndrome/Thrombotic Thrombocytopenic Purpura

This disease is characterized by a microangiopathic hemolytic anemia. It occurs in otherwise uncomplicated pregnancies anywhere from 1 day to several months after delivery. Symptoms are those related to renal insufficiency, such as headache, nausea, and vomiting. The signs include oliguria or anuria, evidence of a bleeding diathesis, and, in many patients, hypertension. Examination of the peripheral blood smear shows the presence of schistocytes and burr cells. Thrombocytopenia is usual. Bleeding times are not usually prolonged, although fibrin degradation products may be increased. Neurologic symptoms, when present, suggest thrombotic thrombocytopenic purpura. The optimal treatment of this condition is uncertain. There has not been substantial experience with plasma exchange; however, based on comparisons with outcomes in the pre–plasma exchange era, this intervention may offer some benefit (see Chapter 15, Microvascular Diseases of the Kidney).

Obstructive Uropathy

Acute renal failure due to bilateral ureteral obstruction from a gravid uterus is extremely unusual. Risk factors include multiple gestation and polyhydramnios. The diagnosis of obstructive uropathy due to ureteral obstruction by the gravid uterus is suggested by the finding of oliguria or anuria in the setting of moderate or severe dilatation of the urinary collecting system, particularly on the left. Amniotomy may be a successful therapy in the patient with polyhydramnios. Alternatively, several patients have been successfully treated by ureteral stenting.

Nephrolithiasis

Pregnancy is associated with absorptive hypercalciuria; however, urinary calculi occur with the same frequency as in nonpregnant women. Ultrasonography is the recommended procedure for detection of urinary calculi to avoid the low risk of radiation required by intravenous pyelography or computed tomography. Pregnancy does not increase the rate of stone formation or the frequency of complications related to stones. In pregnant patients who are unable to pass a ureteral calculus spontaneously, it is possible to place an internal ureteral stent safely and efficaciously. The presence of a ureteral stent does not present complications for subsequent vaginal delivery.

PREGNANCY IN WOMEN WITH RENAL DISEASE

Renal disease can have significant and serious consequences for both maternal health and fetal outcome, and patients with significant renal disease should be managed jointly by an obstetrician experienced in high-risk pregnancies and by a nephrologist.

Risk of Progression of Renal Disease in Pregnancy

The degree of prior renal insufficiency and hypertension largely predict outcome. For the most part, women with renal disease who become pregnant when renal function is normal or minimally depressed tolerate pregnancy without permanent deleterious effects on renal function. Conversely, as many as 40% of women with moderate renal insufficiency (creatinine level of 1.4 to 2.8 mg/dL) experience a more rapid and irreversible decline in renal function after pregnancy than would have been predicted on the basis of the natural history of their disease. Proteinuria may be an independent risk factor for pregnancy-related declines in renal function. Women with severe renal disease (creatinine level > 2.8 mg/dL) should avoid pregnancy because fewer than 50% will have a live birth, and most will have complications including accelerated loss of renal function and severe hypertension.

Although prospective data are not available, it is probable that control of hypertension during pregnancy has protective effects on the kidney, as has been demonstrated in nonpregnant women and in men. An increase in proteinuria, even in the absence of increasing blood pressure, suggests the need for more aggressive blood pressure control. What is more controversial is the precise blood pressure goal for pregnant women. Recalling that pregnancy is a condition associated with afferent arteriolar vasodilatation and greater transmission of systemic blood pressure into the glomerulus, a nephrologist would generally recommend aggressive blood pressure control. However, this goal must be balanced with concerns for fetal well-being.

Effects of Renal Disease on Fetal Outcome

Fertility is greatly diminished by renal insufficiency, particularly when the GFR is less than 50% of normal. Nevertheless, pregnancy occasionally occurs in patients with severe renal insufficiency and even in patients receiving chronic dialysis therapy. The important consequences of maternal renal disease include an increased frequency of fetal loss, intrauterine growth restriction, and prematurity. The major risk factors for poor outcome are uncontrolled hypertension, nephrotic-range proteinuria, and a creatinine level greater than 1.8 mg/dL. In previous studies the presence of all three risk factors resulted in a perinatal mortality rate of approximately 30% versus 5% in the presence of a single risk factor. However, improvements in obstetric care and perinatal support may produce better outcomes in the modern era. As noted, the risk of developing superimposed preeclampsia during pregnancy varies between 20% and 40% in women with some form of underlying renal disease. When preeclampsia is associated with underlying renal insufficiency the disease may manifest earlier than 32 weeks.

TREATMENT OF RENAL FAILURE IN PREGNANCY

Dialysis

The incidence of pregnancy in women of child-bearing age undergoing chronic hemodialysis is less than 1%. With improvements in obstetric and dialytic care approximately 40% to 70% of pregnancies result in a live birth, with the higher figure generally applying to women who initiate dialysis during pregnancy. Most patients experience worsening hypertension and 90% of the infants are small for gestational age. There is no increase in the rate of congenital abnormalities or respiratory distress. The general principle for treatment of patients needing chronic hemodialysis is that more dialysis is better. This dictum has been used empirically in pregnancy. The course of action has included the early institution of dialysis (GFR > 12 mL/min) and treating with more frequent and longer hemodialysis sessions (five to six times weekly for at least 4 hours per session). Anemia should be aggressively treated and hypotension carefully avoided to lessen the chance of fetal hypoperfusion. Chronic peritoneal dialysis has been used as an alternative modality to avoid the risks of intermittent hypotension and anticoagulation associated with hemodialysis. Typically, continuous cycling peritoneal dialysis is used to achieve higher clearance rates.

Transplantation

Kidney transplantation restores fertility in women with chronic kidney disease, and outcomes of pregnancies that occur in women who are recipients of kidney transplants are dramatically better than those experienced by dialysis patients. Two thirds of pregnancies proceed beyond the first trimester and of these more than 90% result in a live birth. Kidney allografts appear to tolerate pregnancy well. There was a fear that pregnancy-induced hyperfiltration could adversely affect long-term survival of allografts; however, adverse effects are not usually apparent unless preexisting chronic allograft dysfunction and/or heavy proteinuria is present. Acute rejection episodes are no more common

Table 17–1: Guidelines for Considering Pregnancy in Renal Transplant Recipients

Good general health for approximately 2 years after transplantation

Stable allograft function (serum creatinine < 2 mg/dL (176 mcmol/L), preferably < 1.5 g/dL (132 mcmol/L)

No recent episodes of acute rejection or evidence of ongoing rejection

Normal blood pressure or minimal antihypertensive regimen (only one drug)

Absence of or minimal proteinuria (< 0.5 g/day)

Normal allograft ultrasound (absence of pelvicaliceal distension)

Recommended immunosuppression:

Prednisone < 15 mg/day

Azathioprine = 2 mg/kg/day

Cyclosporine or tacrolimus at therapeutic levels

Mycophenolate mofetil and sirolimus are contraindicated

Mycophenolate mofetil and sirolimus should be stopped 6 weeks before conception is attempted

Adapted from EBPG Expert Group on Renal Transplantation: Pregnancy in renal transplant recipients. *Nephrol Dial Transplant* 17(Suppl. 4):50, 2002.

than in nonpregnant women. Hypertension or preeclampsia develops in approximately 30% of pregnancies, representing the most important maternal complication. The most significant fetal complication is preterm delivery, which occurs in 45% to 60% of pregnancies, and between 20% and 30% of infants are small for gestational age. Vaginal delivery is not made difficult by the presence of the pelvic kidney. Therefore, cesarean sections should be reserved for the usual obstetric indications. Both cyclosporine and tacrolimus are safe in pregnancy; however, levels usually decline during pregnancy and should be monitored closely. Not all drugs used for the prevention of allograft rejection are acceptable in pregnancy. Mycophenolate mofetil and sirolimus are embryotoxic in animals, and it is recommended that these drugs not be used during pregnancy or while a woman is attempting to conceive. Pregnancy in the renal transplant recipient has become a common enough occurrence that guidelines have emerged to direct the treating transplantation team (Table 17–1).

Inherited Disorders of the Renal Tubule

18

INHERITED DISORDERS ASSOCIATED WITH GENERALIZED DYSFUNCTION OF THE PROXIMAL TUBULE (RENAL FANCONI SYNDROME)

The proximal tubule is responsible for reclaiming almost all of the filtered load of bicarbonate, glucose, and amino acids, as well as most of the filtered load of sodium, chloride, and phosphate. The renal Fanconi syndrome is a generalized dysfunction of the proximal tubule with no primary glomerular involvement. It is usually characterized by variable degrees of phosphate, glucose, amino acid, and bicarbonate wasting. The clinical presentation in children is usually rickets and impaired growth. In adults, the disorder presents as bone disease, manifested as osteomalacia and osteoporosis. In addition, polyuria, renal salt wasting, hypokalemia, acidosis, hypercalciuria, and low-molecular-weight proteinuria can be part of the clinical spectrum. There are both hereditary and acquired forms of the Fanconi syndrome (Table 18–1).

Clinical Presentation

All amino acids are filtered by the glomerulus, and more than 98% are subsequently reabsorbed by multiple transporters in the proximal tubule. In Fanconi syndrome, all amino acids are excreted in excess. Clinically, amino acid losses are relatively modest and do not lead to specific deficiencies, and there is no need for supplementation to affected patients. Phosphate wasting is a cardinal manifestation of the Fanconi syndrome, and serum phosphate levels are usually decreased. Rickets and osteomalacia result from increased urinary losses of phosphate as well as impaired 1α-hydroxylation of 25-hydroxyvitamin D_3 by proximal tubule cells. A hyperchloremic metabolic acidosis (type II) is a

325

Table 18–1: Causes of Inherited and Acquired Fanconi Syndrome

Inherited
  Idiopathic (AD)
  Dent disease (X-linked hypophosphatemic rickets, X-linked
    recessive nephrolithiasis)
  "Sporadic"
  Cystinosis (AR)
  Tyrosinemia type I (AR)
  Galactosemia (AR)
  Glycogen storage disease
  Wilson disease (AR)
  Mitochondrial diseases (cytochrome *c* oxidase deficiency)
  Oculocerebrorenal syndrome of Lowe
  Hereditary fructose intolerance
Acquired
  Paraproteinemias (multiple myeloma)
  Nephrotic syndrome
  Chronic tubulointerstitial nephritis
  Renal transplantation
  Malignancy
Exogenous factors
  Heavy metals (cadmium, mercury, lead, uranium, platinum)
  Drugs (cisplatin, aminoglycosides, 6-mercaptopurine,
    valproate, outdated tetracyclines, methyl-3-chrome,
    ifosfamide)
  Chemical compounds (toluene, maleate, paraquat, Lysol)

AD, autosomal dominant; AR, autosomal recessive.

common finding and is caused by defective bicarbonate reabsorption by the proximal tubule. Distal renal acidification is normal, and the urine pH falls below 5.5 when plasma bicarbonate falls below the urinary reabsorption threshold. Glucosuria is the fourth manifestation of the renal Fanconi syndrome. Serum glucose is normal, and the amount of glucose lost in the urine varies from 0.5 to 10 g/24 hr. Massive glucosuria (and hypoglycemia) may be seen in glycogenosis type I. Renal sodium losses can be significant in the Fanconi syndrome and lead to hypotension, hyponatremia, metabolic alkalosis, and hypokalemia due to increased distal delivery of sodium. Polyuria, polydipsia, and dehydration can be prominent features of the Fanconi syndrome. The decrease in concentrating ability is related to abnormal tubule function of the distal tubule and collecting duct, possibly caused by hypokalemia. Low-molecular-weight proteinuria is almost always present in patients with the renal Fanconi syndrome, and the amount is usually low to moderate. Results of a dipstick test are often positive because of the presence of albuminuria. Hypercalciuria is a common finding in patients with the renal Fanconi syndrome. The pathogenesis is not known. Hypercalciuria is rarely associated with nephrolithiasis in the Fanconi syndrome because of the associated polyuria.

Dent Disease, X-Linked Recessive Hypophosphatemic Rickets, and X-Linked Recessive Nephrolithiasis

Pathogenesis
Dent disease, X-linked recessive hypophosphatemic rickets, and X-linked recessive nephrolithiasis represent the same inherited disorder caused by mutations in the *CLCN5* gene (chromosome Xp11.22) encoding a renal chloride channel, ClC-5. This X-linked recessive disease is associated with a primary renal Fanconi syndrome.

Clinical Presentation
The clinical spectrum of *CLCN5* mutations includes hypercalciuria with calcium phosphate nephrolithiasis, rickets, nephrocalcinosis, low-molecular-weight proteinuria, and renal failure. The same mutation can induce different phenotypes in different families, probably because of genetic or environmental modifiers or both. The disease affects males predominantly, but females often have an attenuated phenotype. The degree of overall proteinuria is relatively constant and amounts to 0.5 to 2 g/day in adults and up to 1 g/day in children. The nephrotic syndrome does not occur, and albumin excretion represents less than half of the proteins excreted. Hypercalciuria is also a hallmark of this disorder and is present in most patients, beginning in childhood. Kidney stones are present in 50% of males and are composed of calcium phosphate or a mixture of calcium phosphate and calcium oxalate. Radiologic nephrocalcinosis of the medullary type is seen in most affected males and occasionally females. Serum phosphate levels are usually below normal values, and rickets or osteomalacia may occur. Systemic acidosis is usually not seen before renal function deteriorates significantly. Spontaneous hypokalemia is common in males, and there is an inability to concentrate urine maximally. Aminoaciduria and glucosuria are also common. Progressive renal failure occurs in 50% of males with end-stage renal failure occurring in the fourth decade on average.

Treatment
Renal stones and hypercalciuria are treated with supportive measures (and, in particular, increased fluid intake). Dietary restriction

of calcium reduces calcium excretion but is not recommended because it may exacerbate bone disease. Thiazide diuretics may trigger hypotension because these patients tend to have a salt-losing nephropathy. Rickets and osteomalacia are treated with small doses of vitamin D, but this should be given with caution because it might increase urine calcium excretion and the risk of nephrolithiasis.

Idiopathic Renal Fanconi Syndrome

Idiopathic renal Fanconi syndrome occurs in the absence of known inborn errors of metabolism or acquired causes of the Fanconi syndrome (see Table 18–1). Most instances are sporadic, although familial cases associated with progressive renal failure have been reported, and the condition can be transmitted as an autosomal dominant trait. No specific loci or genes have been discovered.

Cystinosis

Pathogenesis

Cystinosis is a rare autosomal recessive disease due to defective transport of the disulfide amino acid cystine across lysosomal membranes with consequent intracellular accumulation and cell death (incidence is 1 in 160,000). It is caused by inactivating mutations in *CTNS*, encoding an integral lysosomal membrane protein termed *cystinosin*.

Clinical Presentation

Cystinosis is the most common cause of the renal Fanconi syndrome in children. The clinical spectrum of disease ranges from classic nephropathic cystinosis to a mild adult-onset variant. Nephropathic cystinosis usually presents in the first year of life with failure to thrive, increased thirst, polyuria, poor feeding, and hypophosphatemic rickets. White subjects often have blond hair and blue eyes and are more lightly pigmented. Renal wasting of sodium, calcium, and magnesium is often seen, as well as tubular proteinuria. Progressive renal damage usually culminates in end-stage renal failure by the end of the first decade. The disease does not recur in the donor kidney. However, continued accumulation in tissues results in photophobia, retinal blindness, corneal erosions, diabetes mellitus, distal myopathy, swallowing difficulties, decreased pulmonary function, pancreatic failure, primary hypogonadism in males, and neurologic deterioration in a significant number of renal transplant recipients. Other features of cystinosis include hypothyroidism, insulin-dependent diabetes mellitus, myopathy, and central nervous system involvement in the later stages of the disease.

The diagnosis is usually made by measuring the cystine content of peripheral leukocytes or cultured fibroblasts. Cystinotic patients usually have values higher than 2 nmol of half-cystine/mg of protein (normal < 0.2 nmol of half-cystine/mg of protein). Alternatively, the diagnosis can be made by recognizing the characteristic corneal crystals on slit-lamp examination. Cystinosis can be diagnosed in utero by cystine measurements in amniocytes or chorionic villi or at birth using cystine measurements on the placenta.

Treatment
Early diagnosis and appropriate treatment with dialysis and renal transplantation have improved the outcome of patients with nephropathic cystinosis, and most patients now reach adulthood. Symptomatic treatment involves rehydration, particularly during episodes of gastroenteritis. Replacement of bicarbonate losses with citrate or bicarbonate-containing salts is often indicated. Phosphate losses are replaced with phosphate salts and oral vitamin D therapy. Indomethacin has been used to decrease the renal salt- and water-wasting syndrome. The cystine-letting drug cysteamine, which slows the rate of progression of renal failure and increases growth in affected patients, is now widely used for cystinosis. Kidney function stabilizes upon initiation of therapy and may allow patients treated at an early age to reach adulthood without developing end-stage renal failure. Transplantation is now routinely performed in cystinotic patients.

Lowe Oculocerebrorenal Syndrome

The oculocerebrorenal syndrome of Lowe (ORCL) is an X-linked recessive multisystem disorder characterized by congenital cataracts, mental retardation, and renal Fanconi syndrome. Mutations in the *OCRL1* gene are responsible for OCRL. This gene encodes a 105-kD Golgi protein involved in the inositol phosphate-signaling pathway. Renal dysfunction is a major feature of the disorder and usually occurs within the first year of life. It is characterized by proteinuria, generalized aminoaciduria, carnitine wasting, phosphaturia, and bicarbonaturia. Glomerular function falls with age, with renal failure developing between the second and fourth decade of life. Neurologic findings include infantile hypotonia, mental retardation, and status epilepticus. In the absence of reliable biochemical tests or a confirmed family history, the diagnosis is made clinically on the basis of the cardinal ocular, renal, and neurologic manifestations. Carrier detection can be performed by slit-lamp examination, mutation detection, or linkage analysis of markers if the specific mutation is unknown. Treatment is supportive and includes repletion of bicarbonate, phosphate, and sodium.

Hereditary Fructose Intolerance

Hereditary fructose intolerance caused by aldolase B deficiency (fructose-1,6-bisphosphate aldolase) is an autosomal recessive disorder characterized by severe hypoglycemia and vomiting shortly after fructose ingestion. The disease is associated with proximal tubule dysfunction manifesting as aminoaciduria, bicarbonaturia, and phosphaturia and also lactic acidosis. The incidence is 1 in 23,000. The pathophysiology of the renal Fanconi syndrome is not clear but may be related to impaired acidification and recycling of endosomes similar to that seen in Dent disease. The treatment of hereditary fructose intolerance involves withdrawal of sucrose, fructose, and sorbitol from the diet.

INHERITED DISORDERS OF RENAL AMINO ACID TRANSPORT

Amino acids are freely filtered by the glomerulus; however, the proximal tubule reabsorbs up to 99.9% of the filtered load. Aminoaciduria occurs when a renal transport defect of the proximal tubule decreases the reabsorptive capacity for one or several amino acids or when the threshold for reabsorbing an amino acid is exceeded by elevated plasma levels as a result of a metabolic defect ("overflow aminoaciduria"). Clinically, the most significant renal aminoaciduria is cystinuria. Most of the other disorders are rarely symptomatic.

Cystinuria

Cystinuria is an autosomal recessive disorder associated with defective transport of cystine and the dibasic amino acids ornithine, lysine, and arginine involving the epithelial cells of the renal tubule and gastrointestinal tract. The formation of cystine calculi in the urinary tract, leading to infection and renal failure, is the hallmark of the disorder. The prevalence is approximately 1 in 7000 but varies depending on the geographic location.

Pathogenesis
Cystinuria is caused by mutations in either of two genes implicated in dibasic amino acid luminal transport by the proximal tubule.

Type A cystinuria is an autosomal recessive disease caused by mutations in *SLC3A1* on chromosome 2, which encodes the renal proximal tubule S3 segment and intestinal dibasic amino acid transporter. Jejunal uptake of cystine and dibasic amino acids is absent, and there is no plasma response to an oral cystine load. The risk of nephrolithiasis is very high. *Type B cystinuria* is an incompletely recessive form in which both parents excrete intermediate amounts of cystine (100 to 600 mcmol/g of creatinine). The disease is caused by mutations in the *SLC7A9* gene located on chromosome 19q13, which encodes a protein, BAT1. It belongs to a family of light subunits of amino acid transporters, expressed in the kidney, liver, small intestine, and placenta.

Clinical Presentation

The only known manifestation of cystinuria is nephrolithiasis. Clinical expression of the disease typically starts during the first to third decade. Males tend to be more severely affected than females. Cystine stones are made of a yellow-brown substance, are very hard, and appear radiopaque on roentgenograms due to their sulfur content. Stones are often multiple and staghorn and tend to be smoother than calcium stones. Magnesium ammonium phosphate and calcium stones can also form as a result of infection.

Patients with type A cystinuria can be readily identified because their parents excrete normal amounts of cystine. More than 50% of patients with type A cystinuria will form one or more stones within the first decade of life. Type B heterozygotes show the highest levels of urinary cystine excretion (990 to 1740 mcmol/g of creatinine). The diagnosis is suggested by characteristic hexagonal cystine crystals in the urine of affected patients. Acidification of concentrated urine with acetic acid can precipitate crystals not visible on initial urine microscopy. Diagnosis is ultimately made by measurement of cystine excretion in the urine.

Treatment

Management involves maintaining a high urine flow rate and reducing intake of sodium in the diet, which results in lower urinary cystine concentrations. Fluid intake should be greater than 4 L/day because many patients excrete 1 g or more of cystine daily. Cystine solubility can also be increased by alkalinization of the urine with potassium citrate, but the solubility of cystine does not increase until the pH reaches 7 to 7.5; therefore the requirements for alkali may reach 3 to 4 mmol/kg. Patients who are unable to comply with a regimen of high fluid intake and urine alkalinization, or in whom adequate treatment fails, can be given D-penicillamine in doses of 30 mg/kg up to a maximum of 2 g/day. Through a disulfide exchange reaction D-penicillamine forms the disulfide cysteine-penicillamine, which is much more soluble than cystine. The tolerability to this drug is variable, and the frequent occurrence of side effects such as rash, fever, membranous nephropathy, epidermolysis, and loss of taste complicate therapy. Another drug that may be useful in cystinuria is mercaptopropionylglycine, whose mechanism of action is identical to that of D-penicillamine. This drug is as effective as D-penicillamine in reducing urine cystine excretion, but it also has substantial side effects including skin rash, fever, nausea, proteinuria, and membranous nephropathy.

The introduction of extracorporeal shock wave lithotripsy has not been of great benefit to cystinuric patients because cystine stones are difficult to pulverize. Consequently, percutaneous lithotripsy is more effective. Recent progress in endoscopic urologic treatment of kidney stones has decreased the need for open surgery. Transplantation is sometimes necessary for patients who develop end-stage renal disease from chronic obstruction or infection. A kidney from an unaffected donor will not form cystine stones.

Hartnup Disease

Hartnup disease is an autosomal recessive disorder characterized by excessive urinary excretion of the neutral amino acids alanine, asparagine, glutamine, histidine, isoleucine, leucine, methionine, phenylalanine, serine, threonine, tryptophan, tyrosine, and valine. Its incidence has been estimated in newborn screening programs to be 1 in 26,000. The gene encoding the defective protein responsible for Hartnup disease has not been cloned. The clinical features of this disorder, if any, are due to deficiency of nicotinamide, which is partly derived from tryptophan. These include a photosensitive erythematous skin rash (pellagra-like) clinically identical with niacin deficiency, intermittent cerebellar ataxia, and rarely mental retardation. The diagnosis is easily made by performing a urinary amniogram, which shows increased excretion of neutral amino acids, but not glycine, cystine, dibasic acid, dicarboxylic acid, and imino amino acids. Thus, Hartnup disease can be easily differentiated from the generalized aminoaciduria of Fanconi syndrome. Treatment of symptomatic patients involves the administration of nicotinamide in doses of 50 to 300 mg/day. The value of treating asymptomatic patients is not known, but given the harmlessness of the treatment, this might be a rational choice.

INHERITED DISORDERS OF RENAL PHOSPHATE TRANSPORT

Inherited disorders of renal phosphate transport are characterized by hypophosphatemia due to a reduction in renal tubule reabsorption of inorganic phosphate. These disorders are characterized by metabolic bone disease presenting as rickets in childhood and osteomalacia in adults. The normal phosphate intake in adults varies from 800 to 1600 mg/day, and the average serum phosphate levels remain normal over a wide range of intake. Intestinal phosphate absorption is greatest in the jejunum and ileum and is regulated by vitamin D metabolites. In the normal state, moderate phosphate deprivation that leads to a marginal decrease in serum phosphate levels induces a reduction in urine excretion of phosphate and an increase in 1,25-dihydroxyvitamin D_3 (1,25$[OH]_2D_3$) levels. Renal proximal tubular reabsorption of phosphate is mediated by a Na^+/P_i cotransporter system, which is down-regulated by parathyroid hormone (PTH) and hyperphosphatemia and up-regulated by phosphate deprivation.

X-Linked Hypophosphatemic Rickets

Pathogenesis
X-linked hypophosphatemic rickets is an X-linked dominant disorder characterized by hypophosphatemia with phosphaturia, normal serum calcium and PTH levels, normal to low serum 1,25$(OH)_2D_3$ levels, and elevated levels of serum alkaline phosphatase. The mutated gene, *PHEX*, encodes a large protein of 749 amino acids, which encodes a cell surface–bound protease. Studies suggest that the disease is due to an abnormal circulating factor that results in underexpression of the Na^+/P_i cotransporter in the proximal tubule.

Clinical Presentation
X-linked hypophosphatemic rickets is the most common type of hereditary disorder of renal phosphate metabolism. Its hallmark is an inappropriately normal 1,25$(OH)_2D_3$ level in the presence of hypophosphatemia and rickets. There is no renal wasting of amino acids and glucose. The patients demonstrate growth retardation, femoral or tibial bowing presenting early in life, and evidence of rickets and osteomalacia. Serum phosphate levels are usually lower than 2.5 mg/dL (0.8 mmol/L). The earliest sign of the disease in children can be increased serum alkaline phosphatase levels.

Treatment

Early therapy with $1,25(OH)_2D_3$ (1 to 3 mcg/day) and phosphate (1 to 2 g/day in divided doses) has a beneficial effect on growth and bone disease. Nephrocalcinosis due to vitamin D and phosphate therapy can lead to deterioration of renal function.

Hereditary Hypophosphatemic Rickets with Hypercalciuria

Hereditary hypophosphatemic rickets associated with hypercalciuria is a very rare and apparently autosomal recessive disease. The genetic defect responsible for this disease is not known. The characteristic features are rickets, short stature, increased renal phosphate clearance, hypercalciuria, normal serum calcium levels, increased gastrointestinal absorption of calcium and phosphorus, an elevated serum concentration of $1,25(OH)_2D_3$, and suppressed parathyroid function. The defect in phosphate reabsorption is presumed to be in the proximal tubule. Phosphate deprivation leads to an appropriate increase in $1,25(OH)_2D_3$ production and increased intestinal absorption of calcium and phosphate, leading to hypercalciuria. As a result, PTH is suppressed, and chronic hypophosphatemia leads to a reduction in bone mineralization and growth. Patients respond to daily administration of oral phosphate (1 to 2.5 g/day).

Hereditary Selective Deficiency of 1α,25-Hydroxyvitamin D_3

This rare form of autosomal recessive vitamin D–responsive rickets is not a disease of tubule transport per se, but a 1α-hydroxylation deficiency. It results from inactivating mutations in the P-450 enzyme 1α-hydroxylase on chromosome 12q14. Patients usually appear normal at birth and develop muscle weakness, tetany, convulsions, and rickets starting at 2 months of age. Serum calcium levels are low and PTH levels are high, with low to undetectable levels of $1,25(OH)_2D_3$. Serum levels of 25-hydroxyvitamin D_3 ($25[OH]D_3$) are normal or slightly increased. $1,25(OH)_2D_3$ therapy corrects the rickets and restores the plasma calcium, phosphate, and PTH levels.

Hereditary Generalized Resistance to 1α,25Hydroxyvitamin D_3

This rare autosomal recessive disorder has a phenotype similar to that of selective deficiency of $1α,25(OH)_2D_3$. The salient clinical features include increased serum levels of $25(OH)D_3$ and

$1\alpha,25(OH)_2D_3$ and resistance to exogenous $1\alpha,25(OH)_2D_3$ and $1\alpha,(OH)D_3$. The disease is caused by mutations in the vitamin D receptor gene.

INHERITED DISORDERS OF RENAL GLUCOSE TRANSPORT

Under normal conditions, glucose is almost completely reabsorbed by the proximal tubule through a Na^+-coupled active transport located in the brush border membrane. Only very small amounts of glucose are present in the urine of most normal people. The appearance of glycosuria suggests hyperglycemia (overload glucosuria), and, rarely, abnormal handling of glucose by the kidney. Renal glucosuria may be part of a generalized defect of the proximal tubule (Fanconi syndrome) or present as an isolated defect.

Renal Glucosuria

Renal glucosuria is generally a benign clinical condition that denotes a renal tubular abnormality characterized by variable amounts of glucose in the urine of affected individuals with normal serum glucose levels. Occasionally it is associated with *selective* aminoaciduria, unlike the generalized aminoaciduria seen in the Fanconi syndrome. Renal glucosuria is a rare occurrence when strict diagnostic criteria are applied. These include the following:

1. Oral glucose tolerance test results, levels of plasma insulin and free fatty acids, and glycosylated hemoglobin levels should all be normal.
2. The amount of glucose in the urine (10 to 100 g/day) should be relatively stable except during pregnancy when it may increase.
3. The degree of glucosuria should be largely independent of diet but may fluctuate according to the amount of carbohydrates ingested.
4. The carbohydrate excreted should be glucose.
5. Subjects with renal glucosuria should be able to store and use carbohydrates normally.

There are three subtypes of renal glycosuria. Type A is thought to involve a reduction in the capacity of the glucose transporter in the proximal tubule. Type B glucosuria is thought to be caused by a mutation that decreases the affinity of the transporter for glucose. In type O glucosuria there is no glucose transport in the proximal tubule. Types A and B are benign disorders; however, dehydration and ketosis may complicate type O glucosuria during pregnancy and starvation.

INHERITED HYPOKALEMIC HYPOTENSIVE DISORDERS

Familial hypokalemic, hypochloremic metabolic alkalosis is not a single entity but rather a set of closely related disorders. Bartter syndrome is a genetically heterogeneous disorder manifested by a hypokalemic metabolic alkalosis, hyperreninemic hyperaldosteronism, and normal blood pressure, as well as hyperplasia and hypertrophy of the juxtaglomerular apparatus. It typically presents during the neonatal period and is associated with hypercalciuria and nephrocalcinosis. In contrast, Gitelman syndrome is a disorder affecting the distal tubule that is usually diagnosed at a later stage and is associated with hypocalciuria and hypomagnesemia and predominant muscular signs and symptoms. The features of both disorders are outlined in Table 18–2.

Bartter Syndrome

Pathogenesis

Bartter syndrome is a group of autosomal recessive disorders affecting the function of the thick ascending limb of the loop of Henle, giving a clinical picture of salt-wasting and hypokalemic metabolic alkalosis. It is caused by inactivating mutations in one of at least four genes encoding membrane proteins expressed in this nephron segment:

1. The $Na^+/K^+/2Cl^-$ cotransporter (*NKCC2*)
2. The apical inward-rectifying potassium channel (*ROMK*)
3. ClC-Kb, a basolateral chloride channel (*CLCNKB*)
4. *Barttin*, a protein that acts as an essential activator of the β-subunit of ClC-Kb

Clinical Presentation

Most occurrences of Bartter syndrome present antenatally with polyhydramnios and premature labor. Polyuria and polydipsia are consistently seen. Postnatal findings include failure to thrive, growth retardation, dehydration, low blood pressure, muscle weakness, seizures, and tetany. In contrast to patients with Gitelman syndrome, those with Bartter syndrome are virtually

Table 18–2: Clinical Differences between Bartter and Gitelman Syndromes

	Bartter Syndrome				Gitelman Syndrome
	Type I (NKCC2)	Type II (ROMK)	Type III (CLCNKB)	Type IV (Barttin)	
Polyhydramnios	+	+	+	+	–
Failure to thrive	+	+	+	+	–
Growth retardation	+	+	+	+	–
Polyuria	+	+	+	+	–
Polydipsia	+	+	+	+	–
Muscle cramps/spasms	+	–	–	–	+
Chondrocalcinosis	–	–	–	–	+
Nephrocalcinosis	+	+	–	+	–
Sensorineural deafness	–	–	–	+	–

always hypercalciuric and normomagnesemic. Patients with *ROMK* mutations present with hyperkalemia at birth, which converts to hypokalemia within the first weeks of life. In these patients, Bartter syndrome may be misdiagnosed as pseudohypoaldosteronism type I. In contrast to other patients with Bartter syndrome, they do not need potassium supplementation. Barttin mutations are usually associated with an extremely severe phenotype of intrauterine onset that includes profound renal salt and water wasting, renal failure, sensorineural deafness, and motor retardation.

Treatment
The treatment of Bartter syndrome involves attempts to completely block distal potassium secretion with spironolactone and non-steroidal anti-inflammatory drugs in addition to oral potassium supplementation. Angiotensin-converting enzyme inhibitors have also been used successfully in conjunction with potassium supplements.

Gitelman Syndrome

Pathogenesis
Gitelman syndrome is an autosomal recessive disorder that is usually diagnosed in adults. It results from inactivating mutations in the *SLC12A3* gene encoding the thiazide sensitive Na^+/Cl^- cotransporter, or *NCCT*. This results in sodium and chloride wasting with secondary activation of the renin-angiotensin-aldosterone system. The increased sodium load to the cortical collecting duct leads to increased sodium reabsorption by the epithelial sodium channel, which is counterbalanced by potassium and hydrogen excretion, resulting in hypokalemia and a metabolic alkalosis.

Clinical Presentation
Unlike Bartter syndrome (see Table 18–2), Gitelman syndrome does not present symptomatically in the neonatal period and is often discovered incidentally. Patients have hypokalemic metabolic alkalosis, but in contrast to those with Bartter syndrome, they are hypocalciuric and hypomagnesemic and do not have signs of overt volume depletion. The major differential diagnosis of Gitelman syndrome is diuretic abuse and chronic bulimia. A careful history, as well as measurement of urinary chloride levels (low in patients with surreptitious vomiting) and a urinary diuretic screen, should help differentiate between these conditions.

Treatment
Treatment of Gitelman syndrome includes potassium supplementation and spironolactone. Nonsteroidal anti-inflammatory

drugs are usually not helpful, because prostaglandin levels are normal.

INHERITED HYPOKALEMIC HYPERTENSIVE DISORDERS

Hereditary hypokalemic hypertensive disorders are rare disorders that are due to abnormal biosynthesis, metabolism, or action of steroid hormones and are characterized primarily by low or low-normal plasma renin levels, normal or low serum potassium levels, and salt-sensitive hypertension, suggesting enhanced mineralocorticoid activity. However, most patients with hypokalemia and hypertension have essential hypertension associated with the use of diuretics or secondary aldosteronism from renal artery stenosis or primary hyperaldosteronism from adrenal gland hyperplasia or adenoma.

Congenital Adrenal Hyperplasia

Two of the inherited abnormalities in steroid biosynthesis can result in hypertension: 11β-hydroxylase deficiency and 17α-hydroxylase deficiency. In both deficiencies, overproduction of cortisol precursors results from a loss of negative feedback inhibition of adrenocorticotropic hormone (ACTH) release. These precursors either have intrinsic mineralocorticoid activity or are metabolized to mineralocorticoid agonists. This induces volume- and salt-dependent forms of hypertension with suppressed renin and reduced potassium concentrations.

11β-Hydroxylase Deficiency

Inactivating mutations in the gene encoding 11β-hydroxylase cause 5% of cases of congenital adrenal hyperplasia (90% of cases are caused by 21-hydroxylase deficiency, which is not associated with hypertension). This disease is associated with excess production of deoxycortisone (DOC), 18-deoxycortisol, and androgens. DOC has significant intrinsic mineralocorticoid activity, and high levels trigger hypokalemic hypertension. Because the androgen pathway is unaffected, prenatal masculinization occurs in females and postnatal virilization occurs in both sexes. The diagnosis of 11β-hydroxylase deficiency is made by the detection of increased levels of DOC and 18-deoxycortisol. Treatment consists of exogenous corticoids, which inhibit ACTH secretion. Correction of mild salt wasting from reduced mineralocorticoid production may be necessary.

17α-Hydroxylase Deficiency
17α-Hydroxylase deficiency results in reduced conversion of pregnenolone to progesterone and androgens with absent sex hormone production. The resulting hypogonadism and male pseudohermaphroditism are usually detected in adolescence because of failure to undergo puberty. Elevated glucocorticoid-suppressible levels of DOC and corticosterone, as well as their 18-hydroxylated products, are responsible for hypertension, hypokalemia, and renin and aldosterone suppression. Partial 17α-hydroxylase deficiency occurs and can present as sexual ambiguity in males without hypertension. Corticosteroid replacement corrects ACTH levels and hypertension.

Liddle Syndrome

Pathogenesis
Liddle syndrome is an autosomal dominant form of hypertension characterized by hypokalemia and low levels of plasma renin and aldosterone, resulting from mutations in the β- or γ-subunits of the amiloride-sensitive epithelial sodium channel (ENaC) in the distal convoluted tubule and collecting duct. ENaC activity in the kidney is tightly controlled by several distinct hormonal systems, including aldosterone. In Liddle syndrome, mutations within the cytoplasmic COOH terminus of the β- and γ-subunits of ENaC lead to hyperactivity of the channel. It has not been definitively resolved whether the mutations associated with Liddle syndrome induce constitutive activation of the channel because of an increase in the number of channels or an increased open probability of individual channels. Recent work has supported the hypothesis that the ENaC is removed from the plasma membrane through endocytosis and that Liddle syndrome mutations lead to a failure to remove the channels from the cell membrane.

Clinical Presentation
Constitutive activation of the ENaC causes inappropriate renal Na^+ reabsorption, blunted Na^+ excretion, and low-renin hypertension. Affected individuals have an increased risk of cerebrovascular and cardiovascular accidents, but renal failure is notoriously rare. Liddle syndrome can be differentiated from other rare Mendelian forms of low-renin hypertension with urinary or plasma hormonal profiles (Table 18–3).

Treatment
Hypertension is not rectified by mineralocorticoid receptor inhibitors but can be corrected by a low-salt diet and administration of ENaC antagonists (amiloride or triamterene).

Table 18–3: Urinary Steroid Profiles in Mendelian Forms of Low-Renin Hypertension

	Liddle Syndrome	Glucocorticoid-Remediable Aldosteronism	Apparent Mineralocorticoid Excess
Aldosterone	Decreased	Increased	Decreased
TH-aldo	Decreased	Increased	Decreased
18-Hydroxy-TH-aldo	Decreased	Increased	Decreased
18-Hydroxycortisol-F	Not detected	Increased	Not detected
Tetrahydrocortisol (TH-F)	Normal	Normal	Increased
Tetrahydrocortisone (TH-E)	Normal	Normal	Decreased
TH-F/TH-E	Normal	Normal	Increased

TH-aldo, tetrahydroxyaldosterone.

Data from Wornock DG: Liddle syndrome: An autosomal dominant form of human hypertension. *Kidney Int* 53:18–24, 1998.

341

Apparent Mineralocorticoid Excess

Pathogenesis

Apparent mineralocorticoid excess (AME) is a rare recessive disorder that results in hypokalemic hypertension with low serum levels of renin and aldosterone. It results from a deficiency of the 11β-hydroxysteroid dehydrogenase type 2 enzyme that is responsible for the conversion of cortisol to the inactive metabolite cortisone. In AME, cortisol acts as a potent mineralocorticoid and causes salt retention hypertension and hypokalemia with a suppression of the renin-angiotensin-aldosterone system. In addition, inhibition of 11β-hydroxysteroid dehydrogenase type 2 by licorice (glycyrrhizic acid) or carbenoxolone can result in the development of hypokalemic, hyporeninemic hypertension.

Clinical Presentation

AME is associated with severe juvenile low-renin hypertension, hypokalemic alkalosis, low birth weight, failure to thrive, poor growth, and nephrocalcinosis. The urinary cortisol metabolite tetrahydrocortisol is increased while tetrahydrocortisone is decreased. The milder form of AME (type 2), also due to mutations in the 11β-hydroxysteroid dehydrogenase type 2 gene, has similar clinical features but lacks the typical urinary steroid profile, that is, biochemical analysis reveals a moderately elevated cortisol-to-cortisone metabolite ratio.

Treatment

The treatment of AME is sodium restriction and either triamterene or amiloride. Spironolactone is not effective. Additional antihypertensive agents can be used as needed, particularly in older patients.

Glucocorticoid-Remediable Hyperaldosteronism

Pathogenesis

Glucocorticoid-remediable hyperaldosteronism is an autosomal dominant form of hypertension caused by a chimeric gene duplication arising from unequal crossover between aldosterone synthase and 11β-hydroxylase, two highly similar genes with the same transcriptional orientation lying 45,000 bp apart on chromosome 8. Normally 11β-hydroxylase is expressed at high levels and is regulated by ACTH, whereas aldosterone synthase is expressed at low levels and is regulated by angiotensin II. The genetic defect in this disorder results in the aldosterone synthase gene coming under the control of the regulatory promoter sequences of the 11β-hydroxylase. This leads to increased production of 18-hydroxycortisol and aldosterone metabolites and subsequent hypokalemic, hyporeninemic hypertension.

Clinical Presentation

The phenotypic spectrum of disease is broad, ranging from patients with mild hypertension and normal blood biochemistry to patients with severe hypertension, hypokalemia, and metabolic alkalosis. Glucocorticoid-remediable hyperaldosteronism is associated with high morbidity and mortality from the early onset of hemorrhagic stroke and ruptured intracranial aneurysms (20%). The diagnosis is usually established by measuring 18-hydroxy- or 18-oxocortisol metabolites in the urine or with the dexamethasone suppression test. Patients with glucose-remediable hyperaldosteronism produce high levels of 18-hydroxy- or 18-oxocortisol, steroids that are normally secreted in negligible amounts in normal subjects. In addition, because they secrete aldosterone in response to ACTH, glucocorticoid administration can suppress excessive aldosterone secretion. The diagnosis of glucose-remediable hyperaldosteronism can be definitively established by demonstrating the chimeric gene with molecular techniques.

Treatment

Simple glucocorticoid replacement is the treatment for glucose-remediable hyperaldosteronism. Salt restriction and ENaC inhibition or spironolactone are also effective.

INHERITED HYPERKALEMIC HYPOTENSIVE DISORDERS

Pseudohypoaldosteronism Type I

Pathogenesis

Pseudohypoaldosteronism type I is a rare genetically heterogeneous disorder of which there are two subtypes: an autosomal recessive form with severe manifestations that persist into adulthood and an autosomal dominant form with milder manifestations that lessen with age. The autosomal recessive form is caused by inactivating mutations in ENaC that result in a resistance to the effects of aldosterone. The autosomal dominant form is due to mutations in the mineralocorticoid receptor gene (*MR*).

Clinical Presentation

Autosomal *recessive* pseudohypoaldosteronism type I presents in early life with renal salt wasting, hypotension, hyperkalemia, metabolic acidosis, and, on occasion, failure to thrive. Biochemical features include hyponatremia, high plasma and urinary aldosterone levels, and elevated plasma renin activity. The differential diagnosis includes aldosterone synthase deficiency, salt-wasting forms of congenital adrenal hyperplasia, and Bartter syndrome resulting from mutations in the *ROMK* gene. The manifestations of autosomal *dominant* pseudohypoaldosteronism type I are milder, with remission of the syndrome with age. This is consistent with progressively reduced dependence on aldosterone.

Treatment
Treatment consists of salt supplementation. Administration of aldosterone, fludrocortisone, or deoxycorticosterone is not helpful. Patients with the recessive form usually need lifelong treatment for salt wasting and hyperkalemia, whereas in the dominant form, treatment can usually be withdrawn in adulthood.

INHERITED HYPERKALEMIC HYPERTENSIVE DISORDERS

Pseudohypoaldosteronism Type II

Pathogenesis
Pseudohypoaldosteronism type II, also known as Gordon syndrome, is a volume-dependent low-renin form of hypertension characterized by persistent hyperkalemia despite a normal renal glomerular filtration rate. Hypertension is attributable to increased renal salt reabsorption, hyperkalemia is due to reduced renal K^+ excretion, and metabolic acidosis is due to reduced H^+ excretion. The clinical abnormalities are ameliorated by thiazide diuretics, which inhibit salt reabsorption in the distal nephron. The disease is genetically heterogeneous, and three loci have now been mapped to chromosomes 17, 1, and 12. Two genes that have been identified encode members of the WNK family of serine-threonine kinases: WNK 1 and 4 that localize to the distal nephron. WNK4 negatively regulates surface expression of the thiazide sensitive Na^+/Cl^- cotransporter and mutations result in enhanced surface expression of the cotransporter. Recent data suggest that WNK1 plays a general role in the regulation of epithelial Cl^- flux, and gain of function mutations may lead to enhanced cotransporter activity.

Clinical Presentation
Pseudohypoaldosteronism type II is usually diagnosed in adults. The severity of hyperkalemia varies greatly and is influenced by prior intake of diuretics and salt. In its most severe form, it is associated with muscle weakness (from hyperkalemia), short stature, and intellectual impairment. Mild hyperchloremia, metabolic acidosis, and suppressed plasma renin activity are findings

variably associated with the trait. The plasma renin response to upright posture or to a low-sodium diet is blunted. Aldosterone levels vary from low to high, depending on the level of hyperkalemia. Urinary concentrating ability, acid excretion, and proximal tubular function are all normal.

Treatment
Treatment with thiazide diuretics reverses all the biochemical abnormalities. Lower than average doses can be given if overcorrection is seen.

DIABETES INSIPIDUS

Pathogenesis

The major action of arginine vasopressin (AVP) is to facilitate urinary concentration by allowing water to be transported passively down an osmotic gradient between the tubular fluid and the surrounding interstitium. AVP acts via the vasopressin V_2 receptor located on the basolateral membrane of collecting duct cells. This step initiates a cascade of events that leads to the exocytic insertion of specific water channels, aquaporin-2, into the luminal membrane, thereby increasing the water permeability of this membrane. When AVP is not available, water channels are retrieved by an endocytic process, and the tubule becomes water impermeable.

In nephrogenic diabetes insipidus (NDI), the kidney is unable to concentrate urine despite normal or elevated concentrations of AVP. In congenital NDI, the obvious clinical manifestations of the disease, that is, polyuria and polydipsia, are present at birth and need to be immediately recognized to avoid severe episodes of dehydration. Most (> 90%) patients with congenital NDI have mutations in the *AVPR2* gene, the *Xq28* gene coding for the vasopressin V_2 receptor. In fewer than 10% of the families studied, congenital NDI has an autosomal recessive inheritance, and mutations have been identified in the aquaporin-2 gene (*AQP2*) located in chromosome region 12q13, that is, the vasopressin-sensitive water channel. Other inherited disorders in which mild, moderate, or severe inability to concentrate urine is present include Bartter syndrome, cystinosis, and autosomal dominant hypocalcemia.

Clinical Presentation

Loss-of-Function Mutations of AVPR2
X-linked NDI is caused by *AVPR2* mutations that result in loss of function or dysregulation of the V_2 receptor. Males who have

an *AVPR2* mutation have a phenotype characterized by dehydration episodes, hypernatremia, and hyperthermia as early as the first week of life. Dehydration episodes can be life-threatening. The infants are irritable, cry almost constantly, and, although they are eager to suck, will vomit milk soon after ingestion unless prefed with water. The history given by the mothers often includes persistent constipation, erratic unexplained fever, and failure to gain weight. Heterozygous females exhibit variable degrees of polyuria and polydipsia because of skewed X chromosome inactivation. Early recognition and treatment of X-linked NDI with an abundant intake of water allows a normal life span with normal physical and mental development. A variant of this disorder is autosomal dominant NDI, which results from mutations in the prepro-arginine-vasopressin-neurophysin II gene. Patients with autosomal dominant NDI retain some limited capacity to secrete AVP during severe dehydration, and the polyuria and polydipsia symptoms usually appear after the first year of life when the infant's demand for water is more likely to be understood by adults.

Loss-of-Function Mutations of AQP2
Mutations in the *AQP2* gene that encodes the aquaporin-2 channel results in NDI. The gene is located in chromosome region 12q13 and appears to be inherited in an autosomal recessive fashion. Mutations appear to impair trafficking of aquaporin-2 and/or decrease channel function.

Cystic Diseases of the Kidney

19

Cysts are common renal abnormalities that are composed of a layer of tubular epithelium enclosing a cavity filled with urine-like liquid or semisolid material. They are extremely rare in infants; however, their prevalence increases with age. A relatively large number of clinical conditions are associated with renal cysts (Table 19–1).

Table 19–1: Classification of Renal Cysts

Hereditary polycystic kidney disease
   Autosomal dominant polycystic kidney disease
   Autosomal recessive polycystic kidney disease
Acquired cystic kidney disease (in azotemia and dialysis)
Cystic diseases of the renal medulla
   Medullary cystic disease
      Autosomal recessive
      Autosomal dominant
   Medullary sponge kidney
Simple cysts
Cystic renal dysplasia
Miscellaneous renal cystic disorders
   Hereditary
      Tuberous sclerosis
      von Hippel-Lindau disease
   Nonhereditary
      Solitary multilocular cysts
      Pyelocalyceal cysts
      Renal lymphangiomatosis
      Hilar and perinephric pseudocysts

HEREDITARY POLYCYSTIC KIDNEY DISORDERS

Autosomal dominant polycystic kidney disease (ADPKD) and autosomal recessive polycystic kidney disease (ARPKD) are the principal single-gene disorders that cause polycystic kidney disease. ADPKD is caused by one of two genetic mutations in genes on chromosomes 16 (*PKD1*) and 4 (*PKD2*). *PKD1* and *PKD2* encode proteins polycystin-1 and -2, respectively. The exact mechanism whereby the genetic mutations trigger cystogenesis remains incompletely understood. The gene for ARPKD (*PKHD1*), located on chromosome 6, encodes a relatively large protein called fibrocystin. The cellular location and biologic function of fibrocystin have not been clearly defined.

Autosomal Dominant Polycystic Kidney Disease

ADPKD affects 1 in 500 to 1000 individuals. It is inherited as an autosomal dominant trait with complete penetrance. In about 40% of patients there may be no family history of ADPKD. In most respects, polycystic kidney disease type 1 (PKD1) and type 2 (PKD2) are clinically similar, except that the progression to end-stage renal disease (ESRD) is slower in PKD2. ADPKD may not be clinically apparent until the third or fourth decade of life. There is no way to predict in young patients whether or when renal failure will develop, although several risk factors (hypertension, renal hemorrhage, multiple pregnancies, male sex, and *PKD1* genotype) that are associated with a more rapid course have been identified.

About one half of young adults with ADPKD have cysts of the liver, and the prevalence increases with age. Liver dysfunction and portal hypertension rarely occur, regardless of the size and number of cysts. The liver cysts may continue to grow and to appear de novo after institution of renal replacement therapy. They may become infected and have been the site of origin of cholangiocellular carcinoma. Epithelial cysts occur in organs other than the liver including the pancreas, spleen, and arachnoid layer.

Pathogenesis of Renal Failure

ESRD develops before the end of the seventh decade of life in approximately 50% of individuals with PKD1 or PKD2. Renal failure results from the progressive expansion and encroachment on adjacent parenchyma rather than from loss of function in individual renal tubules. The "pressure" of the expanding

cysts may distort the delicate tubulointerstitial network of capillaries, lymphatics, arterioles, and venules, leading to functional
disturbances of the surrounding parenchyma. Hypertension is
thought to develop due to disturbances in the microvasculature,
leading to activation of the renin-angiotensin system, which in
turn accelerates tubulointerstitial fibrosis. Clinical measurements of glomerular filtration rate (GFR) in ADPKD are poor
predictors of the future course of slowly progressive renal disease.
Indeed, relatively young patients with normal GFR may have
profoundly distorted renal anatomy and extreme renal enlargement, yet the GFR may be within normal limits. This finding
reflects the fact that GFR is maintained within the normal range
in patients with advanced cystic change through compensatory
hyperfiltration in residual glomeruli. Only after the compensatory mechanisms fail is a fall in GFR seen, and this decline can
be relatively precipitous.

Diagnosis
In its fully developed form, ADPKD is not difficult to diagnose
(Table 19–2). Patients present with bilateral renal enlargement
that can be felt on careful palpation. Many patients will have
noticed loin pain, hematuria, and/or increased abdominal girth,
and 60% of patients have a family history of ADPKD. Results
of urinalysis are usually normal early in the disease course.
There may be a defect in maximum concentrating ability, but
urinary dilution remains intact, and urinary acidification is
normal. Massive proteinuria is rare and, if found, should
prompt a search for an additional renal disorder. In the middle

**Table 19–2: Clinical Criteria for Diagnosis of Autosomal
Dominant Polycystic Kidney Disease**

Primary criteria
    More than three fluid-filled cysts scattered diffusely throughout
        renal cortex and medulla of both kidneys
    Definite history of polycystic kidney disease in genetically
        related family members
Secondary criteria
    Polycystic liver
    Renal insufficiency
    Abdominal hernia
    Cardiac valvular lesions
    Cysts of pancreas
    Aneurysms of cerebral arteries
    Seminal vesicle cysts
    Drooping eyelids

to late stages of the disease (20 to 40 years of age), mild persistent proteinuria (>200 mg/day) may be found in 20% to 40% of patients. The hematocrit may be increased above normal, possibly because of abnormal erythropoietin production by cysts, and patients with end-stage ADPKD do not have anemia as profound as that occurring in other types of terminal renal disease.

The diagnosis can be confirmed by radiologic examination. Ultrasonography, the preferred screening method, reveals multiple echo-free areas in both kidneys. Standard criteria for the diagnosis of ADPKD include at least two cysts in at least one kidney in patients younger than 30 years of age. Negative results for radiologic evaluation in a patient older than age 30 effectively excludes the diagnosis of ADPKD. Patients between the ages of 30 and 59 years should have at least two cysts in each kidney, and patients older than 60 years of age should have at least four cysts in each kidney. If the ultrasonography results are equivocal then contrast-enhanced computed tomography (CT) readily distinguishes between solid and cystic renal masses and portrays the diffuse distribution of large and small cysts, a characteristic that is important in differentiating ADPKD from multiple simple cysts. CT scanning also reveals small cysts in the liver, a finding that further helps to differentiate ADPKD from acquired cystic disorders. Gene linkage analysis can be used to determine obligate ADPKD gene carriers, but this method has not gained widespread clinical use. The differential diagnosis of ADPKD includes ARPKD in children, tuberous sclerosis, multiple simple cysts, multicystic dysplastic kidney, von Hippel-Lindau syndrome, and acquired cystic kidney disease.

Therapy
Most patients with ADPKD require no modification in normal physical activity or lifestyle. However, recurrent bouts of gross hematuria, usually related to direct trauma, are associated with a faster decline of renal function; therefore, avoidance of renal trauma seems prudent.

HYPERTENSION Arterial hypertension develops in more than half of patients with ADPKD and is an important risk factor for progression of renal insufficiency. Current recommendations for blood pressure targets derive from studies of renal diseases in general and a target level of less than 120/80 mm Hg is appropriate. Angiotensin-converting enzyme inhibitors and angiotensin receptor blockers are effective in the treatment of hypertension in patients with ADPKD and should be the agents of first choice. Close monitoring of the serum creatinine level is warranted after initiation of therapy and during episodes of cyst hemorrhage or infection. Ca^+ channel blockers, β-adrenergic blockers, and $α_2$-adrenergic agonists may be helpful in refractory disease.

MANAGEMENT OF PAIN Pain, caused by perinephric hemorrhage, is the most common symptom in ADPKD and can lead to analgesic dependence and abuse. Cyst hemorrhage can usually be treated with bed rest and analgesics. Unrelenting pain should be evaluated, especially if it is associated with gross or microscopic hematuria to exclude the possibility of renal infection, stones, or tumors. Pain may also be associated with the enlargement of one or more cysts in a kidney, and some relief may be obtained by percutaneous aspiration of fluid combined with instillation of a sclerosing agent. Alternatively, surgical aspiration and unroofing of cysts has been performed for the treatment of extremely large kidneys filled with cysts. This radical therapy may produce relief that lasts for several years. Percutaneous laparoscopic methods have been developed for cyst unroofing or total nephrectomy with reasonably good outcomes.

HEMATURIA AND INTRARENAL HEMORRHAGE Hematuria is usually caused by the rupture of a cyst into the pelvis of the kidney. It appears suddenly and persists as macroscopic or microscopic bleeding for several days. In addition to vascular rupture into cysts, hematuria may be caused by renal stones, cyst infection, or malignant tumors. Reduced physical activity or bed rest is usually sufficient to control the bleeding. Transcatheter arterial infarction has been used to control recurrent hemorrhage in ADPKD and may be of some value in patients with severe renal blood loss for whom dialysis is imminent or extant.

RENAL INFECTION Parenchymal pyogenic bacterial infection is a major problem for patients with ADPKD, particularly women. Diffuse pyelonephritis is the most common manifestation of parenchymal infection, but one or more cysts may become infected, and, as with any deep-seated abscess, the condition may be difficult to treat. Fever, bacteremia, leukocytosis, bacteriuria, pus casts in the urine, and exquisite tenderness on deep palpation of the kidneys strongly suggest a diagnosis of pyelonephritis. Cyst infection, in contrast, may not be associated with bacteriuria or bacteremia and may be suspected if the infection fails to respond to conventional parenteral therapy. Radiologic studies are not generally useful because the changes induced by infection are similar to those of hemorrhage. Coliform, staphylococcal, and *Bacteroides* organisms have been isolated from cyst fluid aspirates in some patients, but often no organism is isolated.

Pyelonephritis should be treated as for patients without cystic disease. Cyst infections pose a particular problem. Although most cysts are permeable to polar antibiotics, such as cephalosporins and aminoglycosides, some cysts are relatively impermeable, and in these cysts, lipophilic drugs are required to achieve adequate bacteriocidal levels. Parenteral lipid-soluble drugs, such as ciprofloxacin (and newer derivatives), chloramphenicol, erythromycin, tetracyclines, and trimethoprim, may be useful if cephalosporins, penicillin derivatives, and aminoglycosides fail to eradicate the infection.

Once the patient is afebrile, has a normal blood leukocyte count, sterile urine, and no leukocytes in the urine sediment, an oral bacteriocidal antibiotic should be administered until there is no renal pain on deep palpation. Therapy should last for at least 4 to 6 weeks, and if a relapse occurs after this time, then it may be necessary to administer antibiotics for up to 1 year. All patients are advised to refuse urinary tract instrumentation procedures unless absolutely necessary. Nephrectomy is reserved for intractable infection after parenteral antibiotics have been administered unsuccessfully.

ARTERIAL ANEURYSMS Cerebral aneurysms occur in less than 5% of patients. However, in patients with a clear family history of cerebral aneurysm, the risk increases to about 20%. Because most patients with ADPKD do not experience this complication, screening by magnetic resonance angiography is reserved for individuals with a family history of aneurysm and for those who have symptoms consistent with an intracerebral pathologic condition.

NEPHROLITHIASIS The incidence of renal stone formation (uric acid or calcium oxalate) is approximately 20% in ADPKD. The treatment of urinary lithiasis is not different from that in patients without ADPKD (see Chapter 21, Nephrolithiasis.)

PREGNANCY Women who have had more than three pregnancies may experience an earlier onset of renal insufficiency than others. Normotensive women with ADPKD usually have uncomplicated pregnancies; however, those with hypertension have a higher risk for fetal and maternal complications.

END-STAGE DISEASE, DIALYSIS, AND TRANSPLANTATION ADPKD progresses to the end stage in approximately 45% of affected individuals by 60 years of age. Risk factors for progression include hypertension, male sex, *PKD1* as opposed to the *PKD2* genotype, younger age at diagnosis, larger kidneys, episodes of gross and microscopic hematuria, and moderate to severe proteinuria.

CT and magnetic resonance imaging (MRI) studies with radio-contrast material and gadolinium enhancement may provide a tool for judging prognosis in nonazotemic patients. Patients with low degrees of renal volume replacement by cysts may be reassured that they have several years of useful renal function; however, those with extensive cystic change involving over one half of the renal parenchyma are likely to develop ESRD within 8 to 10 years. Aside from control of hypertension, there is no specific therapy targeted to the polycystic disease process that slows progression. Surgical unroofing of surface cysts (the Rovsing procedure) has no beneficial effect on renal function but may provide symptom control.

Patients with ADPKD who are receiving dialysis do as well as or better than others with nondiabetic renal disorders. Patients may have higher hematocrit values, without erythropoietin supplementation, than individuals with other renal diseases. Renal transplantation is used routinely to treat patients with end-stage ADPKD. Post-transplantation patient and kidney survival rates appear to be equal to if not better than those in other renal disorders. Indications for pre- or post-transplantation bilateral nephrectomy include severe pain, unrelenting infection, persistent bacteriuria, recurrent severe urinary tract hemorrhage, renal neoplasm, nephrolithiasis, and extreme kidney size with compression of intra-abdominal vessels and viscera leading to symptoms.

Material to educate patients and their families about ADPKD can be obtained through the Polycystic Kidney Disease Foundation (http://www.PKDcure.org).

Autosomal Recessive Polycystic Kidney Disease

ARPKD is a rare disorder with an incidence of 1 in 10,000 to 50,000 live births. It is inherited as an autosomal recessive trait and because most patients do not have homozygous mutations, there is considerable variability in the clinical expression of the disease. The genetic defect has been localized to a large gene in chromosome 6, *PKHD1,* which encodes a protein called fibrocystin/polyductin. Approximately 50% of individuals with ARPKD die from renal insufficiency and pulmonary maldevelopment within hours or days after birth. The remaining patients have a milder form of disease that may not manifest until later in infancy, childhood, or early adulthood. Those who survive the neonatal period have a 50% to 80% chance of surviving to at least 15 years of age.

Diagnosis

The clinical presentation of ARPKD in the newborn is characterized by a history of oligohydramnios and often by a difficult delivery because of the enlarged fetal kidneys. Severely affected infants also may have Potter facies and respiratory distress diagnosed on the basis of pulmonary hypoplasia and atelectasis. Renal function usually is compromised, but death from renal insufficiency is uncommon in the newborn period. Hypertension often develops in the first several months and may be complicated by cardiac hypertrophy, endocardial fibroelastosis, congestive heart failure, and the onset of renal failure. In older children symptoms and signs referable to hepatic fibrosis and portal hypertension predominate. Ultrasonography is the most important diagnostic tool for initial screening purposes as well as for prenatal diagnosis. Genetic linkage and direct mutational analysis hold promise of more precise diagnosis and characterization of the disease in individual patients.

Therapy

The newborn with pulmonary hypoplasia usually dies of pulmonary insufficiency within the first few days. Nonetheless, until the degree of the pulmonary insufficiency and its cause can be assessed fully, artificial ventilation and aggressive resuscitative measures are indicated. Removal of extremely large kidneys has been necessary in a few infants to improve ventilation. Early institution of dialysis has been used successfully. Patients with less severe ARPKD who survive the newborn period invariably develop progressive renal failure. The management of chronic renal failure in children with ARPKD should follow the same general guidelines used for any child with established chronic renal insufficiency. Parents who give birth to a child with ARPKD can be advised that, on a statistical basis, each of their children will have a 25% chance of having the disease and a 50% chance of being a carrier of the abnormal gene. Emotional support and education of families of patients can be obtained through the Polycystic Kidney Foundation (http://www.PKDcure.org).

ACQUIRED CYSTIC KIDNEY DISEASE

Patients receiving renal replacement therapy for relatively long periods develop multiple cysts in their remnant kidneys—acquired cystic kidney disease (ACKD). It occurs even in patients with chronic renal failure before dialysis, and it has been described in all forms of chronic renal disease. Acquired cysts are found in 7% to 22% of patients with serum creatinine values exceeding 3 mg/dL, in 44% of patients receiving dialysis for less than 3 years, and in 75% of patients after 3 years of dialysis treatment. An important clinical consequence of acquired renal cystic disease is the occurrence of aggressive renal tumors. Renal cell carcinoma in dialysis patients is three times more common in the presence of acquired renal cysts. Overall, the incidence of renal malignancy in dialysis patients has been estimated to be 57 to 134 times greater than that in the general population.

Diagnosis

ACKD develops insidiously. Most patients are asymptomatic, but when symptoms do occur, gross hematuria, flank pain, renal colic, fever, palpable renal mass, and rising hematocrit are the most common. Sonography reveals the bilateral cystic process in advanced disease and is useful in the detection of neoplasms. However, CT, with or without contrast enhancement, is the preferred diagnostic technique and is better for distinguishing between simple cysts and ACKD. MRI, with or without gadolinium enhancement, may also be useful, particularly for the diagnosis of neoplasms, as an alternative to contrast-enhanced CT in patients at risk of contrast nephropathy and when CT findings are indeterminate. Differentiation from ADPKD and from multiple simple cysts usually is suggested by the generally smaller size of the kidneys and of the individual cysts in ACKD, by the usual absence of hepatic cysts, and by the family and patient histories.

Therapy

Bleeding episodes, either intrarenal or perirenal, often may be treated conservatively with bed rest and analgesics. Persistent hemorrhage, however, may require nephrectomy or therapeutic renal embolization and infarction. Because the risk of undetected renal cell carcinoma is high in patients with retroperitoneal hemorrhage, nephrectomy is recommended for those patients in whom carcinoma cannot be ruled out. Because renal cell carcinoma is an important complication of ACKD, CT screening has been recommended after 3 years of dialysis, followed by screening for neoplasm at 1- or 2-year intervals thereafter. Renal masses larger than 3 cm detected in ACKD are treated by excision. For tumors smaller than 3 cm, some physicians advise nephrectomy for the acceptable surgical candidate, whereas others recommend annual CT follow-up with resection if the lesions enlarge. Resection even of small neoplasms seems prudent in preparation for transplantation.

CYSTIC DISEASE OF THE RENAL MEDULLA

Medullary Cystic Disease

Medullary cystic disease (MCD) occurs as both an autosomal dominant and autosomal recessive condition. Disease caused by the different genotypes appears grossly similar with multiple spherical, thin-walled cysts at the corticomedullary junction. The recessive type, called nephronophthisis, appears typically in infants and small children, whereas the dominant form may be detected along the entire spectrum of age.

Diagnosis
The diagnosis of MCD should be suspected in patients with ESRD in childhood and in azotemic adults with a familial history of renal disease. Genetic linkage analysis may be helpful in arriving at a diagnosis in approximately 70% of patients without the need for a renal biopsy. MCD may account for as many as 1% to 5% of all patients who need dialysis or transplantation and for 10% to 20% of cases of renal failure in childhood. Clinical presentation usually occurs in the first or second decade of life but may occur as late as the seventh decade. CT and MRI may be helpful diagnostic procedures, especially for those patients with relatively small medullary cysts that cannot be diagnosed unequivocally by ultrasonography. Open renal biopsy may be the only certain way to make the diagnosis.

Management
Patients who manifest renal insufficiency in childhood usually have the autosomal recessive form of the disease and present with polydipsia, polyuria, pallor, lethargy, and growth retardation. Progression to the end stage of the disease occurs before the age of 20. In the adult form, patients may develop urinary concentration defects sufficient to cause serious Na^+ wastage, hyponatremia, and extracellular fluid volume contraction before the development of ESRD. Some patients require vast quantities of NaCl and water to maintain Na^+ balance. Should oral intake be interrupted for some reason, intravenous salt and water replacement are mandatory. When acidosis occurs (a defect in distal H^+ handling), oral sodium bicarbonate should be given in addition to NaCl. The uncertain pattern of genetic transmission in MCD is a severe obstacle in selecting living related donors for renal transplantation.

Medullary Sponge Kidney

Medullary sponge kidney is typically a benign disorder that may remain asymptomatic throughout life or not be recognized until middle age when secondary calcareous or infective complications emerge. The incidence is approximately 1 in 5000 and progression to renal failure is uncommon. The underlying etiology is unknown, but a genetic predisposition is suggested by reports of a high incidence in family members of affected individuals. Curiously, as many as 25% of patients with medullary sponge kidney have hemihypertrophy of the body, and about 10% of patients with hemihypertrophy also have medullary sponge kidney.

Diagnosis and Management

The disease is associated with hematuria and recurrent urinary tract infections. Nephrolithiasis with renal colic, loin pain, and excretion of small stones is also a prominent feature. The disease seldom progresses to ESRD, although reduced GFRs have been observed, and perhaps 10% of patients have a relatively poor prognosis because of recurring urolithiasis and pyelonephritis. The most commonly recognized functional abnormalities include defective urinary solute concentrating ability and a distal renal tubular acidosis. The diagnosis is made by intravenous urography, which shows radial, linear striations in the papillae or cystic collections of contrast medium in the ectatic collecting ducts.

Renal stones consisting of calcium oxalate, calcium phosphate, and other types of calcium salts commonly form in the ectatic collecting ducts in this disease. This condition accounts for approximately 10% to 20% of occurrences of calcium stones. The nephrolithiasis is largely attributable to absorptive hypercalciuria, hypocitruria, and hyperoxaluria. The defect in renal acidification may also contribute in some patients. The management of the nephrolithiasis is no different from that in the general population with recurrent nephrolithiasis. Because patients with medullary sponge kidney appear to be more susceptible to urinary tract infections, routine preventive measures are warranted, especially in female patients.

Renal abscesses are a rare complication of this disorder that may require prolonged antibiotic therapy or surgical drainage. If the tubule ectasia is unilateral or segmental, a unilateral or partial nephrectomy may be warranted. However, because this is usually a bilateral disorder, partial or complete nephrectomy should be undertaken after careful evaluation indicates that sufficient residual renal function will be preserved.

SIMPLE CYSTS

Simple cysts are the most common cystic abnormality encountered in human kidneys. They are very rare in children and increase in frequency with age so that by age 50 they are found in approximately 50% of the population. Complications are uncommon but include cyst infection, and hypertension due to local compression of intrarenal vessels with subsequent renin release.

Diagnosis

Most simple cysts are found on routine urographic examinations. They are far more common in adults than in children. In most patients simple cysts are asymptomatic, and the major problem is differentiating between a simple cyst and a malignant mass. Occasionally patients may present with a palpable abdominal mass, hematuria after abdominal trauma, an infected cyst, or mild proteinuria.

With lesions as common as simple cysts, it is not surprising that the coincidence of simple cyst and tumor in the same kidney is 2% to 4%. Nonetheless, it is very uncommon to find a neoplasm actually arising within a cyst. Therefore, in asymptomatic patients with a few small and unequivocal simple cysts, further evaluation, except perhaps for periodic follow-up by sonography, is not indicated in the absence of fever, leukocytosis, hematuria, or renal discomfort.

No rigid criteria have been adopted for the use of CT, sonography, arteriography, MRI, and cyst puncture in the evaluation of patients with questionable renal mass lesions; however CT is the most commonly used technique. If the radiologic features are suspicious, then surgical exploration is recommended.

Therapy

The management of symptomatic renal cysts can take several forms. Most intermediate-sized cysts can be aspirated percutaneously, and a sclerosing agent can be instilled into the cavity in an attempt to prevent recurrence. Symptomatic cysts greater than 500 mL in volume are usually drained surgically. Laparoscopic methods are now used routinely.

RENAL DYSPLASIA

The term *renal dysplasia* implies any developmental abnormality resulting from anomalous early development in utero. In general, the most severely dysplastic kidneys are nonfunctional, have no patent connection to the urinary bladder, and remain asymptomatic if unilateral. Less severely dysplastic kidneys may have near-normal function and manifest with clinical symptoms and signs related only to their size or to their increased susceptibility to infection.

MISCELLANEOUS CYSTIC DISORDERS

Tuberous Sclerosis

In this disease complex, hamartomatous tumors may develop in the skin, brain, retina, bone, liver, heart, lung, and kidney. Renal angiomyolipomas are found in as many as 50% of patients, and the combination of cystic kidneys and angiomyolipomas is virtually pathognomonic for tuberous sclerosis. Tuberous sclerosis is an autosomal dominant disorder with an incidence of approximately 1 in 10,000. There are two genotypes: *TSC1* is located on chromosome 9q32p34 and encodes a protein called hamartin; *TSC2* is located next to *PKD1* on chromosome 16p13 and encodes a protein called tuberin. Hamartin and tuberin appear to function together in a tumor-suppressor role. Sonography, CT, MRI, and arteriography are valuable for distinguishing multiple renal cysts from the more common angiomyolipomas in this disease. The cysts may be quite large, and renal impairment, although relatively uncommon, may occur. Hypertension is a major manifestation of the renal abnormality.

von Hippel-Lindau Syndrome

This syndrome includes cerebellar and retinal hemangioblastomas, pancreatic cysts and carcinoma, and renal cysts and tumors. Numerous irregularly distributed renal cysts up to several centimeters in diameter are found in about 65% of the patients and may simulate ADPKD. Malignant tumors complicate cyst development in 25% of patients, metastasize in about one half of those and cause death in about one third. This disease is inherited by autosomal dominant transmission. The gene defect is located at the short arm of chromosome 3 and has been linked to an oncogene locus that is possibly involved in spontaneous renal cell carcinoma. Because of the high risk of development of renal cell carcinoma, annual or semiannual examination by CT or MRI is recommended for patients at risk, beginning in the second decade.

Diabetic Nephropathy

20

Diabetic nephropathy is the single most common cause of end-stage renal disease (ESRD) in Europe and the United States, accounting for 25% to 45% of patients enrolled in ESRD programs. Nephropathy is a major cause of illness and death in diabetes and is associated with strikingly high rates of cardiovascular disease, particularly in type 2 diabetic patients.

Persistent albuminuria (>300 mg/24 hr) is the hallmark of diabetic nephropathy, which can be diagnosed clinically if the following additional criteria are fulfilled: the presence of diabetic retinopathy and the absence of clinical or laboratory evidence of other kidney or renal tract disease. This clinical definition of diabetic nephropathy is valid in both type 1 diabetes and type 2 diabetes. During the last decade longitudinal studies have shown that microalbuminuria strongly predicts the development of diabetic nephropathy in both type 1 and type 2 diabetes. *Microalbuminuria* is defined as urinary albumin excretion greater than 30 mg/24 hr (20 mcg/min) and less than or equal to 300 mg/24 hr (200 mcg/min), irrespective of how the urine is collected.

EPIDEMIOLOGY OF MICROALBUMINURIA AND DIABETIC NEPHROPATHY

Prevalence and Incidence

The overall prevalence of micro- and macroalbuminuria is approximately 30% to 35% in both type 1 and 2 diabetes. The highest prevalence is found in Native Americans with type 2 diabetes followed by black Americans, Mexican Americans, Asian Indians, and European white patients. Diabetic nephropathy rarely develops before 10 years' duration of type 1 diabetes, whereas approximately 3% of patients with newly diagnosed

361

type 2 diabetes have overt nephropathy. The incidence peak (3% per year) is usually found between 10 and 20 years of diabetes, after which a progressive decline in incidence takes place. Thus, the risk of developing diabetic nephropathy for a normoalbuminuric patient with a diabetes duration of greater than 30 years is very low.

Microalbuminuria Predicts Nephropathy

Several longitudinal studies have shown that microalbuminuria strongly predicts the development of diabetic nephropathy in type 1 diabetic patients (risk ratio > 20). The predictive value is somewhat lower in microalbuminuric type 2 diabetic patients (risk ratio 8.5). In addition to microalbuminuria, several other risk factors or markers for development of diabetic nephropathy have been documented including poor glycemic control, hypertension, male sex, familial clustering, smoking, age younger than 20 years at disease onset, and ethnicity.

Prognosis in Microalbuminuria

Microalbuminuria is a strong predictor of total and cardiovascular mortality and cardiovascular morbidity in diabetic patients. The mechanisms linking microalbuminuria and death from cardiovascular disease are poorly understood. Microalbuminuria has been proposed as a marker of widespread endothelial dysfunction that might predispose individuals to enhanced penetrations in the arterial wall of atherogenic lipoprotein particles; has been proposed as a marker of established cardiovascular disease; and is associated with an excess of well-known and potential cardiovascular risk factors. Raised blood pressure, dyslipoproteinemia, increased platelet aggregability, endothelial dysfunction, insulin resistance, and hyperinsulinemia have been demonstrated in microalbuminuria diabetic patients. Recent echocardiographic studies have revealed impaired diastolic function and cardiac hypertrophy in microalbuminuric type 1 and type 2 diabetic patients. Left ventricular hypertrophy predisposes the individual to ischemic heart disease, ventricular arrhythmia, sudden death, and heart failure.

Prognosis in Diabetic Nephropathy

Type 1 diabetic patients without proteinuria have a low and constant relative mortality, whereas patients with proteinuria have a significantly higher relative mortality (> 10-fold).

However, the prognostic importance of proteinuria in type 2 patients is considerably less than that in type 1 diabetes (two-to-fivefold). The cumulative death rate 10 years after onset of abnormally elevated urinary albumin excretion in European type 2 diabetic patients is approximately 70% compared with 45% in normoalbuminuric patients. Indeed much of the excess cardiovascular mortality associated with type 2 diabetes is concentrated in patients with proteinuria.

CLINICAL COURSE AND PATHOPHYSIOLOGY

A preclinical phase consisting of a normo- and a microalbuminuria stage and a clinical phase characterized by albuminuria are well documented in both type 1 and type 2 diabetic patients.

Normoalbuminuria

Approximately one third of type 1 diabetic patients have a glomerular filtration rate (GFR) above the upper normal range of that for age-matched healthy nondiabetic subjects. The degree of hyperfiltration is less in type 2 diabetic patients. The GFR elevation is particularly pronounced in patients with newly diagnosed diabetes and in other patients during intervals with poor metabolic control. Intensified insulin treatment and near-normal blood glucose control reduce GFR toward normal levels after a period of days to weeks in both type 1 and type 2 diabetic patients.

Longitudinal studies suggest that hyperfiltration is a risk factor for subsequent increases in urinary albumin excretion and development of diabetic nephropathy in type 1 diabetic patients, but this has not been conclusively established. The prognostic significance of hyperfiltration in type 2 diabetic patients is unclear.

Microalbuminuria

Subclinical albumin excretion rate has been termed *microalbuminuria,* and it can be normalized by improved glycemic control. In addition to hyperglycemia, many other factors can induce microalbuminuria in diabetic patients such as hypertension, massive obesity, heavy exercise, various acute or chronic illnesses, and cardiac failure. Furthermore, the day-to-day variation in the urinary albumin excretion ratio is high, 30% to 50%, and consequently more than one urine sample is needed to determine whether an individual patient has persistent microalbuminuria. Urinary albumin excretion within the microalbuminuric range (30 to 300 mg/24 hr) in at least two of three consecutive nonketotic sterile urine samples is the generally accepted definition of persistent microalbuminuria. Persistent microalbuminuria is exceptional in the first 5 years of diabetes. The annual rate of rise of urinary albumin excretion is about 20% in both type 2 and type 1 diabetic patients with persistent microalbuminuria. The prevalence of arterial hypertension (= 140/90 mm Hg) in adult type 1 diabetic patients is 42%, 52%, and 79% in subjects with normo-, micro-, and macro-albuminuria, respectively. The prevalence of hypertension in type 2 diabetes is 71%, 90% and 93% in the normo-, micro-, and macroalbuminuria groups, respectively.

Diabetic Nephropathy

Diabetic nephropathy is a clinical syndrome characterized by persistent albuminuria (> 300 mg/24 hr), a relentless decline in GFR, and raised arterial blood pressure. Although albuminuria is the first sign, peripheral edema is the first symptom of diabetic nephropathy. Fluid retention is often observed early in the course of this kidney disease, that is, at a stage with well-preserved renal function and only slight reduction in serum albumin.

The natural history of diabetic nephropathy is a relentless, often linear, but highly variable rate of decline in GFR ranging from 2 to 20 mL/min/yr, with a mean of 12 mL/min/yr. Type 2 diabetic patients suffering from nephropathy display the same degree of loss in GFR. Systemic hypertension accelerates the progression of diabetic nephropathy and a close correlation between blood pressure and the rate of decline in GFR has been documented in type 1 and type 2 diabetic patients. Impaired or abolished renal autoregulation of renal plasma flow as demonstrated in type 1 and type 2 diabetic patients with nephropathy contributes to increased glomerular pressures in diabetic nephropathy—*glomerular hypertension*. Proteinuria itself may contribute to renal damage. Indeed, type 1 diabetic patients with diabetic nephropathy and nephrotic-range proteinuria (> 3 g/24 hr) have the worst prognosis. For many years it was believed that once albuminuria had become persistent, then glycemic control was unimportant because a "point of no return" had been reached. This is a misconception and studies dealing with large numbers of type 1 diabetic patients have documented the important impact of glycemic control on progression of diabetic nephropathy.

Extrarenal Complications in Diabetic Nephropathy
Diabetic retinopathy is present in virtually all type 1 diabetic patients with nephropathy, whereas only 50% to 60% of proteinuric type 2 diabetic patients suffer from retinopathy. Absence of retinopathy should require further investigation for nondiabetic glomerulopathies (see later). Blindness due to severe proliferative retinopathy or maculopathy is approximately five times greater in type 1 and type 2 diabetic patients with nephropathy compared with that in normoalbuminuric patients. Macroangiopathy, for example, stroke, carotid artery stenosis, coronary heart disease, and peripheral vascular disease, is two to five times more common in nephropathic patients. Peripheral neuropathy is present in almost all patients with advanced nephropathy. Foot ulcers with sepsis leading to amputation occur often (>25%), probably owing to a combination of neural and arterial disease. Autonomic neuropathy may be asymptomatic and simply manifest as abnormal cardiovascular reflexes, or it may result in debilitating symptoms. Over one half of patients with advanced nephropathy have symptoms of autonomic neuropathy: gustatory sweating, impotence, postural hypotension, and diarrhea. Diabetic cytopathy is also a common (>30%) problem in these patients.

TREATMENT

Glycemic Control

Primary Prevention
Intensive blood glucose control has a significant beneficial effect on the progression from normo- to microalbuminuria in type 1 diabetic patients. A worsening of diabetic retinopathy may be observed during the initial months of intensive therapy, but in the longer term the rate of deterioration is slower than that in conventionally treated type 1 diabetic patients. Side effects are a major concern with intensive therapy, and the frequency of severe hypoglycemia is higher in intensively treated patients. In the Diabetes Control and Complications trial (DCCT), intensive therapy reduced the occurrence of microalbuminuria by 39% and that of albuminuria by 54%. Despite these impressive results 16% of subjects in the primary prevention cohort and 26% in the secondary prevention cohort developed microalbuminuria during the 9 years of intensive treatment. This finding clearly documents the need for additional treatment modalities to avoid or reduce the burden of diabetic nephropathy. A beneficial effect

on progression of normoalbuminuria to microalbuminuria and macroalbuminuria in type 2 diabetes has been confirmed by the U.K. Prospective Diabetes Study (UKPDS).

Secondary Prevention

Several modifiable risk factors (level of urinary albumin excretion, hemoglobin A_{1c} level, smoking, blood pressure, and serum cholesterol concentration) for progression have been identified in clinical trials with type 1 and type 2 diabetic patients. The renal impact of intensive diabetic treatment versus conventional diabetic treatment on progression or regression of microalbuminuria in type 1 diabetic patients is generally thought to be beneficial. Recently, intensified multifactorial intervention (pharmacologic therapy targeting hyperglycemia, hypertension, dyslipidemia, and microalbuminuria) in patients with type 2 diabetes and microalbuminuria has been demonstrated to substantially slow progression to nephropathy, retinopathy, and autonomic neuropathy. The impact of improved metabolic control on progression of kidney dysfunction in type 1 diabetic patients with overt nephropathy has been disappointing.

Blood Pressure Control

Primary Prevention

Recent laboratory observations are consistent with the concept that glomerular hypertension is a major factor in the pathogenesis of diabetic glomerulopathy and indicate that lowering of systemic blood pressure without a concomitant reduction of glomerular capillary pressure may be insufficient to prevent glomerular injury. Lowering of systemic blood pressure by angiotensin-converting enzyme (ACE) inhibitors or conventional antihypertensive treatment affords significant renoprotection in experimental models of diabetic nephropathy. Three randomized placebo-controlled trials in *normotensive* type 1 and type 2 diabetic patients with normal albumin excretion ratios have suggested a beneficial effect of ACE inhibition on the development of microalbuminuria. In contrast, studies comparing the effect of ACE inhibitors versus a long-acting dihydropyridine calcium antagonist or β-blockade in *hypertensive* type 2 diabetic patients with normoalbuminuria have shown equivalent protection. The UKPDS study reported that by 6 years patients with tight blood pressure control had a 29% reduction in risk of developing microalbuminuria. Beneficial effects of aggressive blood pressure control in normotensive type 2 diabetic patients on albuminuria, retinopathy, and incidence of stroke have recently been demonstrated.

Secondary Prevention

ACE inhibitors significantly reduce the risk of progression to macroalbuminuria compared with placebo in type 1 diabetic patients with microalbuminuria (odds ratio 0.38). In addition, regression to normoalbuminuria occurs more often, and the urinary albumin excretion ratio is 50% lower in patients taking ACE inhibitors. Furthermore, the beneficial effect of ACE inhibitors in preventing progression from microalbuminuria to overt nephropathy is long-lasting and is associated with preservation of a normal GFR. Antihypertensive treatment has a renoprotective effect in hypertensive patients with type 2 diabetes and microalbuminuria, particularly when angiotensin II receptor blockers (ARBs) are used. Based on the trials with ARBs, the American Diabetes Association now recommends: "In hypertensive type 2 diabetic patients with microalbuminuria or clinical albuminuria, ARBs are the initial agents of choice."

Established Nephropathy

Control of hypertension and blockade of the renin-angiotensin system are key therapeutic interventions in established diabetic nephropathy. Indeed, the prognosis of type 1 diabetic patients suffering from diabetic nephropathy has improved during the past decade, largely because of effective antihypertensive treatment with conventional drugs (β-blockers and diuretics) and ACE inhibitors. Early and aggressive antihypertensive treatment reduces albuminuria and the rate of decline in GFR in young men and women with type 1 diabetes and nephropathy. In addition, regression of kidney disease (ΔGFR = 1 mL/min/yr) or remission of proteinuria for at least 1 year (proteinuria = 1 g/24hr) has been documented in up to 20% of type 1 diabetic patients receiving aggressive antihypertensive therapy for diabetic nephropathy. The renoprotective effect of interruption of the renin-angiotensin blockade on the progression of diabetic nephropathy has been conclusively proven in both type 1 (ACE inhibition) and type 2 (ARB) diabetes mellitus. In addition, these agents offer an additional significant mortality benefit in this patient population.

Initiation of antihypertensive treatment usually induces an initial drop in GFR. This phenomenon occurs with conventional antihypertensive treatment with β-blockers and diuretics and when ACE inhibitors or ARBs are used. This initial decline in GFR is due to a functional (hemodynamic) effect of antihypertensive treatment; however, this is accompanied thereafter by a slower decline in kidney function, reflecting the beneficial effect on progression of nephropathy. This is an important clinical point.

Many patients with diabetic nephropathy will experience a modest increment in serum creatinine concentration after initiation of ACE inhibition or ARB therapy. These changes should be anticipated and should not trigger withdrawal of the agent. However, the development of acute renal failure should prompt consideration of the possibility of coexisting bilateral renal artery stenosis or "effective" or actual volume depletion (e.g., congestive heart failure or excessive diuresis).

Lipid Lowering

Hyperlipidemia may promote the progression of chronic renal disease including diabetic nephropathy. However, the renoprotective effect of HMG-CoA reductase inhibitors in patients with type 1 or type 2 diabetes with micro- or macroalbuminuria appears to be highly variable. These agents should only be prescribed if a coexisting indication is present.

Dietary Protein Restriction

Short-term studies in normoalbuminuric, microalbuminuric, and macroalbuminuric type 1 diabetic patients have shown that a low-protein diet (0.6 to 0.8 g/kg/day) reduces urinary albumin excretion and hyperfiltration, independent of changes in glucose control and blood pressure. Longer-term trials in type 1 diabetic patients with diabetic nephropathy suggest that protein restriction reduces the progression of kidney function, but the data are not definitive.

END-STAGE RENAL DISEASE IN DIABETIC PATIENTS

Diabetic nephropathy is the leading cause of ESRD in most Western countries. Survival of diabetic patients receiving hemodialysis is poorer than that of diabetic patients not receiving dialysis whether or not diabetic or primary nondiabetic renal disease accounts for the end-stage renal failure. The diabetic patient with ESRD has several options for renal replacement therapy:

1. Transplantation (kidney only, simultaneous pancreas plus kidney, or pancreas after kidney)
2. Hemodialysis (HD)
3. Continuous ambulatory peritoneal dialysis (CAPD)

The consensus today is that medical rehabilitation and survival are best after transplantation, particularly after transplantation of pancreas plus kidney. The results of CAPD and HD are inferior to those with transplantation, but results between the use of CAPD and HD are comparable.

Management of the Patient with Advanced Renal Failure

The diabetic patient with advanced renal failure usually has a much higher burden of *microvascular* and *macrovascular* complications than the diabetic patient without nephropathy. The diabetic patient with advanced renal impairment, even if he or she is asymptomatic, must therefore be monitored at regular intervals for timely detection of these complications (ophthalmologic examination at half-yearly intervals, cardiac and angiologic status yearly, and foot inspection at each visit). The most vexing clinical problems are related to coronary heart disease and autonomic polyneuropathy.

Hypertension
Blood pressure tends to be higher in diabetic than in nondiabetic patients with renal failure. Because of their beneficial effects on cardiovascular complications and disease progression, treatment with ACE inhibitors or ARBs is obligatory in all patients unless there are contraindications (e.g., renal artery stenosis or resistant hyperkalemia). Patients with diabetic nephropathy retain sodium avidly and have a marked tendency to develop hypervolemia and edema. Therefore, dietary salt restriction and the use of loop diuretics are usually indicated. At least for monotherapy, thiazides are not sufficient once GFR is less than 40 to 50 mL/min. When the creatinine concentration is elevated, multidrug therapy is usually necessary to normalize blood pressure with, on average, three to five antihypertensive agents. In these patients hypertension is also characterized by a wide pulse pressure (as a result of increased aortic stiffness) and by an attenuated nighttime decrease in blood pressure which in itself is a potent risk predictor.

Glycemic Control
The half-life of insulin is prolonged in advanced kidney disease, causing a tendency for patients to develop hypoglycemia. This risk is further compounded by anorexia and by accumulation of most sulfonylurea compounds. Glinides and glitazones do not accumulate, but long-term safety data in renal failure are not available.

Malnutrition
Patients with ESRD due to diabetic nephropathy are typically catabolic and are predisposed to develop malnutrition, particularly during periods of intercurrent illness and fasting.

Therefore, protein-restricted diets are discouraged in patients with advanced renal insufficiency, particularly in anorectic patients. Anorectic obese patients with type 2 diabetes and advanced renal failure often lose massive amounts of weight, leading to normalization of fasting and even postloading glycemia values. Wasting with low muscle mass is an important cause of a physician's misjudging the severity of renal failure, because at any given level of GFR, serum creatinine concentrations are spuriously low.

Acute and "Acute-on-Chronic" Renal Failure
Diabetic patients with nephropathy are particularly prone to develop acute on chronic renal failure. The most common causes include emergency cardiologic interventions involving use of radiocontrast medium, septicemia, low cardiac output, and shock. The high susceptibility of the kidney to ischemic injury may be a contributory factor. Often the acute renal failure is irreversible and necessitates chronic HD. This mode of presentation as irreversible acute renal failure has a particularly poor prognosis.

Vascular Access
Timely creation of vascular access is of overriding importance. It should be considered when the GFR is approximately 20 to 25 mL/min. Although venous runoff problems are not unusual, inadequate arterial inflow is increasingly recognized as the major cause of fistula malfunction. If distal arteries are severely sclerotic, anastomosis at a more proximal level may be necessary. Arteriosclerosis of arm arteries not only jeopardizes fistula flow but also predisposes individuals to the steal phenomenon with digital ischemia.

Initiation of Renal Replacement Therapy
Many nephrologists agree that renal replacement therapy should be started earlier in diabetic than in nondiabetic patients and at a GFR of approximately 15 mL/min. An even earlier start may be justified when hypervolemia and blood pressure become uncontrollable, or when the patient is anorectic and cachectic.

Hemodialysis

In recent years survival of diabetic patients receiving HD has improved and 5-year survival in type 2 diabetic patients receiving HD is approximately 30%.

Intradialytic and Interdialytic Blood Pressure
Diabetic patients receiving HD are more hypertensive than nondiabetic patients, and their blood pressure is exquisitely

volume dependent. The problem is compounded by the fact that patients are predisposed to development of intradialytic hypotension so that it is difficult to reach the target "dry weight" by ultrafiltration. The main causes of intradialytic hypotension are autonomous neuropathy, and diastolic dysfunction so that cardiac output decreases abruptly when left ventricular filling pressure diminishes during ultrafiltration. Longer dialysis sessions, omission of antihypertensive agents immediately before dialysis sessions, and correction of anemia by erythropoietin therapy may lower the incidence of this complication.

Cardiovascular Problems

Cardiovascular mortality accounts for more than half of all deaths in diabetic patients receiving HD. The prevalence of coronary heart disease is significantly higher in diabetic than in nondiabetic patients entering ESRD programs. In addition, the diabetic patient has a higher risk when coronary complications supervene. The impact of ischemic heart disease is amplified by coexisting cardiac abnormalities such as congestive heart failure, left ventricular hypertrophy, and disturbed sympathetic innervation, as well as microvessel disease with diminished coronary reserve. Observational studies suggest that good glycemic control before or during dialysis reduces overall and cardiovascular mortality. It is sensible to reduce afterload (blood pressure control) and preload (hypervolemia). The value of lipid lowering by statins has not been proven but is currently being investigated in type 2 diabetic patients receiving dialysis. Diabetic patients with renal failure are characterized by premature and more pronounced anemia so that timely and effective treatment with recombinant human erythropoietin is advised. Pharmacologic blockade of the renin-angiotensin system using ACE inhibitors or ARBs is also advised, based on an extrapolation of the results of the Heart Outcomes Prevention Evaluation (HOPE) study. In the patient with symptomatic coronary heart disease, active intervention, for example, percutaneous transluminal coronary angioplasty or coronary artery bypass grafting, has been shown to be superior to medical treatment alone. A recent retrospective analysis of diabetic patients receiving dialysis suggested that coronary artery bypass grafts using internal mammary artery grafts (but not coronary artery bypass grafting using venous grafts) yielded superior outcome compared with percutaneous transluminal coronary angioplasty with or without stenting.

Malnutrition

Because of anorexia and prolonged habituation to dietary restriction, the dietary intake of diabetic patients receiving HD often falls short of adequate energy (30 to 35 kcal/kg/day) and protein (1.3 g/kg/day) intake. This is particularly undesirable because malnutrition is a potent predictor of death. The dietary intake of all patients should be reviewed on a regular basis by a clinical nutrition service.

Peritoneal Dialysis

In the United States 7% of all patients with diabetes receiving renal replacement therapy are treated with peritoneal dialysis (PD); however, rates are much higher in Western Europe. There are very good a priori reasons to offer CAPD treatment to diabetic patients initially, including difficulties in vascular access placement with HD, improved survival during the first 2 years in patients treated with PD than with HD (excluding very elderly patients), and avoidance of rapid fluctuations of fluid volumes and electrolyte concentrations. Some evidence suggests that for patients in whom PD is started and then changed to HD when residual renal function had decayed have better long-term survival than patients whose initial treatment was HD. Although protein is lost across the peritoneal membrane, the main nutritional problem is gain of glucose and calories because high glucose concentrations in the dialysate are necessary for osmotic removal of excess body fluid. This leads to weight gain and obesity.

Transplantation

Kidney Transplantation

Although survival of the diabetic patient with a kidney graft is worse than that of a nondiabetic patient receiving a graft, the gain in life expectancy of the diabetic patient with a graft, compared with the diabetic patient on the waiting list who is receiving dialysis, is proportionally much greater than that for the nondiabetic patient, because survival of the diabetic patient receiving dialysis is so much poorer. The higher mortality of the diabetic patient with a kidney graft is mainly explained as the consequence of preexisting vascular disease, left ventricular hypertrophy, and post-transplant hypertension. Diabetic patients must be subjected to a rigorous pretransplantation evaluation, which in most centers includes routine coronary angiography. Pelvic arteries of patients should also be examined by Doppler sonography and, if necessary, angiography, to avoid placement of a renal allograft into an iliac artery with compromised arterial flow at risk of ischemia of the extremity and amputation.

Kidney-Plus-Pancreas Transplantation
Survival of patients with simultaneous pancreas-kidney transplantation (SPK) approaches that of patients receiving transplants for nondiabetic renal disease and is clearly superior to that of diabetic recipients of living donor kidney-only grafts and particularly of cadaver kidney-only grafts. Reversibility of established microvascular complications after SPK is minor at best with the important exception of autonomic polyneuropathy, particularly improved cardiorespiratory reflexes potentially contributing to increased survival, and some improvement in nerve conduction. Further benefits include improved gastric and bladder function, as well as superior quality of life, better metabolic control, and improved survival so that today SPK should be the preferred treatment for the type 1 diabetic patient who meets the selection criteria. There is an increasing tendency for early or even preemptive SPK.

Pancreas-After-Kidney Transplantation
An alternative strategy must be considered in the diabetic patient who has a live kidney donor: to first transplant the living donor kidney and, subsequently, once stable renal function is achieved (GFR > 50 mL/min), to transplant a cadaver donor pancreas. Recent data suggest a poorer outcome in such patients compared with those receiving conventional treatment.

Islet Cell Transplantation
Islet cell transplantation is an area of emerging interest. Successful islet cell transplantation to achieve insulin independence in seven consecutive patients using a steroid-free immunosuppression regimen consisting of sirolimus, tacrolimus, and daclizumab has been reported.

BLADDER DYSFUNCTION

Bladder dysfunction as a sequela of autonomous diabetic polyneuropathy is common in diabetic patients, leading to straining, hesitancy, and the sensation of incomplete emptying of the bladder, but disabling symptoms are rare (with the exception of frail elderly patients). Because of its association with autonomous polyneuropathy, it is not surprising that bladder dysfunction is often associated with postural hypotension, gastroparesis, constipation, and nocturnal diarrhea. Cystometry shows increased bladder volume at the first desire to void and increased maximal bladder capacity associated with decreased detrusor contractility. Cystopathy with residual volume after voiding renders eradication of urinary tract infection (UTI) difficult.

URINARY TRACT INFECTION

It is not absolutely certain whether the frequency of bacteriuria is higher in diabetic patients, but there is no doubt that symptomatic UTIs are more severe and more aggressive. UTIs in patients with diabetes also lead to complications, such as prostatic abscess, emphysematous cystitis and pyelonephritis, intrarenal abscess formation, renal carbuncle, and penile necrosis (Fournier disease). Papillary necrosis should be suspected in diabetic patients with recurrent episodes of UTI, renal colic, hematuria, or obstructive uropathy.

Extrarenal bacterial metastases are common, particularly after UTI with methicillin-resistant staphylococci. In community-acquired UTI, the predominant microbe is *Escherichia coli*, but *Klebsiella* is found more often in diabetic patients than in control subjects. The reasons for the potentially higher frequency and the definitely higher severity of UTI in diabetic patients are not known but may include more favorable conditions for bacterial growth (glucosuria), defective neutrophil function, increased adherence to uroepithelial cells, and impaired bladder evacuation (detrusor paresis). As to the management of UTI, no clear benefits of antibiotic treatment have been demonstrated for treatment of asymptomatic bacteriuria in diabetic patients. Community-acquired symptomatic lower UTIs may be managed with trimethoprim, trimethoprim-sulfamethoxazole, or a quinolone. For nosocomially acquired UTI, sensitivity tests and sensitivity-directed antibiotic intervention are necessary. Invasive candiduria can be managed with amphotericin or by irrigation or systemic administration of fungicidal agents. See Chapter 13, Urinary Tract Infection, Pyelonephritis, and Reflux Nephropathy.

OTHER RENAL DISORDERS IN DIABETIC PATIENTS

It has been reported that renal disorders such as minimal-change disease and membranous nephropathy are more common in the type 1 diabetic patient population than among nondiabetic subjects. In fact, fewer than 1% of type 1 diabetic patients who have had diabetes for 10 or more years, and fewer than 4% of those with proteinuria and long diabetes duration will have conditions other than, or in addition to, diabetic nephropathy. However, type 2 diabetic patients who have proteinuria but not retinopathy or who have unusual features may have a high incidence of other renal diseases. Type 1 diabetic patients with proteinuria who have had diabetes for less than 10 years or type 2 diabetic patients without retinopathy should be thoroughly evaluated for other renal diseases, and renal biopsy for diagnosis and prognosis should be strongly considered.

Nephrolithiasis

21

Renal stones generally consist of calcium salts, uric acid, cystine, or struvite (the triple salt of magnesium, ammonium, and phosphate). Calcium stones predominate and are composed of either calcium oxalate, calcium phosphate crystals, or a combination thereof. The prevalence of kidney stones varies from 4% to 9% in men and from 2% to 4% in women.

CLINICAL PRESENTATION

The clinical presentations of nephrolithiasis include the following:

- Asymptomatic microscopic hematuria/pyuria
- Renal colic (with or without macroscopic hematuria)
- Recurrent urinary tract infection
- Obstructive uropathy

The classic presentation of nephrolithiasis is loin pain in association with hematuria, which may be either macro- or microscopic. Macroscopic hematuria is more common with larger stones or if infection is present. The classic pain of nephrolithiasis is termed *renal colic* and occurs as a result of a stone moving from the renal pelvis into the ureter. The severity of symptoms varies from a mild ache to severe discomfort that requires parenteral opiate administration for relief. Associated symptoms may include nausea, vomiting, and dysuria. Renal pelvic or upper ureteral obstruction triggers flank pain, whereas ureteral obstruction further down triggers pain that radiates to the ipsilateral testicle or labia majora. The pain only resolves with passage of the stone or surgical removal. The absence of pain does not exclude the diagnosis of nephrolithiasis. Indeed, obstructive uropathy due to staghorn calculi is often asymptomatic, and bilateral disease can lead to the development of undetected chronic renal failure.

Special Clinical Problems

Pregnancy

Complications of pregnancy are not increased above those of the general population in patients with nephrolithiasis except for a slightly higher rate of urinary tract infection. Furthermore, the rate of stone formation during pregnancy is no higher than that observed in nongravid stone formers.

Uric Acid and Calcium Stones

A small fraction of patients who form calcium stones also form uric acid stones and occasionally form stones composed of both calcium oxalate and uric acid. These patients display an unusually high recurrence rate; the average recurrence is more than 65 stones per 100 patient-years—nearly twice the average rate for calcium stone formers in general. These patients may have a mixture of metabolic disorders involving both calcium and uric acid, and if they do, both disorders must be treated or else stone recurrence will continue.

MANAGEMENT OF A FIRST URINARY STONE

Investigations

The diagnosis of nephrolithiasis is often suspected in patients presenting with acute flank pain, particularly if it is associated with hematuria. In the absence of the patient passing a stone spontaneously, the diagnosis can be confirmed by radiologic investigation. Specific diagnostic approaches include abdominal plain film, renal ultrasound, intravenous pyelography, and computed tomography. In recent years non–contrast-enhanced computed tomography has emerged as the investigation of choice in this setting because of its superior sensitivity and specificity in identifying ureteric stones. If computed tomography is unavailable, intravenous pyelography or ultrasonography is a suitable alternative, the latter being particularly useful in the setting of pregnancy. A plain film of the abdomen is typically reserved for patients with a documented history of radio-opaque stones.

Renal Colic

Renal colic may be excruciatingly painful, and affected patients often need parenteral therapy for relief of symptoms. In the acute setting therapeutic approaches include nonsteroidal anti-inflammatory drugs and opiates. Ketorlac (30 mg intramuscularly [IM] or intravenously [IV]) has substantial efficacy in this setting, and once pain relief has been achieved, an oral NSAID can be substituted. Other options include morphine (5 mg IM/IV) or meperidine (50 mg IM). Associated nausea may be managed with prochlorperazine (5 to 10 mg orally/IM). If the patient's pain is controlled and he or she is able to drink fluids, then the patient can be discharged to home. All patients should be given a urine strainer to facilitate collection of the stone, which is an essential step in the diagnostic evaluation of the patient with nephrolithiasis.

Indications for Urologic Referral

Emergency urologic referral is required for patients presenting with urosepsis, intractable pain, or bilateral disease manifesting as acute renal failure. Other indications for surgical referral include persistent obstruction, failure to pass a stone (within 4 to 6 weeks), hematuria requiring transfusion, a stone judged to be unlikely to pass spontaneously (>7 mm), staghorn calculi, and stone growth despite optimal medical management. The likelihood of a stone passing spontaneously depends on both its size and anatomic location. Most stones less than 4 to 5 mm will pass spontaneously, but passage of a stone greater than 7 mm in diameter is uncommon. Proximal ureteric stones are less likely to pass than stones located more distally. Current surgical management options include cystoscopic placement of ureteral stents, nephrostomy with urine drainage, extracorporeal shock wave lithotripsy (which many require ureteral stent placement if the patient is symptomatic), and ureteroscopy with stone fragmentation (usually with laser lithotripsy). Large renal stones can be fragmented through nephrostomy. These newer approaches have all but eliminated the need for open surgical procedures. A complete discussion of the optimal surgical approach to renal stone disease is beyond the scope of this chapter, and readers are referred to Nephrolithiasis: Lithotripsy and Surgery in *Therapy in Nephrology and Hypertension,* companion to *Brenner and Rector's The Kidney,* 2nd ed.

Evaluation of the Patient with Nephrolithiasis

All patients with nephrolithiasis should undergo a basic evaluation upon first presentation. Patients with evidence suggesting an underlying metabolic disorder should undergo a more

Table 21–1: Basic Metabolic Evaluation of Nephrolithiasis

Analysis of stone composition
Urinalysis (including sediment examination)
Urine culture
Serum chemistry analysis
Blood urea nitrogen/creatinine
Total CO_2
Uric acid
Calcium (repeat if high normal)
Intact parathyroid hormone level if calcium level is high
   or high normal

thorough evaluation. The appropriate baseline investigations are outlined in Table 21–1. All evaluations should include an analysis of the stone composition if possible. Blood testing should include a routine chemistry profile including measurement of the serum calcium, total CO_2, and uric acid concentrations. The serum calcium measurement should be repeated if the calcium level is in the high normal range to exclude hyperparathyroidism, and the parathyroid hormone (PTH) level should be measured in selected patients. Routine urinalysis will typically reveal hematuria if stones are present. Importantly, an alkaline urine is a risk factor for calcium-phosphate stones and may also point to the presence of a urea-splitting organism. A urine pH greater than 5.4 in the presence of a metabolic acidosis suggests a defect in distal tubular acidification, which is associated with recurrent nephrolithiasis (classic distal renal tubular acidosis). Urine microscopy may reveal the characteristic hexagonal crystals of cystinuria. Whether or not all patients require a more complete evaluation is controversial; however, the following patient groups clearly require a more complete metabolic evaluation as outlined in Table 21–2: children; patients with recurrent stones or multiple stones on first presentation; patients with non–calcium-based stones; and African American patients.

A 24-hour urine collection should be obtained for the evaluation of the excretion of calcium, oxalate, sodium, uric acid, and citrate. A 24-hour creatinine collection should also be performed to ensure the adequacy of the collection. Commercially available collection kits now allow the simultaneous measurement of all these factors and measurement of the urinary supersaturation from a single 24-hour collection (http://www.litholink.com). Because there is significant day-to-day variation in the excretion of calcium, oxalate, etc., two or more collections may be required.

Table 21–2: Complete Metabolic Evaluation of Nephrolithiasis*

24-Hour Urine Collections	Normal Values
Total volume	>2 L
Calcium	<4 mg/kg (0.1 mmol)
Oxalate	<45 mg (0.4 mmol)
Phosphorous	<1100 mg (35 mmol)
Citrate	>320 mg (17 mmol)
Uric acid	<800 mg (4.7 mmol)
Sodium	<3 g (130 mmol)
Urine Supersaturation Values	
Calcium oxalate	<5
Calcium phosphate	<0.5–2
Uric acid	0–1

*The 24-hour urinary creatinine excretion should also be measured to ensure the adequacy of the collection. The normal rate of urinary creatinine excretion in patients younger than age 50 is 20 to 25 mg/kg (177 to 221 mcmol/kg) lean body weight in men and 15 to 20 mg/kg (133 to 177 mcmol/kg) lean body weight in women.

CALCIUM STONES

Calcium oxalate and calcium phosphate stones account for most renal stones, and because they are so common, much is known about their natural history and pathogenesis.

Epidemiology and Natural History

The annual incidence of kidney stones in the industrialized world is 1 in 1000 persons with a peak incidence in the third decade. White race and male sex are significant risk factors. Unfortunately, recurrence rates are high: 40% to 50% by 5 years and more than 50% to 60% by 10 years. Patients at risk of stone recurrence cannot be identified prospectively by laboratory evaluation. In dealing with patients who have had a single stone, it is important for the clinician to emphasize that the natural history of stone disease is one of chronic recurrence and that although effective interventions exist to decrease the incidence of new stone formation, the treatment is lifelong and a "cure" is an unrealistic expectation.

Etiology

Primary Hyperparathyroidism

Approximately 20% of patients with hyperparathyroidism will develop nephrolithiasis, usually calcium oxalate stones. Despite the fact that PTH stimulates distal tubule calcium reabsorption, urinary calcium excretion may be greatly elevated in those patients with primary hyperparathyroidism who form renal stones even when hypercalcemia is slight. Stones often recur and become bilateral if the diagnosis is not made early in the course of the disease. Nephrocalcinosis may be the only renal manifestation of hyperparathyroidism. Less commonly, parenchymal calcification may be accompanied by calculi in the renal pelvis and ureters. The presence of nephrocalcinosis should prompt a diagnostic evaluation to exclude hyperparathyroidism, but there are other causes of that syndrome.

DIAGNOSIS   Immunometric assays distinguish hyperparathyroidism and hypercalcemia of malignancy with a high level of reliability and show high (or absence of suppression) PTH levels in 90% of patients with hyperparathyroidism. Despite advances in the measurement of immunoreactive PTH, the diagnosis of primary hyperparathyroidism still requires the demonstration of hypercalcemia and the exclusion of other causes. In general, multiple serum samples should be studied, and even modest elevations of calcium concentration should be accorded considerable weight, if consistent. Humoral hypercalcemia of malignancy may be difficult to distinguish from hyperparathyroidism, because both present as hypercalcemia with hypercalciuria. PTH-related peptide has been identified as a mediator of humoral hypercalcemia of malignancy and the diagnosis of humoral hypercalcemia of malignancy can be confirmed by demonstration of a high serum concentration of parathyroid hormone–related protein. This finding is present in most hypercalcemic patients with solid tumors.

TREATMENT   Removal of the adenoma or hyperplastic glands is indicated in patients with renal stone disease. Medical therapy may be used for patients deemed not to be surgical candidates. Dietary salt restriction reduces urine calcium excretion and may be helpful in preventing stones in patients not having surgery. Bisphosphonates, which inhibit osteoclast function, are effective in controlling hypercalcemia with short-term use. However, hypercalciuria does not improve with these agents. After successful surgery, the serum calcium level becomes normal and cessation of hypercalciuria presumably accounts for the marked decrease in the rate of stone formation compared with that observed in the preoperative period. Patients with osteitis fibrosa appear to suffer more severe renal damage than those presenting with renal calculi alone.

Idiopathic Hypercalciuria

Between 30% and 50% of calcium stone formers excrete more calcium in their urine than normal people customarily do—more than 300 mg/24 hr (men), 250 mg/24 hr (women), or 4 mg/kg body weight/24 hr (either sex)—and are therefore labeled as being hypercalciuric. Hypercalciuria is termed "idiopathic" if the serum calcium level is normal and if sarcoidosis, renal tubular acidosis (RTA), hyperthyroidism, malignant tumors, rapidly progressive bone disease, immobilization, Paget disease, Cushing disease (or syndrome), and furosemide administration—the usual causes of normocalcemic hypercalciuria—can be excluded. Virtually all normocalcemic hypercalciuria encountered in patients with nephrolithiasis is idiopathic. The etiology of idiopathic hypercalciuria involves one or all of the following events: enhanced intestinal calcium adsorption, reduced renal tubular adsorption, increased calcium mobilization from bone, or a renal phosphate leak.

TREATMENT Unfortunately, identification of the pathogenesis of any single patient's hypercalciuria is not easily achieved, restricting the ability of the practicing physician to carefully tailor therapy.

DIET

As with any type of stone, high water intake is always the cornerstone of the therapeutic regimen. A high fluid intake (2 to 2.5 L/day) results in a greater than 50% reduction in stone recurrence over 5 years. Dietary sodium restriction reduces urine calcium excretion lowering the risk of stone formation. A high protein intake increases urine calcium excretion and causes negative calcium balance, so dietary protein restriction would also seem to be a prudent recommendation. A low-calcium diet has long been advocated for the treatment of hypercalciuric stone disease and has been shown to be effective in reducing urine calcium excretion. However, given the risks of osteopenia and the absence of compelling prospective data suggesting that calcium restriction reduces stone frequency, this therapeutic approach should be avoided. A recent study compared the effectiveness of a low-calcium diet to a low-sodium, low-protein, normal-calcium diet. One hundred twenty male hypercalciuric recurrent calcium stone formers were randomly assigned to receive either a low-calcium (400 mg/day) diet with no sodium or protein restriction or a 1200-mg calcium, low-sodium, low-protein diet. The patients were followed for 5 years. In the low-salt, low-protein diet group, the urinary calcium oxalate supersaturation fell, and stone recurrence was significantly lower compared with that in the calcium-restricted group. Based on this study sodium restriction is now favored over calcium restriction in the prevention of recurrent nephrolithiasis.

THIAZIDE DIURETICS

Thiazide diuretics are the first-line therapy for idiopathic hypercalciuria. They inhibit tubule resorption of NaCl, stimulate calcium reabsorption by the distal convoluted tubule, and trigger a fall in urine supersaturation of calcium salts. Multiple randomized studies show a benefit for the use of thiazide diuretics in the treatment of recurrent calcium oxalate nephrolithiasis with respect to the incidence of recurrent stones. Chlorthalidone 25 to 50 mg daily is usually sufficient. Diuretic-induced hypokalemia can predispose to hypocitraturia, a known risk factor for stone pathogenesis; therefore, serum potassium levels should be checked after several days and if hypokalemia develops, then potassium citrate supplements (e.g., Uro-cit K 20 to 40 mmol daily) can be administered.

Hyperuricosuria

The usual upper limits of daily urine uric acid excretion, 800 mg (men) and 750 mg (women), are exceeded more often by calcium stone formers than by normal people. In hyperuricosuric patients who form calcium stones, stone disease begins at a later age and is unusually active and severe. The pathogenetic link between hyperuricosuria and the tendency to develop calcium stones probably involves seed crystals of urate initiating calcium oxalate precipitation from the urine. Urinary uric acid crystals are commonly found in the setting of volume depletion, emphasizing the need to maintain a brisk urine flow in patients with a risk of stone formation. Low urine pH is also a risk factor. A reduction in new stone formation during allopurinol administration is the most compelling evidence for the role of hyperuricosuria in calcium oxalate stone disease. Allopurinol dramatically reduces new stone formation in patients with combined uric acid-calcium stones and may be combined with a thiazide diuretic in patients with idiopathic hypercalciuria and hyperuricosuria. Allopurinol should begin at a dosage of 100 mg/day, gradually increasing to 300 mg/day. A low-protein, low-purine diet can decrease uric acid secretion and raise urinary pH; however, compliance with this diet if often poor. All patients should maintain a brisk oral fluid intake and alkalinization of the urine with potassium citrate to achieve a urine pH of 6.5 to 7 is also helpful. The urine pH should not exceed 7 because this may trigger precipitation of calcium-phosphate salts.

Hypocitraturia

Citrate inhibits stone formation and hypocitraturia is found in 15% to 60% of stone formers. Hypocitraturia may occur as an isolated abnormality or be associated with hypercalciuria, distal RTA (see later), chronic diarrheal states, and diuretic-induced hypokalemia. The management of hypocitraturia involves correction of any underlying disorder that reduces urine citrate, such as acidosis or hypokalemia, or, if the patient has idiopathic hypocitraturia, induction of a mild metabolic alkalosis to increase urine citrate excretion. Any alkali supplement will raise urine citrate levels; potassium bicarbonate, or preferably, potassium citrate may be used. Potassium citrate therapy is generally well tolerated, but some patients note significant gastrointestinal side effects, particularly dyspepsia. These side effects may be lessened by taking potassium citrate with meals, which will not affect intestinal absorption of the drug. Because alkali will not only increase urine citrate but may also raise urine pH, urine calcium phosphate supersaturation may occur. Clinicians should watch for the potential conversion of calcium oxalate stones to calcium phosphate stones if urine pH increases substantially during therapy. In addition, in patients with renal insufficiency, serum potassium levels should be monitored closely after initiation of therapy.

Renal Tubular Acidosis

Classic hypokalemic distal RTA is a cause of nephrocalcinosis and renal stone formation (calcium phosphate > calcium oxalate). When distal RTA is acquired as a drug- or toxin-induced nephropathy, it usually does not cause stones, possibly because of the associated concentrating deficit. Proximal RTA or any other form of renal acidosis associated with renal disease is not usually associated with stones. Hypercalciuria and elevated urine phosphorus excretion both tend to raise urine saturation with respect to calcium phosphate, but alkaline urine pH and hypocitruria are the most important etiologic factors. The hypocitruria and metabolic acidosis should be treated with either potassium citrate or potassium bicarbonate. High doses are often required (1 to 2 mmol/kg in two to three divided doses), and although this treatment may increase the urine pH, the increase is offset by the fall in calcium oxalate supersaturation.

Idiopathic Calcium Lithiasis

Despite a thorough evaluation, a remediable cause of stones will not be found in up to 10% of patients. However, it should be recognized that risk factors for urinary stone formation are continuous variables, and the normal limits are somewhat arbitrary. Many patients with idiopathic calcium lithiasis have urine chemistry measurements at the border of the normal limits, which increases urine supersaturation and contributes to stone formation. Identification of the urine chemistry values closest to the stone-forming range will allow the clinician to plan rational therapy for most patients. Hydration, restriction of dietary protein and sodium, and avoidance of foods that contain excessive oxalate are prudent management measures. Pharmacologic therapy to further reduce urine supersaturation may be useful if hydration and diet fail to control stone formation. However, small-scale studies suggest that thiazide diuretics and allopurinol are significantly less effective in patients with idiopathic calcium stones than in patients with established hypercalciuria or hyperuricosuria. In this setting citrate supplementation has also been used with some success.

Hyperoxaluria

Hyperoxaluria causes stones by raising the saturation of the urine with respect to calcium oxalate and is found in 5% to 25% of stone formers. The upper limit of normal for oxalate excretion is usually considered to be 45 mg/day in an adult. Hyperoxaluria can result from one of the following problems:

- Excessive dietary intake
- Overabsorption (enteric oxaluria)
- Crohn disease/ileal resection/celiac disease/pancreatic insufficiency
- Metabolic overproduction
- Primary oxaluria types I and II
- Ethylene glycol intoxication

Oxalate is an end product of several metabolic pathways; the amount of oxalate in the urine reflects the sum total of intestinal absorption plus de novo synthesis. Dietary oxalate intake is estimated to be 50 to 200 mg/day with about 10% being absorbed and a liberal intake of high-oxalate foods can cause frank hyperoxaluria. Calcium and magnesium complex oxalate in the intestinal tract, and diets low in calcium have been shown to increase urine oxalate excretion even when oxalate intake is fixed. Increased luminal free fatty acids may promote oxalate overabsorption by increasing the permeability of colon epithelium to oxalate

(Crohn disease, celiac sprue, pancreatic insufficiency, and small intestinal bypass surgery for obesity). In general, a low-fat, low-oxalate diet should be tried first, followed by oral calcium carbonate or cholestyramine, which both bind intestinal oxalate if dietary manipulation proves unsuccessful. Treatment needs to be aggressive because patients can develop renal failure and systemic oxalosis from severe enteric hyperoxaluria.

Hyperoxaluria may also be inherited as an autosomal recessive trait. Primary hyperoxaluria is characterized by urinary oxalate excretion of 100 to 300 mg/day, recurrent calcium oxalate calculi, progressive renal failure, and oxalosis, beginning as early as childhood. Treatment of primary hyperoxaluria focuses on reducing oxalate excretion and maintaining a high urine flow. In some cases pyridoxine has been used successfully to treat patients with primary hyperoxaluria.

URIC ACID STONES

Uric acid crystal formation in the urinary tract may manifest itself as crystalluria, stones, or obstruction. In addition, uric acid and its salt, sodium hydrogen urate, may produce intrarenal disease by initiating an inflammatory response to interstitial deposition as a consequence of hyperuricemia. Crystalluria often occurs in uric acid stone formers and is accompanied by dysuria and hematuria. It may occur in the absence of hyperuricemia or hyperuricosuria, and crystals may be present in the urine of normal subjects whenever urine pH is low.

Natural History

Uric acid stones account for 5% to 10% of all renal stones in the United States, but this figure varies in other parts of the globe. The chance of stone formation increases with increasing serum urate levels and urine excretion rates.

Clinical Classification of Uric Acid Nephrolithiasis

Uric acid stone–forming conditions include a variety of disorders involving disturbances in purine metabolism, renal urate handling, and urine pH.

Idiopathic Uric Acid Stones
Both sporadic and familial forms of idiopathic uric acid stones occur. The familial form is inherited as an autosomal dominant

trait, and stones are formed at an earlier age than in the sporadic form and are more likely to cause obstruction and subsequent loss of renal function. Men and women are affected equally, and an ethnic predilection (Jews and Italians) has been suggested. In the sporadic variety, stone formation or crystalluria usually begins in middle age, with predictable recurrence if the disorder is not treated. Serum and urine uric acid levels are normal in both forms, and the urine pH is invariably low. The mechanism for stone formation is related to the low urine pH. Most uric acid stone formers appear to have reduced ammonium excretion as the cause of the low urine pH.

Gout

Patients with primary gout may also have uric acid stones. The frequency of uric acid stones is directly related to the degree of uricosuria. The disease may be heterogeneous, because uric acid overexcretion persists despite a low-purine diet in some 21% to 28% of gouty subjects. In addition, urine pH tends to be low, suggesting a defect in ammonium production. Most patients also have a defect in renal urate excretion such that hyperuricemia is required for excretion of even normal amounts of uric acid.

Malignant Disease

Myeloproliferative disease and chronic granulocytic leukemia in adults and acute leukemia in childhood are the common neoplastic disorders that cause hyperuricosuria. Massive cell necrosis in response to chemotherapy abruptly increases urine uric acid excretion, which may cause extensive precipitation and urinary tract obstruction. In the absence of chemotherapy, less marked uricosuria may cause uric acid stones.

Gastrointestinal Diseases

Acute diarrheal states and chronic inflammatory bowel disease may increase urine uric acid concentration through excessive water loss and dehydration. Urine pH tends to fall with extra-cellular volume contraction, increasing the possibility of stone formation. Patients with ileostomy are particularly at risk, and associated small bowel disease (proximal ileum) may contribute to the lowered urine pH through significant bicarbonate loss. Hyperoxaluria may also be present in patients with ileal resection, leading to mixed stones composed of both uric acid and calcium oxalate.

Drug-Induced Stones

Probenecid and aspirin in large doses are both common uricosuric drugs. Hyperuricemic patients respond to these agents with a transient increase in uric acid excretion. Excretion then falls but remains higher than pretreatment levels, owing to reduced intestinal uricolysis. In patients with high dietary purine intake, the efficient excretion of uric acid induced by the drugs may increase the risk of uric acid stone formation or calcium oxalate stone formation.

Treatment

The goals of therapy are a regression in the size of preformed stones and the prevention of new ones. The available therapeutic tools include fluids, alkali, diet, and allopurinol. Urine volume can be increased to about 2 L/day with minimal inconvenience. Urine pH should be maintained within the range of 6 to 6.5. During the day, this can be achieved by ingestion of alkali, as either bicarbonate or citrate. Citrate may be preferred over bicarbonate because it requires less frequent dosing. If nocturnal urine pH falls and stone formation persists, a single dose of 250 mg of acetazolamide at bedtime will usually maintain an alkaline urine. Dietary purine may be reduced to avoid periods of transient excessive uric acid excretion. Allopurinol should be used if stones recur despite fluid and alkali, or if the patient has gout. Allopurinol is also indicated for the dissolution or reduction in size of existing stones and when large, nonobstructing renal pelvic stones are too large to pass. If given before chemotherapy for myeloproliferative or lymphoproliferative malignant disease, allopurinol prevents widespread uric acid precipitation. When allopurinol is used for treatment of patients with massive uric acid overproduction, excellent hydration must be maintained.

CYSTINURIA

See Chapter 18, Inherited Disorders of the Renal Tubule.

STRUVITE (INFECTION) STONES

Struvite ($MgNH_4PO_4 \cdot 6H_2O$) stones form in the renal pelvis and calices only when the urinary tract is infected by a urea-splitting bacterium, usually a *Proteus* species. Struvite stones tend to branch and enlarge, and their growth is rapid. Often, they fill the renal collecting systems and assume a staghorn configuration. They often grow back after surgical removal because infected chalky fragments have been left behind. Renal injury occurs as a result of a combination of obstruction and infection.

Because of the large size of these calculi, pyelolithotomy is often difficult. Struvite stones are very destructive and difficult to control.

Bacteriology

Proteus and *Providencia* species possess urease in more than 90% of isolates. Other common urinary pathogens that usually contain urease include *Klebsiella, Pseudomonas,* and enterococci. *Escherichia coli* rarely possesses urease activity. *Ureaplasma urealyticum,* a fastidious bacterium that requires special culture techniques for isolation, has been shown to cause struvite stones. Every fragment of the stone is infected and therefore can enlarge in urine.

Predisposing Factors

Calcium, uric acid, or cystine stones can become infected, especially as a result of instrumentation of the urinary tract. Chronic bladder catheterization promotes infection, and *Proteus* or *Pseudomonas* species can predominate despite the use of antimicrobial agents. Patients with spinal cord injury or any other form of neurogenic bladder or in whom ileal diversion of the ureter has been performed are especially prone to formation of struvite stones. However, struvite stones also occur without any predisposing cause. They are three times more common in women than in men, presumably because urinary tract infection is much more common in women. Often, they grow silently. Radiographic studies performed because of recurrent symptoms of urinary infection, hematuria, or pyuria or because of symptoms not related to the urinary system can disclose a staghorn calculus so large that it fills the renal collecting system and provokes amazement that its symptoms could be so meager.

Treatment

The preferred treatment of a struvite staghorn stone is surgical removal. Untreated staghorn calculi ultimately require nephrectomy in 50% of patients. Open surgical removal had been the procedure of choice and often led to improved renal function if obstruction was present. However, in the past, recurrence rates approached 30%. Percutaneous nephrolithotomy can completely remove struvite stones in 85% to 90% of kidneys with only a 10% relapse rate in those kidneys rendered stone-free. Extracorporeal shock wave lithotripsy with ureteral stenting has been used as monotherapy for large-volume struvite stones, resulting in stone-free rates of 50% to 75%. The American Urologic Association clinical guidelines recommend use of a combined approach of percutaneous nephrolithotomy and shock wave lithotripsy to give the best stone-free rates with the least patient morbidity in patients with struvite staghorn stones. No matter which approach is taken, the best long-term results depend on clearing the urinary tract of stones and sterilizing the urine. Monthly urine cultures should be obtained, and antibiotic therapy should be continued until the urine culture is negative on three consecutive occasions. Antibiotic treatment and conservative measures may be preferable to surgery in selected patients. Any metabolic disorder should be treated. Antibiotic use should be based on antibiotic resistance patterns of the infecting organism. Culture of stone material may allow more specific antibiotic therapy directed against the organism producing the stone. Although hope of cure is remote, stone growth can be slowed by reducing the bacterial population. Struvite stones often recur and patients need long-term follow-up and surveillance for urinary tract infections.

Urinary Tract Obstruction

22

In obstructive nephropathy the extent of recovery of renal function is inversely related to the duration and extent of obstruction; therefore prompt diagnosis and relief of obstruction are the cornerstones of effective management. Several terms with varying definitions have been used to describe urinary tract obstruction. It should be noted that they are not interchangeable:

- *Hydronephrosis:* Dilation of the renal pelvis and calices proximal to the point of obstruction
- *Obstructive uropathy:* A blockage to urine flow due to a structural or functional derangement anywhere from the tip of the urethra back to the renal pelvis that increases pressure proximal to the site of obstruction
- *Obstructive nephropathy:* The functional or pathologic damage to the renal parenchyma resulting from the obstruction anywhere along the urinary tract

PREVALENCE AND INCIDENCE

The frequency of urinary tract obstruction varies widely among different patient populations and depends on age, sex, and concurrent medical conditions. In autopsy subjects less than 10 years of age, the principal causes of urinary tract obstruction are neurologic abnormalities or ureteral and urethral strictures. Between the ages of 20 and 60, the frequency of urinary obstruction is higher among women than among men, mainly because of the effects of pregnancy and uterine cancer. After age 60, the frequency of urinary tract obstruction among men increases above that among women because of prostatic disease.

ETIOLOGY

Congenital Causes of Obstruction

Any level along the urinary tract from the ureteropelvic junction to the tip of urethra can be obstructed because of congenital anomalies (Table 22–1). Congenital causes of urinary tract obstruction are important because in younger patients they often lead to severe renal impairment and may result in end-stage renal disease. There is considerable controversy as to whether all obstructions early in life are clinically significant. The widespread use of fetal ultrasound has resulted in detection of many obstructions that remain asymptomatic and may resolve spontaneously with prospective follow-up. Because operative complications may be high, the use of fetal or neonatal surgery for the relief of obstruction remains controversial. Although bilateral obstruction requires intervention, the simple presence of unilateral hydronephrosis does not. Indications for surgery in patients with unilateral hydronephrosis include symptoms of obstruction or impaired renal function in a salvageable hydronephrotic kidney.

Table 22–1: Congenital Causes of Urinary Tract Obstruction

Ureteropelvic junction
   Ureteropelvic junction obstruction
Proximal and middle ureter
   Ureteral folds
   Ureteral valves
   Strictures
   Benign fibroepithelial polyps
   Retrocaval ureter
Distal ureter
   Ureterovesical junction obstruction
   Vesicoureteral reflux
   Prune-belly syndrome
   Ureteroceles
Bladder
   Bladder diverticula
   Neurologic conditions (e.g., spina bifida)
Urethra
   Posterior urethral valves
   Urethral diverticula
   Anterior urethral valves
   Urethral atresia
   Labial fusion

Acquired Causes of Obstruction

Intrinsic Causes
Acquired causes of obstruction may be intrinsic or extrinsic to the urinary tract (Table 22–2). Nephrolithiasis represents the most common cause of ureteral obstruction in younger men. A symptomatic stone is formed in 12% of the U.S. population

Table 22–2: Acquired Causes of Urinary Tract Obstruction

Intrinsic Processes	Extrinsic Processes
Intraluminal	**Reproductive tract**
Intrarenal	Female
Uric acid nephropathy	Uterus
Sulfonamides	Pregnancy
Acyclovir	Tumor (fibroids, endometrial
Indinavir	or cervical cancer)
Multiple myeloma	Endometriosis
Intraureteral	Uterine prolapse
Nephrolithiasis	Ureteral ligation (surgical)
Papillary necrosis	Ovary
Blood clots	Tubo-ovarian abscess
Fungus balls	Tumor
Intramural	Cyst
Functional	Male
Diseases	Benign prostatic hyperplasia
Diabetes mellitus	Prostate cancer
Multiple sclerosis	**Malignant neoplasms**
Cerebrovascular disease	Genitourinary tract
Spinal cord injury	Tumors of kidney, ureter,
Parkinson disease	bladder, urethra
Anticholinergic agents	Other sites
Levodopa (α-adrenergic	Metastatic spread
properties)	Direct extension
Anatomic	**Gastrointestinal system**
Ureteral strictures	Crohn disease
Schistosomiasis	Appendicitis
Tuberculosis	Diverticulosis
Drugs (e.g., nonsteroidal	Chronic pancreatitis with
anti-inflammatory agents)	pseudocyst formation
Ureteral instrumentation	Acute pancreatitis
Urethral strictures	**Vascular system**
	Arterial aneurysms
	Abdominal aortic aneurysm
	Iliac artery aneurysm

Continued

Table 22–2: (cont'd)

Intrinsic Processes	Extrinsic Processes

Benign or malignant tumors of the renal pelvis, ureter, bladder	Venous
	  Ovarian vein
	    thrombophlebitis
	Vasculitides
	  Systemic lupus
	    erythematosus
	  Polyarteritis nodosa
	  Wegener granulomatosis
	  Schönlein-Henoch purpura
	Retroperitoneal processes
	  Fibrosis
	    Idiopathic
	    Drug-induced
	    Inflammatory
	    Ascending lymphangitis
	      of the lower extremities
	    Chronic urinary tract
	      infection
	    Tuberculosis
	    Sarcoidosis
	    Iatrogenic (multiple
	      abdominal surgical
	      procedures)
	    Enlarged retroperitoneal
	      nodes
	    Tumor invasion
	    Tumor mass
	    Hemorrhage
	    Urinoma
	Biologic agents
	  Actinomycosis

at some time in their lives, with a male-to-female predominance of 3:1. When these stones cause obstruction, it tends to be acute, unilateral, and intermittent, usually without a long-term impact on renal function. Less common types of stones, such as struvite (ammonium-magnesium-sulfate) and cystine stones, are more often associated with renal damage because these substances accumulate over time and often form staghorn calculi.

Intrinsic intramural processes that cause obstruction include functional abnormalities, such as those associated with the neurologic

dysfunction of diabetes mellitus, multiple sclerosis, and spinal cord injury. Lower spinal tract injury may result in a flaccid, atonic bladder and failure of micturition. When the bladder does not void normally, renal damage may develop as a consequence of recurrent urinary tract infections and back pressure produced by the accumulation of residual urine. Various drugs can cause intrinsic intramural obstruction by disrupting the normal function of the smooth muscle of the urinary tract (see Table 22–2).

Acquired anatomic abnormalities of the wall of the urinary tract include ureteral strictures and benign as well as malignant tumors of the renal pelvis, ureter, bladder, and urethra. Ureteral strictures may occur as a result of radiation therapy for local cancers, such as cervical cancer, or as a result of analgesic abuse. In addition, strictures may develop as a complication of ureteral instrumentation or surgery. Certain infectious organisms may produce intrinsic obstruction of the urinary tract as well. *Schistosoma haematobium* infects nearly 100 million people worldwide. Although active infection can be treated and obstructive uropathy may resolve, chronic schistosomiasis ("bilharziasis") may develop in untreated patients, leading to irreversible ureteral or bladder fibrosis and obstruction.

Extrinsic Causes

A wide variety of diseases cause acquired extrinsic urinary tract obstruction. Because processes affecting the female reproductive tract such as pregnancy and pelvic neoplasms often cause obstructive uropathy, urinary tract obstruction occurs more often in younger women than in younger men. Noninvasive imaging studies have shown that more than two thirds of women entering their third trimester of pregnancy demonstrate some degree of dilation of the collecting system. Most of these occurrences are subclinical and appear to resolve completely soon after delivery. Pelvic malignant neoplasms represent the second most common cause of extrinsic obstructive uropathy in women. In older women, uterine prolapse may cause obstruction, with hydronephrosis developing in 5% of patients. Pelvic inflammatory disease, particularly a tuboovarian abscess, can also cause obstruction. Although endometriosis only rarely results in ureteral obstruction, it should be excluded in all premenopausal woman presenting with unilateral obstruction. The onset of obstruction may be insidious, and the process is usually confined to the pelvic portion of the ureter. Inadvertent ligation of the ureter in abdominal and retroperitoneal operations during gynecologic procedures is also a cause of ureteral obstruction.

Benign prostatic hyperplasia, the most common cause of urinary tract obstruction in men, produces some symptoms of bladder outlet obstruction in 75% of men aged 50 years and older. Presenting symptoms include urgency, difficulty initiating micturition, dribbling at the end of micturition, incomplete bladder emptying, and nocturia. The diagnosis may be established by history and urodynamic studies. Malignant genitourinary tumors occasionally result in urinary tract obstruction. Bladder cancer is the second most common cause (after cervical cancer) of malignant obstruction of the ureter. Prostate cancer may cause obstruction by compression of the bladder neck, invasion of the ureteral orifices, or metastatic involvement of the ureter or pelvic nodes. Although urothelial tumors of the renal pelvis, ureter, and urethra are rare, they also may lead to urinary obstruction.

Several gastrointestinal processes including Crohn disease may extend into the retroperitoneum, leading to ureteric obstruction, usually on the right side. Abdominal aortic aneurysms are the most common vascular cause of urinary obstruction. Obstruction occurs either because of direct pressure from the aneurysmal aorta on the ureter or because of associated retroperitoneal fibrosis. Aneurysms of the iliac vessels may also cause obstruction. Retroperitoneal processes, such as tumor invasion leading to compression and fibrosis, can produce obstruction. The major extrinsic causes of retroperitoneal obstruction, accounting for 70% of all cases, are tumors of the cervix, prostate, bladder, colon, ovary, or uterus. Retroperitoneal fibrosis usually involves the middle third of the ureter, typically in the fifth and sixth decade of life. It may be drug-induced (e.g., methysergide), or it may occur as a consequence of multiple abdominal surgical procedures. It may also be associated with conditions as varied as sarcoidosis, gonorrhea, chronic urinary tract infections, Schönlein-Henoch purpura, biliary tract disease, tuberculosis, and inflammatory processes of the lower extremities with ascending lymphangitis.

CLINICAL ASPECTS

Patients with urinary tract obstruction may or may not exhibit symptoms referable to the urinary tract. The clinical presentation depends on the rate of onset of the obstruction (acute or chronic), the degree of obstruction (partial or complete), whether the obstruction is unilateral or bilateral, and whether the obstruction is intrinsic or extrinsic. Pain is usually associated with obstruction of sudden onset and appears to result from abrupt stretching of the renal capsule or collecting system.

The severity of the pain correlates with the rate, rather than the degree, of distention. With ureteropelvic junction obstruction, flank pain may develop when the patient ingests large quantities of fluids or receives diuretics.

Sometimes, symptoms of obstruction include changes in urine output. Bilateral urinary tract obstruction is one of the few conditions that can result in anuria; however, obstruction may coexist with no change in urine output. Recurrent urinary tract infections may be the only sign of obstruction, particularly in children. As mentioned earlier, difficulty initiating urination, decreased size or force of the urine stream, postvoiding dribbling, and incomplete emptying are signs of bladder outlet obstruction in patients with prostatic disease. Spastic bladder or irritative symptoms such as dysuria, frequency, and urgency may result from urinary tract infection. The cyclical appearance of obstructive symptoms may also be a sign of endometriosis.

On physical examination, several signs may suggest urinary obstruction. A palpable abdominal mass, especially in neonates, may represent hydronephrosis. A palpable suprapubic mass may represent a distended bladder. On laboratory examination, proteinuria, if present, is generally less than 2 g/day. Microscopic hematuria is a common finding, but gross hematuria may develop occasionally as well. The urine sediment is often normal.

DIAGNOSIS

History and Physical Examination

A careful history and a well-directed and complete physical examination often reveal the specific cause of urinary obstruction. Important information in the history includes the type and duration of symptoms (voiding difficulties, flank pain, and decreased urine output), number of urinary tract infections (especially in children), pattern of fluid intake and urine output, history of stone disease, malignancies, gynecologic diseases, history of recent surgery, and prescription medication use. The abdominal examination may reveal hydronephrosis, presenting as a flank mass or a distended bladder. A pelvic examination in women and a rectal examination in all patients are mandatory.

Laboratory Evaluation

Unexplained renal failure with a benign urinary sediment should suggest urinary tract obstruction. Microscopic hematuria without proteinuria or casts suggests a calculus or tumor. Pyuria and bacteriuria may indicate pyelonephritis; bacteriuria alone may suggest stasis. Serum electrolytes, blood urea nitrogen concentration, and creatinine, Ca^{2+}, phosphorus, Mg^{2+}, uric acid, and albumin levels should be measured. These will help identify disorders of distal nephron function (impaired osmoregulation or acid excretion) and uremia. Urinary chemistry values may also suggest distal tubular dysfunction (isosthenuric urine or high urine pH), an inability to reabsorb sodium normally (urinary Na^+ >20 mEq/L, fractional excretion of Na^+ [FE_{Na}] >1%, and osmolality <350 mOsm). Alternatively, in acute obstruction urinary chemistry values may be consistent with prerenal azotemia (urinary Na^+ <20 mEq/L, FE_{Na} <1%, and osmolality >500 mOsm).

Radiologic Evaluation

A variety of radiologic techniques are used in the evaluation of obstructive uropathy. The risk of use of radiocontrast material in the setting of renal insufficiency, as well as that of exposure to radiation in pregnant women, must always be taken into consideration.

Plain Film Imaging of the Abdomen

If a renal calculus is suspected, it may be detected along the course of ureter or in the bladder by a plain film of the abdomen (kidney, ureter, and bladder) because 90% of calculi are radio-opaque. The plain film can also provide information on the size and overall contour of the kidneys.

Ultrasonography

When obstruction is suspected, ultrasonography is the preferred screening modality because it is safe and cost effective and lacks ionizing radiation, making it ideal for pregnant patients. Moreover, because no contrast material is involved, it is well suited to patients with an elevated or rising serum creatinine level. Ultrasonography can be used to determine the size and shape of the kidney and dilation of the pelvis and calices and may demonstrate thinned cortex in severe long-standing hydronephrosis. It has both high sensitivity and specificity for detecting hydronephrosis. However, it may fail to detect obstruction in the first 48 hours when hydronephrosis has not, as yet, developed. False-positive conclusions may be the result of a large extrarenal pelvis, parapelvic cysts, vesicoureteral reflux, or a high urine flow rate.

Antenatal Ultrasonography

Prenatal hydronephrosis is diagnosed with an incidence of 1 in 100 to 500 maternal-fetal ultrasonographic studies. Both obstructive and nonobstructive processes can cause dilation of the urinary tract (see earlier). The long-term morbidity of mild hydronephrosis (pelviectasis without calyceal dilation) is low. Severe hydronephrosis (pelvicaliceal dilation with parenchymal thinning) may require postnatal surgical intervention because of declining renal function, infection, or symptoms. Overall, approximately 5% to 25% of patients with antenatal hydronephrosis will ultimately require surgical intervention. Therefore, long-term follow-up of these patients is required. Functional imaging is required for patients with persistent postnatal hydronephrosis. All infants with prenatally detected hydronephrosis that is confirmed with postnatal studies should be given antibiotic prophylaxis pending the outcome of further evaluation. An infection in the setting of ureteral obstruction can cause significant morbidity in the uroseptic infant, and renal damage is a potential comorbidity. Oral amoxicillin (10 mg/kg/day) is the most commonly used prophylactic antibiotic.

Intravenous Urography

Intravenous urography (IVU) (also known as intravenous pyelography [IVP]) provides both functional and anatomic data, particularly for the ureter. Until recently it was considered to be the gold standard for imaging in acute renal colic. However, the procedure has significant drawbacks, including the risk of contrast nephrotoxicity and the fact that it is contraindicated in pregnancy. Furthermore, kidneys may not be visualized in patients with severe obstruction because the suppressed glomerular filtration rate may not allow excretion of the contrast material. All of these concerns have led to replacement of IVU with computed tomography (CT), ultrasound, and magnetic resonance imaging (MRI) in many patients.

Computed Tomography

A distinct advantage of CT is that it can visualize a dilated collecting system, even without contrast enhancement and can also be performed more quickly than IVU. Non–contrast-enhanced CT is more effective than IVU in precisely identifying ureteral stones and as effective as IVU in determining the presence or absence of ureteral obstruction. Even radiolucent stones can be identified. CT is useful in identifying extrinsic causes of obstruction (e.g., retroperitoneal fibrosis, lymphadenopathy, and hematoma). CT can also detect extraurinary pathologic conditions and can establish nonurogenital causes of pain. All of these advantages establish non–contrast-enhanced helical CT as the diagnostic study of choice for the evaluation of the patient with acute flank pain.

Isotopic Renography

Isotopic renography, or renal scintigraphy, can be used to diagnose upper urinary tract obstruction while avoiding the risks associated with radiocontrast agents. Although it provides a functional assessment of the obstructed kidney, anatomic definition is poor. Isotopic renography is typically used to estimate the fractional contribution of each kidney to overall renal function and repeat studies can gauge the extent to which relief of the obstruction has restored renal function.

Magnetic Resonance Imaging

MRI can be used to explore the urinary tract when obstruction is suspected. Because MRI does not use ionizing radiation and because gadolinium contrast agents are essentially nonnephrotoxic, MRI is especially useful in children, women of child-bearing age, and patients with renal insufficiency or renal allografts. However, MRI provides no substantial diagnostic advantages compared with the combination of ultrasound and CT.

Retrograde and Antegrade Pyelography

When standard radiographic methods fail to produce a diagnosis or when obstruction must be promptly relieved (e.g., bilateral obstruction, obstruction of solitary kidney, or symptomatic infection in the obstructed system), more invasive investigation, with a combination of treatments, may be necessary. Retrograde pyelography is performed by cystoscopically guided cannulation of the ureteral orifice and injection of contrast material. The procedure can be combined with placement of a ureteral stent to relieve an obstruction or possibly with stone extraction. Antegrade pyelography is performed by percutaneous cannulation of the kidney and injection of the contrast material into the kidney and ureter. This procedure should establish the proximal level of obstruction and may also serve as a first step in relieving obstruction by means of percutaneous nephrostomy.

TREATMENT OF URINARY TRACT OBSTRUCTION AND RECOVERY OF RENAL FUNCTION

Once the presence of obstruction is established, intervention is usually indicated to relieve it. The type of intervention depends on the location of the obstruction, its degree, and its etiology, as well as the presence or absence of concomitant diseases and complications and the general condition of the patient. The first step usually involves prompt relief of the obstruction, followed by the definitive treatment. Infravesical obstruction (e.g., benign prostatic hyperplasia or urethral stricture) can be easily relieved with placement of a urethral catheter. If the urethra is impassable, suprapubic cystostomy may be necessary. Alternatively, insertion of a nephrostomy tube or ureteral stent may be indicated when supravesical urinary obstruction is present. The urgency of the intervention depends on the degree of renal impairment, the presence or absence of infection, and the overall risk of the procedure. The presence of the infection in an obstructed urinary tract, or urosepsis, is a urologic emergency that requires prompt relief of the obstruction and antibiotic therapy. Acute renal failure, associated with bilateral ureteral obstruction or with the obstruction of a single functioning kidney, also calls for emergency intervention.

Calculi, the most common form of acute unilateral urinary obstruction, can usually be managed conservatively with analgesics to control pain and intravenous fluids to increase urine flow. Ninety percent of stones smaller than 5 mm pass spontaneously, but as stones get larger, the possibility that they will pass spontaneously becomes progressively less likely. Surgery or instrumentation is indicated for persistent obstruction, uncontrollable pain, or urinary tract infection. Current treatment options include cystoscopic placement of ureteral stents, nephrostomy with urine drainage, extracorporeal shock wave lithotripsy (which may require ureteral stent placement if the patient is symptomatic), and ureteroscopy with stone fragmentation (usually with laser lithotripsy). Large renal stones can be fragmented through nephrostomy. These newer approaches have all but eliminated the need for open surgical procedures.

Intramural or extrinsic ureteral obstruction may be relieved by placement of a ureteral stent through the cystoscope. If this cannot be accomplished or if the procedure is ineffective (especially for extrinsic ureteral compression by tumors), then nephrostomy tubes will need to be inserted to effect prompt relief of the obstruction. For infravesical obstruction due to benign prostatic hyperplasia, surgery can be safely delayed or completely avoided in patients with minimal symptoms, lack of infection, and an anatomically normal upper urinary tract. If needed, transurethral resection of the prostate, laser ablation, or other techniques can be used for definitive treatment. Internal urethrotomy with direct visualization may be effective in the treatment of urethral strictures, because dilation usually has only a temporary effect. In patients with impassable urethral strictures, suprapubic cystostomy may be necessary followed by open urethroplasty to restore urinary tract continuity, when possible. Patients with a neurogenic bladder require a variety of approaches, including frequent voiding, often by external compression, medications to stimulate bladder activity or relax the urethral sphincter, and intermittent catheterization using meticulous technique to avoid infection. Long-term indwelling bladder catheters should be avoided because they increase the risk of infection and renal damage. If more conservative measures such as frequent voiding or intermittent catheterization are not effective, ileovesicostomy or another form of urinary diversion should be considered.

In many forms of obstruction, initial stabilization of the patient's condition is followed by a decision as to whether to continue observation or to move on to definitive surgery or nephrectomy. The actual course chosen depends on the likelihood that renal function will improve with the relief of obstruction. Factors that affect the decision of whether to operate and what form of surgical intervention to use include the age and general condition of the patient, the appearance and function of the obstructed kidney and the contralateral one, the cause of the obstruction, and the presence of infection. The extent of recovery of renal function depends on the extent and duration of the obstruction.

Estimating Renal Damage and Potential for Recovery

As noted earlier, when a clinician decides whether to bypass or reconstruct drainage of an obstructed kidney rather than excise it, the potential for meaningful recovery of function in the affected kidney represents a critical issue. Isotopic renography with a variety of isotopes can be used to examine renal function, as outlined earlier. This approach is a far more reliable indicator of potential renal function when applied well after temporary drainage of the obstructed kidney (e.g., by nephrostomy tubes) has been achieved than if it is performed while the obstruction is still present. Of course, anatomic studies will reveal the remaining size and volume of the kidney and can provide some idea of the extent to which the tissue remains viable. All of these considerations contribute to the final clinical judgment as to whether attempts should be made to salvage the kidney.

Recovery of Renal Function after Prolonged Obstruction

The potential for recovery of renal function depends primarily on the extent and duration of the obstruction, but other factors, such as the presence of other illnesses and the presence or absence of urinary tract infection, play an important role as well. Recovery of renal function in humans has been documented after release of obstruction of more than 60 days' duration. Because it is difficult to predict whether renal function will recover when temporary relief of obstruction has been achieved, it makes sense to measure function repeatedly with isotopic renography over time, before deciding on a definitive surgical course. Chronic bilateral obstruction, as seen in benign prostatic hyperplasia, can cause chronic renal failure, especially when the obstruction is of prolonged duration and when it is accompanied by urinary tract infections. Progressive loss of renal function can be slowed or halted by relieving the obstruction and treating the infection. When obstruction has been relieved and there is poor return of renal function, interstitial fibrosis and inflammation may have supervened.

POSTOBSTRUCTIVE DIURESIS

Release of obstruction can lead to marked natriuresis and diuresis with the wasting of potassium, phosphate, and divalent cations. It is notable that clinically significant postobstructive diuresis usually occurs only in the setting of prior bilateral obstruction or unilateral obstruction of a solitary functioning kidney. The mechanisms involved include a combination of intrinsic damage to tubular salt, solute, and water reabsorption, as well as the effects of volume expansion, solute (e.g., urea) accumulation, and attendant increases in natriuretic substances such as atrial natriuretic peptide. Management of the patient with postobstructive diuresis focuses on avoidance of severe volume depletion due to salt wasting and other electrolyte imbalances, such as hypokalemia, hyponatremia, hypernatremia, and hypomagnesemia. Postobstructive diuresis is usually self-limited and lasts for several days to a week, but may, in rare patients, persist for months. Volume or free water replacement is appropriate only when the salt and water losses result in volume depletion or a disturbance of osmolality. In many patients, excessive volume or fluid replacement prolongs the diuresis and natriuresis. Because the initial urine is isosthenuric, with a Na^+ concentration of approximately 80 mEq/L, an appropriate starting fluid for replacement may be 0.45% saline, given at a rate somewhat slower than that of the urine output. During this period, meticulous monitoring of vital signs, volume status, urine output, and serum and urine chemistry values and osmolality is imperative. This will determine the need for ongoing replacement of salt, free water, and other electrolytes. With massive diuresis, these measurements will need to be repeated often, up to four times daily, with frequent adjustment of replacement fluids as needed.

Renal Neoplasia | *23*

Malignant neoplasms involving the renal parenchyma and renal pelvis may be primary or secondary in origin, although the latter are typically of little clinical consequence. The main primary renal tumors are the following:

- Renal cell carcinomas (80% to 85%)
- Transitional carcinomas (7% to 8%)
- Nephroblastoma (Wilms tumor) in children (5% to 6%)
- Other parenchymal epithelial tumors. These include oncocytomas, collecting duct tumors, and renal sarcomas, which are uncommon but are being recognized more often with pathologic findings

RENAL CELL CARCINOMA

Epidemiology

Renal cell carcinoma (RCC) is responsible for 2% to 3% of all cancers and 2% of all cancer deaths. The incidence varies widely from country to country, with the highest rates being found in northern Europe and North America. RCC occurs predominantly in the sixth to eighth decade of life and is uncommon in patients younger than 40 years of age. The 5-year survival rate has improved in recent years and is now approximately 60%. Risk factors for the development of RCC include tobacco use; urbanization and exposure to cadmium, asbestos, and petroleum by-products; analgesic abuse; and acquired cystic disease of the kidney in end-stage renal failure. Genetic factors have been implicated in the etiology of RCC; inherited disorders associated with RCC include tuberous sclerosis, autosomal dominant adult polycystic kidney disease, and von Hippel-Lindau disease.

Clinical and Laboratory Features

The clinical manifestations of RCC are extremely varied. Many tumors are clinically silent, and 25% to 30% of patients present with distant metastases, with an additional 25% having locally advanced disease at diagnosis. The most common presenting symptom is hematuria, followed by abdominal mass, pain, and weight loss. The classic triad of flank pain, hematuria, and a palpable abdominal renal mass occurs in only about 10% of patients. Hematuria, gross or microscopic, is usually observed only if the tumor has invaded the collecting system. The sudden onset of a scrotal varicocele is indicative of obstruction of the gonadal vein at its entry point into the left renal vein by tumor thrombus, and this finding should always raise the possibility of a neoplasm within the kidney. Of patients initially seen with metastatic disease, 75% have lung involvement. Other common sites for metastasis include lymph nodes, bone, and liver. A number of patients with RCC experience systemic symptoms or a paraneoplastic syndrome (Table 23–1). Fever, accompanied by night sweats, anorexia, weight loss, and fatigue, is one of the more common manifestations of RCC. Hormones produced by RCCs include parathyroid-like hormone, gonadotropins, placental lactogen, adrenocorticotropic hormone–like substance, renin, erythropoietin, glucagon, and insulin. Several of these hormones have been associated with specific paraneoplastic phenomena. Erythrocytosis, defined as a hematocrit greater than 55 mL/dL, occurs in almost 4% of patients with RCC. Hypercalcemia occurs in up to 15% of all patients with RCC and is an independent negative prognostic factor in patients with metastatic RCC. Hypercalcemia can occur in the absence of osseous metastases, and ectopic production of parathyroid hormone–related peptide by the primary tumor has been documented in these patients.

Radiologic Diagnosis

For patients with symptoms suggestive of RCC, the radiologic approaches available for evaluation of the kidney include computed tomography (CT), magnetic resonance imaging, and ultrasonography. Although intravenous pyelography remains useful in the evaluation of hematuria, CT and ultrasonography are the mainstays of evaluation of a suspected renal mass. As seen on CT, the typical RCC is generally larger than 4 cm in diameter, has a heterogeneous density, and enhances with contrast material. Ultrasonography, although less sensitive than CT, is particularly useful in differentiating between a simple benign cyst

Table 23–1: Paraneoplastic Syndromes Associated with Renal Cell Cancer Syndrome

Syndrome	Incidence (%)
Anemia	20–40
Cachexia, fatigue, weight loss	33
Fever	30
Hypertension	24
Hypercalcemia	10–15
Hepatic dysfunction (Stauffer syndrome)	3–6
Amyloidosis	3–5
Erythrocytosis	3–4
Enteropathy	3
Neuromyopathy	3

From McDougal WS, Garnick MB: Clinical signs and symptoms of kidney cancer. In Vogelzang NJ, Scardino PT, Shipley WU, et al (eds): *Comprehensive Textbook of Genitourinary Oncology.* Baltimore, Williams & Wilkins, 1996.

and a more complex cyst or a solid tumor. It has a sensitivity of 97%, a specificity of 97%, and a false-negative rate of only 1% in differentiating a benign cyst from a potentially malignant tumor. Magnetic resonance imaging with gadolinium as the contrast material is superior to CT for evaluating the inferior vena cava if tumor extension into this vessel is suspected. Magnetic resonance imaging is also a useful adjunct to ultrasonography in the evaluation of renal masses if radiographic contrast material cannot be used because of allergy or inadequate renal function. Although most solid renal masses are RCCs, some lesions are benign and complicate the diagnosis. These include angiomyolipomas and renal oncocytomas. Selective renal arteriography, a mainstay of diagnosis in the past, is now rarely used. Renal arteriography is generally reserved for selected patients in whom preoperative mapping of the vasculature is necessary, such as when nephron-sparing surgery is contemplated.

Staging and Prognosis

After the presumptive diagnosis of renal carcinoma has been made, an evaluation of the extent of involvement of regional and distant metastatic sites should be made. Renal carcinomas can grow locally into very large masses and invade through surrounding fascia into adjacent organs. The most common sites of metastasis are the regional lymphatics, lungs, bone, liver, brain, ipsilateral adrenal gland, and contralateral kidney. Metastases to unusual sites, such as the thyroid gland, pancreas, mucosal surfaces, skin, and soft tissue, are not uncommon in this disease. CT scanning of the abdomen is the principal radiologic tool for defining the local/regional extent of RCC. Staging evaluation should also include CT scans of the chest and a bone scan. Of note, approximately 2% of patients present with bilateral tumors, and 25% to 30% of patients have overt metastases at initial evaluation. The TNM (tumor-node-metastasis) system is used for staging of RCC and includes most consistent prognostic variables that influence survival (Table 23–2). Survival based on stage is displayed in Table 23–3. Other factors that have a bearing on prognosis include the histologic subtype (see earlier), the patient's performance status, and the presence of paraneoplastic signs or symptoms such as anemia, hypercalcemia, hepatopathy, fever, or weight loss.

Table 23–2: TNM Staging for Renal Cell Carcinoma

Primary tumor (T)
    TX Primary tumor cannot be assessed
    T0 No evidence of primary tumor
    T1 Tumor 7 cm or less in greatest dimension, limited to the kidney
    T2 Tumor more than 7 cm in greatest dimension, limited to the kidney
    T3 Tumor extends into major veins or invades adrenal gland or perinephric tissue, but not beyond Gerota fascia
    T3a Tumor invades adrenal gland or perinephric tissue, but not beyond Gerota fascia
    T3b Tumor grossly extends into renal vein(s) or vena cava below diaphragm
    T3c Tumor grossly extends into vena cava above diaphragm
    T4 Tumor invades beyond Gerota fascia
Regional lymph nodes (N)*
    NX Regional lymph nodes cannot be assessed
    N0 No regional lymph node metastasis
    N1 Metastasis in a single regional lymph node
    N2 Metastasis in more than one regional lymph node
Distant metastasis (M)
    MX Distant metastasis cannot be assessed
    M0 No distant metastasis
    M1 Distant metastasis

*Laterality does not affect the N classification.

Table 23–3: Correlation of Stage Grouping with Survival in Patients with Renal Cell Cancer

	Stage Grouping			*5-Year Survival (%)*
I	T1	N0	M0	90–95
II	T2	N0	M0	70–85
III	T3a	N0	M0	50–65
	T3b	N0	M0	50–65
	T3c	N0	M0	45–50
	T1	N1	M0	25–30
	T2	N1	M0	25–30
	T3	N1	M0	15–20
IV	T4	Any N	M0	10
	Any T	N2	M0	10
Any T	Any N	Any N	M1	<5

Surgical Management

Nephrectomy

The mainstay of treatment of primary RCC is surgical excision or nephrectomy. This may involve a radical nephrectomy, which includes early ligation of the renal artery and renal vein and en bloc excision of the kidney with the surrounding Gerota fascia and ipsilateral adrenal gland. The early ligation of the vascular pedicle is important to prevent dissemination of tumor at the time of surgery. In recent years the value of radical nephrectomy is being reassessed. Involvement of the ipsilateral adrenal gland occurs only 4% of the time, and in most instances, this is associated with either direct extension from an upper pole lesion or the presence of metastatic disease. Therefore, adrenalectomy is often reserved for patients with large upper pole lesions or those with solitary ipsilateral adrenal metastases. The benefit of performing regional lymph node dissection in conjunction with radical nephrectomy is controversial. With improved preoperative CT staging, the incidence of unsuspected nodal metastases is low. The benefit of lymphadenectomy is largely prognostic, and regional lymph node dissection should only be performed in patients being considered for adjuvant treatment protocols (see later).

Nephron-Sparing Surgery

The generally accepted criteria for consideration of nephron-sparing or partial nephrectomy include bilateral tumors, tumor in a solitary kidney, or compromised renal function. The rate of recurrence in the partially resected kidney ranges from 4% to 10%.

Complications of nephron-sparing surgery include urinary fistulas, acute tubular necrosis, the need for temporary or permanent dialysis, and hemorrhage. Because of the favorable results seen with nephron-sparing surgery and the increasing number of smaller, incidentally discovered tumors, nephron-sparing surgery has been increasingly used to treat patients with small (<4 cm), polar tumors and a normal contralateral kidney. The primary concern with this approach is that a multicentric tumor would go unrecognized and result in recurrent disease in the salvaged kidney. With highly sensitive preoperative staging, the increasing use of three-dimensional reconstruction of CT images, and the use of intraoperative ultrasound, such an occurrence should be rare.

Laparoscopic Nephrectomy
Although no randomized study has been conducted, clinical data to date suggest that laparoscopic radical nephrectomy may be a viable alternative to an open procedure, with equivalent surgical efficacy and safety and substantially reduced postoperative recovery time.

Vena Caval Involvement
Inferior vena caval involvement with tumor thrombus is found in about 5% of patients undergoing radical nephrectomy. Vena caval obstruction may produce various clinical manifestations, including abdominal distention with ascites, hepatic dysfunction (possibly related to Budd-Chiari syndrome), nephrotic syndrome, caput medusa, varicocele, malabsorption, and pulmonary emboli. Survival rates in patients with subdiaphragmatic lesions approach 50%; patients with supradiaphragmatic thrombi do considerably worse. A team of specialists is usually required for the surgical management of these patients because operative mortality may be as high as 5% to 10%, particularly if thrombectomy of an intracardiac tumor is contemplated.

Radiofrequency Ablation
Efforts to develop less invasive therapeutic techniques have led to the use of radiofrequency ablation in patients with small renal tumors, multiple lesions, impaired renal function, solitary kidneys, or significant surgical risks (or any combination of these factors). Although this is a safe procedure, pathologic analysis has demonstrated small foci of viable tumor present in several patients, raising concerns about local recurrence and the potential for metastatic spread.

Angioinfarction
Angioinfarction is performed with or without nephrectomy for the treatment of patients with metastatic or locally advanced RCC.

This approach has been used to reduce vascularity and the consequent risk of hemorrhage during nephrectomy in patients with large, marginally resectable primary tumors and to control symptoms such as bleeding or pain in patients with unresectable tumors or distant metastases. Most patients experience pain, fever, and nausea after the procedure that may last for several days.

Debulking Nephrectomy

Patients with RCC who present with metastatic disease typically have a poor prognosis, with no 5-year survivors reported in some series. Regression of distant metastases after removal of the primary tumor is an infrequent event (<1%) and is unlikely to yield a survival advantage in patients presenting with metastatic disease. However, responses to immunotherapy are uncommon in patients with primary tumors in place. Consequently, some groups have advocated that patients presenting with metastatic disease undergo debulking nephrectomy before immunotherapy commences. Indeed, some prospective evidence exists to support a role for nephrectomy in patients with metastatic or locally advanced disease who do not have liver, bone, or central nervous system involvement and have good performance status.

Palliative Surgery

Palliative nephrectomy is rarely necessary. Pain and bleeding can be controlled with systemic pain medication and angioinfarction, clot colic can be minimized with ureteral stents and hydration, and hypercalcemia, fatigue, fever, and other systemic symptoms can often be controlled with nonsteroidal anti-inflammatory drugs, bisphosphonates, hydration, and appetite stimulants such as medroxyprogesterone.

Resection of Metastatic Disease

Surgical resection of metastatic disease has been actively pursued in certain clinical situations. Resection of solitary metastases or oligometastases, often in the ipsilateral lung or adrenal gland, in conjunction with nephrectomy, occasionally provides long-term survival. Another situation in which resection of metastases has been considered is after effective systemic therapy.

Radiation Therapy

The major sites of systemic metastases include the lung, bone, and brain. Radiation treatment of disease in these areas can provide palliation of bone pain, prevent cord compression or fracture, trigger regression of central nervous system metastases, or provide control of hemoptysis or airway obstruction.

Objective responses occur in about 50% of patients. Palliation of large renal bed recurrences by external beam irradiation has been unsatisfactory.

Systemic Therapy

Although surgical resection of localized disease can be curative, many patients later experience recurrence, and 50% of patients present with either regional or metastatic disease. In these patients the median survival is only 12 months, emphasizing the need for more effective adjuvant therapies. Treatment options include chemotherapy, immunotherapy, and, more recently, molecular biology–based targeted therapeutic approaches.

Chemotherapy

Single-agent chemotherapy has minimal or no activity against RCC. Response rates with combination chemotherapy regimens are slightly better, but these regimens are associated with increased toxicity and may not produce a survival benefit compared with single-agent chemotherapy. Emerging options include the use of gemcitabine in combination with 5-fluorouracil.

Immunotherapy

The most successful immunotherapeutic strategies for RCC involve the administration of interferon-α (IFN-α) and interleukin-2 (IL-2). The mechanism of action of these cytokines is incompletely understood but may involve the direct killing of tumor cells by activated T and natural killer cells, as well as an antiangiogenic effects.

INTERFERON-α   IFN-α has undergone extensive clinical evaluation for the treatment of metastatic RCC over the past two decades. Most studies have demonstrated some antitumor effect, with the overall response rate being approximately 15%. The median time to response is approximately 4 months. However, most responses are partial and short lived (median response duration of 6 to 7 months) and only about 2% of patients have had complete responses. The toxicity of IFN-α includes flulike symptoms, such as fever, chills, myalgia, and fatigue, as well as weight loss, altered taste, depression, anemia, leukopenia, and elevated liver function test results. Most side effects, especially the flulike symptoms, tend to diminish with time during chronic therapy. Efforts to improve the clinical activity of IFN-α have included combinations with 5-fluorouracil, *cis*-retinoic acid, IFN-γ, thalidomide, and IL-2.

INTERLEUKIN-2 High-dose bolus IL-2 has received U.S. Food and Drug Administration approval for metastatic RCC. Because of the considerable toxicity associated with high-dose IL-2 regimens (e.g., hypotension and capillary leak syndrome), treatment should be administered in a setting in which a level of care comparable to that provided in an intensive care unit is available. In addition, such treatment should be restricted to carefully selected patients with excellent organ function in centers with personnel who have experience with this treatment. The clinical result of this approach is a complete response in approximately 7% of patients and a partial response in 8%. Although the overall response rates are low, a large percentage of patients who have a response, particularly those remaining free of progression for longer than 2 years or those who undergo resection to achieve disease-free status after a response to high-dose IL-2, appear unlikely to have progression of RCC and may actually be "cured."

Nonmyeloablative Allogeneic Transplantation

Allogeneic bone marrow transplantation has evolved from a means to achieve chemotherapeutic dose escalation to a form of adoptive immunotherapy. Preliminary experience with nonmyeloablative allogeneic transplantation in patients with RCC has been reported by a number of centers. However, substantial hematologic toxicities, as well as graft-versus host disease may occur, and such adverse outcomes are associated with poorer pretransplant performance status. Although promising, nonmyeloablative transplantation requires substantial further development before it can be considered in a larger number of patients.

RENAL PELVIC TUMORS

Uroepithelial tumors account for approximately 10% of all primary renal cancers. Tumors of the upper urinary tract are twice as common in men, usually occur in patients older than 65 years of age, and are generally unilateral. Risk factors for the development of urothelial tumors include exposure to cigarettes, certain chemicals, plastics, coal, tar, and asphalt. Long-term exposure to the analgesic phenacetin, usually ingested over years by women for headache relief, has been associated with the development of renal pelvic tumors. These tumors are often multicentric and have a high rate of recurrence. Although most tumors of the upper urinary tract are transitional cell carcinomas (>90% of lesions), squamous cell carcinomas also occur, usually in the setting of chronic infection with kidney stones. Adenocarcinomas and other miscellaneous subtypes are rare.

Initial Features and Diagnostic Evaluation

The most common initial feature is gross hematuria, which occurs in 75% of patients, followed by flank pain in 30%. Radiologic evaluation may reveal either a nonfunctioning kidney and nonvisualization of the collecting system or, more commonly, a filling defect of the caliceal system, or renal pelvis, on intravenous pyelography. Results of exfoliative cytologic examination are usually positive, as they are in bladder cancers. A positive cytologic test result in the presence of a filling defect of the renal pelvis or ureter confirms the diagnosis. If the diagnosis is still uncertain after pyelography, ureteroscopy may facilitate it.

Staging and Grading

Transitional cell carcinomas are graded on a scale of I, representing a well-differentiated lesion, to IV, anaplastic and undifferentiated lesions. In a staging system similar to that used for urinary bladder cancer, stage 0 is limited to the mucosa, stage A indicates invasion into the lamina propria without muscularis invasion, stage B indicates invasion into the muscularis, stage C indicates invasion into the serosa, and stage D represents metastatic disease. Lymphatic metastases usually indicate that more widespread metastatic disease is or will be present.

Management

For low-grade, low-stage transitional cancers, the general approach to treatment is conservative and consists of local excision and preservation of the kidney parenchyma. Five-year survival rates are usually in excess of 60%. For high-stage and high-grade lesions that have infiltrated into the renal parenchyma, the surgical treatment of choice is nephroureterectomy and removal of a cuff of bladder that encompasses the ipsilateral ureteral orifice. In patients with regionally advanced or metastatic renal pelvic tumors, systemic chemotherapy is often used. Standard first-line regimens for patients with locally advanced or metastatic transitional cell carcinoma include methotrexate, vinblastine, doxorubicin (Adriamycin), and cisplatin (MVAC); gemcitabine and cisplatin; or paclitaxel and cisplatin. Initial response rates vary, depending on prognostic factors, but long-term survival is poor.

OTHER KIDNEY TUMORS

Renal Sarcomas

Renal sarcomas account for approximately 1% to 2% of primary renal cancers. Fibrosarcomas are the most common and prognosis is poor as a result of late diagnosis and the presence of locally advanced involvement into the renal vein or metastatic disease at initial evaluation. Five-year survival rates are less than 20%. Other, rarer, sarcoma variants may occur and include leiomyosarcoma, rhabdomyosarcoma, osteogenic sarcoma, and liposarcoma.

Wilms Tumor

In children, Wilms tumor (nephroblastoma) is the most common cancer of the kidney and accounts for approximately 400 new cases per year in the United States. Several well-described genetic abnormalities are associated with Wilms tumor. Patients with Wilms tumor may also manifest other abnormalities, including aniridia, WAGR syndrome (Wilms tumor, aniridia, other genitourinary abnormalities, and mental retardation), Denys-Drash syndrome (Wilms tumor, glomerulitis, and pseudohermaphroditism), hemihypertrophy, trisomy 21, other rare physical abnormalities of macroglossia, and developmental sexual disorders. Abnormalities in *WT1* (chromosome 11p13) and *WT2* (11p15) and mutations at 16q have all been implicated in the molecular genetics of Wilms tumor. Loss of heterozygosity in *WT1* and 16q occur in 20% of patients; inactivation of *WT2* has also been described. Other genetic abnormalities have suggested the presence of additional abnormal chromosomal locations. Patients with trisomy 21 and XX/XY mosaicisms have been reported to have an increased incidence of Wilms tumor.

Initial Features

An abdominal mass, with or without abdominal pain, is the most common finding and occurs in 80% and 40% of patients, respectively. Other physical abnormalities, including aniridia, genitourinary abnormalities, and hemihypertrophy, may occasionally be detected. Hematuria, anemia, hypertension, or acute severe abdominal pain may also be present. Abdominal ultrasound is an important diagnostic test to further evaluate the mass and its anatomic extension, which may include inferior or superior extension into the vena cava. Intravenous pyelography and CT are also warranted. Metastatic evaluation of liver, chest, and bone complement the evaluation. The diagnosis is usually established by surgery. If the diagnostic tests and clinical features suggest the presence of a Wilms tumor, preoperative needle biopsy should be avoided because of the attendant risk of tumor spillage.

Multimodality Management
High cure rates have been achieved with the concerted effort of multimodality teams performing surgery, radiation therapy, and chemotherapy. Removal of all gross tumor by radical resection should be attempted. Most patients receive radiation therapy as an adjunct to surgical removal. Chemotherapy is an important component of therapy in Wilms tumors. In addition to being used after surgery in conjunction with radiation therapy, neoadjuvant chemotherapy can diminish the size of the primary tumor and induce regression of metastatic lesions. Agents that have activity against Wilms tumor include vincristine, dactinomycin, doxorubicin, etoposide, ifosfamide, and cisplatin. Cure rates approach 80% to 90% with survival rates of 92% to 97% in early stage disease. For patients who experience relapse or for those with poor prognostic features, bone marrow transplantation has been offered with good results.

IV

Hypertension

Essential Hypertension

24

High blood pressure (BP) is a leading risk factor for heart disease, stroke, and kidney failure. It is estimated that 45 million people in the United States are hypertensive. Nevertheless, fewer than 30% of all hypertensive patients have adequate BP control. In general, the upper limits of normal BP in older persons have been considered to be a systolic value of 140 mm Hg and a diastolic value of 90 mm Hg. These figures may be adjusted downward for younger patients to the point that readings in excess of 120/80 mm Hg may be considered hypertensive.

Clinical studies indicate that relatively higher BPs that are casually recorded, even those that are within the normal range, are statistically associated with increased mortality from cardiovascular complications. It is well established that antihypertensive treatment provides a significant degree of protection against complications such as congestive heart failure (CHF), renal failure, and stroke but not coronary artery disease. Nonetheless, the risks of death and disability associated with hypertension are increased only in the broad statistical sense; most patients with hypertension live lives of normal longevity and health. Thus, risks are apparently not distributed randomly but are concentrated in subgroups of patients that have been proven difficult to identify accurately. For these and other reasons, hypertension cannot be considered a discrete disease entity but must be considered a factor common to the development of several pathologic events. Thus, hypertension is a physical sign and a risk factor to be assessed in conjunction with other physiologic and environmental factors.

NOMENCLATURE

In an attempt to clarify the nomenclature, recent guidelines have designated a classification system for BP for adults. Hypertension is stratified as follows:

- Prehypertension (120 to 139 mm Hg or 80 to 89 mm Hg)
- Stage 1 (140 to 159 mm Hg or 90 to 99 mm Hg)

- Stage 2 (160 to 179 mm Hg or 100 to 109 mm Hg)
- Stage 3 (=180 mm Hg or =110 mm Hg)

Essential hypertension: The pathophysiologic mechanism underlying hypertension is unknown in approximately 90% of patients. Members of this group are classified as having *primary hypertension* or *essential hypertension,* signifying that no cause for their disorder has been found.

Secondary hypertension: This implies a discrete cause for the hypertension, which may or may not be curable (Table 24–1).

Isolated systolic hypertension: Hypertension may be purely systolic and accompanied by a normal or even lowered diastolic pressure.

Table 24–1: Known Causes of Secondary Hypertension
Renal Disorders

Renal
  Renal parenchymal
    Acute and chronic glomerulonephritis, pyelonephritis,
      nephrocalcinosis, neoplasms, glomerulosclerosis
    Obstructive uropathies and hydronephrosis
    Renin-secreting renal tumors
    Congenital defect in renal sodium transport
      (Liddle syndrome)
  Renovascular
    Renal arterial lesions, occlusions, stenoses, aneurysms,
      thromboses
    Coarctation of the aorta with renal ischemia
Adrenocortical disorders
  Cushing syndrome (cortisol excess)
  Primary aldosteronism (Conn syndrome)
  Pseudoprimary aldosteronism (bilateral adrenocortical
    hyperplasia)
  Congenital or acquired enzymatic defects with excess
    Na^+-retaining steroids (11β-hydroxylase deficiency,
    11β-hydroxysteroid dehydrogenase deficiency,
    17-hydroxylase deficiency)
  Adrenal carcinoma
  Ectopic corticotropin-secreting tumor
Pheochromocytoma
Other endocrine causes
  Hypothyroidism (diastolic hypertension)
  Hyperthyroidism (systolic hypertension)
  Hypercalcemic states
  Acromegaly

Continued

Table 24–1: (cont'd)

Toxemias of pregnancy
Neurogenic factors
  Increased intracranial pressure
  Familial dysautonomia
  Acute porphyria, buffer denervation, poliomyelitis, spinal cord
    injuries
Iatrogenic and other causes
  Oral contraceptive or estrogen therapy
  Mineralocorticoid or glucocorticoid therapies, licorice
    ingestion (i.e., acquired 11β-hydroxysteroid dehydrogenase
    deficiency)
  Sympathomimetic drugs (decongestants)
  Antidepressants
  Alcohol abuse
  Lead toxicity
  Monoamine oxidase inhibitors (interactions with other agents)
  Excessive salt appetite?

From Blumenfeld JD, Mann SJ, Laragh JH: Clinical evaluation and differential diagnosis of the individual hypertensive patient. In Laragh JH, Brenner BM (eds): *Hypertension: Pathophysiology, Diagnosis, and Management,* 2nd ed. New York, Raven Press, 1995, pp 1897–1911.

This is usually observed in elderly patients and is a manifestation of decreased arterial elasticity.

Labile hypertension: This describes an intermittent form of hypertension. It is unclear whether such patients develop sustained hypertension with consequent secondary cardiovascular damage.

Borderline hypertension: BP readings close to the upper limits of the normal range or only slightly elevated.

Malignant hypertension: A syndrome characterized clinically by severe accelerating hypertension with neuroretinopathy or papilledema and by evidence of renal damage. Clinically, it is almost always associated with massive oversecretion of renin and aldosterone and is relieved by bilateral nephrectomy or anti-renin drugs. This syndrome can occur de novo, but most often it follows preexisting hypertension.

Accelerated hypertension: A term often used synonymously with malignant hypertension, but sometimes only used to imply a significant increase in the pace or severity of the hypertensive process.

DEFINING THE RISK OF HYPERTENSIVE COMPLICATIONS

Traditionally, practice guidelines for the treatment of hypertension have been based on the premise that a discrete cut point separates normotension and hypertension. However, there is, in fact, a continuous, graded, and independent relationship between the height of the BP and the incidence of cardiovascular disease and stroke. Hypertension is not the sole determinant of cardiovascular risk and whether or how soon these complications occur in an individual hypertensive patient appears to be strongly determined by the concurrence of other risk factors, such as left ventricular hypertrophy (LVH), glucose intolerance, smoking, hypercholesterolemia, and obesity. In fact, only some hypertensive individuals will have a heart attack or stroke even with BP at the highest end of the range, and more than half of all heart attacks and almost half of all strokes occur in normotensive individuals. Thus, there is no threshold BP that distinguishes patients at risk.

COMPLICATIONS OF HYPERTENSION

Coronary Heart Disease and Left Ventricular Hypertrophy

Life insurance statistics and the Framingham Heart Study have established the fact that hypertensive individuals, as a population, have shortened survival and that this vulnerability correlates broadly with increasing levels of arterial BP. At ages younger than 50, diastolic BP is the strongest predictor of cardiovascular risk. Between ages 50 and 59, all three BP components are comparable predictors (systolic, diastolic mean BP). However, from age 60 onward, systolic BP best predicts all-cause mortality and cardiac death. Electrocardiographic evidence of LVH is present in about 3% to 8% of hypertensive patients and in 12% to 30% of hypertensive patients examined by echocardiography. Compared with patients with a normal left ventricular (LV) mass, patients with concentric LVH have a 10-fold greater mortality and a 5-fold higher rate of cardiovascular events, especially stroke and heart failure.

Stroke

Stroke is the most feared and devastating complication of hypertension. Atherothrombotic brain infarction accounts for most strokes in those with hypertension. The risk of stroke is positively associated with BP, and there is no critical level below which stroke does not occur. Systolic BP is more closely associated with atherothrombotic infarction than other factors such as diastolic BP or pulse pressure.

Heart Failure

Hypertension is the most common condition antedating heart failure. Hypertensive patients have a threefold higher risk of heart failure than normotensive subjects. The risk is further amplified further when LVH is present, and although myocardial infarction (MI) is a principal cause of systolic dysfunction, diastolic dysfunction plays an important role in the pathogenesis of heart failure in hypertensive patients.

Chronic Renal Insufficiency

Hypertension is the second most common cause of end-stage renal disease (ESRD). However, this statistic is probably inaccurate because the cause of ESRD is often uncertain. In many patients, hypertension is applied as a diagnosis by default because BP is elevated in most patients when dialysis is initiated. The relatively low incidence of ESRD in patients with essential hypertension is a barrier to assessing a relationship with hypertension and assessing benefits from treatment. Nevertheless, an independent graded relationship of the incidence of ESRD with both systolic and diastolic BP has been reported in men.

Microalbuminuria

Microalbuminuria (30 to 150 mg/day) is caused by impaired permselectivity of the glomerular capillary and is a clinical marker of glomerular hyperfiltration. In patients with diabetes mellitus, microalbuminuria predicts the onset of progressive renal failure and cardiovascular disease. These complications can be attenuated by effective treatment of hypertension, particularly with regimens that include an angiotensin-converting enzyme (ACE) inhibitor or angiotensin receptor blocker (ARB). The increased risk of cardiovascular and peripheral vascular disease associated with microalbuminuria also applies to nondiabetic hypertensive patients. Patients with essential hypertension and LVH have higher glomerular filtration rate and filtration fraction than those without ventricular hypertrophy, and effective BP reduction with antihypertensive agents can decrease albumin excretion. There is compelling evidence that ACE inhibitors or ARBs are the most effective agents in accomplishing this goal. It has not been clearly established whether the treatment-related reduction in albumin excretion per se is associated with a decline in cardiovascular risk in patients with essential hypertension or whether this change simply reflects the decline in BP.

Benefits of Treating Hypertension

The Veterans Administration Cooperative trial of the 1960s was the first major American study to demonstrate an improvement in cardiovascular morbidity and mortality in patients with diastolic BPs of 105 to 129 mm Hg. The benefit was manifested by a reduced frequency of strokes, CHF, and dissection of the aorta but not of ischemic cardiac events. Notably, no benefit was achieved among the patients with diastolic BP less than 105 mm Hg. Furthermore, a particularly relevant finding was that the major benefit in the group with diastolic BP between 105 and 115 mm Hg was realized by those patients who had displayed evidence of preexisting cardiovascular disease on entering the study. Subsequent trials have confirmed the benefit of antihypertensive treatment in patients with milder forms of hypertension. Once again the primary benefit is a reduction in stroke incidence, but beneficial effects on the development of CHF and ischemic cardiac events have also been demonstrated.

Several large, randomized, placebo-controlled treatment trials have also confirmed the benefits of treating elderly patients with isolated systolic hypertension. Antihypertensive treatment (diuretics or β-blockers) significantly reduces overall and cardiovascular mortality in elderly patients. These benefits are greater in male patients with higher baseline risk status, such as preexisting cardiovascular disease.

Benefits and Limitations of Treating Hypertension in Specific Clinical Settings

Left Ventricular Hypertrophy
Regression of echocardiographic LVH has been reported during treatment with several classes of antihypertensive medications. ACE inhibitors have been shown to both prevent and reverse LVH in patients with essential hypertension. In the Heart Outcomes Prevention Evaluation (HOPE) study, these beneficial effects were independent of BP changes and were associated with a reduced risk of death, myocardial infarction, and CHF. In the Losartan Intervention for Endpoint Reduction (LIFE) study, losartan treatment was associated with a significant reduction in stroke compared with atenolol treatment in hypertensive patients with electrocardiographic evidence of LVH.

Medical History

Evaluation of the severity and time course of the hypertensive disorder is important to allow planning of the pace of the medical workup and treatment. Accordingly, after learning of any current symptoms, the clinician should record the duration of the hypertension, the circumstances of its onset, and the highest known readings. Was the BP elevation merely discovered on routine examination? Does the patient have symptoms that suggest sleep apnea? Which drugs has the patient tried, and what effect have they produced? Has the patient taken any agents that may raise BP, such as oral contraceptives, diet pills, antidepressants, or cocaine or other illicit drugs or had a high intake of alcohol?

Classically, headaches in hypertensive patients are said to be occipital and pulsatile, most prominent on awakening and gradually lessening during the day. Other neurologic symptoms may include blurred vision, unsteadiness of gait, sluggishness, and in some patients, a decreased libido. Whereas some of these symptoms may be nonspecific, blurred vision may reflect vascular changes in the fundi. More advanced hypertensive disease may also be accompanied by more defined focal sensory or motor neurologic changes, occurring paroxysmally and associated with either transient ischemic attacks or more sustained attacks presaging the onset of hypertensive encephalopathy or stroke.

Early symptoms of cardiac dysfunction are expressed by increased fatigability or by shortness of breath on effort, which probably reflect the increased cardiac work of hypertension or impending heart failure. Young patients with labile pressure or largely systolic hypertension may exhibit tachycardia and signs of an unstable or hyperdynamic circulation. Palpitations may reflect an arrhythmia, which is more common in hypertensive than in normotensive people, especially in the presence of demonstrable LVH. Because coronary artery disease and myocardial infarction are more prevalent in hypertensive patients, a history of angina pectoris or documented myocardial infarction may be elicited.

The renal history may reveal antecedent acute glomerulonephritis, proteinuria, hematuria, nocturia, polyuria, or recurrent urinary tract infections. Renal colic or renal trauma should be noted, and the physician should suspect that the hypertension has a renal basis whenever it can be established that the urinary tract symptoms or the proteinuria preceded the hypertension. An abrupt onset of hypertension with rapid progression, especially in young or old patients, should lead the physician to strongly suspect renovascular hypertension due to either fibromuscular hyperplasia or an atherosclerotic plaque, respectively. This suspicion is reinforced by retinopathy or by cardiac or renal involvement, all of which are likely to be more prominent in patients with renovascular hypertension. Polyuria or nocturia may indicate more severe renal hypertension or a metabolic abnormality such as hypokalemia or hypercalcemia. An inability to concentrate the urine, with polydipsia, polyuria, and nocturia, commonly occurs in patients with primary aldosteronism or malignant hypertension or chronic renal disorders, including glomerulonephritis, tubulointerstitial nephropathy, or obstructive uropathy. Muscle weakness may accompany hypokalemia or hypercalcemia.

Patients should be asked about their smoking, drinking, exercise, and dietary habits. Obesity can be an important factor in producing or amplifying hypertension. Excessive regular consumption of alcohol can also induce or aggravate hypertension, and, in some patients, cessation of the habit may correct the hypertensive process. Tobacco, because it is a known vasoconstrictor, is especially contraindicated in hypertensive subjects, even though no causal relationship between smoking and the development of essential hypertension has been defined. The risk factor analysis is completed by the identification of any target organ damage and of any other coexisting diseases.

Physical Examination

Special Aspects
The general appearance is unrevealing in most patients with hypertension. However, a florid facies—with or without a tendency for rapid color changes, which would suggest vasomotor instability—may signify an underlying metabolic process, perhaps pheochromocytoma, a hyperdynamic circulation, or hyperthyroidism. A ruddy complexion with a bluish tinge characterizes some patients with essential hypertension and reactive polycythemia (Gaisböck syndrome). Truncal obesity with moon facies, frontal baldness, atrophic extremities with abdominal striae, atrophy of the skin, and spontaneous ecchymoses suggests Cushing syndrome.

Blood Pressure
In most hypertensive patients, elevated BP is the only abnormal finding. Hence, the way in which the BP is measured assumes great importance. The patient should be seated quietly, and a cuff size appropriate to the arm diameter should be chosen. Several readings should be taken, and it is generally recommended that phase 5

of Korotkoff sounds (disappearance) be taken as diastolic pressure. Establishing a diagnosis of hypertension often requires more than one visit, because the pressure tends to fall with repeated measurement. Even after several visits, however, a fairly sizable group of patients exhibit a persistently elevated pressure in the clinic although they are normotensive at other times. This phenomenon, often referred to as *white coat hypertension,* can be detected only by including measurements made outside the clinic. These measurements can be obtained by having the patient measure his or her BP at home or by ambulatory monitoring.

Fundus
Ophthalmoscopic examination of the optic fundi is one of the most valuable clinical tools for assessing target organ damage, the severity and duration of the hypertension, and the urgency for applying treatment.

Heart
A forceful apical thrust is common even in early hypertensive disease and may be exaggerated in the so-called hyperdynamic state. In contrast, a sustained, heaving LV pulse indicates significant hypertrophy due to pressure overload. Probably the earliest physical sign of cardiac involvement is the fourth heart sound (S_4), the atrial gallop occasionally heard in normal patients; it is usually audible before cardiac enlargement is detectable, and it is said to reflect reduced ventricular compliance, leading to a more forceful atrial contraction. The third heart sound may be a late manifestation of hypertensive heart disease and reflects the early diastolic compliance abnormality of LV failure. In severe hypertension, an accentuated aortic second sound may be accompanied by an aortic insufficiency murmur. It suggests dilation of the aortic root and may indicate the need for more urgent therapy.

Vascular System
Bruits and thrills, indicative of occlusive disease, are more prevalent in hypertensive patients and may occur throughout the arterial tree. Accordingly, the physician should examine the carotid arteries, abdominal aorta, renal arteries, and femoral arteries. A diastolic component to a bruit or palpable thrill over a peripheral vessel usually suggests a higher-grade stenosis. When pulses in the lower extremities are absent or dampened, coarctation of the aorta should be suspected in a young person, and occlusive aortic femoral disease should be suspected in an older one.

Abdomen
The aorta should be palpated carefully in all patients inasmuch as aortic dilation or aneurysm is a highly treatable condition best identified at the initial physical examination. A systolic and diastolic bruit in the upper epigastrium or in one or both upper quadrants of the abdomen suggests renal artery stenosis. A palpable enlargement of one or both kidneys may suggest polycystic renal disease, hydronephrosis, or a renal tumor.

Neurologic Examination
Gross neurologic deficits in sensory or motor function, mentation, or mood are not likely to be ignored. More subtle deficits suggesting transient cerebral ischemia or autonomic dysfunction may be overlooked and should be sought clinically, especially when the history is suggestive.

Initial Laboratory Evaluation

The initial laboratory evaluation should include a complete blood count and hematocrit together with a complete urinalysis; blood urea nitrogen, serum creatinine, serum uric acid, fasting blood glucose, and serum electrolyte measurements; and a lipid profile. If the serum K^+ level is borderline or low (i.e., 3.6 mEq/L), the test should be repeated on two or three separate occasions. The serum K^+ concentration serves as a baseline value for the subsequent response to thiazide diuretics and often provides the first laboratory clue to the presence of primary or secondary aldosterone excess. Serum Ca^{2+} and circulating thyroid hormone levels may point to parathyroid or thyroid disease, which often exists without clear-cut clinical evidence. Measurement of serum cholesterol, high- and low-density lipoprotein cholesterol, and triglyceride levels are important in the analysis of coexistent risk factors. Optional tests include a urine albumin-to-creatinine ratio.

Electrocardiogram and Echocardiography

A routine electrocardiogram to identify signs of LVH is highly desirable for all patients with newly established high BP. Manifestations of LVH include T-wave abnormalities, expressed either by notching or by a biphasic form, particularly in the precordial leads. As LVH progresses, voltage of the R waves increases, and then a characteristic strain pattern involving ST-segment depressions and T-wave inversion occurs. With the advent of echocardiography and its application to the development of highly sensitive methods for examining cardiac structure and function, investigators have been able to study the evolution of cardiac hypertrophy in hypertensive patients with greater precision than before (see "Left Ventricular Hypertrophy").

Ambulatory and Home Blood Pressure Monitoring

Ambulatory BP monitoring, whereby multiple indirect BP readings are obtained automatically over 1 or more days, is being used to investigate BP patterns in normal individuals and in hypertensive patients. Studies of normotensive subjects show that BP is characterized by a circadian rhythm with peaks during the daytime hours. Patients who have "office" or white coat hypertension can be successfully identified with ambulatory BP monitoring and thus may not require medication. Home BP monitoring is used increasingly in the evaluation and treatment of patients with hypertension. Although BP readings are generally higher in the medical office setting, these measurements do not correlate as well as home readings to the presence of abnormal markers for cardiovascular risk (e.g., LVH). Although home BP monitors are generally accurate, the patient's technique and the precision and reproducibility of the measurements should be validated during an office visit by the clinician.

Searching for Remediable Causes of Hypertension

The clinical features suggestive of secondary hypertension are outlined above. When a pheochromocytoma is suspected, measurements of catecholamines in plasma or in urine, or in both, and measurement of metanephrines, their urinary metabolites, are essential. Cushing syndrome can be diagnosed by an elevated 24-hour urinary free cortisol level. Urinary aldosterone levels, when combined with measurements of urinary Na^+ and K^+ excretion, are valuable for establishing the diagnosis of primary aldosteronism and other hypertensive conditions associated with either low-renin levels or hypokalemia. A plasma aldosterone-to-renin ratio greater than 50 (ng/dL to ng/mL per hour) has been suggested as a simple screening test for this disorder. However, there is some concern that this test may be misleading in patients with low-renin essential hypertension or when measurements are made during antihypertensive treatment with agents that affect renin secretion. If results of a biochemical analysis suggest a primary aldosterone excess, then a thin slice adrenal computed tomography scan can help identify an adenoma. The approach to the patient with suspected renovascular hypertension is outlined in Chapter 25, Renovascular Hypertension and Ischemic Nephropathy.

Therapy for Essential Hypertension

The goal for BP in the patient with uncomplicated hypertension is less than 140/80 mm Hg because this level of BP control has been associated with a significant decrease in the incidence of cardiovascular events. In patients with diabetes or renal disease the goal should be less than 130/80 mm Hg. After performing the initial evaluation, in which the diagnosis of secondary forms of hypertension has been excluded, the clinician is then faced with the treatment of essential hypertension. All patients should undertake nonpharmacologic interventions, including the following:

- Dietary sodium restriction (<2.4 g or 100 mEq of sodium per day)
- Maintenance of normal body weight (body mass index <25.0)
- Moderation of alcohol intake (<2 drinks/day in men, <1 drink/day in women)
- Aerobic exercise (e.g., brisk walking) 30 minutes per day most days of the week

The effect of dietary composition on BP was evaluated in the Dietary Approaches to Stop Hypertension (DASH) study. In that study, a diet rich in fruits, vegetables, and low-fat dairy products in addition to dietary sodium restriction intake significantly lowered systolic BP (8 to 14 mm Hg). These BP-lowering effects were observed in both black and white subjects and were comparable in obese and nonobese subjects. However, only a relatively small percentage of patients will achieve a goal BP of less than 140/90 mm Hg with nonpharmacologic intervention; therefore, pharmacologic therapy is required in most patients.

Drug treatment of the hypertensive patient is a complex decision-making process. It is complicated by the fact that many pharmacologically distinct drug classes are available, all of which effectively lower the BP and have been demonstrated to reduce the complications of hypertension. In patients with uncomplicated hypertension, the initial drug of choice according to JNC (Joint National Committee on Prevention, Detection, Evaluation, and Treatment of High Blood Pressure) VII guidelines should be a thiazide diuretic either alone or in combination with an agent previously demonstrated to have a beneficial affect on cardiovascular outcomes (an ACE-inhibitor, ARB, β-blocker, or calcium channel blocker). If the BP is considerably above the goal (greater than 160/100 mm Hg), consideration should be given to use of two agents from the outset. Indeed, most patients will require at least two medications to achieve adequate control. In certain clinical circumstances, specific antihypertensive agents are indicated (Table 24–2). An algorithm outlining the approach to the treatment

Table 24–2: Indications for Specific Subclasses of Antihypertensive Agents

Congestive heart failure	ACE-inhibitor
	ARB
	β-Blocker
	Aldosterone antagonist
Angina pectoris	β-Blocker
	Long-acting CCB
After myocardial infarction	ACE-inhibitor
	β-Blocker
	Aldosterone antagonist
Left ventricular hypertrophy	All classes except α-blockers and hydralazine
Diabetes mellitus	ACE-inhibitor
	ARB
	CCB
	Thiazide diuretic
	β-Blocker
Diabetic microalbuminuria	ACE-inhibitor (type I)
	ARB (type 2)
Chronic kidney disease (especially if proteinuric)	ACE-inhibitor
	ARB

ACE, angiotensin-converting enzyme; ARB, angiotensin receptor blocker; CCB, calcium channel blocker.

of essential hypertension is given in Figure 24–1. The class effects and side effects of the individual agents are discussed in Chapter 33, Diuretics, and Chapter 34, Antihypertensive Drugs. The management of hypertensive emergencies is discussed in Chapter 34, Antihypertensive Drugs.

Specific Patient Populations

Hypertension in African Americans

The prevalence of hypertension is higher in people of African-American ancestry, and the degree of hypertension is typically more severe. Several studies have noted a relative resistance to monotherapy with agents that interrupt the renin-angiotensin-aldosterone system in African Americans (ACE inhibitors, ARBs, and β-blockers). In contrast, diuretics and calcium channel blockers are usually quite effective. If specific indications exist, the resistance to ACE inhibitor and ARB therapy can usually be abrogated if these agents are administered concomitantly with an appropriate diuretic.

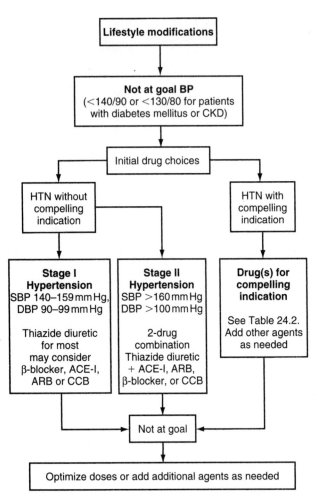

Figure 24–1. Algorithm for treatment of hypertension. ACE-I, angiotensin converting enzyme inhibitor; ARB, angiotensin receptor blocker; BP, blood pressure; CCB, calcium channel blocker; CKD, chronic kidney disease; DBP, diastolic blood pressure; SBP, systolic blood pressure. Modified from JNC VII report. *JAMA* 289:2560–2572, 2003.

Hypertension in the Elderly

Hypertension is common in elderly persons, and despite the fact that they benefit most from antihypertensive therapy (more baseline risk = greater risk reduction with therapy), control of hypertension in this population tends to be poorer than that in younger subjects. The goal BP in elderly patients is the same as that in younger subjects (<140/90 mm Hg). Postural hypotension can be problematic, and therefore lower initial doses of medication should be considered and incremental increases in dosing need to be undertaken with appropriate caution. Despite these considerations, most elderly hypertensive patients will require more than one medication for appropriate BP control.

Refractory Hypertension

See Chapter 34, Antihypertensive Drugs.

Renovascular Hypertension and Ischemic Nephropathy

25

The clinical manifestations of renovascular disease include the following:

- Asymptomatic "incidental" renal artery stenosis (RAS)
- Renovascular hypertension
- Ischemic nephropathy
- Accelerated cardiovascular disease
- Congestive heart failure/stroke/secondary hyperaldosteronism

Each of these clinical manifestations presents different comorbid and risk factor management issues. Whereas RAS can accelerate cardiovascular disease and threaten the viability of the kidney, renal revascularization, either surgical or percutaneous, is not always indicated. The benefits of renal artery interventional procedures include the potential to improve systemic blood pressure and to preserve or salvage renal function. However, the procedures themselves may threaten the viability of the affected kidney through vascular thrombosis, dissection, restenosis, or atheroemboli and can precipitate the need for lifelong renal replacement therapy. It is therefore important that clinicians understand the risks and benefits of both medical management and interventions to restore renal perfusion pressure.

PATHOPHYSIOLOGY

Renal Artery Stenosis versus Renovascular Hypertension

RAS is identified in 20% to 45% of patients undergoing vascular imaging for other reasons, such as coronary heart disease or lower extremity peripheral vascular disease. However, most of the

Table 25–1: Examples of Vascular Lesions Producing Renal Hypoperfusion and the Syndrome of Renovascular Hypertension

Unilateral disease
    Unilateral atherosclerotic renal artery stenosis
    Unilateral fibromuscular dysplasia
    Medial fibroplasia
    Perimedial fibroplasia
    Intimal fibroplasia
    Medial hyperplasia
    Renal artery aneurysm
    Arterial embolus
    Arteriovenous fistula (congenital/traumatic)
    Segmental arterial occlusion (post-traumatic)
    Extrinsic compression of renal artery (e.g., pheochromocytoma)
    Renal compression (e.g., metastatic tumor)
Bilateral disease or solitary functioning kidney
    Stenosis to a solitary functioning kidney
    Bilateral renal arterial stenosis
    Aortic coarctation
    Systemic vasculitis (e.g., Takayasu arteritis, polyarteritis)
    Atheroembolic disease

observed stenoses are of little or no hemodynamic significance. The term *renovascular hypertension* refers to a rise in arterial pressure induced by a reduction in renal perfusion that can be triggered by a variety of lesions (Table 25–1). Luminal narrowing must approach 70% to 80% before hemodynamically significant changes occur. When renal artery lesions reach these critical dimensions, a series of integrated renal responses leads to a rise in systemic arterial pressure and restoration of renal perfusion pressure. Foremost among these pathways is the release of renin with subsequent generation of angiotensin II and release of aldosterone. If the renal artery lesion progresses further, a cycle of reduced perfusion and rising arterial pressures recurs until malignant-phase hypertension develops.

Mechanisms of Ischemic Nephropathy

Patients with stenosis affecting the entire renal mass can develop reduced blood flow and glomerular filtration when poststenotic pressures fall below the range of autoregulation. This process is reversible if pressure is restored or the vascular lesion is removed. However, if the lesion is allowed to progress, the recurrent reduction in kidney blood flow can result in a pathologic cascade that produces irreversible renal fibrosis.

EPIDEMIOLOGY OF RENAL ARTERY STENOSIS

Most stenotic lesions are caused by "fibromuscular diseases" or atherosclerotic plaques. The prevalence of renovascular disease varies widely depending on the population studied. In unselected populations with mild to moderate hypertension, the frequency of renovascular disease is only between 0.6% and 3%, whereas in a referral clinic of elderly patients, the prevalence may exceed 30%.

Fibromuscular Disease

The term *fibromuscular disease* (FMD) commonly refers to one of several conditions affecting the intima or fibrous layers of the vessel wall. Approximately 3% to 5% of the population (female > male) have FMD. In many of these individuals, FMD is present at an early age and does not affect either renal blood flow or arterial pressure. Previous estimates derived from hypertension referral clinics suggested that 25% of patients with renovascular hypertension had FMD; more recent studies suggest that the rate is less than 20%. Smoking is a risk factor for disease progression. Medial fibroplasia is the most common subtype, often associated with a "string-of-beads" appearance on arteriography. Such lesions consist primarily of intravascular "webs," each of which may have only a moderate hemodynamic effect. The combination of multiple webs in series, however, can impede blood flow characteristics and activate responses within the kidney to reduced perfusion. FMD lesions are classically located away from the origin of the renal artery, often in the midportion of the vessel or at the first arterial bifurcation. Some of these expand to develop small vascular aneurysms. Occasionally intimal hyperplasia can progress and lead to renal ischemia and atrophy. Although these are commonly considered a disorder of younger women, they can present at older ages, sometimes combined with atherosclerotic lesions, which magnify the hemodynamic effects.

Atherosclerosis

Atherosclerosis affecting the renal arteries is the most common cause of renovascular disease (75% to 85% of patients). Atherosclerotic RAS is commonly associated with vascular disease in other vascular beds. Approximately 20% of patients undergoing coronary angiography and up to 50% of patients undergoing aortography for peripheral vascular disease have renal artery lesions of some degree. The prevalence of such lesions increases with age and with the presence of atherosclerotic risk factors such as elevated cholesterol levels, smoking, and hypertension. Indeed the probability of identifying high-grade RAS in hypertensive patients with chronic renal failure rises from 3.2% in the sixth decade to more than 25% in the eighth decade. Atherosclerotic disease is most often located at the origin of the artery, usually representing a direct extension of an aortic plaque into the renal arterial segment.

CLINICAL FEATURES OF RENOVASCULAR HYPERTENSION

Changing Population Demographics

As a result of recent decreases in mortality rates from coronary and cerebrovascular events, the incidence of RAS is increasing in the elderly population. The prevalence of advanced coronary disease, congestive heart failure, previous stroke or transient ischemic attack, and aortic disease, as well as impaired renal function, is high in patients with atherosclerotic renal artery disease.

Clinical Presentation of Renal Artery Stenosis

Manifestations of renal artery disease vary widely across a spectrum as illustrated in Table 25–2. The spectrum of disease may range from a purely incidental finding noted during angiography for other indications to advancing renal failure leading to the need for dialytic support. Clinical features of patients with renovascular hypertension differ from those of patients with essential hypertension. Many features, including duration of hypertension, age of onset (>55 years), funduscopic findings, hypokalemia, and so on, are more common with renovascular hypertension, but they have limited discriminating or predictive value. If renal artery lesions progress to critical stenosis, they can produce a rapidly developing form of hypertension, which may be severe and associated with neuroretinopathy or papilledema and accompanied by evidence of renal damage. Such patients are most often seen with acute renovascular events, such as sudden occlusion of a renal artery or branch vessel. More commonly, RAS presents as a progressive worsening of preexisting hypertension, often with a modest rise in the serum creatinine level. Because the prevalence of both hypertension and atherosclerosis rises with age, this disorder must be considered, particularly in older patients with progression of blood pressure elevation. As patients age, some of the most striking examples of renovascular hypertension are seen in those in whom previous good control of hypertension has deteriorated, causing an accelerated

Table 25–2: Clinical Features of Patients with Renovascular Hypertension

Clinical Feature	Essential Hypertension (%)	Renovascular Hypertension (%)
Duration < 1 yr	12	24
Age of onset older than 50 yr	9	15
Family history of hypertension	71	46
Grade 3 or 4 fundi	7	15
Abdominal bruit	9	46
Blood urea nitrogen > 20 mg/dL (7 mmol/L)	8	16
Potassium < 3.4 mEq/L	8	16
Urinary casts	9	20
Proteinuria	32	46

Syndromes associated with renovascular hypertension
1. Early- or late-onset hypertension (younger than 30 yr or older than 50 yr)
2. Acceleration of treated essential hypertension
3. Deterioration of renal function in treated essential hypertension
4. Acute renal failure during treatment of hypertension
5. "Flash" pulmonary edema
6. Progressive renal failure

rise in systolic blood pressure and target organ injury, such as stroke. Declining renal function during antihypertensive therapy is a common manifestation of progressive renal arterial disease. In critical renal arterial stenosis, blood flow and perfusion pressures to the kidney depend on an elevated systemic blood pressure. Any reduction in systemic arterial pressure induced by any antihypertensive regimen can precipitate acute falls in renal perfusion pressure and hence glomerular filtration rate (GFR). This phenomenon has become particularly common since the introduction of angiotensin-converting enzyme (ACE) inhibitors and, more recently, of angiotensin receptor blockers (ARB), which specifically interrupt angiotensin II–mediated efferent arteriolar vasoconstriction. A sudden rise in serum creatinine soon after these agents are started suggests bilateral RAS or stenosis to a solitary functioning kidney.

Other syndromes heralding occult RAS include rapidly developing episodes of circulatory congestion (so-called flash pulmonary edema). This usually occurs in patients with hypertension and with left ventricular systolic function that may be well preserved. Renovascular disease causes volume retention and resistance to diuretics in such patients. Further volume expansion (e.g., a high-salt diet or diuretic withdrawal) triggers a rapid rise in arterial pressure and this in turn impairs cardiac function owing to rapidly developing diastolic dysfunction that leads to an abrupt onset of pulmonary edema. Such episodes tend to be rapid both in onset and in resolution. A similar sequence of events may produce symptoms of crescendo angina from otherwise stable coronary disease. When the role of RAS is identified, renal revascularization can prevent its recurrence.

Another clinical presentation of RAS is advanced renal failure, occasionally at end stage and requiring renal replacement therapy. Some estimates indicate that between 12% and 14% of patients reaching end-stage renal disease with no other identifiable primary renal disease may have occult, bilateral RAS. Unfortunately, most patients with advanced renal dysfunction and RAS typically have multiple comorbid diseases and commonly have irreversible renal injury on biopsy. Those with declining renal function have a poor survival rate regardless of intervention, the strongest predictor of which is a low baseline GFR. The likely benefit of revascularization for salvage, or at least stabilization, of renal function is greatest when the GFR is relatively well preserved. Remarkably, RAS can be associated with proteinuria, occasionally to nephrotic levels. Such proteinuria can diminish or resolve entirely after renal revascularization.

Clinical manifestations and prognosis differ when renovascular disease affects one of two kidneys or affects the entire functioning renal mass. Although blood pressure levels may be similar, response to renal revascularization leads to a greater decrease in bilateral disease. Most patients with episodic pulmonary edema have bilateral disease or a solitary functional kidney. Long-term mortality during follow-up is higher when bilateral disease is present, regardless of whether renal revascularization is undertaken, reflecting an overall higher atherosclerotic disease burden. The causes of death in patients with atherosclerotic RAS are due mainly to cardiovascular disease, including stroke and congestive heart failure.

Progressive Vascular Occlusion

Atherosclerosis is a progressive disorder, and the impetus to intervene in RAS depends many times on predicting the likelihood of progression in the individual patient. Importantly, clinical events such as detectable changes in renal function or accelerating hypertension bear only a limited relationship to vascular atherosclerotic lesion progression. Retrospective angiographic studies from the 1970s indicate that atherosclerotic lesions progress to more severe levels in 40% to 60% of patients followed from 2 to 5 years with up to 16% of renal arteries developing total occlusion. More recent prospective studies suggest that current rates of progression are approximately 20% over 3 years with less than 10% of patients developing complete occlusion. The improved management of cardiovascular risk factors including the widespread use of statin-class drugs and aspirin, diminishing of tobacco use, and more intensive antihypertensive therapy may have resulted a change in the natural history of this disorder; however, this hypothesis remains unproven.

DIAGNOSTIC TESTING FOR RENOVASCULAR HYPERTENSION AND ISCHEMIC NEPHROPATHY

Goals of Evaluation

The goals of the diagnostic evaluation in the patient with suspected renovascular disease are outlined in Table 25–3.

Table 25–3: Goals of Diagnostic Evaluation and Therapeutic Intervention in Renovascular Hypertension and Ischemic Nephropathy

Goals of diagnostic evaluation
- Establish presence of renal artery stenosis: location and type of lesion
- Establish whether unilateral or bilateral stenosis (or stenosis to a solitary kidney) is present
- Establish presence and function of stenotic and nonstenotic kidneys
- Establish hemodynamic severity of renal arterial disease
- Plan vascular intervention: degree and location of atherosclerotic disease

Goals of therapy
- I. Improved blood pressure control:
  - Prevent morbidity and mortality of high blood pressure
  - Improve blood pressure control and reduce medication requirement
- II. Preservation of renal function:
  - Reduce risk of renal-adverse perfusion from use of antihypertensive agents
  - Reduce episodes of circulatory congestion ("flash" pulmonary edema)
  - Reduce risk of progressive vascular occlusion causing loss of renal function: "preservation of renal function"
  - Salvage renal function, i.e., recover glomerular filtration rate

Diagnostic tests in renovascular disease fall into three general categories:

1. Functional studies to evaluate the role of stenotic lesions particularly related to activation of the renin-angiotensin system
2. Imaging studies to identify the presence and degree of vascular stenosis
3. Studies to predict the likelihood of benefit from renal revascularization

Physiologic and Functional Studies of the Renin-Angiotensin System

Peripheral plasma renin activity and its response to administration of an ACE inhibitor such as captopril have been proposed as a marker of renovascular disease. Although these studies are promising for patients with known renovascular hypertension, they have lower performance as diagnostic tests when applied to wider populations and their sensitivity and specificity are too low for them to be used as major determinants in clinical decision making. In contrast, measurement of renal vein renin levels has been widely applied in planning surgical revascularization. These measurements are obtained by sampling renal vein and inferior vena cava blood individually. The renin level of the vena cava is taken as being comparable to the arterial levels in each kidney and allows estimation of the contribution of each kidney to total circulating levels of plasma renin activity. Lateralization is defined usually as a ratio exceeding 1.5 between the renin activity of the stenotic kidney and the nonstenotic kidney. In general, the greater the degree of lateralization, the more probable that a clinical blood pressure benefit will be seen from revascularization on that side. In recent years the shift away from revascularization for control of blood pressure toward revascularization for preservation of renal function has led to a decline in the use of renal vein assays. However, in patients for whom it is important to establish the degree of pressor effect of a specific kidney before considering nephrectomy, measurement of renal vein renin levels remains a useful diagnostic test.

Studies of Individual Renal Function

Separate renal function measurements can be obtained with radionuclide techniques. These methods use a variety of radioisotopes (e.g., technetium-99m [^{99m}Tc] mertiatide or ^{99m}Tc pentetate) to estimate fractional blood flow to each kidney and estimate single-kidney GFR. Administration of captopril beforehand magnifies differences between both kidneys, primarily by delaying excretion of the filtered isotope due to removal of the efferent arteriolar effects of angiotensin-II. Some authors rely upon such measurements to follow progressive renal artery disease and its effect on unilateral kidney function as a guide to consider revascularization. Serial measurement of individual renal function by radionuclide studies may allow more precise identification of progressive ischemic injury to the affected kidney in unilateral renal artery disease than can be determined from the overall GFR.

Noninvasive Imaging and Assessment of the Renal Vasculature

Current practice is to limit invasive arteriography to endovascular intervention, for example, the placement of stents or angioplasty. Although renal arteriography remains the gold standard for evaluation of the renal vasculature, its invasive nature, potential hazards (e.g., contrast nephropathy and atheroembolism) make it most suitable for those in whom intervention is planned, often during the same procedure. As a result, most clinicians favor preliminary noninvasive studies beforehand.

Captopril Renography

Imaging the kidneys using the radiopharmaceuticals ^{99m}Tc pentetate and ^{99m}Tc mertiatide provides useful information about the size and GFRs of both kidneys. The change in glomerular filtration characteristics after ACE inhibition allows inferences on the dependence of glomerular filtration upon angiotensin II. Captopril renography has a reasonably high specificity and thus can be used in populations having a low pretest probability with an expectation that a normal study will exclude significant renovascular hypertension in more than 95% of patients. Important considerations in the use of captopril renography include its lower sensitivity and specificity in the presence of renal insufficiency (usually defined as creatinine concentration > 2 mg/dL [175 mcmol/L]) and the need to withdraw diuretics and ACE inhibitors for 4 to 14 days before the study. It should be emphasized that renography provides functional information but no direct anatomic information, that is, the location of renal arterial disease, the number of renal arteries, or associated aortic or ostial disease.

Doppler Ultrasound of the Renal Arteries

Duplex interrogation of the renal arteries provides measurements of localized velocities of blood flow with a sensitivity and specificity as high as 90% in experienced hands. This provides an inexpensive means for measuring vascular occlusive disease to establish the diagnosis of RAS, follow its progression, and monitor for restenosis after endovascular intervention. Its main drawbacks relate to the difficulties of obtaining adequate studies in obese patients and interoperator variability. Recent studies emphasize the potential for Doppler ultrasound to characterize small vessel flow characteristics within the kidney. The resistive index provides an estimate of the relative flow velocities in diastole and systole. A resistive index greater than 80 is suggested as a means of identifying irreversible parenchymal disease that will not respond to renal vascularization. In contrast, a resistive index less than 80 is proposed to reliably predict a favorable blood pressure response and GFR response to revascularization.

Magnetic Resonance Angiography

Gadolinium-enhanced magnetic resonance angiography of the abdominal and renal vasculature is becoming a mainstay of evaluation of renovascular disease in many institutions. Comparative studies indicate that its sensitivity ranges from 83% to 100% and specificity from 92% to 97%. This technique is suitable for patients with impaired renal function because gadolinium is not nephrotoxic. Other advantages include the avoidance of radiation and the ability to estimate parenchymal volume and relative function from the nephrogram. Drawbacks include the expense, a tendency to overestimate the severity of atherosclerotic lesions, and an inability to perform follow-up studies of metallic stents because of signal degradation.

Computed Tomography Angiography

Computed tomography angiography using "helical" or multiple head scanners and intravenous contrast material can provide excellent images of both kidneys and the vascular tree. Resolution and reconstruction techniques render this modality capable of identifying smaller vessels, vascular lesions, and parenchymal characteristics, including stones. When used for detection of RAS, computed tomography angiography correlates well with conventional arteriography and sensitivity may reach 98% and specificity 94%. Although this technique offers a noninvasive examination of the main renal vessels, it has the drawback of requiring a considerable amount of contrast material. As a result, it is less ideally suited for evaluation of renovascular hypertension or ischemic nephropathy in patients with impaired renal function.

MANAGEMENT OF RENAL ARTERY STENOSIS AND ISCHEMIC NEPHROPATHY

In most cases the management of the patient with renovascular disease represents a balance between the pharmacologic management of hypertension and cardiovascular risk factors and the decision whether or not to proceed with renal revascularization. What should not be taken for granted is the premise that renal revascularization prolongs life or prevents end-stage renal disease in all patients. Indeed, risks are substantial with both endovascular and surgical intervention in the aorta and renal vasculature and include irreversible loss of renal function.

The goals of therapy in renovascular disease can be divided into three categories:

- Prevention of morbidity and mortality associated with hypertension
- Preservation of kidney function
- Facilitation of volume management in congestive cardiac failure

Newer antihypertensive agents and the expanding use of agents that block the renin-angiotensin system for indications other than hypertension have fundamentally changed the presentation and clinical management of renovascular disease. "Uncontrollable" hypertension is now rarely the main reason for considering renal revascularization. Rather, the hazards of underperfusion of kidney tissue leading to irreversible renal failure have led many to consider revascularization for "preservation" of renal function. Thus, it is important to emphasize that long-term clinical outcomes in patients with atherosclerotic renovascular disease are commonly determined by other disease entities (termed *competing risk*), which has significant implications for decisions about invasive therapy. The burden of atherosclerotic disease associated with RAS is often widespread, and the causes of death include a broad array of cardiovascular events. Therefore, the management of comorbid cardiovascular risk factors, including cessation of smoking, lipid control, and treatment of diabetes and obesity, is an essential component of the treatment plan for affected patients. An algorithm for managing these patients is illustrated in Figure 25–1.

Management of Unilateral Renal Artery Stenosis

Since the introduction of agents that block the renin-angiotensin system, most patients (86% to 92%) with unilateral renal artery disease can achieve blood pressure levels of less than

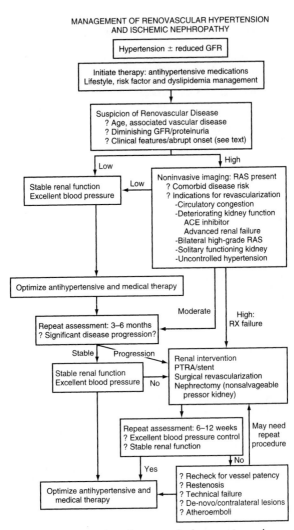

MANAGEMENT OF RENOVASCULAR HYPERTENSION
AND ISCHEMIC NEPHROPATHY

Figure 25–1. Management of renovascular hypertension and ischemic nephropathy. ACE, angiotensin-converting enzyme; GFR, glomerular filtration rate; PTRA, percutaneous renal artery angioplasty; RAS, renal artery stenosis.

140/90 mm Hg with medical regimens based upon these agents. Indeed the widespread use of ACE inhibitors and ARBs ensures that subcritical instances of renovascular disease are treated without being identified. Extrapolating from the experience of ACE inhibition in trials of congestive cardiac failure is reassuring in regard to the use of ACE inhibition in patients with diffuse vascular disease including renovascular disease. Thousands of patients with marginal arterial pressures and clinical heart failure have been treated with blockade of the renin-angiotensin system over many years. Many of these patients have undetected renal artery lesions and although minor changes in serum creatinine levels are observed in approximately 10% of patients, a rise sufficient to lead to withdrawal of these agents under trial monitoring conditions occurs in only 1% to 2%. More importantly, patients with congestive heart failure and moderate chronic renal failure (creatinine levels of 1.4 to 2.3 mg/dL [120 to 200 mcmol/L]), many of whom have RAS, have a major survival benefit from ACE inhibition.

It follows therefore that many patients with unilateral RAS can be managed without restoration of blood flow for a long period, sometimes indefinitely. The judgment on endovascular intervention in the individual patient depends on the clinical response to conservative management and the anticipated outcome of revascularization. In trials addressing the relative value of endovascular repair, specifically angioplasty compared with medical therapy in atherosclerotic RAS, endovascular intervention was demonstrated to have little or no advantage over antihypertensive drug therapy in patients whose blood pressure was controlled adequately by pharmacologic intervention, albeit that patients conservatively managed usually required a greater number of antihypertensive medications. The benefits of angioplasty, even in the short term, are moderate compared with those of effective antihypertensive therapy. However, hypertension that fails to respond to medical therapy often improves after revascularization, and many clinicians support a role for endovascular intervention in the management of patients with refractory hypertension and RAS.

Progressive Renal Artery Stenosis in Medically Treated Patients

As noted earlier, the potential for progressive vascular occlusion is central to management of patients with renovascular disease. It may be argued that failure to revascularize the kidneys exposes the patient to the hazard of undetected, progressive occlusion, potentially leading to total occlusion and irreversible loss of renal function. However, prospective studies indicate that rates of progression of renovascular disease are moderate and occur at widely varying rates. Often, such patients can be managed well without revascularization for many years. The clinical issue in a specific patient often hinges on whether the risks of revascularization are truly less than the risks of progression. It is clear that for many patients with progressive disease, optimal long-term stability of kidney function and blood pressure control can be achieved by successful surgical or endovascular restoration of the renal blood supply.

Surgical Treatment of Renovascular Hypertension and Ischemic Nephropathy

With the advent of endovascular techniques, surgical intervention is less commonly performed in the current era. Several of the options developed for renal artery reconstruction are endarterectomy and aortorenal, splenorenal, and hepatorenal bypass grafting. Most of these methods focus on reconstruction of the vascular supply for preservation of nephron mass. Benefits of surgical intervention include excellent long-term patency (>90%), both for renal artery procedures alone and when combined with aortic reconstruction. This leads some clinicians to favor this approach for younger patients with a longer life expectancy. Risk factors for poor outcome include advanced age, an elevated creatinine level (>3 mg/dL [265 mcmol/L]), and associated aortic or other vascular disease.

Endovascular Renal Procedures

The ability to restore renal perfusion in high-risk patients with endovascular methods represents a major advance in the management of renovascular hypertension and ischemic nephropathy. The past two decades have been characterized by a major shift from surgical reconstruction toward preferential application of endovascular procedures particularly, in elderly patients and in those with high levels of comorbidity. The introduction of endovascular stents has accelerated the trend away from surgical intervention, in part because of the improved patency rates achieved for ostial atherosclerotic lesions compared with rates for angioplasty alone. However, it is often difficult to ascertain the risk and benefit ratio of these procedures from the published literature.

Angioplasty for Fibromuscular Disease

Most lesions of medial fibroplasia are located at a distance away from the renal artery ostium. Many of these have multiple webs within the vessel, which can be successfully traversed and opened by balloon angioplasty; stents are rarely required. A clinical benefit for blood pressure control has been reported in observational outcome studies in 65% to 75% of patients. Cure of hypertension, defined as sustained blood pressure levels less than 140/90 mm Hg with no antihypertensive medications, may be obtained in between 35% and 50% of patients. Predictors of cure include lower systolic blood pressures, younger age, and shorter duration of hypertension. In general, such patients have relatively less aortic disease and have less risk for the major complications of angioplasty than patients with atherosclerotic renal disease. Because the risk for major procedural complications is low, most clinicians advocate early intervention for patients with FMD with the hope of a reduced requirement for antihypertensive medications after successful angioplasty.

Angioplasty and Stent Placement for Atherosclerotic Renal Artery Stenosis

Few advances in renovascular disease treatment have been associated with the level of controversy as that over the use of endovascular stent placement for atherosclerotic renovascular disease. Ostial lesions commonly fail to respond to angioplasty alone in part because of extensive recoil of the plaque, which typically extends into the main portion of the aorta. Endovascular stents represent a major technical advance in this area. Intermediate (6 to 12 months) vessel patency is significantly better after stent placement compared with that seen with angioplasty alone (29% versus 75%), and restenosis rates are less than 15% compared with almost 50% with angioplasty. The demographic features of patients undergoing renal revascularization have been changing during the last decades. The mean age of patients undergoing either surgery or angioplasty (with or without stents) has climbed from 55 years to more than 75 years because many patients who otherwise would not be considered candidates for major surgical procedures, such as aortic or renal reconstruction, are now being offered endovascular procedures. The outcomes of patients undergoing placement of renal artery stenting are considered in terms of (1) blood pressure control and (2) preservation or salvage of renal function in ischemic nephropathy. Although "cures" are rare, typical falls in standardized blood pressure measurement are in the range of 5 to 10 mm Hg (systolic), which may result in a decrease in the number of medications needed. Other reported benefits include improvement in anginal and congestive cardiac failure symptoms presumably because of amelioration of diastolic dysfunction and improvements in natriuretic capacity. The ambiguity in outcome of many clinical trials may reflect the problem of patient selection, which probably contributes to an understatement of the benefit of revascularization. Most trials have excluded patients with accelerated hypertension, advancing renal dysfunction, or recent congestive cardiac failure, for whom successful revascularization can offer a major benefit. Importantly, the crossover rate from medical therapy ranged from 26% to 44% in the prospective trial, indicating that medical therapy alone simply does not succeed in a subset of patients with renovascular hypertension.

In general, changes in renal function for atherosclerotic RAS after endovascular intervention, as reflected by serum creatinine levels, have been small. Careful evaluation of the literature indicates that three distinctly different clinical outcomes are routinely observed. In some instances (approximately 27%), revascularization results in a distinct improvement in kidney function. There can be no doubt that such patients benefit from the procedure and the major morbidity (and probably mortality) associated with advanced renal failure is avoided. The bulk of patients, however, have no measurable change in renal function (approximately 52%). Whether such patients benefit much depends upon the true clinical likelihood of progressive renal injury if the stenotic lesion were managed without revascularization, as discussed earlier. Those without the risk of progression probably gain little. The most significant concern, however, is the group of patients whose renal function deteriorates further after a revascularization procedure. In most reports, the number of patients in this group ranges from 19% to 25%. In some instances, this progression represent the presence of atheroembolic disease or a variety of complications, including vessel dissection with thrombosis. Hence, nearly 20% of patients face a relatively rapid progression of renal insufficiency and the potential for requiring renal replacement therapy, including dialysis or renal transplantation. Possible mechanisms of deterioration include atheroembolic injury, which may be nearly universal after any vascular intervention, and acceleration of oxidative stress producing interstitial fibrosis.

Few studies have compared endovascular intervention (percutaneous transluminal renal angioplasty [PTRA] without stents) and surgical repair. A single study of nonstial, unilateral atherosclerotic disease in which patients were randomly assigned to undergo surgery or PTRA indicate that whereas surgical success rates were higher and PTRA was needed on a repeat basis in several patients, the 2-year patency rates were 90% for PTRA and 97% for surgery.

Predictors of Possible Benefit for Renal Revascularization

Identification of patients most likely to obtain improved blood pressure or renal function after renal revascularization remains an elusive task. As noted, functional tests of renin release, such as measurement of renal vein renin levels, have not performed universally well as predictors of outcome. These studies are most useful when results are positive; for example, the likelihood of benefit improves with more evident lateralization. However, they have relatively poor negative predictive value; that is, when results of such studies are negative, outcomes of vessel repair may still be beneficial. As a clinical matter, recent progression of hypertension remains one of the most consistent predictors of improved blood pressure after intervention. Predicting favorable renal functional outcomes is also difficult. As with hypertension, a recent deterioration of kidney function portends more likely improvement with reconstruction. Several series indicate that surgical or endovascular procedures are least likely to benefit those with advanced renal insufficiency, usually characterized by serum creatinine levels greater than 3 mg/dL (265 mcmol/L). Small kidneys, as identified by length less than 8 cm, are less likely to recover function, particularly when little function can be identified on radionuclide renography. Reports on measurement of the renal resistance index by Doppler ultrasound indicate that identification of lower resistance was a favorable marker for improvement in both GFR and blood pressure, whereas an elevated resistance index was an independent marker for poor outcomes; however, none of these criteria are absolute.

SUMMARY

Renovascular disease is common, particularly in older people with atherosclerotic disease elsewhere. It can produce a wide array of clinical effects, ranging from asymptomatic "incidental" disease to accelerated hypertension and progressive renal failure. With improved imaging and an older population, significant renal artery disease is detected more often than ever before. Management of cardiovascular risk and hypertension is the primary objective of medical management. It is incumbent upon clinicians to evaluate both the role of renal artery disease in the individual patient and the potential risk-to-benefit ratio for timing of renal revascularization. For most patients, the realistic goals of renal revascularization are to reduce medication requirements and to stabilize renal function over time. Patients with bilateral disease or stenosis to a solitary functioning kidney may achieve a lower risk of circulatory congestion (flash pulmonary edema or its equivalent) and a lower risk for advancing renal failure.

Hypertension in Renal Parenchymal Disease

26

Hypertension and its partner disorder, diabetes, are the principal reasons for the initiation of renal replacement therapy with dialysis or transplantation. Hypertension remains extremely common in patients with end-stage renal disease (ESRD), occurring in at least 80% of dialysis patients, and chronic kidney disease is the most common cause of secondary hypertension. Together, hypertension and renal disease increase the risk for cardiovascular disease (CVD). Even a modest degree of renal impairment (e.g., a 30% decline in glomerular filtration rate [GFR] or albuminuria >200 mg/g of creatinine) dramatically increases the risk for CVD. The fact that only a small minority of people with hypertension develop ESRD is probably best explained by the time interval necessary for renal failure to develop; most hypertensive patients die of CVD before ESRD occurs. The progression of hypertension and renal disease involves an interacting series of dysregulatory relationships among several basic physiologic mechanisms, the ultimate result of which is a "vicious cycle" in which worsening hypertension and nephron loss mutually reinforce each other's contribution to "accelerated aging," with premature death from cardiovascular or renal disease.

The main groups of pathogenetic factors in the development of both hypertension and renal disease include the following:

1. Neurohumoral factors (principally the sympathetic nervous system)
2. The renin-angiotensin-aldosterone system (RAAS)
3. Metabolic factors (the metabolic syndrome and reactive oxygen species)
4. Vascular factors (e.g., calcium-mediated vasoconstriction and arterial stiffening)
5. Disordered renal salt and water excretion
6. Exogenous factors (mainly drugs)

457

A complete discussion of the relative contribution of these factors is found in Chapter 47, Hypertension and Renal Disease, in *Brenner and Rector's The Kidney.*

CLINICAL STUDIES

Age and Systolic Hypertension

Age strongly affects the relationship between systolic blood pressure (SBP) and diastolic blood pressure (DBP), both within and between individuals. From 20 to 50 years of age, SBP and DBP increase with age in a parallel manner. After 50 years of age, DBP decreases whereas SBP continues to rise in both men and women and in all demographic groups. This pattern accounts for the increase in pulse pressure (PP) (PP = SBP – DBP) that is driven by the age-related increase in stiffness of the aorta and central arteries. Some investigators have suggested that PP is superior to SBP as a risk marker for coronary events. However, closer scrutiny reveals that the more robust association between PP and coronary events occurs only in people older than 60 years of age.

Systolic Hypertension and Cardiovascular Disease Risk

In the general population, both SBP and DBP are continuously related to morbidity and mortality from CVD. It is almost universally accepted that elevated SBP is the more robust predictor of poor cardiovascular and renal outcomes, and SBP has become the principal end point for the classification and treatment of hypertension. DBP cannot be completely disregarded, however, because it remains a useful predictor of risk in those younger than 50 years of age, especially in African-American men, who have an increased risk for ESRD. The continuous nature of the relationship between SBP and CVD risk has been well established in longitudinal studies; for men or women ages 40 to 70, each 20 mm Hg increase in SBP (or each 10 mm Hg increase in DBP) doubles the risk of CVD at any level of SBP from 115 to 175 mm Hg (or DBP from 75 to 115 mm Hg). Furthermore, randomized clinical trials have shown unequivocally that lowering SBP lowers cardiovascular morbidity and mortality.

Aging, Hypertension, and Loss of Renal Function

Increased SBP is a more robust predictor of ESRD than DBP. In addition, SBP and PP are also related to proteinuria, an important marker of chronic kidney disease. With advancing age in industrialized societies, there is a steady decrease in GFR that is accelerated by the presence of hypertension. A meta-regression analysis of recent treatment trials in middle-aged people at risk for progressive kidney disease (largely due to diabetes or hypertension) found that the rate of decline in GFR was inversely related to the baseline SBP; with a baseline SBP of 130 to 140 mm Hg, the rate of decline in GFR was about 2 mL/min/yr, but it was twofold to threefold higher when the baseline SBP was between 150 and 160 mm Hg. Although death from CVD often supervenes before chronic kidney disease becomes the patient's primary medical condition, current trends toward increased longevity and improved CVD prevalence and outcome rates suggests a continuing increase in the number of elderly people who develop hypertension-related chronic kidney disease.

Cardiovascular Disease Risk and Renal Failure

Renal failure is a major risk factor for premature CVD and death. Elevations in the serum creatinine level are independent predictors of poor outcomes in acute coronary syndromes. A reduced GFR or an estimated creatinine clearance of less than 60 mL/min is a risk factor for congestive heart failure, and moderate renal impairment has been associated with a 40% increased risk in all-cause mortality in patients with congestive heart failure. Albuminuria is also a major cardiovascular risk factor, at least in patients with diabetes. In patients with ESRD, hypertension is strongly associated with increased death from CVD, and it is the single most important predictor of coronary artery disease in these patients, even more so than cigarette smoking or hyperlipidemia. Controlled studies on the benefits of antihypertensive therapy for patients receiving hemodialysis or peritoneal dialysis are not available. However, maintaining a controlled blood pressure (BP) is considered to be of great importance for long-term survival.

Hypotension as a Risk Factor

Although it is increasingly being recognized that maintenance of optimal BP (120/80 mm Hg or less) is desirable, hypotension is also potentially dangerous. In individuals with hypotensive episodes, increased lability of BP is a common finding, with extremely high values present as well. This pattern of exaggerated BP variability exposes the individual to risks from both hypertension and hypotension. Postural hypotension (usually defined as a drop of 20 mm Hg in SBP or 10 mm Hg in DBP on standing) is associated with cerebrovascular disease and with premature death. In patients with ESRD, the relationship between BP and CVD risk is a J-shaped or U-shaped curve. Low mean arterial pressure is independently associated with increased mortality. There are obvious pathophysiologic reasons why low BP may be associated with adverse outcomes in patients with ESRD, the most prominent of which is that exposure to hypertension for several years causes these patients to develop cardiac failure, which lowers BP (so-called *reverse causality*).

The Metabolic Syndrome and Risk Factor Interactions

Certain traits, including obesity, hypertension, impaired glucose tolerance, and dyslipidemia, occur together more often than would be predicted by chance. This cluster, originally termed the *insulin resistance syndrome* is now known as the *metabolic syndrome* and has been defined as the presence of three or more of the following: increased waist circumference (>40 inches in men or >35 inches in women), increased fasting glucose concentration (>110 mg/dL [6.1 mmol/L]), increased triglyceride concentration (>150 mg/dL [1.7 mmol/L]), and a low concentration of high-density lipoprotein cholesterol (<50 mg/dL [1.3 mmol/L] in women or <40 mg/dL [1 mmol/L] in men). The long-term impact of the metabolic syndrome is a progressive increase in overall CVD and renal disease risk proportional to the number of components present. The nature of the interaction is mostly additive in the context of renal disease. Given the high prevalence of hyperglycemia and dyslipidemia in patients with ESRD, extremely aggressive management of these risk factors along with hypertension in this population is needed.

AMBULATORY BLOOD PRESSURE MONITORING

It has become apparent that assessment of hypertension and its consequences is more reliably and fully accomplished by ambulatory BP monitoring (ABPM) techniques than by casual office readings.

Blood Pressure Variability

ABPM is more valuable than clinic readings because ABPM gives a better representation of BP responses to many different situations.

The overall waking or sleeping BP is also more representative of an individual's average BP. ABPM is particularly useful in assessing the presence of "white coat hypertension" and in judging responses to antihypertensive medications. Although the overall prognostic significance of the phenomenon is still debated, it is clear that the pattern of target organ damage in patients with white coat hypertension is substantially less than that observed in individuals with sustained hypertension. In patients with ESRD, ABPM is useful to assess the wide variation in BP caused by dialysis treatments and interdialytic salt and water retention. The average of predialysis and postdialysis BP readings may be a reasonable predictor of mean interdialytic BP, but ABPM or self-measured home BPs may be better markers of interdialytic BP load than BPs obtained at dialysis centers.

Diurnal Rhythms

Another important phenomenon described by ABPM is the diurnal rhythm of BP. Normally, SBP and DBP tend to be highest during the morning, followed by a gradual decrease during the course of the day, and an abrupt fall-off during sleep. Approximately 10% to 25% of patients with essential hypertension fail to manifest normal nocturnal dipping of BP (defined as a nighttime BP fall of more than 10%); these patients are called *nondippers*, and those with a normal circadian rhythm are called *dippers*. Correlations between urinary albumin excretion, 24-hour DBP, and nighttime DBP are present in nondippers. Patients with advanced renal disease and up to 80% of those receiving maintenance hemodialysis fail to exhibit nocturnal BP dipping. At times, nocturnal BP can be greater than daytime BP in these individuals. Because BP is usually measured during the day, failure to obtain nocturnal readings may lead to the erroneous impression of good BP control.

Target Organ Damage

A large body of evidence from subjects with essential hypertension has shown that ABPM values correlate more closely than office BPs with overall morbidity and with the incidence and timing of cardiovascular complications. There is also a significant correlation between nighttime SBP or DBP and urinary albumin excretion and between 24-hour SBP and albumin excretion in hypertensive patients. Among hemodialysis patients, the absence of normal BP dipping also predicts adverse cardiovascular events.

TREATMENT OF HYPERTENSION IN CHRONIC KIDNEY DISEASE

As listed earlier, a number of interacting factors contribute to the accelerated age-related downward spiral of increased BP and decreased renal function. Although this process is relatively slow, it ultimately results in CVD and renal deterioration. The most important part of this downward cycle is certainly the direct effect of hypertension on loss of renal function and the simultaneous ability of renal dysfunction to raise BP. The speed with which the downward spiral proceeds is related to individual pathogenetic factors and interactions with other cardiovascular risk factors such as dyslipidemia, cigarette smoking, and glucose intolerance. Therefore, disease prevention via fastidious lifestyle modification is an important overall component of any treatment strategy (Table 26–1).

In patients with kidney disease, BP control is more complex to manage in that they not only have an increase in vascular resistance but also often have increased blood volume, which

Table 26–1: Considerations for Initial Therapy in Patients with Renal Disease

Increased blood volume (common in glomerular diseases)	Reduce blood volume (salt restriction, HCTZ, loop diuretic if creatinine > 2)
Decreased blood volume (common in tubular diseases)	May need salt supplementation
Increased peripheral vascular resistance	Vasodilation (ACEI, CCB, ARB)
Proteinuria	Reduce proteinuria (ACEI, ARB, NDCCB) (goal systolic blood pressure < 125 mm Hg if more than 1 g/day)
Diabetes with proteinuria	Control blood pressure and glycemia (ACEI if type 1, ARB if type 2 (blood pressure systolic < 130 mm Hg)
More than 20 mm Hg from systolic goal	Fixed-dose combination therapy (ACEI/HCTZ, BB/HCTZ, ACEI/CCB, ARB/HCTZ); use of HCTZ depends on renal function

ACEI, angiotensin-converting enzyme inhibitor; ARB, adrenergic receptor blocker; BB, β-blocker; CCB, calcium channel blocker; HCTZ, hydrochlorothiazide; NDCCB, nondihydropyridine calcium channel blocker.

contributes to the hypertensive process. Understandings about renal autoregulation provide some insight into appropriate levels of BP control and the relative importance of different kinds of antihypertensive drugs in preserving renal function. The glomerular circulation operates optimally at one half to two thirds of the systemic BP. Preglomerular vasoconstriction is necessary to step systemic pressure down to glomerular capillary pressure levels that are optimal for filtration yet low enough to avoid mechanical injury to the filtering apparatus. The efferent glomerular arteriole also serves an important purpose. It vasoconstricts during situations of diminished effective arterial blood volume to maintain adequate pressure for glomerular filtration. With the development of vascular disease, the afferent glomerular arteriole does not vasoconstrict properly, allowing transmission of systemic BP into the glomerulus. A clinical clue pointing to the failure of autoregulation is the presence of microalbumin or protein in the urine. Under these circumstances, systemic BP should be reduced more substantially to minimize the risk of mechanical injury to the glomerulus.

Hypertension with Diabetic and Nondiabetic Renal Disease

Treatment of hypertension to retard the rate of renal deterioration is now firmly established as a core principle of management. The threshold BP of 130/80 mm Hg is recommended for antihypertensive drug treatment in hypertensive people with diabetes or renal impairment, defined by either reduced GFR (<60 mL/min) or serum creatinine concentration (>1.5 mg/dL [130 mcmol/L] in men or >1.3 mg/dL [115 mcmol/L] in women) or albuminuria (urinary albumin excretion >300 mg/day or albumin concentration >200 mg/g of creatinine). In the Sixth Report of the Joint National Committee on Prevention, Detection, Evaluation, and Treatment of High Blood Pressure (JNC VI), the recommended goal for SBP is less than 130 mm Hg in patients with renal disease and less than 125 mm Hg if proteinuria greater than 1 g/24 hr is present. It is possible that even lower BPs may be necessary for optimal delay of progression of renal disease, particularly in the presence of proteinuria and in patients with diabetes.

Drugs that block the RAAS such as angiotensin-converting enzyme (ACE) inhibitors and angiotensin receptor blockers (ARBs) provide a more consistent opportunity to reduce progression of renal disease as part of an intensive BP-lowering strategy compared with other commonly used antihypertensive drugs. The benefit of these drugs is seen, in part, in their facilitation of efferent glomerular arteriolar dilation by antagonizing the effects of angiotensin II as they lower blood pressure. Thus, there is a more consistent reduction in both systemic and glomerular capillary pressure. Special attention should be paid to adequate dosing of these agents, as in the IRMA2 (Irbesartan in Patients with Type 2 Diabetes and Microalbuminuria Study) study, in which the higher dose of irbesartan (300 versus 150 mg/day) was clearly superior in protecting the kidney. Individual response rates vary widely and are strongly influenced by drug dose and changes in dietary sodium. Notably the effect of ACE inhibitors on reduction of proteinuria is abolished with high salt intake. In using either ACE inhibitors or an ARB (or indeed a combination thereof), the following should be the goal of therapy:

- BP less than 130/85 (proteinuria < 1 g); BP less than 125/75 (proteinuria > 1 g)
- Proteinuria less than 300 mg/dL
- Decline in GFR of less than 2 mL/min/yr

Many patients with chronic kidney disease exhibit a reversible fall in GFR with ACE inhibitor or ARB therapy that is not detrimental. This fall in GFR occurs because of hemodynamic changes, but the long-term reduction in perfusion pressure is renoprotective. Indeed, type 1 diabetic patients with the greatest initial decline in GFR have the slowest rate of loss of renal function over time. This predicted fall in GFR and the potential for hyperkalemia mandate measurement of the serum creatinine and potassium concentrations within 5 to 10 days after initiation of treatment with an ACE inhibitor or ARB or after a significant dose augmentation. It should be emphasized that ACE inhibitors should not be withdrawn immediately if a modest increase in serum creatinine is noted; a 20% to 30% decline in GFR can be expected and close monitoring is warranted. Hyperkalemia can be managed in most patients by dietary restriction. Additional medications can be added to these drugs to facilitate better BP control and also help reduce glomerular capillary pressure and proteinuria. Sufficient diuretic treatment to control blood volume should also be used, and concomitant administration of a loop diuretic may aid in the control of hyperkalemia. When the serum creatinine level reaches 2 mg/dL (176 mmol/L), volume reduction is better with the use of loop diuretics as opposed to thiazide diuretics, which are more effective as peripheral vasodilators. In advanced chronic kidney disease high-dose loop diuretic therapy (furosemide 100 to 200 mg twice a day or torsemide 100 to 200 mg every day) with or without the thiazide diuretic metolazone (2.5 to 5 mg three times weekly or every day) can be a useful therapeutic option. However, close clinical surveillance is imperative when combination therapy is initiated because of a high incidence of hypokalemia, excessive extracellular volume depletion, and azotemia.

Some investigators have questioned the safety of using calcium channel blockers in patients with kidney disease because of their preferential effects on dilating the afferent glomerular arteriole. Some studies have demonstrated that they can increase proteinuria despite lowering blood pressure. However, if these drugs are given with either ACE inhibitors or ARBs, which dilate the efferent glomerular arteriole, there is no clinical evidence that they are detrimental and worsen progression of renal disease. If anything, lower BP achieved with these drugs in combination may provide a better opportunity to protect against the loss of kidney function. BP control often becomes substantially more difficult as GFR declines, and four- or five-drug regimens (including increasing doses of loop diuretics, adrenergic inhibitors, vasodilators, and anti-RAAS drugs) are often needed. This subject is discussed further in Chapter 32, Specific Pharmacologic Approaches to Clinical Renoprotection.

Hypertension in End-Stage Renal Disease

An ideal goal BP has not been established for patients with ESRD. In the only prospective study performed so far in dialysis patients, a BP of 140/90 mm Hg was associated with reduced occurrence of left ventricular hypertrophy and death. Varying recommendations reflect the existing confusion in the literature as to what level of BP predicts better outcome in this patient population.

Dialysis
As renal mass declines further, dialysis therapy replaces diuretics for control of extracellular volume, although wide interdialytic fluctuations in BP complicate therapy. In most dialysis patients, BP rises during the interdialytic period in proportion to the amount of sodium and water ingested. To achieve dry weight, there should be a progressive reduction in each postdialysis weight over 4 to 8 weeks, to a point at which BP is reduced during each treatment to acceptable values (SBP < 140 mm Hg if possible) but not to levels at which the patient experiences symptoms of excessive sodium depletion (e.g., fatigue, cramps, or nausea). When dry weight is achieved and maintained, postdialysis BP becomes normal in most patients and antihypertensive drug treatment can be reduced. During the initiation of dialysis treatment in patients with SBP greater than 140 to 159 mm Hg and DBP greater than 90 to 99 mm Hg who have no major cardiovascular complications, antihypertensive medications are sometimes withheld until dry weight is achieved. If BP remains lower than 150/95 mm Hg between dialysis treatments in lower-risk patients, consideration can be given to controlling BP by

dialysis alone, especially in patients who experience intradialytic hypotensive episodes.

A comment on the use of vigorous dialysis instead of drug therapy is warranted. In addition to reducing quality of life through symptoms (e.g., weakness, malaise, nausea, and fatigue), overzealous ultrafiltration may cause a more serious group of untoward consequences, including hypotension, compromise of residual renal function, cerebral or coronary ischemic events, and paradoxical hypertension. In contrast, more vigorous ultrafiltration may be necessary in patients with left ventricular failure, acute pulmonary edema, pericardial effusion, or a dissecting aneurysm of the aorta. All of these are complex problems that are dependent on the (somewhat arbitrary) assignment of a particular dry weight and the associated choice of vasoactive drugs. Because of potential adverse consequences, the attending physician and staff must pay close attention to the balance between the dry weight assigned by the nursing staff and the cardiovascular drugs needed to optimize the risk profile. In some patients, a small degree of liberalization of dry weight and a concomitant increase in the use of antithypertensive drugs will improve quality of life.

Drug Therapy

If BP remains greater than 160/100 mm Hg, antihypertensive drug therapy is definitely necessary, usually with combinations of two or more drugs. For patients who are already taking antihypertensive medications at the beginning of dialysis, the same drugs should be continued, and the dose should be tapered as BP decreases with ultrafiltration. Severe hypertension (>180/110 mm Hg) or clinically significant target organ damage (e.g., symptoms of cardiac ischemia, heart failure, cerebrovascular disease, retinopathy, and aneurysms) should prompt even more vigorous drug therapy with multidrug regimens.

At some point during the progression to ESRD, vascular and neural sensitivity to angiotensin II diminishes. Therefore, ACE inhibitors and ARBs become less effective in most dialysis patients. The ongoing role of the sympathetic nervous system is demonstrated by the continuing utility of clonidine and labetalol to control BP in these patients. In those with more severe hypertension, the role of cellular calcium in perpetuating ongoing vasoconstriction is consistent with the utility of calcium antagonists to lower BP, especially in combination with sympatholytic drugs. If no cause for resistant hypertension is found, continuous ambulatory peritoneal dialysis should be considered, because it is generally more effective than hemodialysis for BP control. Given the effectiveness of appropriate dialytic therapy and the power of antihypertensive drug combinations, it is rarely (if ever) necessary to consider renal ablation with surgical or embolic nephrectomy. Loop diuretics have a role in limiting interdialytic weight gain in those few dialysis patients with residual renal function.

Paradoxical Hypertension during Hemodialysis
Hypertension induced by hemodialysis is a topic that has received little attention. It occurs in a small number of patients, and its causes have not been well delineated. In a few patients, increases in BP late in dialysis may represent dialytic removal of certain water-soluble antihypertensive drugs, including certain ACE inhibitors, minoxidil, and some β-blockers. A more common cause is probably excessive reflex activation of the sympathetic nervous system and the RAAS caused by rapid or exaggerated reductions in venous return and cardiac preload, activating the cardiopulmonary baroreflexes, which in turn cause central sympathetic stimulation. In patients with ESRD with native kidneys still present, a favorable response to anti-RAAS drugs is occasionally seen. Volume overload and cardiac distention may play a role as well.

V

Chronic Renal Failure

Hematologic Consequences of Renal Failure

27

ANEMIA OF RENAL FAILURE

The anemia of renal failure is characterized by normocytic and normochromic red blood cells (RBCs), an inappropriately low reticulocyte count for the degree of anemia, and a hypoplastic erythroid bone marrow, with normal leukopoiesis and megakaryocytopoiesis. Anemia is a constant feature of chronic renal failure and the hematocrit typically declines in parallel with the fall in the glomerular filtration rate.

Pathophysiology of Renal Anemia

The anemia of renal failure is a complex disorder determined by a variety of factors. Although the primary defect is decreased erythropoiesis, a number of other factors play contributory roles. These include increased blood loss during hemodialysis (HD), occult gastrointestinal losses, a shortened RBC half-life, superimposed iron or folic acid deficiency, and possibly a direct suppressive effect of uremic toxins on erythropoiesis, although this last point remains controversial. RBCs from uremic patients are intrinsically normal, and the RBC life span may become nearly normal or normal in patients undergoing carefully controlled dialysis who are also receiving recombinant human erythropoietin (rhEPO) therapy.

Erythropoiesis

Erythropoiesis is the dynamic process of RBC production. The transformation of a multipotential stem cell into a mature RBC occurs in two morphologically distinct stages, of which only the first is responsive to EPO. The latter stages of erythropoiesis are EPO independent but require adequate supplies of iron, vitamin B_{12}, and folic acid.

Erythropoietin

EPO is a sialylglycoprotein composed of 165 amino acids 18 with an estimated molecular mass of 34,000 D. Serum concentrations of EPO normally range from 8 to 18 mU/mL ($\approx$0.1 mg/mL [5 pmol/L]) and, in anemia, may increase 100- to 1000-fold. EPO messenger RNA levels are highly sensitive to changes in tissue oxygenation. The site of production within the kidney is in the interstitial cells of the renal cortex near the base of the proximal tubule cells.

Anemia can develop relatively early in the course of chronic renal failure (at creatinine clearances between 50 and 60 mL/min/1.73 m^2). The impairment of EPO production parallels the progressive reduction of nephron mass such that the plasma concentration of EPO becomes disproportionately low for the degree of reduction of hemoglobin concentration. Although the kidney is the major source of EPO production, detectable levels have been noted in anephric patients due to hepatic production. Indeed approximately 7% of patients receiving dialysis require no EPO supplementation. In autosomal dominant polycystic disease, the degree of anemia is less than and the serum level of EPO is greater than those usually accounted for by increased serum creatinine concentrations, because cystic kidneys may maintain EPO production despite advancing renal failure. Cobalt, androgens, and insulin-derived growth factor favor erythropoiesis, and inflammatory cytokines antagonize the effects of EPO.

Recombinant Human Erythropoietin

The cloning and expression of the human *EPO* gene were achieved in 1984, and the clinical efficacy of rhEPO in reversing the anemia of uremia was rapidly established. Anemia in end-stage renal failure (ESRD) responded well to rhEPO, and the need for transfusion was soon eliminated. Concerns that the effectiveness of rhEPO might depend on concomitant HD were dispelled by the equally favorable results obtained in predialysis patients and patients receiving continuous ambulatory peritoneal dialysis (CAPD).

There are two forms of rhEPO: epoetin alfa and epoetin beta. They differ from each other in the oligosaccharide component. Both forms of rhEPO are available for clinical use and demonstrate similar pharmacokinetics and efficacy profiles. The half-life ranges from 4 to 13 hours after intravenous administration and is approximately 24 hours after subcutaneous administration. Both rhEPO preparations appear to be eliminated by primarily nonrenal routes. In recent years the novel erythropoiesis stimulating protein (Aranesp), a molecule that stimulates erythropoiesis by the same mechanism as erythropoietin has emerged for clinical use. Aranesp, also named darbepoetin alfa, has an approximately threefold longer serum half-life, allowing less frequent administration (weekly or alternate weekly) than rhEPO with equal outcome and safety profiles.

MANAGEMENT OF RENAL ANEMIA

Treatment with Recombinant Erythropoietin

Renal anemia is rapidly corrected by rhEPO therapy, but the dose required can vary greatly. Within the therapeutic range of approximately 50 to 300 international units/kg three times per week, the rate of hemoglobin increase depends on the dose of rhEPO. Evidence exists that not all patients who could benefit are receiving rhEPO therapy, and, of those who are, many are not being treated adequately. The guidelines for patient management with rhEPO are outlined in Table 27–1. Dosages exceeding 300 international units/kg three times per week do not enhance the erythropoietic response. Current recommendations are as follows:

- 80 to 120 units/kg/wk subcutaneously or 120 to 180 units/kg/wk intravenously per National Kidney Foundation Kidney Disease Outcomes Quality Initiative (K/DOQI) guidelines
- 50 to 150 units/kg/wk subcutaneously or intravenously per European best-practices guidelines
- 100 to 200 units/kg/wk per Canadian guidelines

Higher starting doses are used when there is a need to rapidly increase the level of hemoglobin. Suggested rates of hemoglobin correction range from 1 to 2 g/dL/mo and should be less than 2 to 3 g/dL/mo. Concern has been raised about blood pressure control with more rapid rates of correction, potential induction of access clotting, and prolonged oscillation of hemoglobin values around the desired target, causing a delay in attainment of stable levels. In patients with a slow initial response over the first month of treatment, the dose of rhEPO may be increased by up to 50%. A dose reduction of 25% or extension of the interval between doses (the latter in particular for subcutaneous administration) is appropriate for patients experiencing rapid increases in hemoglobin. During the correction phase, the dosage of rhEPO must be adjusted monthly until the target is attained; the response to any change of dosage requires 4 weeks to be completely assessed. Each time a dosage needs to be increased, the increment

Table 27–1: Guidelines for Treatment with Recombinant Human Erythropoietin (rhEPO) in Patients with Chronic Kidney Disease

Anemia workup should be initiated when:
- Hemoglobin < 11 g/dL (hematocrit < 33%) in premenopausal women and prepubertal patients
- Hemoglobin < 12 g/dL (hematocrit < 37%) in adult males and postmenopausal women

Anemia workup should include a test for occult blood in the stool and measurement of iron parameters.
- Serum iron
- Total iron binding capacity
- Transferrin saturation
- Ferritin

Patients with microcytic anemia and normal iron stores should be evaluated for aluminum toxicity and thalassemia.

Uncontrolled hypertension is a contraindication to the initiation of rhEPO therapy.

The hemoglobin level or hematocrit should be measured each week during induction of therapy and every 2 wk thereafter.

Serum iron, TIBC, and serum ferritin should be measured monthly for 3 mo and every 2 to 3 mo thereafter.

The target range for hemoglobin (hematocrit) should be 11 g/dL (33%) to 12 g/dL (36%).

Adapted from Ad Hoc Committee for the National Kidney Foundation: Statement of the clinical use of recombinant erythropoietin in anemia of end-stage renal disease. *Am J Kidney Dis* 14:163–169, 1989; and National Kidney Foundation—K/DOQI Clinical Practice Guidelines for Anemia of Chronic Kidney Disease, 2000. *Am J Kidney Dis* 37(Suppl 1):S182–S238, 2001.

should not exceed 30 international units/kg three times per week. When the target hemoglobin is about to be reached and in rapid responders, the dosage should be decreased by approximately 25 international units/kg three times per week to avoid overshooting the target. Thereafter, the dose should be titrated down gradually by making adjustments at convenient intervals (8 weeks). In general, the higher the target, the greater the maintenance dose. The median intravenous maintenance dose necessary for maintaining the target hemoglobin-hematocrit value at approximately 12 g/dL is on average 75 international units/kg three times per week. However, some patients may only need 25 international units/kg three times per week, whereas others may require more than 200 international units/kg three times per week. The subcutaneous route of administration may be more effective and is the route of choice in predialysis and CAPD patients. There is no role for intraperitoneal administration of rhEPO. The suggested initial dose of Aranesp is 0.45 mcg/kg once a week either subcutaneously or intravenously. When the target hemoglobin level is reached, the maintenance dose of Aranesp is determined for the individual patient. To change from rhEPO to Aranesp, a rule of thumb is to divide the rhEPO dose by a factor of 200.

After treatment has begun, provided that iron stores and essential cofactors are either adequate or being replenished, hemoglobin should be checked weekly or biweekly. After a stable hemoglobin concentration is attained, it should be checked at least monthly, with follow-up at shorter intervals (weekly or biweekly) for dosage instability such as intercurrent illnesses or hospitalization. Iron stores should be evaluated a minimum of every 3 months by measurement of transferrin saturation and ferritin, with evaluations timed appropriately around periods of iron repletion to avoid artifactually elevated values.

Predialysis

RhEPO therapy should be started for patients with uncomplicated anemia of chronic renal disease before ESRD has developed. The progression of renal disease is not significantly altered and may be slowed, provided that hypertension is treated adequately. In most published studies, the rhEPO doses used in this setting were lower than those in dialysis patients, that is, 50 to 100 international units/kg week subcutaneously.

Dialysis

There has long been an impression that removal of more small or toxic middle molecules results in higher hemoglobin levels. However, the data are controversial. Studies show that in patients with inadequate responses to anemia and suboptimal urea reduction ratios increasing the level of dialysis results in an increase in the hematocrit. The effect of a higher delivered dose of dialysis on the response to rhEPO, apart from the specific effect of better removal of uremic toxins, may be to ameliorate the anemia as a result of improvements in RBC survival, blood coagulation, nutritional status, and well-being.

Transplant

With immediate kidney graft function, the EPO serum levels will double within 7 days after transplantation and will remain elevated until the anemia is corrected. The gradual increase of EPO is accompanied, after a lag period of some weeks, by an increase in hematocrit. With adequate graft function, hematocrit should normalize within months. In some transplant recipients, iron deficiency due to increased iron utilization may occur, but this should correct spontaneously.

In the first weeks after renal transplantation, some patients present with marked anemia due to blood loss, bone marrow suppressive effects of medication, intercurrent inflammatory and infectious diseases, graft rejection, and inadequate EPO production by the transplanted kidney. Post-transplant erythrocytosis (hemoglobin 16 to 17 g/dL) is seen in up to 10% of patients. Angiotensin-converting enzyme inhibitors and angiotensin receptor blockers diminish post-transplant erythrocytosis without altering EPO plasma levels probably by reversibly preventing the recruitment of pluripotent hematopoietic stem cells.

Side Effects

The most commonly reported adverse events with rhEPO use include arterial hypertension, clotted vascular access, and hyperkalemia. The relationship of rhEPO therapy to seizures is uncertain. However, the rate of seizures during the first 90 days of rhEPO therapy appears to be higher than that during the subsequent 90 days; therefore, strict control of the rate of hemoglobin rise (no more than 1.5 g/dL in any 4-week period) and close monitoring of the blood pressure appear warranted.

CLOTTING Clotting of the vascular access and the artificial kidney are often reported. In patients treated with rhEPO, increases in factor VIII, von Willebrand factor antigen, fibrinogen, and whole-blood platelet aggregation are observed. These effects, together with other transient but significant changes occurring in tissue plasminogen activator antigen, plasminogen activator inhibitor, and antithrombin III, and combined with reduction of fibrinolytic activity, all favor a tendency for thrombosis. Increased anticoagulation with heparin may be required during HD to prevent filter clotting. A statistically significant relationship has not been established between the rate of rise in hemoglobin and the incidence of cerebrovascular accidents, transient ischemic attacks, and myocardial infarction.

LOSS OF DIALYTIC EFFICIENCY The initial concerns when rhEPO was introduced that increases in red cell mass might result in worsening azotemia and hyperkalemia have not materialized as clinically significant issues. Although decrements in solute clearance have been reported with successful treatment, they are small (10% to 15%), and when the delivered dialysis dose is closely monitored, shortfalls in delivered clearance can be investigated and rectified prospectively.

ARTERIAL HYPERTENSION New onset or worsening of hypertension is the most commonly reported side effect of rhEPO therapy in patients with ESRD and occurs in up to one third of patients. The following risk factors have been identified: pre-existing hypertension, rapid correction of anemia, and high doses of rhEPO. Enhanced vascular reactivity associated with an increased RBC mass, enhanced vascular responsiveness to norepinephrine and direct effects on vascular smooth cells via a specific EPO receptor are all postulated causes. In most cases, arterial hypertension can be effectively managed by reducing dry body weight, starting or increasing antihypertensive therapy, and reducing the dose of rhEPO. Regression of left ventricular hypertrophy and normalization of cardiac index and other hemodynamic and functional parameters are evident during treatment with rhEPO and are maintained afterward, providing an adequate control of blood pressure.

PURE RED CELL APLASIA An alarming side effect of EPO use is the development of anti-EPO antibodies, which is associated with severe transfusion-dependent anemia, caused by a pure red cell (bone marrow) aplasia. In a study in 2002, 13 patients with pure red cell aplasia who had developed antibodies able to block the formation of erythroid colonies by normal bone marrow cells were described and characterized, and subsequently more than 100 patients with this condition have been reported worldwide with a substantial proportion demonstrating anti-EPO antibodies. The red cell aplasia developed, on average, 10 months after initiation of therapy, with a range of 1 to 92 months. Although the data are too scanty for a firm conclusion, it seems that the incidence of pure red cell aplasia is higher in patients who are taking EPO subcutaneously than in those who are taking the drug intravenously. When pure red cell aplasia is suspected, EPO administration should be immediately interrupted. It is also recommended that patients not be switched to another form of EPO or to darbepoetin, because the anti-EPO antibodies cross-react with all commercially available recombinant erythropoietic products. A role for immunosuppressive treatment has yet to be confirmed.

Causes for Inadequate Response

Hyporesponsiveness to rhEPO has been defined as a failure to achieve the target hematocrit in the presence of adequate iron stores at a dose of 450 international units/kg/wk intravenously within 4 to 6 months or failure to maintain it subsequently at that dose. Several conditions have been associated with inadequate responses to rhEPO. Iron deficiency (both absolute and functional) is the most common cause. Other factors are inadequate dialysis, protein malnutrition, severe hyperparathyroidism, aluminium overload, underlying infections, inflammatory or malignant

Table 27–2: Causes of Inadequate Response to Recombinant Human Erythropoietin Therapy

Iron deficiency
Chronic blood loss (dialysis circuit/gastrointestinal tract)
Iron malabsorption
Infection/inflammation
Malnutrition: folate or vitamin B_{12} deficiency
Aluminum toxicity
Osteitis fibrosa
Hemoglobinopathies (e.g., α- and β-thalassemia, sickle cell anemia)
Malignancies
Hemolysis
Pure red cell aplasia

diseases, occult blood loss, and hemoglobinopathies (e.g., thalassemias) (Table 27–2).

IRON DEFICIENCY A suboptimal response to rhEPO most commonly results from failure of delivery of an adequate amount of iron to the erythron. Enhanced iron utilization due to rhEPO-induced RBC formation can quickly deplete iron stores previously reduced by poor iron absorption, occult gastrointestinal bleeding, or dialysis-related blood losses. Most treated patients develop iron deficiency and therefore require more rhEPO to maintain the same rate of RBC production. If the iron balance is not restored by oral or parenteral iron replacement and iron deficiency worsens, an initial good response may then abate. The most accurate assessment of iron stores is given by staining of the bone marrow aspirate for iron with Perl Prussian blue stain; however, in clinical practice the iron status is commonly assessed by serum iron concentration, serum ferritin (SF), transferrin saturation, and RBC indices. Serum iron concentration fluctuates during rhEPO administration, but SF, a protein secreted into the plasma by the reticuloendothelial cells under the regulation of intracellular iron concentration, is a good indicator of iron stores. The transferrin saturation index (calculated according to the formula: saturation percent = serum iron/total iron capacity)—that means transferrin-bound iron—has an even higher sensitivity and similar specificity. Iron deficiency due to the consumption of iron deposits by rhEPO-stimulated erythropoiesis may be concealed by the persistence of apparently adequate ferritin levels, but it is disclosed by both a transferrin saturation index less than 20% and prompt erythropoietic response to intravenous administration of iron dextran.

The failure to make enough iron available to meet the demands of enhanced erythropoiesis despite the presence of adequate iron stores, as reflected by the level of SF, has been defined as *functional iron deficiency* (compared with *absolute iron deficiency* or *iron storage deficiency*). The RBCs appear hypochromic (with mean corpuscular hemoglobin concentration < 28 g/dL) when mobilization of iron from stores and its transport to the erythron become inadequate. A percentage of circulating hypochromic RBCs greater than 10% (normal range: < 2.5% of circulating RBCs) in the presence of adequate iron stores and the absence of hemoglobinopathies or inflammatory diseases should be diagnostic of functional iron deficiency. In the presence of an adequate response to rhEPO, the amount of iron supplementation should be targeted to keeping the level of SF greater than 100 ng/mL, the transferrin saturation index more than 20%, and hypochromic RBCs less than 10%.

Iron Treatment

Oral Iron

EPO therapy is most successful when adequate iron stores are present, and this usually requires iron supplementation. Oral supplementation of iron offers the benefits of simplicity, low cost, and safety, but its efficacy is limited. K/DOQI guidelines recommend that when oral iron is used in adults, 200 mg of elemental iron should be administered daily in two to three divided doses. Most iron salts, of which ferrous sulfate is the most popular agent, cause gastrointestinal side effects, including dyspepsia, constipation, and bloating. The efficacy of oral iron supplementation in patients with kidney disease has been rigorously studied only in patients treated by HD. In this patient subgroup oral iron is typically ineffective for improving the response to rhEPO. The reasons for failure of oral iron treatment in HD patients include poor compliance due to gastrointestinal side effects and diminished gastrointestinal iron absorption. This latter point is obtained in large part from the fact that if oral iron is taken at the same time as food, phosphate binders, or other medications that directly interfere with its absorption, adequate intake will not be achieved. In contrast, in patients with chronic kidney disease and in those being treated by peritoneal dialysis (PD), ongoing iron losses are less than those experienced by HD patients. Accordingly, they have less of a need for iron supplementation and may derive greater benefit from oral iron treatment. The efficacy of oral iron in patients with kidney disease may be enhanced through several simple practices: first, the dose should provide at least 200 mg of elemental iron per day (for ferrous sulfate, this goal would be achieved by taking approximately three 325-mg tablets per day); second, iron administration should occur between meals and should be spaced at least 1 hour apart from the ingestion of phosphate binders, which may also interfere with iron absorption; and third, because iron is absorbed proximally in the gastrointestinal tract, delayed-release iron supplements should be avoided.

Intravenous Iron

The efficacy of intravenous iron treatment has been widely studied in HD patients. Studies have consistently demonstrated that intravenous iron treatment results in higher hemoglobin levels or a reduced requirement for EPO (up to 40%), or both. The available formulations are iron dextran, iron sucrose, and ferric gluconate. Iron dextran has been used for several decades and although it is clearly effective, its safety profile remains problematic with severe adverse reactions observed in approximately 0.6% of patients treated. Anaphylactic reactions are believed to be related to the drug's dextran component. The mechanism of iron dextran–related anaphylaxis is incompletely understood but may be related to direct release of vasoactive mediators by mast cells. Alternative agents include iron sucrose and ferric gluconate. Because these agents do not contain a dextran moiety, they have a far lower risk of anaphylaxis, serious adverse events are no more common than with placebo, and they have largely replaced iron dextran in clinical practice.

Two strategies for administering intravenous iron to HD patients are in common use. The first entails surveillance for the presence of iron deficiency every 3 months and, if detected, treatment with a short, repletion course of intravenous iron. Typically 1000 mg of either iron sucrose or ferric gluconate can be given in divided doses over a period of 2 to 3 weeks. Patients will generally demonstrate a significant improvement in responsiveness to rhEPO thereafter. Many, however, will remain iron deficient, so assessment of iron stores should be repeated after completion of such a course of treatment. A second strategy is to anticipate iron deficiency by administering small weekly doses to maintain stable iron stores. Weekly doses of 12.5 to 100 mg of intravenous iron may improve responsiveness to rhEPO. The potential advantage of such an approach lies in linking iron replacement temporally with ongoing iron losses. Assessment of iron stores should be performed quarterly, however, to ensure the adequacy of this approach.

In patients being treated by PD or those with chronic kidney disease who are not yet undergoing dialysis, iron deficiency develops less often than in patients being treated by HD because the former patients do not sustain the chronic ongoing losses of iron experienced by those receiving HD. Iron still plays a central role in the maintenance of responsiveness to rhEPO, however, and deficiency states refractory to oral iron replacement may develop during the course of treatment. When these patients develop iron deficiency, a course of oral iron should be attempted. If this does not successfully replete iron stores, intravenous iron can be administered. Because of the inconvenience of needing to obtain sequential intravenous access in these patients, a larger infusion of iron is often used; for example, 200 to 300 mg of diluted iron sucrose or ferric gluconate may be infused over a 2-hour period. Such an approach appears to be effective and well tolerated.

Aluminum Overload

In HD patients, aluminum toxicity may cause microcytic anemia despite normal iron deposits. Aluminum and iron use common pathways for intestinal absorption, transport in the plasma, and binding to transferrin; aluminum overload may interfere with iron utilization in the response to rhEPO. The sources of aluminum accumulation are primarily both gastrointestinal absorption from antacids used to bind dietary phosphorus and improperly processed water for dialysate. The best way of diagnosing aluminum overload is bone biopsy. Basal serum aluminum concentrations greater than 50 ng/mL and aluminium levels after a deferoxamine challenge test (a single dose of 500 to 1000 mg intravenously) higher than 175 ng/mL suggest aluminium overload. Treatment with intravenous deferoxamine should improve not only the aluminium-induced microcytic anemia but also the normocytic anemia with questionable aluminum accumulation; it may help also restore responsiveness to rhEPO.

Infectious and Inflammatory Chronic Diseases and Malignancies

Erythropoiesis is negatively regulated by several macrophage-derived cytokines, including tumor necrosis factor-α, interleukin-1 and -6, and transforming growth factor-β, all factors that are elevated in inflammatory processes. These cytokines have inhibitory effects, either directly or mediated, on the erythroid progenitor cells, and they may also impair iron metabolism by sequestering iron inside the macrophages ("inflammatory iron block"). The anemia that occurs with inflammation, infection, and malignancies is normocytic and normochromic in most patients but, not uncommonly, may be microcytic and hypochromic despite normal or raised levels of SF. This is because in addition to reflecting iron stores, ferritin is also an acute-phase protein. The association of chronic inflammatory disease with chronic renal failure creates a therapeutic challenge, because the anemia may possibly become resistant to rhEPO at the usual dosage but may respond, at least partially, to high doses. In dialysis patients, the dose of rhEPO required to maintain the target hematocrit is higher when baseline plasma fibrinogen and serum transferrin concentrations and the serum C-reactive protein concentration are also high. Both rhEPO dose and serum C-reactive protein are inversely correlated with serum albumin and serum iron levels, suggesting that the mechanisms by which inflammatory cytokines inhibit erythropoiesis are coupled to iron metabolism. Hyporesponsiveness to rhEPO has been reported in HD patients with severe hyperparathyroidism; a dramatic improvement has been observed after surgical parathyroidectomy. A direct toxic effect of parathyroid hormone on erythropoietic bone marrow has been suggested, but the osteitis fibrosa induced by hyperparathyroidism, with the consequent bone marrow fibrosis and reduction of the erythroid cell mass, appears to be the main cause of the poor response to rhEPO.

Other Therapies
Blood transfusions do not represent an optimal therapy: the target hematocrit is markedly lower than that for rhEPO therapy, and they do not prevent or retard the development of heart disease. The risks of repeated blood transfusions are as follows: iron overload (suppression of erythroid marrow); blood-borne viral infections; and human leukocyte antigen (HLA) immunization (production of cytotoxic antibodies to HLA antigens). Androgens have been used with moderate success. Their erythrogenic action appears to be mediated through increased EPO production.

Quality of Life and Survival Outcomes

The correction of anemia with rhEPO has virtually eliminated the need for transfusion in most patients with the anemia of chronic renal failure. It has also improved the quality of life as measured by several different parameters. Exercise capacity and tolerance have been measurably increased, and surveys of both objective and subjective quality-of-life indicators have shown significant improvement. Anemia is an independent predictor of both heart failure and overall mortality in ESRD; anemia is also independently predictive of heart failure. The relative risk of death is significantly increased in patients with hematocrit values less than 33%.

Target Hematocrit

The appropriate target hematocrit is a matter of controversy. Significant relief of symptoms, with a low risk of side effect profile, has been observed when the hematocrit value in HD patients is between 29% and 33%. However, additional improvements in quality of life, cardiac function, physical work capacity, cognitive function, and sexual function have been reported at a hematocrit of 36% to 39%, and the K/DOQI guidelines suggest a target hematocrit of 33% to 36%. The benefits and risks of complete correction of anemia (hematocrit 38% to 42%) and the optimal target concentration have not yet been established. Clinicians are reluctant to totally correct anemia in patients with ESRD because (1) the morbidity of anemia is not well understood, (2) there is a bias that moderate anemia is acceptable for dialysis patients, (3) the principles of rhEPO therapy are not followed, (4) there is an inordinate amount of concern about the side effects of therapy, and (5) the cost of the treatment is high. The safety of long-term maintenance of a normal hematocrit has been questioned, as a consequence, in part, of the early termination of the Normal Hematocrit Cardiac Trial, in which the patients randomly assigned to the normal hematocrit group had higher mortality and a higher incidence of nonfatal myocardial infarction.

EFFECT OF RENAL FAILURE ON HEMOSTASIS

Uremic patients have an underlying bleeding diathesis and have a significant risk for bleeding during surgery or invasive procedures. Subepidermal and submucosal bleeding are the major manifestations observed; gastrointestinal bleeding, hemopericardium, or subdural hematoma are seen only occasionally. The skin bleeding time is the best predictor of clinical bleeding.

Causes of Uremic Bleeding

Over the past 20 years, research has partially clarified the nature of uremic bleeding. The pathogenesis is multifactorial, and the major defects involve anemia and platelet-vessel wall and platelet-platelet interactions. Anemia is a significant contributor and hemostatic improvement can be achieved with rhEPO therapy. The presence of "uremic toxins" impairs platelet thrombi formation by inhibiting the activity of the glycoprotein adhesion receptor IIb-IIIa, which results in diminished von Willebrand factor-induced platelet-platelet adhesion. HD removes these toxins and partially reverses the prolongation of the bleeding time.

Consequences of the Bleeding Tendency in Uremia

Gastrointestinal bleeding occurs with greater frequency and higher mortality in uremic patients than in the general population. Upper gastrointestinal bleeding is the second leading cause of death in patients with acute renal failure. The most common causes of bleeding are peptic ulcers, hemorrhagic esophagitis, gastritis, duodenitis, and gastric telangiectasias. Angiodysplasia with gastrointestinal bleeding has been observed in the stomach, duodenum, jejunum, and colon. This abnormality, affecting the microcirculation of the gastrointestinal mucosa and submucosa, occurs most often in HD patients. Although now rare, hemorrhagic pericarditis with cardiac tamponade can occur in uremic patients. The clinical features of this condition include a normal cardiac shadow, increased jugular venous distension with hypotension, shortness of breath, and a pericardial friction rub. Deaths due to hemorrhagic pericarditis have been reported to be as high as 3% to 5% among dialysis patients.

Subdural hematoma has been reported to occur in 5% to 15% of HD patients. It usually overlies the frontal or parietal lobe and is bilateral in approximately 15% of patients. Headache, vomiting, seizures, hypertension, drowsiness, confusion, and coma are the usual symptoms. Head trauma, hypertension, and systemic anticoagulation are risk factors. Spontaneous retroperitoneal bleeding is a rare complication in patients receiving chronic HD. Trauma, anticoagulation, and the presence of polycystic kidneys are predisposing factors. The symptoms and signs include sudden onset of pain in the abdomen, flank, back, or hip, with an associated drop in blood pressure. Spontaneous subcapsular hematoma of the liver is a newly recognized complication in uremic patients. Typically, patients have right upper quadrant pain, fever, and sometimes elevated bilirubin and alkaline phosphate levels accompanied by a falling hematocrit. Intraocular bleeding with only temporary visual loss has also been reported in a large percentage of transplant and dialysis patients after cataract surgery. Another risk of bleeding in uremic patients is associated with aspirin given to prevent vascular access thrombosis or platelet activation on dialyzer membranes. The beneficial effect of aspirin on vascular access thrombosis can be achieved with a moderate dosage of aspirin (160 mg/day), which inhibits platelet thromboxane A_2 generation without affecting vascular prostacyclin formation. However, even a moderate dosage of aspirin prolongs the bleeding time, and this fact may explain the higher frequency of gastrointestinal bleeding observed in uremic patients receiving aspirin. Thus, the use of aspirin in uremic patients treated with rhEPO to prevent the thrombotic complications associated with an increasing hematocrit requires a judicious evaluation of the risk-benefit profile.

Thrombotic Complications

Thrombosis of the arteriovenous shunt is a common occurrence in uremic patients undergoing HD. Reduced levels of antithrombin III, protein C, and protein S may contribute to a thrombotic tendency in some patients. Because platelet aggregation plays a major role in thrombus formation, antiplatelet agents have been used; however, thrombosis in an arteriovenous graft usually reflects an anatomic stenosis at the venous anastomosis due to fibrointimal hyperplasia rather than spontaneous thrombosis related to a prothrombotic tendency. Fibrinolytic agents, such as streptokinase or urokinase, are occasionally used by interventional radiologists to thrombolyse acutely occluded grafts with reasonable success rates when combined with balloon angioplasty of the venous stenosis.

Therapeutic Strategies

Although some investigators have found that both HD and PD partially improve the hemostatic abnormality of uremia, both forms of dialysis can potentially produce adverse effects on hemostasis (Table 27–3). For all patients with hemorrhagic complications or who are undergoing major surgery, the adequacy of dialysis should be appropriately checked. It is also advisable to change the dialysis schedule for 1 or 2 months in patients who have experienced severe hemorrhages (such as major gastrointestinal bleeding, hemorrhagic pericarditis, or subdural hematomas) or who have undergone recent cardiovascular surgery so that heparin can be avoided. Acute bleeding episodes may be treated with desmopressin at a dose of 0.3 mcg/kg intravenously (added to 50 mL of saline over 30 minutes) or subcutaneously. Intranasal administration of this drug at a dose of 3 mcg/kg is also effective and is well tolerated. The effect of desmopressin lasts only a few hours, a major limitation to its use in treating severe hemorrhage, and it appears to lose efficacy when administered repeatedly. Because the favorable effect of cryoprecipitate on bleeding time has not been uniformly observed, its use is

Table 27–3: Guidelines for the Management of Hemorrhagic Complications of Uremia

For patients with hemorrhagic complications or undergoing major surgery, dialysis adequacy should be assessed.

Acute anemia should be promptly corrected, and hematocrit should be increased to 30% or more, by infusion of packed red blood cells.

For long-term correction of anemia erythropoietin is administered.

Acute bleeding episodes may be treated by intravenous infusion of desmopressin at a dose of 0.3 mcg/kg body weight in 50 mL of saline over 30 min, or by subcutaneous injection at the same dose. Intranasal administration of desmopressin at a dose of 3 mcg/kg body weight is also effective. The effect of desmopressin is short-lasting, and repeated doses are associated with loss of effect.

Persistent chronic bleeding may be effectively treated with intravenous infusion of conjugated estrogen. The usual dose schedule is 0.6 mg/kg body weight a day for 5 days.

not recommended. Conjugated estrogen treatment given by intravenous infusion in a cumulative dose of 3 mg/kg as daily divided doses (i.e., 0.6 mg/kg for 5 consecutive days) is the most appropriate way of achieving long-lasting hemostatic competence. Severely anemic patients should receive blood or RBC transfusions to improve hematocrit values. RBC transfusions are hemostatically effective only when the hematocrit rises above 30%. As an alternative, bleeding in patients with renal failure and hematocrit less than 30% can be treated successfully with erythropoietin.

HD is accompanied by a transient form of platelet activation related to the interaction of platelets with artificial membranes and vascular access itself. Dialysis patients have accelerated platelet turnover, supporting the concept that platelets are chronically activated by dialytic treatment. Repeated platelet activation on dialysis membranes may induce refractoriness to further platelet stimulation, possibly contributing to clinical bleeding that can occur at termination of the dialysis procedure. In addition, heparin may also present a problem. "Regional" heparinization has been used to minimize the effects of systemic anticoagulation. Heparin is given by constant infusion through the inlet line of the dialyzer. Simultaneously, protamine sulfate is infused into the outlet port before the blood returns to the patient. Even this schedule of heparin administration, however, may be associated with a high incidence of bleeding. As an alternative, frequent injections of low-dose heparin can be given during dialysis to maintain a lower and more constant level. Usually, 40 to 50 international units/kg of heparin is given at the beginning of HD, followed by 60% of the initial dose after 1 hour and 2 hours, and 30% of the initial dose after 3 hours. The activated partial thromboplastin time is measured hourly and should be maintained at 1.5 to 2 times the basal value. For patients with a high risk for bleeding an ethylene-vinyl alcohol copolymer hollow-fiber dialysis membrane that does not require systemic anticoagulation can be used, provided that blood flow is maintained at more than 200 mL/min. Low-molecular-weight heparin has been proposed as an alternative to unfractionated heparin in patients receiving chronic HD who have a high risk for bleeding. Prostacyclin shows some promise as an alternative. Given in a continuous infusion during dialysis at a mean dose of 5 ng/kg/min, prostacyclin completely inhibits platelet aggregation without causing bleeding. However, it is expensive; is associated with headache, flushing, tachycardia, and chest and abdominal pain; and requires careful monitoring and a physician's supervision. Thus, the use of prostacyclin should be limited to patients with a high risk for hemorrhage. With PD, when applicable, the risk of bleeding associated with heparin or anticoagulants is avoided.

The anecdotal observation of diminished gastrointestinal bleeding in uremic patients treated with conjugated estrogens and the improved hemostasis in von Willebrand disease in pregnant patients led to investigations of the effect of estrogens on bleeding in uremia. One oral dose of 25 mg of conjugated estrogen normalizes the bleeding time for 3 to 10 days, with no apparent ill effects. A controlled study showed that conjugated estrogens, given intravenously at a cumulative dose of 3 mg/kg divided over 5 consecutive days, produced a long-lasting reduction in the bleeding time in uremic patients. At least 0.6 mg/kg of estrogen was needed to reduce the bleeding time, and four or five infusions spaced 24 hours apart were needed to reduce the bleeding time by at least 50%. Thus, estrogens may be a reasonable alternative to desmopressin in the treatment of uremic bleeding, especially when a long-lasting effect is required.

EFFECT OF RENAL FAILURE ON GRANULOCYTES AND MONOCYTES

Renal failure is associated with an increased susceptibility to infections. In cell-mediated defense against infectious agents, granulocytes and monocytes move by chemotaxis to the site of injury. Cells then phagocytose microorganisms through complex processes that include cell adhesion and the formation of oxygen free radicals (particularly H_2O_2 from O_2. Many studies have found that leukocyte chemotaxis is impaired in uremia, possibly because of a circulating inhibitor of chemotaxis, a decreased intracellular cyclic guanosine monophosphate-to-cyclic adenosine monophosphate ratio, or a plasma factor blocking granulocyte membrane receptors. Interestingly, the chemotactic activity of granulocytes is diminished further, rather than corrected, by HD. Studies of granulocyte phagocytosis and respiratory burst in uremia are conflicting. HD has a profound effect on granulocyte kinetics. During the first 2 hours of HD, all patients develop peripheral neutropenia mediated by complement activation on the dialysis membrane and sequestration of granulocytes in the lung. In the hours after HD, the release of neutrophils from the bone marrow and sites of sequestration produces rebound neutrophilia. Thus, pulmonary dysfunction occurring within the first hours of HD may be the result of endothelial injury caused by massive granulocyte adherence to pulmonary vessels. During HD with nonbiocompatible membranes (e.g., cuprophane), there is a rapid increase in the surface expression of phagocyte adhesion receptors, leading to cell aggregation and sequestration in the pulmonary vasculature. These effects are observed to a lesser degree with newer biocompatible membranes.

Monocytes are also markedly activated by contact with dialysis membranes, as documented by transient increases in plasma levels of interleukin-1 and tumor necrosis factor during HD. The functional consequences of monocyte activation during HD may include the possibility that cytokine release might trigger hypotension or augment susceptibility to infections and atherosclerosis. It has been known for many years that uremic patients suffer from an acquired form of immunodeficiency characterized by abnormal T-cell proliferation in response to antigenic challenges. This defect could well be the consequence of monocyte dysfunction, because T-cell activation is monocyte-dependent. The monocytes in uremic patients who do not respond to hepatitis B vaccination are unable to deliver the necessary signal required for triggering interleukin-2 synthesis to T lymphocytes. However, further studies are needed to clarify the true clinical impact of these changes on the immunodeficiency of uremic patients.

Cardiovascular Aspects of Chronic Kidney Disease

28

BACKGROUND

Cardiovascular Disease

Cardiovascular disease is the predominant cause of death in patients with chronic kidney disease (CKD). Heart disease accounts for 40% to 45% of all deaths among both dialysis patients and transplant recipients. Most clinical consequences of cardiac disease result from either cardiomyopathy (systolic or diastolic) or ischemic heart disease. Although myocardial infarction and angina are usually attributable to the presence of critical coronary artery disease (CAD), they may also result from decreased perfusion of the myocardium due to nonatherosclerotic small vessel disease and left ventricular (LV) hypertrophy. Valvular heart disease due to dystrophic calcification of the aortic and mitral valves is another significant cause of cardiac morbidity.

Cardiovascular Disease and Stage of Chronic Kidney Disease

It is important to recognize that the time of presentation of cardiovascular disease depends not only on prevailing cardiovascular abnormalities but also on the duration, severity, and type of renal disease.

Chronic Renal Insufficiency

LV hypertrophy is present in 40% of those with moderate chronic renal insufficiency. Risk factors that accelerate the development of symptomatic cardiomyopathy in patients with CKD include diabetes, hypertension, tobacco use, and anemia.

End-Stage Renal Disease

Only 15% of patients commencing dialysis have a normal echocardiogram and a substantial minority of patients have already developed systolic dysfunction. Over time many patients with LV hypertrophy with preserved systolic function develop LV dilatation and symptomatic heart failure.

Renal Transplant Recipients

Mortality rates, including those from cardiovascular death, in transplant recipients are lower than those for dialysis patients. There is evidence that systolic dysfunction, LV hypertrophy, and concentric hypertrophy all improve after renal transplantation. Improvements in extracellular volume control, anemia, and calcium and phosphate abnormalities, as well as normalization of the uremic environment undoubtedly could account for the enhanced longevity after transplantation. However, cardiovascular disease remains the leading cause of death and it should be remembered that these patients still may have a wide variety of cardiovascular risks after transplantation.

PATHOLOGY AND PATHOPHYSIOLOGY

Cardiac Disease

Left Ventricular Hypertrophy

LV hypertrophy is an adaptive process that occurs in response to a long-term increase in myocardial work caused by LV pressure or volume overload. The initial effects of LV hypertrophy are beneficial; however, LV hypertrophy in response to chronic pressure and volume overload in CKD/end-stage renal disease (ESRD) eventually becomes maladaptive because continuing pressure and volume overload ultimately lead first to LV dilatation and eventually to systolic dysfunction. The principal factors contributing to the pressure and volume overload characteristic of patients with CKD include the following:

Pressure Overload	Volume Overload
• Hypertension	• Increased extracellular volume
• Arteriosclerosis	• Arteriovenous fistulas
• Aortic stenosis	• Anemia

Reduced arterial wall compliance is a key component of LV afterload. Arterial stiffness due to arteriosclerosis is common in patients with CKD and is characterized clinically by increased systolic pressure and widening of the pulse pressure. Because the peripheral resistance in most dialysis patients is within the normal range, it is likely that the effects of arterial stiffening contribute more significantly to cardiovascular morbidity than does an elevation in mean blood pressure. Indeed the systolic pressure and pulse pressure more closely correlate with LV hypertrophy than does diastolic blood pressure. In addition to the dominant influence of pressure and volume overload, other factors may also contribute to the development of the cardiomyopathy of CKD/ESRD, including raised sympathetic activity, homocysteine, and endothelin.

Cardiac Failure

DIASTOLIC DYSFUNCTION Hemodialysis patients with LV hypertrophy often have some impairment in LV diastolic function. The increased LV stiffness means that small increases in extracellular volume trigger large rises in LV pressure, predisposing to symptomatic pulmonary edema. The reverse is also true: Volume depletion results in a large fall in LV pressure with symptomatic hypotension and hemodynamic instability, as is often observed following rapid ultrafiltration in hemodialysis. This is often a clinical clue to the presence of diastolic dysfunction in a hemodialysis patient.

SYSTOLIC DYSFUNCTION Decreased systolic function is often observed in patients in whom cardiac disease was present before the onset of dialysis therapy and in patients who have experienced prolonged and marked hemodynamic overload. Diminished myocardial contractility may also be a result of overload cardiomyopathy, in which the myocardium relies on Starling forces to maintain a normal output. This manifestation of cardiomyopathy has a substantially worse prognosis than that for either concentric LV hypertrophy or LV dilatation with normal systolic function. In dialysis patients, systolic dysfunction is strongly associated with the presence of ischemic heart disease or sustained biomechanical stress or both. However, it can also be a reversible manifestation of severe uremia, improving when the uremic environment is managed. Renal transplantation has also been shown to normalize systolic function in dialysis patients with systolic dysfunction and subsequently to reduce but not normalize the LV mass index.

SYMPTOMATIC CARDIAC FAILURE If left untreated, both LV hypertrophy and LV dilatation will ultimately progress to dilated cardiomyopathy. The clinical presentation is symptomatic heart failure, with dyspnea and pulmonary venous congestion, ultimately resulting in acute pulmonary edema. This end-stage clinical manifestation of cardiac disease may result from systolic failure, usually caused by dilated cardiomyopathy or ischemia or both or from diastolic dysfunction in association with LV hypertrophy.

Ischemic Heart Disease

ATHEROMATOUS ISCHEMIC HEART DISEASE The uremic milieu and/or its associated comorbidities provide hemodynamic and metabolic perturbations that lead to coronary artery wall damage. CAD is highly prevalent in the population with CKD, because of both the demographic characteristics of the patient population and their underlying disease states (e.g., hypertension and diabetes mellitus). The prevalence of CAD in patients entering dialysis programs varies, depending on associated comorbidities, but ranges from 15% to 73%. Of these, it is estimated that more than 50%, particularly diabetic patients, are asymptomatic. Both mechanical and humoral factors predispose to atheroma formation. Arterial hypertension causes increased tensile stress, which results in endothelial cell activation and injury. In addition to endothelial injury and activation, vascular pathologic changes with chronic uremia include autocrine and endocrine sequelae from a diverse range of seemingly unrelated factors. These include the following:

- Dyslipidemias and disturbances of glucose metabolism
- Derangement of platelet function associated with high levels of prothrombotic factors
- Increased oxidant stress
- Hyperhomocysteinemia

Two factors have received particular attention recently for their contribution to the development of atheroma in CKD: inflammation and vascular calcification. Evidence from clinical studies has shown that C-reactive protein levels are a powerful predictor of mortality in both hemodialysis and peritoneal dialysis patients. Epidemiologic studies support its pathogenetic role as a cardiovascular risk factor in the general community, a situation that may be amenable to intervention by agents such as aspirin and pravastatin. Coronary atherosclerotic plaque morphology in patients with CKD is distinguished by severe calcium deposition, and such deposits may contribute substantially to the high rate of complications seen in CKD. Markers of coronary and carotid calcification include longer duration of dialysis, hyperparathyroidism, estimates of calcium and phosphate load, C-reactive protein levels, elevated homocysteine levels, and age. The etiology of such changes almost certainly relates to the positive calcium and phosphate balances to which CKD patients are exposed, through both increased intake and inadequate excretion. Calcium-containing phosphate binders, together with hyperparathyroidism and vitamin D use contribute to vessel calcification. Although coronary artery calcification predicts subsequent coronary events in the general population, its clinical significance in patients with CKD is unknown. It is possible that the more generalized arterial calcification observed in dialysis patients does not predict atherosclerotic coronary events but rather is a marker for arteriosclerosis and diminished vascular compliance and a risk factor for LV hypertrophy.

NONATHEROMATOUS ISCHEMIC HEART DISEASE About 25% of dialysis patients with ischemic symptoms do not have critical coronary artery stenosis. It is likely that their symptoms result from microvascular disease and an underlying cardiomyopathy. In LV hypertrophy, increases in myocardial oxygen demand may not be met with adequate increases in coronary flow, especially if there are pathologic changes in the large coronary arteries or in the small coronary vessels. Decreased arterial compliance and volume overload probably reduce cardiac transmural perfusion and aggravate subendocardial ischemia.

Dialysis Hypotension

The pathophysiology of the clinical manifestations of dialysis hypotension is multifactorial and not fully understood. It may occur in the presence of systolic failure, diastolic dysfunction, or ischemic disease. In the latter, it is usually associated with chest pain, whether atherosclerotic or nonatherosclerotic in origin. In dilated cardiomyopathy, hypotension during dialysis occurs only in patients in whom resting cardiac output does not increase in response to plasma volume depletion. Such patients usually have severe systolic failure, because the dialysis procedure actually improves myocardial performance in most patients with depressed LV function. LV hypertrophy, which is highly prevalent in this population, may also be a contributing factor to dialysis hypotension. Because of diminished LV compliance, the relationship between LV end-diastolic pressure and volume is exaggerated. As a result, during dialysis, relative hypovolemia may result in a disproportionately large decrease in LV end-diastolic pressure, which in turn leads to hypotension if a compensatory increase in peripheral resistance does not occur.

Arrhythmias

LV hypertrophy and coronary heart disease are associated with an increased risk of arrhythmias. In addition, serum electrolyte levels that can affect cardiac conduction, including potassium, calcium, magnesium, and hydrogen, are often abnormal or undergo rapid fluctuations during hemodialysis. For all these reasons, arrhythmias (or sudden death) are of particular concern in patients undergoing dialysis. High-grade ventricular arrhythmias such as multiple premature ventricular contractions, ventricular couplets, and ventricular tachycardia have been observed in up to 30% of dialysis patients by 24-hour Holter monitoring. Older age, dialysis-associated hypotension, preexisting heart disease, LV hypertrophy, and digoxin therapy are associated with a higher prevalence and greater severity of cardiac arrhythmias. A considerable variation in the frequency and severity of arrhythmias is seen during hemodialysis, as well as in the interdialytic period. Because of these factors, there is no consensus on the frequency of arrhythmias in these patients or their clinical significance. There are also conflicting data about the effect of dialysis and of various dialysis compositions and dialysis protocols on the occurrence of rhythm disturbances. Most atrial arrhythmias have low clinical significance, although sustained, rate-related (fast or slow) impairment of LV filling can trigger hypotension. Arrhythmias in peritoneal dialysis patients consist mainly of atrial and/or ventricular premature beats and peritoneal dialysis by itself does not appear to provoke or aggravate arrhythmias. The arrhythmias seen in these patients are more a reflection of the patient's age, underlying ischemic heart disease, or an association with LV hypertrophy. The use of digoxin in hemodialysis patients has also raised concern about precipitation of arrhythmias, especially in the immediate postdialysis period, when both hypokalemia and relative hypercalcemia may occur. However, no increase in the incidence of arrhythmias after dialysis is observed in patients taking digoxin.

Valvular Disease
Most valvular lesions observed in patients with CKD are acquired and develop from dystrophic calcification of the valvular annulus and leaflets, particularly the aortic and mitral valves. The prevalence of aortic valve calcification in dialysis patients is as high as 55%, similar to that in the elderly general population, although it occurs 10 to 20 years earlier and it has also been associated with rhythm and cardiac conduction defects. Aortic valve orifice stenosis in CKD can evolve rapidly from valve sclerosis (within 6 months) to hemodynamically significant stenosis, with a worsening of LV hypertrophy and rapidly evolving symptomatology. Age, duration of dialysis, a raised phosphate level, and an elevated calcium phosphate product appear to be the most important risk factors for the development of aortic stenosis. Mitral valve calcification is not as common as aortic valve disease in CKD and the pathogenetic factors are not as well defined.

EPIDEMIOLOGY AND CARDIAC RISK FACTORS

Although there is undoubtedly a higher incidence of cardiovascular disease in the pre-ESRD than in the general population, the major burden of ill health in CKD occurs once the patient has commenced renal replacement therapy. Risk factors for cardiovascular death include echocardiographic abnormalities (LV hypertrophy or systolic dysfunction), diabetes mellitus, congestive heart failure, and a recent myocardial infarction. Interestingly the presence of CAD is not a significant risk factor for death when examined independently of age, diabetes, and heart failure, suggesting that CAD exerts its effects through compromise of LV function.

Uremia as an Independent Cardiovascular Risk Factor

The uremic state is cardiomyopathic because of its hemodynamic milieu (hypertension, volume overload, and reduced arterial compliance). However, the evidence for uremia itself as an independent risk factor for atherogenic disease is less certain. Large-scale longitudinal studies of community-derived cohorts have failed to identify renal insufficiency as an independent cardiac risk factor. In contrast, similar studies of cohorts with higher degrees of comorbidity, including elderly, hypertensive, and cardiac patients, consistently identified renal insufficiency as a predictor of adverse cardiovascular outcomes independent of the traditional risk factors outlined later.

MANAGEMENT

Diagnosis

The diagnostic tools discussed in this section can often be applied across the spectrum of CKD; they can be used to investigate both ischemic and cardiomyopathic disease, and they are limited by the same clinical considerations, both renal and cardiovascular. In a practical context, it is, of course, assumed that careful clinical assessment will always precede further diagnostic endeavors.

Cardiac Disease
ELECTROCARDIOGRAPHY   The increasing prevalence of LV hypertrophy as renal function worsens predisposes to abnormalities in resting and exercise electrocardiographic findings in patients with CKD. In dialysis patients, minor incremental changes in the PR

and QRS intervals, together with nonspecific ST-T wave changes, are often seen in the resting electrocardiogram, and these may be more prominent during dialysis because of substantial intracellular and extracellular electrolyte shifts. However, in episodes of acute coronary ischemia (unstable angina and myocardial infarction), classic electrocardiographic changes seem to occur as expected. Exercise-related electrocardiographic changes should be interpreted with caution. Resting abnormalities, a restricted maximal pulse rate (autonomic neuropathy), and limited exercise capacity in patients with CKD may either mask or erroneously predict underlying ischemia.

BIOCHEMICAL MARKERS OF ISCHEMIA Serial estimates of levels of standard myocardial enzymes (creatine phosphokinase and lactate dehydrogenase), when elevated, reliably diagnose acute myocardial infarction in CKD, although single estimates have poor specificity. Recently, attention has focused on the role of troponin levels in predicting outcome in acute ischemia. In CKD concerns about impaired troponin clearance as renal function worsened exist; however, third-generation cardiac troponin T assays are reliable independent predictors of death at all glomerular filtration rates (GFR).

ECHOCARDIOGRAPHY Two-dimensional and M-mode echocardiographic studies provide a noninvasive assessment of LV structure and function, together with imaging of valves and pericardium. Because LV mass varies over the course of a hemodialysis session owing to the effects of fluid removal, whenever possible imaging should be carried out when the patient has achieved so-called *dry weight*. Dobutamine stress echocardiography is being recognized as a screening tool for ischemic heart disease in patients with CKD, particularly for those patients who are unable to exercise adequately. It can also be used in patients with valvular disease or impaired systolic function to assess underlying systolic reserve. For dialysis patients, negative predictive values in excess of 95% have been reported with reasonable patient numbers and follow-up times, and the sensitivity may be broadly comparable to that of exercise-related scintigraphic scanning.

NUCLEAR SCINTIGRAPHIC SCANNING Nuclear scintigraphy can be used for assessment of both myocardial systolic function and ischemia. The predominant role for nuclear scanning techniques in CKD, however, is in the assessment of myocardial ischemia, particularly as a screening tool in the workup for transplantation. Exercise-based studies and dipyridamole to enhance vasodilatation are commonly used, together with technetium-labeled thallium, methoxyisobutylisonitrile, or metaiodobenzylguanidine.

Inherent problems with scintigraphy need to be taken into consideration: blood pressure may be too high or too low to permit safe administration of a vasodilatory agent; high endogenous circulating levels of adenosine may blunt the efficacy of dipyridamole; coronary flow reserve may be reduced due to LV hypertrophy and small vessel disease; and symmetrical coronary disease or a blunted tachycardic response due to autonomic neuropathy, or both, can mask significant pathologic conditions.

ELECTRON-BEAM ULTRAFAST COMPUTED TOMOGRAPHY–DERIVED CORONARY ARTERY CALCIFICATION The relatively new technique of electron-beam ultrafast computed tomography relies on the principle that coronary artery calcification is a reliable surrogate for significant coronary atherosclerosis although this is far from certain. Widespread vessel wall calcification is common in uremia, and evidence is accumulating that increased calcium content per se portends a poor prognosis. The role of electron-beam ultrafast computed tomography in evaluating risk or disease in patients undergoing transplantation is unknown.

CORONARY ANGIOGRAPHY Patients with CKD who have CAD are often asymptomatic. Despite the availability of newer diagnostic tools, the sensitivity and specificity of most noninvasive techniques are limited, and the gold standard for diagnosis of CAD remains coronary angiography. Given the risks of contrast nephropathy and cholesterol embolization, coronary angiography should be reserved for patients with CKD who have unstable angina and/or myocardial infarction who are receiving maximal therapy and in whom coronary revascularization is a viable therapeutic modality. For reasons of cost, access, demand, and possible deterioration in renal function, it is not possible to screen all patients with CKD by formal angiography. This limitation is of particular significance in patients being evaluated for transplantation, and some effort has been directed to establishing guidelines to determine which patients have the most risk and hence may benefit from coronary catheterization. Most units now have a predefined strategy to determine which patients require more intensive cardiac workup in this context, usually stratified into diabetic and nondiabetic patients, and all patients except those with the lowest risk for ischemic heart disease should receive some form of screening.

Treatment

Cardiac Disease
CARDIOMYOPATHY AND CARDIAC FAILURE A reversible precipitating or aggravating factor is often found in patients with CKD

who present with cardiac failure. Arrhythmias, underlying myocardial ischemia, anemia, uncontrolled hypertension, and the use of drugs that may adversely affect cardiac performance can all precipitate a clinical presentation of cardiac failure and should be addressed. A careful and ongoing assessment of the optimal target weight is a central component of dialysis care.

PHARMACOTHERAPY In most patients with cardiac failure and CKD, combination pharmacotherapy is required, and dosing considerations and interactions among medications need careful consideration. Other issues, such as effects on comorbid conditions (e.g., diabetes, peripheral vascular disease, glaucoma, and chronic airflow obstruction), compliance, and potential interactions with other drugs (e.g., immunosuppression, anticoagulants, and statin therapy) can be important.

Loop diuretics are indispensable for achieving and maintaining euvolemia in all patients with cardiac failure, including those with CKD. Dose augmentation is typically required as GFR falls. Although thiazide diuretics become ineffective with a GFR lower than 30 mL/min, the synergistic diuretic effect of loop diuretics and metolazone persists even at relatively advanced stages of renal insufficiency and can be a useful therapeutic option with close supervision.

The effects of aldosterone antagonists are unpredictable in patients with CKD. The primary reason for consideration of their use is their recently reported benefit in cardiac disease or reduction of proteinuria in patients with CKD. Hyperkalemia in particular can result when these drugs are combined with blockade of the renin-angiotensin system or β-receptor antagonists in the setting of CKD. Dose reduction or avoidance is advised in such circumstances.

Angiotensin-converting enzyme (ACE) inhibitors or angiotensin receptor antagonists improve symptoms, morbidity, and survival in nonuremic individuals with heart failure, and it is reasonable to extrapolate these results to the population with CKD. ACE inhibitors should be used in patients with symptomatic cardiac failure, to prevent cardiac failure in asymptomatic patients whose LV ejection fraction is less than 35%, and in patients with an ejection fraction of 40% or less after a myocardial infarction. Although these drugs have not been well studied in patients with CKD, it is reasonable to consider using them if there is no contraindication. They should be used cautiously in patients not yet receiving dialysis with a GFR lower than 25 mL/min, and avoidance may be advisable in this group as well as in patients with severe renovascular disease, in patients with acute renal dysfunction, or in those who have recently received a transplant. Hyperkalemia in moderately advanced CKD (GFR <60 mL/min) and renal artery stenosis in a transplanted kidney are additional concerns requiring monitoring after treatment is started.

The use of β-receptor antagonists improves the prognosis of individuals with asymptomatic systolic dysfunction, regardless of whether they have had a myocardial infarction. Chronic activation of the adrenergic nervous system contributes to the development of LV hypertrophy, ischemia, and myocyte damage and exerts a maladaptive role in chronic heart failure in patients receiving hemodialysis. In recommending increased use of β-receptor antagonists in dialysis patients, one should remember that contraindications to their use (reactive airway disease, sinus-node dysfunction, and cardiac conduction abnormalities) occur often in patients with CKD. Furthermore, the dose of some drugs (e.g., atenolol) often needs to be reduced according to the degree of renal impairment.

The use of digoxin is controversial. It has not been found to reduce mortality in the general population, and its use is associated with a variety of risks in patients with severe impairment of kidney function. These risks include a predisposition to toxicity because of impaired clearance as renal function declines and an increased risk of arrhythmia in association with hypokalemia, which can occur especially during or after dialysis. On the basis of these results, digoxin should not be considered a first-line drug in the management of heart failure in CKD. It is reasonable to consider its use for rate control in atrial fibrillation and for patients with substantial systolic dysfunction or symptoms despite the use of other agents, with or without atrial fibrillation.

The treatment of diastolic dysfunction is less well defined. Attempts to eliminate the cause are usually the focus of therapy, which includes aggressive control of hypertension, treatment of anemia, and control of other factors responsible for the development of LV hypertrophy. The drugs of choice in diastolic failure are probably verapamil and diltiazem, which enhance LV diastolic relaxation. Excessive diuresis should be avoided, as should the use of digoxin and direct vasodilators, such as prazosin, hydralazine, or minoxidil.

Ischemic Heart Disease

The treatment of both the acute (unstable angina and acute myocardial infarction) and the nonacute (stable angina and cardiac failure) presentations of CAD in patients with CKD is the same as that in the general population.

PHARMACOTHERAPY Patients with CKD and stable angina who have not had an infarct should be treated with standard anti-anginal agents for relief of symptoms. For those who have had an infarct, β-receptor blockade should be prescribed, as should an ACE inhibitor for patients with LV dysfunction. Although the benefit of aspirin therapy in nonuremic patients is substantial, the risk of complications probably increases as renal function declines; however, the benefits still probably outweigh the risks for patients with acute presentations of ischemia and for those who have a high risk for ischemia.

CORONARY REVASCULARIZATION Despite the relatively high incidence of asymptomatic ischemia in CKD, there is no evidence to suggest that aggressive investigation and treatment result in improved mortality statistics. For patients who have had an infarction, angiography is indicated if there are symptoms of myocardial ischemia at rest or after minimal exertion or if there is early, severe ischemia during a stress test. For other patients, the use of coronary angiography should be limited to those with symptoms refractory to medical therapy. As in the general population, coronary arteriography should be reserved for patients in whom revascularization (angioplasty, stenting, or bypass grafting) would be undertaken if critical CAD were identified on the basis of an assessment of the significance of the lesion, the operative risk, and overall life expectancy. Initial success rates for coronary angioplasty in patients with CKD are similar to those in the general population; however, the restenosis rate may be higher. In addition, one-year mortality rates after angioplasty vary proportionately with renal function, with the higher rates in those with the lowest GFRs.

Among hemodialysis patients, the in-hospital mortality rate for coronary artery bypass grafting is four times higher than that for the general population. Hence, there is a consensus favoring the use of bypass surgery only for left main or extensive three-vessel disease and the use of angioplasty for single-vessel disease. In the remaining patients with multivessel disease, it appears that angioplasty with stents has clinical outcomes similar to those for coronary artery bypass grafting , but more repeat revascularization procedures are needed. In view of the propensity for restenosis after angioplasty in dialysis patients, coronary artery bypass grafting is probably the revascularization procedure of choice, although angioplasty with stenting may be useful in multivessel disease with culprit lesions.

In summary, evidence suggests that patients with CKD in general have a higher risk for complications and have poorer long-term outcomes, regardless of the revascularization procedure used. Effectively, the decision to use a particular procedure will be based on the specific cardiac and overall clinical condition of the patient, together with available resources.

Arrhythmias and Valvular Disease
A discussion of the specific and detailed management of cardiac arrhythmias is largely beyond the scope of this text. An awareness of the potential for and types of arrhythmias likely to be encountered is advocated, and they should be managed in accordance with general principles. Perhaps the most important practical consideration is to solicit the advice and support of a cardiologist for patients with resistant or troublesome arrhythmias and/or poor cardiac function. Consideration of the renal metabolism of drugs (such as digoxin and β-receptor antagonists) in patients with impaired renal function is necessary, as is the disturbed homeostasis of monovalent and divalent ions in the population with CKD.

In patients with CKD who have mitral or aortic valve disease, primary control of potentiating factors, frequent monitoring once valve aperture is encroached, and appraisal of the individual patient and associated comorbidities once surgery is considered would appear, in the absence of evidence, to be a reasonable approach to treatment.

Risk Factor Intervention

Table 28–1 lists pharmacologic and nonpharmacologic interventions to minimize cardiovascular disease in patients with CKD.

Hypertension
PREDIALYSIS ACE inhibitors or angiotensin II antagonists are considered to be the first-line agents in most patients owing to their documented benefit in delaying the progression of proteinuric CKD. Other beneficial effects include improved cardiovascular disease outcomes in patients with at least one cardiovascular disease risk factor in addition to either diabetes or manifest vascular disease and reduced hospitalization for heart failure in diabetic patients with overt nephropathy. Concerns about hyperkalemia and the use of these agents in patients with renovascular disease mandate the close monitoring of renal function and serum potassium. The effects of calcium channel blockers, particularly the dihydropyridines, have not compared well against those of ACE inhibitors and angiotensin II antagonists in reduction of proteinuria, a delay in progression of renal function, or

Table 28–1: Risk Factor Intervention to Minimize Cardiovascular Disease in Patients with Chronic Kidney Disease

Nonpharmacologic interventions
- Stop tobacco use
- Minimize excess extracellular fluid to target blood pressure < 140/90 mm Hg
- Awareness and prevention of inflammation and hypoalbuminemia
- Dietary modification to target low-density lipoprotein cholesterol < 100 mg/dL (2.6 mmol/L)
- Renal transplantation when appropriate
- Coronary revascularization for secondary prevention of ischemic vascular disease

Pharmacologic interventions
- Drug therapy to target blood pressure < 140/90 mm Hg
- Epoetin and iron therapy to target hemoglobin concentration > 11 g/dL (upper limits not clearly defined)
- Treatment with HMG-CoA reductase inhibitor (statin) therapy to target LDL cholesterol < 100 mg/dL (2.6 mmol/L)
- Treat abnormal divalent ion levels to target serum calcium 9.2 to 9.6 mg/dL (2.3 to 2.4 mmol/L), serum phosphate 2.5 to 4.5 mg/dL (0.8 to 1.45 mmol/L), and intact parathyroid hormone 100 to 200 pg/mL (22 to 33 pmol/L)
- Antiplatelet agents in patients with coronary disease, vascular disease, or diabetes
- Appropriate use of ACE inhibitors (or ARA in predialysis patients) for treatment of proteinuria and arteriosclerosis
- Use of ACE inhibitors and β-receptor antagonists in patients with known ischemic vascular disease

ACE, angiotensin-converting enzyme; ARA, angiotensin receptor antagonist; HMG-CoA, 3-hydroxy-3-methylglutaryl coenzyme A; LDL, low-density lipoprotein.

prevention of cardiovascular events. The use of β-receptor antagonists, diuretics, and other vasodilators depends on the response to treatment and underlying comorbidities. The aim of treatment of hypertension should generally be blood pressure levels lower than 130/85 mm Hg for individuals with parenchymal disease, 125/75 mm Hg if there is more than 1 g/day of proteinuria, and 130/80 mm Hg for patients with diabetes and less than 1 g/day of proteinuria.

DIALYSIS The mainstay of therapy in dialysis patients is maintenance of normal extracellular fluid volume. A reasonable target blood pressure for antihypertensive treatment is less than 140/90 mm Hg before dialysis, unless the patient develops symptomatic hypotension or low blood pressure during or after dialysis. Antihypertensive drugs should be prescribed for patients whose blood pressure is higher than 140/90 mm Hg after achievement of dry weight. Selection of antihypertensive agents is best guided by the presence of associated comorbidities.

TRANSPLANTATION   Limited data are available on the optimal antihypertensive regimens in transplant recipients. Calcium channel blockers are widely used because they are well tolerated and because of their effects in counteracting calcineurin-mediated vasoconstriction. The use of ACE inhibitors or angiotensin II antagonists is probably justified in most patients, although they are best avoided in the first 6 months after transplantation when concerns about hyperkalemia, anemia, and abrupt rises in serum creatinine are greatest. The goal blood pressure is 130/80 mm Hg or lower in line with the Sixth Report of the Joint National Committee on Prevention, Detection, Evaluation, and Treatment of High Blood Pressure (JNC VI) for patients with kidney disease.

DYSLIPIDEMIA   In short-term studies, statins have been recognized as being safe and efficient for patients with CKD/ESRD, although their benefit in reducing adverse cardiovascular outcomes has not yet been proved. Target low-density lipoprotein cholesterol levels are less than 100 mg/dL (2.6 mmol/L) for pharmacologic and diet therapy. The statins are the most effective drugs for lowering low-density lipoprotein cholesterol levels in CKD and should be the agents of first choice. Dose reduction should be instituted when statins are used in combination with calcineurin inhibitors and may be required in individual patients as GFR declines. Clinicians should be alert to the finding that dialysis patients appear to have a higher risk of myositis from statin use than the general population.

SMOKING   There are no studies demonstrating that cessation of smoking improves the outcome of CKD at any stage. Nevertheless, it is reasonable to extrapolate data from the general population that indicate a reduction in cardiovascular risk over time after smoking cessation.

DIABETES   Strict glycemic control reduces microvascular but not necessarily macrovascular complications of type 1 and type 2 diabetes. Tight glycemic control would seem to be an appropriate aim in predialysis patients, unless hypoglycemic episodes are troublesome or unpredictable. In transplant recipients, tight control may be difficult because of the hyperglycemic tendency of immunosuppressive agents; however, strict glycemic control after transplantation may reduce the development of new diabetic changes in the transplanted kidney and is a worthy goal.

Uremia-Related Risk Factors

ANEMIA   LV mass increases significantly in patients with CKD as the level of hemoglobin falls below 10 g/dL. Anemia correction by erythropoietin can prevent or reverse early echocardiographic changes in CKD but has little effect after LV hypertrophy has progressed to LV dilatation.

INFLAMMATION   The source of elevated C-reactive protein levels in patients with CKD is uncertain. Both statins and aspirin have been studied for their effects on reducing inflammation in patients with CKD and in the general population. The suggestion is that each agent modifies the inflammatory response beyond the effects for which it was designed and the use of these agents should be considered in patients who have evidence of or have a high risk for cardiovascular disease.

HYPERHOMOCYSTEINEMIA   A combination of high-dose folic acid, vitamin B_{12}, and vitamin B_6 lowers homocysteine levels by 25%, which may restore normal levels in patients with chronic renal insufficiency or in renal transplant recipients but not in dialysis patients. However, no trials have yet shown that lowering homocysteine levels improves cardiovascular outcome. Thus, screening for homocysteine levels would appear to have only a limited role and currently cannot be advocated as part of a general management strategy.

OXIDATIVE STRESS   Although evidence of increased oxidative stress in CKD exists, there are no longitudinal studies examining the impact of oxidative stress on subsequent de novo cardiac events. On the basis of current evidence for dialysis patients, it is possible only to suggest replacement of vitamins C and E lost to dialysis or metabolism rather than increased intake for antioxidant purposes.

ABNORMAL DIVALENT ION METABOLISM   Patients with CKD are in a substantial positive calcium balance from an early stage of disease, and attempts to minimize the calcium load in the context of parathyroid hormone and phosphate control are assuming increasing importance. The target concentration for serum calcium is between 9.2 and 9.6 mg/dL (2.3 to 2.4 mmol/L) and for serum phosphate it is 2.5 to 4.5 mg/dL (0.8 to 1.45 mmol/L) to achieve a calcium-phosphate product of less than 55 mg^2/dL^2. The target range for intact parathyroid hormone levels is suggested to be between 200 and 300 pg/mL (22 to 33 pmol/L). Renagel (Sevelamer hydrochloride) is a noncalcium, nonaluminum agent that is an effective, albeit costly, phosphate binder and is not associated with hypercalcemia.

Neurologic Complications of Renal Insufficiency

29

End-stage renal disease (ESRD) is associated with at least five well-described disorders of the nervous system including the following:

- Uremic encephalopathy
- Dialysis dysequilibrium syndrome (DDS)
- Dialysis dementia
- Stroke
- Sexual dysfunction

In addition to the manifestations of neurologic dysfunction just described, which are specifically related to renal insufficiency, dialysis, or both, a number of other neurologic disorders occur with increased frequency in patients who have ESRD and are being treated with chronic hemodialysis. Subdural hematoma, certain electrolyte disorders (e.g., hyponatremia, hypernatremia, hyperkalemia, phosphate depletion, and hypercalcemia), vitamin deficiencies, Wernicke encephalopathy, drug intoxication, hypertensive encephalopathy, and acute trace element intoxication must be considered in patients with chronic renal failure (CRF) who manifest an altered mental state. Patients with renal failure also are at risk for development of the same varieties of organic brain disease and metabolic encephalopathy that can affect the general population. Therefore, when a patient with ESRD presents with altered mental status, a thorough and complete evaluation is necessary.

UREMIC ENCEPHALOPATHY

The term *uremic encephalopathy* is used to describe the early appearance and dialysis responsiveness of the nonspecific neurologic symptoms of uremia. It is an acute or subacute organic brain syndrome that regularly occurs in patients with acute renal failure (ARF) or CRF when the glomerular filtration rate declines to less than 10% of normal. The exact nature of the "uremic toxins" involved in the development of uremic encephalopathy remains unclear. As with other organic brain syndromes, these patients display variable disorders of consciousness, psychomotor behavior, thinking, memory, speech, perception, and emotion. The symptoms of uremic encephalopathy are shown in Table 29–1. Key early clinical features include daytime drowsiness and insomnia with a tendency for sleep inversion, itching, and "restless legs." Symptoms of uremia are generally more severe and progress more rapidly in patients with ARF than in those with CRF. In more slowly progressive CRF, the number and severity of symptoms also typically vary cyclically, with intervals of acceptable well-being in an otherwise inexorable downhill course toward increasing disability. The symptoms are readily ameliorated by dialysis procedures and suppressed by maintenance dialysis regimens and are also usually eliminated entirely after successful renal transplantation. Therefore, the early recognition of the encephalopathy of renal failure is important because it is decisively treatable by renal replacement therapy. In addition, since the widespread introduction of recombinant human erythropoietin as a therapeutic agent in patients with ESRD treated with hemodialysis, it is now clear that brain function and quality of life are significantly improved by correction of the anemia with erythropoietin.

Table 29–1: Signs and Symptoms of Uremic Encephalopathy

Early uremia
    Anorexia
    Malaise
    Insomnia
    Diminished attention span
    Decreased libido
Moderate uremia
    Emesis
    Decreased activity
    Easy fatigability
    Decreased cognition
    Impotence
Advanced uremia
    Severe weakness and fatigue
    Pruritus
    Disorientation
    Confusion
    Asterixis
    Stupor, seizures, coma

Diagnosis of Uremic Encephalopathy

The diagnosis of uremic encephalopathy in most patients is suspected if there is a constellation of clinical signs and symptoms that indicate renal or urologic disease or injury. However, the presenting symptoms of uremia are similar to those of many other encephalopathic states (e.g., drug intoxication or hepatic encephalopathy). There is a risk of misdiagnosis and mistreatment because patients with renal failure are subject to other intercurrent illnesses that may also induce other encephalopathic effects. Moreover, if a drug with potential central nervous system (CNS) toxicity is excreted or significantly metabolized by the kidney, the ensuing encephalopathic symptoms may be attributable to the fact that the drug has reached toxic CNS levels at dose rates inappropriate for a suppressed glomerular filtration rate. Despite the possibilities that such multiple causes of encephalopathy might occur simultaneously, uremic encephalopathy may be successfully differentiated in most instances by means of standard clinical and laboratory methods and, if necessary, a trial of dialysis.

Uremic Encephalopathy in Patients with Hepatic Insufficiency

In patients who have advanced liver disease with hepatic insufficiency, it is often difficult to differentiate whether the cause of encephalopathy is hepatic or renal. Under normal conditions most urea generated in the liver is excreted in the urine with a small percentage being excreted into the gastrointestinal tract, where it is metabolized by colonic bacteria to form ammonia. However, in patients with renal failure caused by an increase in the blood urea concentration, the amount of urea entering the colon rises, leading to enhanced ammonia generation, which in the setting of hepatic dysfunction triggers an increase in plasma ammonia levels. Plasma ammonia levels have been shown to correlate well with the severity of hepatic encephalopathy. Therefore, patients with liver damage and ESRD have a particular risk for development of encephalopathy, because both conditions act synergistically to increase blood ammonia and hence the risk of encephalopathy.

To further complicate the assessment, it should also be noted that plasma urea and serum creatinine levels are poor markers of renal function in patients with severe liver disease. Many patients who have liver disease, with normal or near-normal plasma urea and creatinine values, may in fact have severe renal impairment.

Restless Leg Syndrome

Restless leg syndrome is found in up to 50% of patients receiving maintenance renal replacement therapy. It is characterized by an urge to move the legs, usually accompanied or caused by uncomfortable and unpleasant sensations in the legs, which worsen during rest/inactivity, particularly at night. The etiology is unclear and does not appear to be related to inadequate clearance on dialysis. Treatment with antiparkinsonian therapies, such as ropinirole hydrochloride, have been somewhat successful; carbidopa/levodopa therapy has proven to be successful.

CHRONIC RENAL FAILURE

Cognitive functions impaired in uremia include sustained and selective attention capacity, speed of decision making, short-term memory, and mental manipulation of symbols.

Electroencephalogram in Patients with Chronic Kidney Disease

Findings on an encephalogram (EEG) in patients with CKD are usually less severe than those observed in patients with ARF. Several investigations have shown good correlation between the slow delta wave activity and the decline of renal function as estimated by the serum creatinine level. After the initiation of dialysis, there may be an initial period of clinical stabilization during which time the EEG deteriorates (up to 6 months), but it then approaches normal values. Significant improvement is seen in the EEG abnormalities after renal transplantation.

Psychologic Testing in Patients with Chronic Kidney Disease

Several different types of psychologic tests have been applied to subjects with CRF. These have been designed to measure the effects of dialysis, renal transplantation, or parathyroidectomy. In general, performance outcomes are poorer in patients with CKD than in normal subjects, and there appears to be a consensus, based on psychologic testing, that CKD results in organic-like losses of intellectual function, particularly information-processing capacities. Psychologic testing scores typically improve with treatment by dialysis or renal transplantation. Supporting a role for hyperparathyroidism in the development of uremic encephalopathy in patients who underwent parathyroidectomy for other medical reasons is the fact that they have shown significant improvements in several areas of psychologic testing including general cognitive function, nonverbal problem solving, and visual-motor or visual-spatial skills.

ACUTE RENAL FAILURE

The clinical manifestations of ARF include abnormalities of mental status that can progress rapidly to disorientation and confusion. Fixed attitudes, torpor, and other signs of toxic psychosis are common, and if they are untreated, uremic coma often supervenes. Other clinical findings include cranial nerve signs such as nystagmus, transient mild facial asymmetries, visual field defects, and papilledema of the optic fundi. About one half of the patients have dysarthria, and many have diffuse weakness and fasciculations. Marked asymmetrical variation of deep tendon reflexes is noted in most patients. Progression of hyperreflexia, with sustained clonus at the patella or ankle, is common and is an absolute indication for renal replacement therapy. The EEG is usually grossly abnormal with marked enhancement of delta slow wave activity. Although many factors contribute to uremic encephalopathy, investigators have shown no correlation between encephalopathy and any of the commonly measured indicators of renal failure (e.g., blood urea nitrogen, creatinine, bicarbonate, arterial pH, and potassium). Parathyroid hormone has been postulated to be a possible mediator of uremic brain dysfunction.

NEUROLOGIC COMPLICATIONS OF END-STAGE RENAL DISEASE AND ITS THERAPY

Dialysis Dysequilibrium Syndrome

In patients with ESRD, several CNS disorders may occur as a consequence of dialysis therapy. DDS is a clinical syndrome that typically occurs in patients with severe uremia who are undergoing an initial hemodialysis treatment. The classic symptoms include headache, nausea, emesis, blurring of vision, muscular twitching, disorientation, hypertension, tremors, and seizures. However, milder symptoms, such as muscle cramps, anorexia, restlessness, and dizziness, may occur. Although DDS has been reported in all age-groups, it is more common among younger patients, particularly the pediatric age-group. The syndrome is most often associated with rapid hemodialysis of patients with ARF and rapid correction of serum osmolality, but it also has occasionally been reported after maintenance hemodialysis of patients with CRF. The symptoms are usually self-limited, but recovery may take several days.

The key to avoiding DDS is the gradual institution of dialysis. The target reduction in blood urea nitrogen levels after the first dialysis treatment should not exceed 40%. The precise prescription of dialysis to achieve this outcome includes consideration of variables such as membrane size, blood flow rate, and duration of treatment. Isolated ultrafiltration can continue for a longer period if volume removal is the critical management issue. Other less widely used options include the intravenous infusion of mannitol or glycerol. Administration of 50 mL of 50% mannitol at the initiation and after 2 hours of the initial three hemodialysis treatments has generally been successful in preventing symptoms of DDS. The use of lower clearance targets in initial hemodialysis treatments has led to a sharp decline in reports of seizures, coma, and death, and most presentations of DDS are generally mild, consisting of nausea, weakness, headache, fatigue, and muscle cramps. It is important to recognize that the diagnosis of DDS should be one of exclusion, and a differential diagnosis of patients presenting with these symptoms is shown in Table 29–2.

Dialysis Dementia

Dialysis dementia (also called dialysis encephalopathy) is a progressive, often fatal neurologic disease that has been reported almost exclusively in patients being treated with chronic hemodialysis. The syndrome is not alleviated by increased frequency of dialysis or by renal transplantation. The etiology has not been elucidated and although an increase in brain aluminum

Table 29–2: Differential Diagnosis of Dialysis Disequilibrium Syndrome

Subdural hematoma
Uremia
Acute cerebrovascular accident
Dialysis dementia
Cardiac arrhythmia
Malfunction of fluid-proportioning system
Hypoglycemia
Hypercalcemia
Hyponatremia

content has been strongly implicated in some patients with dialysis dementia, it is not the sole etiologic factor. Additional possible causes of dialysis dementia include other trace element contaminants, normal-pressure hydrocephalus, slow viral infection of the CNS, and regional alterations in cerebral blood flow. There are at least three subgroups, and in two of them the etiology of dialysis encephalopathy must be regarded as unknown:

- An epidemic form that is related to aluminum contamination of the dialysate
- Sporadic endemic cases in which aluminum intoxication is unlikely to be a contributory factor
- Dementia associated with congenital or early childhood renal disease that may represent developmental neurologic defects resulting from exposure of the growing brain to a uremic environment

At this time, there is no known satisfactory treatment for patients with dialysis encephalopathy. Most patients reported on in the literature have not survived, usually dying within 18 months from the time of diagnosis.

Clinical Manifestations of Dialysis Dementia

Dialysis dementia is not usually seen before 2 years of hemodialysis treatment. Early clinical manifestations consist of a mixed dysarthria-apraxia of speech with slurring, stuttering, and hesitancy. Personality changes include psychoses, progressing to dementia, myoclonus, and seizures. Symptoms initially are intermittent and are often worse during dialysis, but eventually become constant. In most patients, the disease progresses to death within 12 to 18 months. Early in the disease, the EEG shows multifocal bursts of high-amplitude delta activity with spikes and sharp waves, intermixed with runs of more normal-appearing background activity. These EEG abnormalities may precede overt clinical symptoms by 6 months. The EEG has been said to be pathognomonic, but a similar pattern may also be seen in other metabolic encephalopathies. The diagnosis depends on the presence of the typical clinical picture and is confirmed by the characteristic EEG.

Aluminum and Dialysis Dementia

Aluminum intoxication was first implicated in the development of this disorder in the mid-1970s. The aluminum content of brain gray matter in patients with dialysis dementia is 11 times that of normal individuals and 4 times that of unaffected patients receiving chronic hemodialysis. This was a significant finding because in Alzheimer's disease aluminum accumulates in protein moieties of neurofibrillary tangles and in amyloid cores of senile plaques. Senile plaques and neurofibrillary tangles, diagnostic features of Alzheimer's disease, are also observed in most patients with dialysis dementia. However, in contrast to Alzheimer's disease, the aluminum is located not in the neurons but rather in glial cells and the walls of blood vessels. Oral phosphate binders containing aluminum were originally suspected as the source of aluminum. Subsequent reports of outbreaks of dementia in dialysis patients in association with significant aluminum contamination of the local water supply identified the dialysate as another potential source. The increased total body burden of aluminum is not restricted to neural tissue, and high levels are also found in bone and other soft tissues. It is unclear how aluminum enters the brain. Even with high blood aluminum levels, most is bound to transferrin and therefore cannot bind to the cerebral transferrin receptors. Thus, perhaps patients who develop dialysis dementia have less transferrin-binding capacity, less transferrin, or a greater density of transferrin receptors in the brain. The plasma aluminum level is poorly correlated with the degree of tissue aluminum deposition, and the diagnosis of aluminum toxicity is usually suggested by a rise in plasma aluminum concentration (>200 ng/mL) after intravenous infusion of desferrioxamine (40 mg/kg).

Prevention and Treatment of Dialysis Dementia

Measures to limit aluminum exposure are the cornerstone of the prevention and treatment of dialysis dementia. The use of aluminum-based phosphate binders should be restricted to short courses in patients with refractory hyperphosphatemia and avoided completely in those suspected of having early clinical changes consistent with dialysis dementia. Lowering the dialysate aluminum to less than 20 mcg/L by deionization appears to prevent onset of the disease in patients, and it is now the standard of care. Among patients with overt disease, eliminating the source of aluminum has resulted in improvement in some but not all patients. The use of desferrioxamine to chelate aluminum or other trace elements is an experimental treatment and is currently under extensive investigation. There have been several reports of improvement in patients with dialysis dementia treated with deferoxamine, but these results have not been confirmed, and its current role is limited to the treatment of acute intoxication. Renal transplantation has generally not been helpful in patients with established dialysis dementia. Diazepam or clonazepam are useful in controlling seizure activity associated with the disease but become ineffective later on and do not alter the final outcome. Treatment of sporadic cases, in which

Table 29–3: Differential Diagnosis of Dialysis Dementia

Metabolic encephalopathies
   Hypercalcemia
   Hypophosphatemia
   Hypoglycemia
   Hyperosmolality
   Hyponatremia
   Symptomatic uremia
   Drug intoxications
   Trace metal intoxications
   Hyperparathyroidism
Hypertensive encephalopathy
Dialysis disequilibrium
Structural lesions of the brain
   Subdural hematoma
   Normal-pressure hydrocephalus
   Stroke

the etiology is not clear, is more difficult. Every effort should be made to identify a treatable cause. Dialysis dementia must be differentiated from other metabolic encephalopathies such as hypercalcemia and hypophosphatemia, hyperparathyroidism, acute heavy metal intoxications, and structural neurologic lesions such as subdural hematoma (Table 29–3).

Chronic Dialysis-Dependent Encephalopathy

It is currently not usual for patients receiving hemodialysis to survive for 25 years. However, among patients who have been undergoing hemodialysis for longer than 10 years, there is often mental deterioration, with markedly decreased intellectual capability, even without medical evidence of stroke. The collective syndrome of *chronic dialysis–dependent encephalopathy* is a combination of probable organic mental disorders plus psychiatric disorders commonly associated with hemodialysis. Although the exact etiology is unknown, the clinical manifestations include depression, impaired cognition, and visual deterioration. The recent use of advanced neuroimaging techniques has led to increased understanding of the changes in the human brain caused by uremia. Acute and subacute movement disorders have been observed in patients with ESRD. These have been associated with bilateral basal ganglia and internal capsule lesions. Cerebral atrophy has been observed in chronic hemodialysis patients, and it tends to worsen as dialysis therapy continues. Cerebral atrophy was previously thought to be associated with dialysis dementia, but this is apparently not the case. ESRD has also been reported to lead to deterioration of vision. Some cases are associated with uremic pseudotumor cerebri, and in these selected patients, surgical optic nerve fenestration may improve visual loss. There is probably a loss of neurons that is not detectable by techniques currently in common use, and several well-studied pathophysiologic mechanisms probably contribute to the potential loss of brain tissue in patients with chronic dialysis–dependent encephalopathy including oxidative stress, inflammation, hyperhomocysteinemia, and neuronal apoptosis.

OTHER CENTRAL NERVOUS SYSTEM COMPLICATIONS OF DIALYSIS

Subdural Hematoma

Subdural hematoma is a rare cause of death in patients maintained with chronic hemodialysis. This condition presents with headache, drowsiness, nausea, and vomiting and may proceed to loss of consciousness with clinical signs of increased intracranial pressure. On physical examination, evidence of localized neurologic disease is often seen; there may be signs of meningeal irritation, and somnolence and focal seizures may be observed. The diagnosis of a subdural hematoma can usually be made by computed tomography or magnetic resonance imaging, and this diagnosis should be entertained as a possible cause of altered mental status, particularly in dialysis patients taking anticoagulants. Rapid diagnosis and operative intervention are required if a fatal outcome is to be averted.

Technical Dialysis Errors

Improper proportioning of dialysate, due to human or mechanical error, is an important cause of neurologic abnormality in dialysis patients. The usual effect of such mistakes is the production of hyponatremia or hypernatremia. Either of these abnormalities of body fluid osmolality can lead to seizures and coma, although different mechanisms are involved. In acute hypernatremia, there is excessive thirst, lethargy, irritability, seizures, and coma, with spasticity and muscle rigidity. In acute hyponatremia, there is weakness, fatigue, and dulled sensorium, which may also progress to seizures and coma, respiratory arrest, and death. Such symptoms developing soon after initiation of hemodialysis should alert the physician to the possibility of an error. A check of the dialysate osmolality or sodium concentration is the most rapid means of detecting this problem. Overly aggressive ultrafiltration in dialysis patients, particularly in those with diastolic dysfunction and large vessel arteriolosclerosis, may trigger overt hypotension. This can manifest as seizures which, although actually caused by cerebrovascular insufficiency, may be mistaken for DDS, particularly in diabetic subjects.

Stroke

Key to the high incidence of stroke in patients with ESRD is the coincidence of many of the known risk factors for stroke in this population including hypertension, cigarette use, diabetes mellitus, and hyperlipidemia. As with the general population, most preventive interventions in patients with CKD focus on cardiovascular risk factor minimization. More specific interventions include screening of patients who have renal failure for the presence of carotid stenosis or for the presence of large atherosclerotic plaques (>4 mm thick), which are important predictors for the possibility of stroke in the future. Clinical examination and electrocardiography can diagnose the presence of atrial fibrillation, another major risk factor for stroke. Migraine is a common clinical disorder, often characterized by an aura, headache, and autonomic dysfunction. In patients with ESRD, headache is common, and the possible association with impending stroke may not be recognized. Transient ischemic attacks are often associated with numbness, weakness, or partial blindness. Such symptoms occur in patients with ESRD, particularly if they also have diabetes mellitus, and it may not be generally recognized that they are often the harbinger of stroke. The presence of such a symptom complex should trigger a workup that includes evaluation of the carotid arteries (ultrasound, computed tomography, or magnetic resonance imaging).

Therapy for Stroke in CKD/ESRD

As in patients without renal dysfunction, in many patients, acute stroke can be successfully treated if timely therapy is initiated. An initial computed tomography scan usually reveals acute stroke and serves to differentiate occlusive from hemorrhagic stroke. If a nonhemorrhagic stroke is present, treatment prospects can be examined with magnetic resonance angiography, which is noninvasive and avoids the nephrotoxicity of intravenous radiocontrast material. If acute stroke is diagnosed within an appropriate time window (within 3 hours after onset of symptoms), current treatments may include the administration of thrombolytic therapy, antithrombotic and antiplatelet drugs, defibrinating agents, and neuroprotective drugs. Importantly, some cases of apparent acute stroke in dialysis patients are caused by subdural hematoma, which must always be considered in the differential diagnosis of stroke in dialysis patients.

SEXUAL DYSFUNCTION IN UREMIA

Pathogenesis of Uremic Sexual Dysfunction

Disturbances in sexual function including erectile dysfunction, decreased libido, and decreased frequency of intercourse are common complications of CKD. Sexual dysfunction is observed in at least 50% of male patients receiving maintenance hemodialysis. A number of abnormalities associated with renal failure appear to be important in the genesis of impotence, including autonomic nervous system dysfunction, impairment in arterial and venous systems of the penis, hypertension, drug-related side effects, and other associated endocrine abnormalities.

Therapy for Sexual Dysfunction in Uremia

The management of sexual dysfunction in the patient with renal disease must address the underlying cause and exacerbating factors. Many drugs used to treat hypertension can lead to impotence, including calcium channel blockers and β-blockers, and this should be considered in any evaluation. It is also important to exclude undiagnosed depression because the incidence of mood disturbance is considerably higher in patients with advancing renal disease than in the general population. If these etiologic factors have been addressed and the problem persists, then treatment options include the use of sildenafil (Viagra), which is highly effective in men with ESRD. If this is unsuccessful, then other treatment options for impotence in men with ESRD include penile prostheses, direct injection of alprostadil into the penis, and vacuum constrictive devices.

UREMIC NEUROPATHY

Clinical Manifestations

Peripheral neuropathy is probably present in more than one half of patients with ESRD at the time of institution of dialysis. Many patients with CRF who are neurologically asymptomatic may exhibit abnormalities on physical examination including evidence of autonomic neuropathy, such as postural hypotension.

Moreover, in patients who have renal insufficiency, abnormal nerve conduction may be present in the absence of symptoms or abnormal findings on physical examination although the routine application of this examination is limited due to patient discomfort.

Uremic neuropathy is usually a distal, symmetrical, mixed polyneuropathy. In general, motor and sensory modalities are both affected, and lower extremities are more severely involved than are the upper extremities. Clinically, uremic polyneuropathy cannot be distinguished from the neuropathies associated with certain other metabolic disorders, such as diabetes mellitus, chronic alcoholism, and various deficiency states. The occurrence of neuropathy bears no relation to the type of underlying disease process (i.e., glomerulonephritis or pyelonephritis). However, certain diseases that can lead to renal failure may simultaneously affect peripheral nerve function in a manner separate from the manifestations of uremia. Such diseases include amyloidosis, multiple myeloma, systemic lupus erythematosus, polyarteritis, nodosa, diabetes mellitus, and hepatic failure. The clinical manifestations of uremic neuropathy usually appears when the glomerular filtration rate falls below 12 mL/min.

Peripheral Nerves

The restless leg syndrome is a common early manifestation of CRF. Clinically, patients experience sensations in the lower extremities such as crawling, prickling, and pruritus. The sensations are worse distally than proximally and are generally more prominent in the evening. Another symptom experienced by patients with early uremic neuropathy is the burning foot syndrome, which is present in fewer than 10% of patients with CRF. Rather than "burning," the actual symptoms consist of swelling sensations, constriction, and tenderness of the distal lower extremities. The physical signs of peripheral nerve dysfunction often begin with loss of deep tendon reflexes, particularly knee and ankle jerks. Impaired vibratory sensation is also an early sign of uremic neuropathy. Loss of sensation in the lower leg is common and often takes the form of "stocking glove" anesthesia of the lower leg. The sensory loss includes pain, light touch, vibration, and pressure.

Metabolic Neuropathy

Uremic neuropathy is one of a group of central-peripheral axonopathies, also known as dying-back polyneuropathies, which include neuropathies associated with diabetes, multiple myeloma, and certain hereditary polyneuropathies. There is also an associated degeneration of the spinal cord, particularly involving posterior columns, as well as other portions of the CNS. The clinical characteristics of such distal axonopathies include the following:

1. Insidious onset
2. Onset in legs
3. Stocking-glove sensory loss
4. Early loss of Achilles reflex
5. Moderate slowing of motor nerve conduction
6. Normal cerebrospinal fluid protein content
7. Slow recovery
8. Residual disability

In addition to uremic neuropathy, uremic myopathy is a common cause of weakness, exercise limitation, and rapid-onset tiredness in dialysis patients. Later on, muscle wasting occurs, particularly in the limb muscles.

Renal Osteodystrophy

30

Renal osteodystrophy is the term used to describe the many different patterns of skeletal abnormalities that can occur in the course of chronic kidney disease (CKD). The abnormalities include the following:

- Osteitis fibrosa
- Adynamic bone disease
- Osteomalacia related to aluminum accumulation
- Mixed renal osteodystrophy

Osteitis fibrosa is a manifestation of the effects of high levels of parathyroid hormone (PTH) on bone and is associated with a high rate of bone turnover, whereas adynamic bone is characterized by an extremely low bone turnover rate. These patterns of bony abnormalities may occur together, leading to the designation of mixed renal osteodystrophy, a disorder with some signs of secondary hyperparathyroidism associated with mineralization defects. In addition, the skeleton may be affected by other processes associated with the management of end-stage renal disease, such as amyloidosis, postmenopausal osteoporosis, or osteoporosis resulting from corticosteroid therapy.

PATHOGENESIS OF RENAL OSTEODYSTROPHY

Secondary Hyperparathyroidism (High Bone Turnover Renal Osteodystrophy)

Hyperplasia of the parathyroid glands and increased levels of PTH in blood occur early in the course of CKD and are associated with histologic bone changes even in patients with mild to moderate CKD. Under normal circumstances, the concentration of ionized calcium in blood is the principal determinant of the rate of PTH secretion. In the presence of kidney disease, however, a constellation of factors contribute to altering the regulation of PTH secretion including hyperphosphatemia, hypocalcemia, low 1,25-dihydroxyvitamin D_3 (calcitriol) levels, and intrinsic abnormalities of the parathyroid gland.

Adynamic Bone and Osteomalacia (Low Bone Turnover Renal Osteodystrophy)

The low bone turnover skeletal disorders in patients with renal failure include adynamic bone, which is characterized by an extremely slow rate of bone formation, and osteomalacia, which is characterized by a slow rate of bone formation with marked defects in bone mineralization, reflected by an increased volume of nonmineralized bone matrix.

Adynamic Bone
The pathogenesis of adynamic bone probably includes a number of factors. However, primary among these factors is relative hypoparathyroidism. Although PTH levels are higher than those in subjects with normal renal function, they are significantly lower in patients with adynamic bone disease than in patients with other types of renal osteodystrophy. A variety of factors may contribute to this relative degree of hypoparathyroidism, such as better phosphate control with the use of calcium-containing phosphate binders, treatment with vitamin D, older age, and the presence of diabetes, which appears to be associated with low bone turnover even in the absence of renal failure.

Low-Turnover Osteomalacia
Substantial epidemiologic and experimental evidence indicates that low-turnover osteomalacia is related to aluminum intoxication. The incidence of aluminum-related bone disease has decreased markedly in recent years, as water purification standards for hemodialysis have been improved. Although many patients with aluminum-related bone disease have osteomalacia, some also appear to have adynamic bone, possibly related to the toxic effects of aluminum on osteoblast function, as well as the inhibitory effects of aluminum on the parathyroid gland.

Other Factors That May Affect the Skeleton in Chronic Renal Failure

Metabolic Acidosis
Metabolic acidosis is common in advanced CKD and may affect bone by liberation of bone mineral as hydrogen ions are buffered

by bone carbonate. In addition, acidosis may enhance osteoclast-mediated bone resorption and inhibit osteoblast-mediated bone formation.

Corticosteroids

It is well recognized that the use of glucocorticoids, which have a suppressive effect on bone formation, is associated with loss of bone and an increased risk of fracture. In the course of chronic renal disease, many patients have received corticosteroid therapy, and its use complicates the manifestation of renal osteodystrophy.

CLINICAL SIGNS AND SYMPTOMS OF RENAL OSTEODYSTROPHY

Bone disease in patients with CKD is usually asymptomatic and symptoms appear only late in the course of renal failure. Symptoms are insidious in onset and nonspecific in nature at first. By the time symptoms appear, significant biochemical abnormalities and severe histologic changes are usually present.

Bone Pain

With advances in the management of hyperphosphatemia and hyperparathyroidism, bone pain is no longer a prominent symptom of renal osteodystrophy. If present, it often develops insidiously and may present as a nonspecific ache. The most severe bone pain occurs with osteomalacia, particularly when it is associated with aluminum deposition. The pain is usually vague and may be diffuse or localized to the low back, hips, knees, and legs. Back pain may represent vertebral collapse and fractures with minimal trauma. Physical findings are usually absent, but occasionally localized bone tenderness may be demonstrated.

Myopathy and Muscle Weakness

Proximal muscle weakness is associated with secondary hyper-parathyroidism, phosphate depletion, and, potentially, vitamin D deficiency. This can be a serious and debilitating problem in patients with advanced renal failure. Some clinical improvement has been demonstrated after vitamin D repletion.

Spontaneous Tendon Rupture

Spontaneous rupture of tendons has been noted in patients with long-standing renal disease undergoing dialysis, and it usually has been associated with evidence of severe secondary hyperparathyroidism. The quadriceps or triceps tendons and the Achilles tendon have been the tendons most commonly described, but the condition may also involve the extensor tendons of the fingers.

Pruritus

Itching is a common symptom in patients with renal failure. It may reflect the presence of a high level of PTH, hypercalcemia, and a high calcium-phosphorus product ($Ca \times P$) or metastatic calcifications. The mechanism whereby secondary hyperparathyroidism leads to pruritus is not fully understood; however, rapid improvement after surgery in some patients suggests a direct effect of PTH.

Metastatic and Extraskeletal Calcifications

Extraskeletal calcifications have been observed in patients with CKD for many years and may occur either in damaged tissue (dystrophic calcification) or in apparently normal tissue. In recent years, the potential clinical consequences of soft tissue calcification, particularly those involving the cardiovascular system, have received increased focus (see Chapter 28, Cardiovascular Aspects of Chronic Kidney Disease).

Clinical Manifestations

CALCIFICATION OF THE SKIN AND CALCIPHYLAXIS Calcification in the skin may result in severe pruritus, which is believed to be associated with an elevated $Ca \times P$ value. Skin arteriolar calcification may also manifest as acute skin necrosis, calciphylaxis, which can result in gangrene and has a poor prognosis. This syndrome is better termed *calcific uremic arteriolopathy* and manifests with the development of painful areas on the lower extremities, trunk, or buttocks that become violaceous, mottled, and indurated and subsequently ulcerate. Skin biopsy demonstrates calcification within the arterioles, and fat necrosis may be evident. The exact etiology of this disorder is unclear. Risk factors include hyperparathyroidism, the use of vitamin D analogs, obesity, and diabetes mellitus. Although this disorder had been associated with severe hyperparathyroidism, many cases occur in the absence of hyperparathyroidism at the time of diagnosis. The clinical appearance of these lesions is similar to that seen with warfarin skin necrosis, which suggests a role for altered coagulation, particularly in the protein C and protein S pathways, in the final manifestations of this problem. The management of calciphylaxis is discussed later.

OCULAR CALCIFICATION Calcifications are often found in the cornea and conjunctiva and rarely produce symptoms. However, they may lead to complaints of dry or gritty eyes or erythema of the conjunctiva.

CALCIFICATION OF JOINTS The periarticular structures are often involved in calcification in patients with renal failure. The articular cartilage may become calcified, which may lead to significant symptoms and is manifested as pseudogout.

CALCIFICATION OF THE CARDIOVASCULAR SYSTEM Cardiovascular calcification is extremely common in patients with end-stage renal disease and may contribute to the higher mortality rate in this patient group by adding to peripheral ischemia, impaired myocardial function, coronary artery disease, cardiac valvular dysfunction, sudden death, and other cardiovascular events such as stroke. Vascular calcifications appear to be associated with hyperphosphatemia and an elevated $Ca \times P$ value. Calcification of coronary arteries is best visualized and quantitated by electron-beam computed tomography. High electron-beam computed tomography scores, indicating severe coronary artery calcification in young dialysis patients, are associated with high calcium intake, an elevated $Ca \times P$ product, and a low bone turnover state. The clinical implications of this condition have not been fully elucidated.

Dialysis-Associated Amyloidosis

Amyloid deposition in articular and periarticular tissues can result in a disabling arthropathy in patients who have been receiving dialysis for a long period. The amyloid deposition is composed of β_2-microglobulin fibrils. Although amyloid deposits may be present for a number of years before the onset of symptoms, the clinical manifestations of β_2-microglobulin amyloidosis usually occur after 8 to 12 years of hemodialysis, and it affects more than 50% of patients. Clinical manifestations are typically insidious in onset and include carpal tunnel syndrome, shoulder arthralgia, chronic tenosynovitis of the finger flexors, and chronic swelling of the knees, shoulders, wrists, fingers, and elbows.

Destructive arthropathies may also be part of the β_2-microglobulin amyloid syndrome and are manifested by subchondral bone erosions, often in locations such as hip, knee, or spine. These are often asymptomatic and remain undiagnosed for many years, but they can result in pain or even spontaneous fractures.

β_2-Microglobulin amyloid may be suspected when radiographic examination reveals subchondral bone cysts or erosions that increase in size or number over time and appear to have a symmetrical distribution. The diagnosis of β_2-microglobulin amyloidosis is made by its characteristic histologic appearance with Congo red stain, which can be followed with precise typing of the amyloid by immunohistochemical analysis.

BIOCHEMICAL FEATURES OF RENAL OSTEODYSTROPHY

Histologic examination of undecalcified sections of bone is the gold standard for the diagnosis of renal osteodystrophy, but this is rarely performed. Imaging studies have limited clinical utility for the diagnosis of renal osteodystrophy. Therefore, it becomes important to evaluate biochemical parameters related to bone and mineral metabolism early in the course of CKD.

Serum Calcium and Phosphorus Levels

Serum Phosphorus
The progressive reduction in glomerular filtration rate (GFR) observed during the course of CKD results in phosphate retention. However, hyperphosphatemia is not a prominent metabolic abnormality early in the course of CKD, owing to the phosphaturic action of PTH. Hyperphosphatemia has a tendency to occur once the GFR has decreased to 20% of normal at which time the renal excretory capacity becomes inadequate to handle dietary intake of phosphorus. Treatment of secondary hyperparathyroidism with vitamin D compounds may adversely affect serum phosphorus levels by enhancing phosphate absorption by the intestine as well as through the actions of PTH on bone remodeling. Monitoring of the serum phosphorus concentration is not very helpful in establishing the diagnosis of a specific type of renal osteodystrophy. However, ensuring adequate phosphate control is a crucial therapeutic intervention because hyperphosphatemia may aggravate hyperparathyroidism by decreasing the levels of ionized calcium, decreasing the synthesis of calcitriol, and directly increasing PTH secretion.

Serum Calcium
In advanced CKD, the total serum calcium concentration may decrease below the normal range; however, this is not a universal finding. Regardless of the etiology of hypocalcemia, it is important

to correct the serum calcium concentration during the course of CKD, because it is a very important stimulus for PTH secretion. Hypercalcemia in patients with CKD may suggest low bone turnover osteodystrophy (osteomalacia and adynamic bone disease). In these patients, the hypercalcemia often becomes manifest after administration of low doses of vitamin D compounds or calcium supplements. As a result of the low bone turnover, the excess calcium absorbed from the intestine may not be deposited in the bone, leading to the development of hypercalcemia. Severe secondary hyperparathyroidism is also associated with hypercalcemia, as is persistent hyperparathyroidism after successful renal transplantation. Although elevations in serum calcium may suggest abnormal bone turnover, hypercalcemia in CKD is often the result of therapeutic strategies used in the management of renal osteodystrophy. The intestinal absorption of calcium may increase after the administration of calcium-containing phosphate binders, because oral calcium administration increases calcium absorption by ionic diffusion. The increase in serum calcium level may be more pronounced when calcium salts are administered in conjunction with vitamin D compounds, because the latter increase calcium transport by the intestinal cells. Elevated serum calcium concentrations may suppress PTH secretion, leading to relative hypoparathyroidism, which may in turn contribute to the development of low-turnover osteodystrophy.

Assay for Parathyroid Hormone

Accurate assessment of the activity of the parathyroid glands is essential for the monitoring and management of hyperparathyroidism. Interpretation of early immunoassays for PTH was complicated by the fact that PTH circulates not only in the form of the intact 84-amino acid peptide but also as multiple fragments of the hormone, particularly from the middle and COOH-terminal regions of the PTH molecule. More recently, this problem has been largely overcome by two-site immunoradiometric assays, and therefore the threshold for initiation of calcitriol therapy in CKD has been lowered.

Biologic Markers of Bone Formation

Total Alkaline Phosphatase

Measurement of total alkaline phosphatase may provide an index of osteoblastic bone formation, because increased total alkaline phosphatase in this patient population is often the result of increases in the bone-specific isoform. Although high levels of alkaline phosphatase have been shown to correlate with PTH levels and histologic findings of hyperparathyroid bone disease, wide variation has been seen in most studies examining the correlation of total alkaline phosphatase with levels of PTH and histologic parameters of bone formation. However, the total alkaline phosphatase level may be useful for monitoring the progression of bone disease as well as the response to therapy.

Bone-Specific Alkaline Phosphatase

The development of monoclonal antibodies specific for bone alkaline phosphatase has allowed the opportunity to evaluate its usefulness as an index of bone formation. Preliminary studies in hemodialysis patients have demonstrated that bone-specific alkaline phosphatase is better correlated than PTH or total alkaline phosphatase with histomorphometric parameters of bone formation and bone resorption and may in the future be helpful in the diagnosis of both high- and low-turnover renal osteodystrophy, especially when examined in conjunction with PTH levels.

Aluminum Levels and the Desferrioxamine Test

The measurement of basal serum aluminum levels is of limited diagnostic value in identifying patients with aluminum-related bone disease, because these levels are affected by recent aluminum load and are less indicative of aluminum toxicity. Because aluminum is deposited in several organs including bone, brain, heart, and liver, the measurement of the increment in serum aluminum level after a standardized infusion of desferrioxamine has been used to assess tissue stores of aluminum and to identify patients who have a high risk for aluminum-related bone disease. However, the desferrioxamine test has been shown not to be a reliable indicator of aluminum-related bone disease in the absence of determinations of PTH levels. An increase in serum aluminum level of more than 50 mcg/L after the infusion of desferrioxamine (5 mg/kg) combined with a PTH level greater than 650 pg/mL (70 pmol/L) is consistent with aluminum overload but not with aluminum-related bone disease. On the other hand, the same increment in serum aluminum level accompanied by a PTH level lower than 650 pg/mL (70 pmol/L) points to the presence of aluminum-related bone disease. The combination of an increment in serum aluminum level of greater than 50 mcg/L (1.9 mcmol/L) and an intact PTH level of less than 150 pg/mL (16.5 pmol/L) has a sensitivity and specificity of 87% and 95% for detecting aluminum bone disease.

RADIOGRAPHIC FEATURES OF RENAL OSTEODYSTROPHY

Considerable amounts of bone mineral can be lost before there is obvious radiologic change and radiologic features do not correlate well with histologic appearance. Therefore, routine use of skeletal radiographs for screening of bone disease in patients with CKD has limited value.

Hyperparathyroid Bone Disease

One of the principal radiologic features of secondary hyperparathyroidism is evidence of subperiosteal bone resorption. The earliest lesions often appear in the middle phalanges of the second or third digits. As the lesions progress, the erosions may extend along the bone and involve other sites. These erosions are asymptomatic but are occasionally associated with synovitis or symptoms of joint pain. Subperiosteal erosions may also be seen in the tibia, the neck of the femur, the humerus, the pelvic bones, and the distal ends of the clavicles. Bone resorption in the skull produces a mottled, lucent appearance commonly associated with areas of osteosclerosis, giving the appearance of a "pepper-pot skull." These erosions usually do not heal rapidly after therapy for high-turnover bone disease, and remineralization may be extremely slow, even after successful therapy for the underlying metabolic abnormality.

Hyperparathyroidism can also be associated with cystic lesions of bone that may represent brown tumors (osteoclastomas). These may be accompanied by pain, and there is a need to distinguish these lesions from malignant tumors, metastases, or cysts associated with amyloidosis. With correction of the underlying metabolic abnormality, these cystic areas may be replaced by areas of sclerosis. Alteration of trabecular volume of spongy bone may lead to osteosclerosis. This is generally apparent in vertebrae, pelvis, skull, clavicle, humerus, and proximal and distal femur and tibia. These areas of osteosclerosis in the spine lead to the characteristic "rugger-jersey" appearance on lateral view. Osteosclerosis also contribute to the salt-and-pepper appearance of the skull.

Osteomalacia

The pathognomonic feature of osteomalacia in adults is pseudofractures or Looser zones. These are straight bands of radiolucency that are usually perpendicular to the long axis of the bone. They may be bilateral, and they are sometimes associated with a small, poorly mineralizing callus. Pseudofractures may also be seen in the pubic rami, scapulae, or ribs. Spontaneous stress fractures occur in the metatarsals and ribs and are often painful. Deformities of the long bones, characteristic of rickets, may also be seen, especially in children and young adults. The features of secondary hyperparathyroidism may also be associated with these features of osteomalacia.

Osteopenia

A common radiographic feature of renal bone disease is decreased bone mineral density. This is a nonspecific finding that can be seen in either high- or low-turnover bone disease. Osteopenia may result in fractures, particularly in the vertebrae; crush fractures can result in deformities of the vertebrae.

Metastatic Calcification

Radiographs may reveal extraskeletal calcifications in patients with CKD. Calcification may be manifested in organs such as the heart, lungs, and skeletal muscle. Metastatic calcification is more commonly observed in large blood vessels such as the aorta, iliac, and femoral arteries and in the arteries of the extremities. Calcification can also be found in periarticular sites such as the hips or shoulders.

Dialysis-Related Amyloidosis

The radiologic features of dialysis-related amyloidosis are present long before the onset of symptoms. They are usually manifested as bone cysts, and periarticular cystic bone lesions may be seen in the wrist or tarsal bone, femoral or humeral head, distal radius, acetabulum, pubic symphysis, or tibial plateau. These lesions are characteristic but are not pathognomonic for dialysis-related amyloidosis, and they need to be differentiated from other cystic lesions. Amyloid-related cysts often involve the large synovial joints, and subchondral cysts are more characteristic of amyloidosis. These cysts may also be demonstrated by computed tomography or magnetic resonance imaging techniques, which can be useful for evaluating the extent of disease, particularly in the spine and femoral neck.

Destructive Spondyloarthropathy

Spondyloarthropathy, usually affecting the cervical spine, may be seen in patients who have been receiving dialysis for a prolonged period. A reduction in the disc space with destruction or sclerosis of the adjacent vertebral end plates are seen. These findings need to be distinguished from infective osteomyelitis, and other imaging techniques (e.g., magnetic resonance imaging) may be helpful.

Quantitative Measurements of Bone Mineral Content

Dual radiograph absorptiometry, quantitative ultrasonography, and quantitative computed tomography scanning are noninvasive methods used for the quantification of bone mineral density that have been widely applied in patient populations without renal disease. Their role in the diagnosis and management of renal osteodystrophy remains limited because they only measure bone density and provide no information about bone structure or bone cell activity and they have not, as yet, been shown to predict clinical outcomes in patients with renal bone disease.

Bone Biopsy

Bone biopsy is the gold standard for the classification and diagnosis of renal osteodystrophy. Because it is an invasive technique, it is not in widespread clinical use. However, if a diagnosis cannot be made with the use of noninvasive parameters, a bone biopsy should be considered.

PREVENTION AND MANAGEMENT OF RENAL OSTEODYSTROPHY

The objectives for the management of abnormal divalent ion metabolism and bone disease in patients with kidney failure are as follows:

1. To maintain the blood levels of calcium and phosphorus as close to normal as possible
2. To prevent the development of parathyroid hyperplasia, or if secondary hyperparathyroidism has already developed, to suppress the secretion of PTH
3. To prevent extraskeletal deposition of calcium
4. To prevent or reverse the accumulation of substances such as aluminum and iron, which can adversely affect the skeleton

Management of Phosphorus

The dietary phosphorus intake can be lowered in proportion to the decrease in GFR in patients with mild renal insufficiency primarily by restricting the intake of dairy products and by adherence to a low-phosphate diet. In patients with advanced CKD or end-stage renal disease, dietary restriction alone is typically ineffective. Consequently, most dialysis patients use phosphate binders to reduce the amount of phosphorus absorbed and achieve a normal serum phosphorus concentration (3.5 to 4.5 mg/dL [1.13 to 1.45 mmol/L]). A $Ca \times P$ exceeding 60 mg^2/dL^2 is associated with a higher mortality in patients with end-stage renal disease. Therefore, it is critical that serum phosphorus be controlled within the normal range and that attempts are made to maintain a $Ca \times P$ of less than 55 mg^2/dL^2. At the same time, it is important that the total amount of calcium ingested by the patient (dietary calcium plus calcium-containing phosphate binders) is no greater than 2 g/day, because high calcium intake has been associated with cardiovascular complications.

Aluminum as a Phosphate Binder

Aluminum-containing compounds that bind phosphorus in the intestinal tract include aluminum hydroxide and aluminum carbonate gels. However, the use of large amounts of aluminum for long periods is associated with significant bone, hematologic, and neurologic toxicity. Therefore, the administration of aluminum-based binders should be restricted to brief courses (<1 week) when control of severe hyperphosphatemia cannot be achieved using non–aluminum-based binders and dialysis alone. The serum aluminum level in dialysis patients should always be maintained at less than 20 mcg/L (0.74 mcmol/L).

Calcium Carbonate as a Phosphate Binder

Calcium carbonate is an effective phosphate binder. It should be taken with meals, both to increase its efficiency as a phosphate binder and to minimize the absorption of calcium and the risk of hypercalcemia. Transient episodes of hypercalcemia are often observed during therapy with calcium carbonate, and the administration of large amounts of calcium carbonate may increase the risk of hypercalcemia and extraskeletal cardiovascular calcification. The risk of hypercalcemia in hemodialysis patients taking calcium-based binders may be reduced by using a dialysate calcium concentration of 2.5 mEq/L. Importantly, calcium carbonate dissolves only in acid media, and administration of proton pump inhibitors or H_2-receptor antagonists may limit its efficiency.

Calcium Acetate as a Phosphate Binder

Calcium acetate binds phosphorus more efficiently than calcium carbonate or calcium citrate. However, the overall incidence of hypercalcemia is the same with each formulation. The solubility of calcium acetate is not pH dependent.

Calcium Citrate as a Phosphate Binder
Calcium citrate has also been shown to be an effective phosphate-binding agent, but it increases aluminum absorption. Therefore, calcium citrate should not be given to patients with renal failure, especially if there is a possibility that they may also ingest aluminum-containing drugs.

Sevelamer Hydrochloride as a Phosphate Binder
Sevelamer hydrochloride (Renagel) is a novel phosphate binder that is now widely available. It is completely resistant to intestinal digestion and is not absorbed in the gastrointestinal tract. Sevelamer effectively and safely lowers the serum phosphate concentration without changing the serum calcium level. Long-term studies have also shown a decrease in low-density lipoprotein and an increase in high-density lipoprotein cholesterol in patients treated with sevelamer. The mechanism may be similar to that of cholestyramine (i.e., binding of bile salts). Of great potential clinical importance is the finding that control of phosphorus with sevelamer is associated with a lower incidence of iatrogenic hypercalcemia and vascular calcification (coronary artery/aortic) than treatment with calcium-based binders. This finding strongly suggests that calcium load is an important factor associated with vascular calcification.

Management of Calcium

Dietary Calcium Supplements
Oral calcium supplementation is usually required in patients with advanced CKD because of a combination of impaired calcium absorption and suboptimal dietary quantities of calcium. In patients with advanced renal failure who have creatinine clearances lower than 10 mL/min and in patients undergoing regular dialysis, calcium supplementation is recommended to provide a maximum of 1.5 g of elemental calcium/day. The calcium supplements should be taken in several small doses throughout the day, rather than in one or two large doses. Also, ingestion of calcium supplements with meals that are high in phosphate should be limited if the goal is to augment intestinal absorption of calcium rather than to bind calcium phosphate in the intestine. The monitoring of serum calcium and phosphorus at biweekly or monthly intervals is important because of the variability in response of individual patients to a given amount of calcium.

Treatment with oral calcium supplements is not without risk. Patients with advanced renal failure who are given dietary supplements of calcium may develop hypercalcemia because they lack the mechanisms for increased urinary calcium excretion if calcium absorption increases more than expected. Calcium supplements should be given cautiously to patients with marked hyperphosphatemia because of the risk of increasing $Ca \times P$ and predisposing the patient to extraskeletal and cardiovascular calcifications. Hypercalcemia is more common in patients whose serum phosphorus levels are decreased to less than 2 to 3 mg/dL (0.65 to 1 mmol/L). Most uremic patients with moderate to advanced kidney failure and mild hypercalcemia are asymptomatic. However, these patients can develop pruritus and hypertension, in addition to the more common symptoms of nausea, anorexia, vomiting, mental confusion, and lethargy.

Dialysate Calcium Concentration

The level of calcium in the dialysate can affect serum calcium levels in patients treated with maintenance hemodialysis. In the past it was generally recommended that the dialysate calcium concentration be 3 to 3.5 mEq/L. However, these recommendations were for patients who ingested aluminum-containing phosphate-binding agents. In patients who use calcium carbonate or acetate as a phosphate binder or who use vitamin D preparations, there is considerable risk of hypercalcemia with the use of dialysate containing calcium concentrations greater than 2.5 mEq/L. A dialysate containing 2.5 mEq/L of calcium is now the standard of care. Lower calcium concentrations (1.5 to 2 mEq/L) may be indicated in patients with overt hypercalcemia or adynamic bone disease with a suppressed intact PTH level (<100 pg/mL). However, this course of action mandates close follow-up of the intact PTH and serum calcium levels and an aggressive search for the underlying cause of the hypercalcemia.

Use of Vitamin D Sterols

Decreases in calcitriol production play a major role in the generation and maintenance of secondary hyperparathyroidism, and, accordingly, the use of vitamin D sterols is a rational approach to its treatment. Because hyperparathyroidism begins relatively early in the course of CKD, it is important to assess patients for vitamin D deficiency early in the disease course. Relatively large amounts of vitamin D-binding protein may be lost in the urine of proteinuric patients, and this, coupled with poor dietary intake and lack of exposure to sunlight, may result in vitamin D deficiency. The overall vitamin D status is best assessed with measurements of 25-hydroxyvitamin D; if values are found to be less than 30 ng/mL, supplementation should be undertaken. Although it would be desirable to administer vitamin D, such as ergocalciferol, at a dose of 1000 to 2000 units/day, such preparations are not readily available in the United States; accordingly, a reasonable dose would be 50,000 units taken once a month.

Use of Calcitriol

As CKD progresses, hyperparathyroidism may require the use of active vitamin D sterols. The occurrence of hypercalcemia or aggravation of hyperphosphatemia (or both) by the use of active vitamin D sterols may be detrimental to residual renal function, so these drugs should be used with caution and monitored closely. Calcitriol (1,25-dihydroxyvitamin D_3) is the most active metabolite of vitamin D and it is an effective agent both orally and intravenously for the treatment of secondary hyperparathyroidism. The goal intact PTH level varies, depending on the level of residual renal function:

- Stage III CKD (GFR 30 to 59 mL/min); goal PTH is 35 to 70 pg/mL
- Stage IV CKD (GFR 15 to 29 mL/min); goal PTH is 70 to 110 pg/mL
- Stage V CKD (GFR < 15 mL/min); goal PTH is 150 to 300 pg/mL

The principal toxicities of calcitriol are hypercalcemia and hyperphosphatemia or both. These are common complications of therapy that may limit its use at doses that effectively suppress PTH levels. Treatment with an active calcitriol or any active vitamin D sterol should be undertaken only in patients with serum levels of corrected total calcium less than 9.5 mg/dL and serum phosphorus less than 4.6 mg/dL. The hypercalcemic toxicity of calcitriol is aggravated by the concomitant use of large doses of calcium-containing phosphate-binding antacids. Although in the United States most calcitriol therapy is administered by intermittent intravenous injection (0.5 to 3 mcg at dialysis), oral therapy (0.25 to 1 mcg/day) can also be used, and therapy with oral calcitriol in an intermittent fashion (oral pulse) can produce good results.

Vitamin D Prohormones

1α-Hydroxyvitamin D_3 or (α-calcidiol) is widely used outside the United States for the control of hyperparathyroidism. This vitamin D sterol becomes hydroxylated in the 25 position by the hepatic 25-hydroxylase, resulting in the production of 1,25-dihydroxyvitamin D_3. This sterol has been shown to be active in patients with CKD, and it has been used both orally and intravenously with good clinical effects, similar to those with calcitriol. 1αHydroxyvitamin D_2 is a similar prohormone, based on the vitamin D_2 structure, which also requires hydroxylation in the 25 position in the liver before it becomes an active vitamin D sterol.

Control of Metabolic Acidosis

A chronic metabolic acidosis is characteristic of stage IV to V CKD and is implicated in the loss of bone mineral. Patients with advanced CKD should have their serum levels of total CO_2 monitored often. Although the clinical data are not conclusive, National Kidney Foundation Kidney Disease Outcomes Quality Initiative (K/DOQI) guidelines suggest that total CO_2 should be maintained at greater than 22 mmol/L to prevent bone demineralization. As alluded to earlier, exogenous alkali salts containing citrate can increase the absorption of dietary aluminum in patients with CKD; therefore, citrate alkali salts should be avoided in patients with CKD who are exposed to aluminum salts.

Parathyroidectomy

Surgical removal of parathyroid tissue should be considered for patients with severe hyperparathyroidism manifested by very high levels of PTH (e.g., intact PTH >800 pg/mL), who have hypercalcemia and/or hyperphosphatemia or an elevated $Ca \times P$ that is resistant to or precludes medical therapy. Several surgical procedures have been described, including subtotal parathyroidectomy, subtotal parathyroidectomy with parathyroid tissue autotransplantation, and total parathyroidectomy. All of these approaches result in satisfactory reductions in PTH. Preoperative imaging of the parathyroid glands by technetium 99m-sestamibi, computed tomography, magnetic resonance imaging, or ultrasonography is not routinely performed by most surgeons and is usually reserved for reoperation.

Total parathyroidectomy is not widely performed, because there is a risk of inducing a low bone turnover state with this procedure. Persistent hyperparathyroidism immediately after surgery occurs in up to one fourth of patients and is usually due to a missed gland. Even after initially successful surgery, the recurrence of hyperparathyroidism may be as high as 30% after 5 years. Postoperatively, it is imperative to monitor the levels of calcium closely (e.g., every 6 hours for a few days), and a calcium infusion should be given, if necessary, to maintain the levels of ionized calcium between 4.6 and 5.4 mg/dL (1.15 to 1.36 mmol/L). Patients may require high doses of oral calcium supplementation (up to 4 g of elemental calcium or higher per day). Calcitriol should be continued either orally or intravenously, and up to 5 mcg/day may be required to normalize serum calcium levels. Phosphate supplementation may also be necessary if hypophosphatemia occurs.

Integrated Management of Renal Osteodystrophy

Hyperparathyroidism begins early in the course of renal insufficiency, and, accordingly, monitoring of parathyroid activity should begin when the GFR is initially decreased. If PTH levels are elevated, it is reasonable to evaluate vitamin D status by measurement of 25-hydroxyvitamin D levels; if the result is less than 30 ng/mL, vitamin D supplementation should be prescribed to provide 1,000 to 2,000 units/day or 50,000 units once a month. The degree of elevation in PTH before active therapy is begun and the lower limit of PTH that is desired are uncertain in early to moderate renal insufficiency. It seems reasonable that, at a GFR of 50 to 80 mL/min, a target range from the upper half of the normal range to 50% above the upper limit of normal in the intact PTH assay would be appropriate. Values higher than this range should be treated to prevent parathyroid growth. After vitamin D status is demonstrated to be adequate, dietary phosphorus restriction should be instituted, and the effect on PTH levels should be monitored. If this does not result in a satisfactory decrease in PTH, phosphate binders should be prescribed with meals, and the resultant effect on PTH should be monitored. Initially, calcium-containing salts (e.g., 1.5 g of elemental calcium/day) can be used because the calcium load can be handled by the kidneys, but if large doses are required, consideration should be given to non–calcium-containing phosphate binders. If acidosis is present, it should be treated with sodium bicarbonate. If PTH levels remain elevated despite these measures, the use of vitamin D sterols should be considered. Calcitriol or 1α-hydroxyvitamin D_3 may be used in initial doses of 0.25 to 0.5 mcg/day, respectively, with the patient being monitored closely for hypercalcemia. Increased doses should be used with appropriate caution, and dosing two to three times per week may be considered. As renal failure advances, these measures need to be intensified. PTH values may be tolerated up to twice the upper limit of normal as GFR becomes less than 20 mL/min.

Once dialysis is required, consideration should be given to the use of higher doses of vitamin D sterols because monitoring is easier in the dialysis setting. Adequate control of serum levels of phosphorus continues to be of paramount importance, and every effort should be made to achieve predialysis values no higher than 5.5 mg/dL, with calcium values in the lower half of the normal range if possible. Target values for PTH are now believed to range from 150 to 300 pg/mL (17 to 43 pmol/L) (in the intact PTH assay and 30% to 50% lower than this when using assays that are specific for PTH 1-84). Consideration should be given to the choice of dialysate calcium in light of the total calcium intake of the patient.

To prevent and manage aluminum-related bone disease, it is important to avoid aluminum exposure. The water used for dialysis should be monitored for aluminum content, and aluminum-containing phosphate binders as well as citrate-containing compounds should be avoided. In patients with severe hyperparathyroidism and significant aluminum accumulation in bone, aluminum removal should be considered before parathyroidectomy, because aluminum accumulation may increase rapidly after removal of the parathyroid glands. Chelation therapy with desferrioxamine has been used for many years; however, this therapy is associated with significant side effects, and the use of regimens with low-dose desferrioxamine is advised.

Management of Calciphylaxis

The management of calciphylaxis is a difficult clinical problem. Attempts should be made to lower the $Ca \times P$ value. Serum phosphorus may be lowered by the use of non–calcium-containing phosphate binders and by intensifying hemodialysis to increase removal of phosphorus. Calcium supplements and vitamin D compounds should be avoided, because they are known risk factors for the development of calciphylaxis. In addition, the use of dialysate containing a low calcium concentration has been recommended. Parathyroidectomy should be considered only in patients whose PTH levels are elevated, although the evidence for this treatment is poor. Aggressive control of infections with local care and antibiotic therapy is central in the management of calciphylaxis. Other measures that have been described in the management of this disorder include hyperbaric oxygen, glucocorticoids, cimetidine, and bisphosphonates.

Management of Dialysis-Associated Amyloidosis

The options for management of dialysis-associated amyloidosis are rather limited. The use of biocompatible, high-flux dialysis membranes may be useful to delay the development of this disorder by removing β_2-microglobulin. Hemofiltration may be more effective than hemodialysis for this removal. Renal transplantation controls the symptoms of dialysis-associated amyloidosis, which may be related to the use of immunosuppressive agents, and it also stops the progression of this disorder.

BONE DISEASE AFTER RENAL TRANSPLANTATION

See Chapter 40, Clinical Aspects of Renal Transplantation.

Nutritional Therapy in Renal Disease

31

Nutritional management is a central component of the care of patients with chronic kidney disease (CKD) and end-stage renal disease (ESRD). In contrast to fat and carbohydrate, excess protein cannot be stored and therefore must be broken down and eliminated in the form of nitrogenous waste. In renal failure, the excretion of nitrogenous waste is limited, and the accumulation of the metabolic by-products of protein catabolism produces the clinical syndrome of uremia. In addition, malnutrition is common in advanced CKD/ESRD and is a significant risk factor for adverse patient outcomes. The goals of nutritional management for patients with CKD/ESRD are the following:

- Prevention of malnutrition
- Limitation of nitrogenous waste accumulation
- Normalization of metabolic disturbance
- Prevention of progressive renal disease
- Minimization of cardiovascular risk

Because of the complexity of the medical and nutritional concerns encountered in this patient population, a consultation with a dietitian experienced in the care of patients with CKD is essential in most cases.

MALNUTRITION IN RENAL DISEASE

Protein-energy malnutrition (PEM) and inflammation are common in patients with CKD, and both typically worsen as the CKD progresses to ESRD. Approximately 40% of hemodialysis (HD) patients in the United States have PEM, with 8% to 10% having severe malnutrition. The consequences of malnutrition include increased overall mortality, increased hospitalization rates, poor wound healing, and increased susceptibility to infection. The major contributing factor to the development of PEM is poor dietary intake. This results from a multitude of factors including anorexia (uremia), dietary restrictions, depression, altered taste sensation, and gastroparesis. Metabolic disturbances such as acidemia and intercurrent catabolic illness also contribute to ongoing net body protein losses. Metabolic acidosis is a major factor causing excessive catabolism of amino acids and protein in patients with CKD/ESRD, and correction of metabolic acidosis in predialysis patients, as well as those treated by HD or peritoneal dialysis (PD), sharply decreases the degradation of body protein stores. More recently, chronic inflammatory responses have been implicated in the development of PEM and cardiovascular disease in CKD/ESRD.

ASSESSMENT OF PROTEIN STORES IN CHRONIC RENAL FAILURE

The gold standard for evaluating whether protein stores are being maintained is nitrogen balance. Unfortunately, measurement of nitrogen balance is difficult and requires careful measurement of the food eaten and all routes of nitrogen excretion. It also does not provide rates of protein turnover and, hence, rarely gives insight into mechanisms that cause loss of protein stores. For these reasons measurement of nitrogen balance has largely been supplanted by a number of anthropometric and biochemical markers of nutritional status.

History and Physical Examination

The clinical assessment of nutritional status should begin with a thorough history focusing on recent changes in dietary intake, weight, and gastrointestinal symptoms. Height and weight measurement should be compared with historical records for evidence of weight loss. However, the clinician must be acutely aware of the confounding effects of salt and water retention in advancing CKD, which can mask the loss of lean body mass. Symptoms of depression should also be identified because depressive illness can result in a significant fall in caloric intake.

Anthropometrics

These include patient weight, height, body mass index, skin fold thickness, and mid-arm muscle circumference measurements. Skin fold thickness in the triceps or subscapular area can be used to assess body fat stores, and mid-arm circumference can be used to assess lean body mass. There is significant interpatient variation, depending on factors such as age, sex, and race, and the lack of accurate population-specific reference values limits the utility of these measurements. However, measurements less than 70% of age- and sex-matched "normal" values are highly suggestive of malnutrition. Virtually all cross-sectional studies of dialysis patients have found a high incidence of anthropometric abnormalities suggestive of malnutrition. Serial changes in anthropometric measurements are best used to monitor the response to intervention in an individual patient over time.

Biochemical Markers

The concentration of serum albumin is often cited as an index of the adequacy of the diet, with a low value being equated with malnutrition. Although the serum albumin concentration is a reasonable marker of body protein stores and a reliable predictor of mortality in dialysis patients, the conclusion that a low serum albumin concentration is simply due to a low-protein diet can be very misleading. The serum albumin concentration is the result of a balance between synthesis and degradation of albumin. The serum albumin concentration responds relatively slowly to changes in protein stores because the half-life of albumin is approximately 20 days. A fall in plasma albumin levels may lag behind the development of malnutrition by several months and in malnourished patients albumin levels are only slowly restored to normal during protein refeeding. In contrast, during states of volume expansion, the serum albumin concentration falls due to dilutional effects. Despite these drawbacks, because of the strength of the association of hypoalbuminemia with poor outcomes, this remains a widely used marker in nutritional assessment and should be measured monthly in all dialysis patients.

Other serum markers of malnutrition in renal disease include serum transferrin and prealbumin concentrations. The serum transferrin level may be a more reliable marker than the albumin level as an estimate of protein nutrition because transferrin is more sensitive to protein deficiency and has a shorter half-life ($\approx$10 days). Unfortunately, serum transferrin levels, like those of serum albumin, change with factors other than nutritional status. The serum transferrin level may rise when iron stores are depleted and diminish by as much as 50% with chronic inflammatory disorders such as malignant tumors, rheumatoid arthritis, and infections. The serum concentration of prealbumin also has been touted as an index of nutritional status. It has a half-life of about two days and therefore changes more rapidly with variations in nutritional status. However, the problem of other factors causing changes in serum albumin levels (e.g., inflammation) undoubtedly applies to serum prealbumin. Compared with serum albumin and transferrin concentrations, prealbumin concentrations in HD patients appear to have a special advantage as markers because they are more highly correlated with complications (at a level less than 0.3 g/L, a higher incidence of complications is observed, including infections and mortality). Results from other studies of HD or chronic ambulatory peritoneal dialysis (CAPD) patients concur; however, the usefulness of the prealbumin concentration as a nutritional marker has not been extensively evaluated in predialysis patients. Other markers of malnutrition in renal disease include inappropriately low phosphate, potassium, or blood urea nitrogen levels, all of which can result from diminished protein intake. Hypocholesterolemia has been suggested to reflect diminished caloric intake.

Albumin synthesis falls sharply in subjects with inflammatory illnesses (i.e., albumin functions as a "negative" acute-phase reactant), whereas levels of the acute-phase reactant proteins such as C-reactive protein rise. Some investigators have equated the high level of C-reactive protein with inflammation and have suggested a link between this inflammation and cardiovascular disease in dialysis patients that may be responsive to treatment with 3-hydroxy-3-methylglutaryl-coenzyme A reductase inhibitors.

ROLE OF SPECIFIC DIETARY CONSTITUENTS IN RENAL DISEASE

Energy Requirements of Uremic Patients

Patients with CKD do not have any special ability to adapt to a low-calorie intake. Consequently, if energy intake is inadequate, calorie malnutrition and negative nitrogen balance develop, especially when protein intake is restricted. In many patients with CKD, the daily caloric intake falls below the recommended levels of 30 to 35 kcal/kg/day even with intensive dietary counseling. In general, the recommended caloric intake in patients with CKD/ESRD is 35 kcal/kg/day for those patients younger than 65 years of age, especially if they are on a protein-restricted diet or are underweight. For patients older than 65 years of age, 30 to 35 kcal/kg/day should suffice. It is important to remember that in CAPD patients the absorption of glucose from the dialysate may contribute 700 kcal/day to the patient's daily caloric requirements.

Protein

In normal healthy adults, the minimum dietary protein intake to prevent net nitrogen loss is approximately 0.6 g/kg/day. Most individuals eating a typical Western diet consume an amount considerably in excess of this figure (1 to 2 g/day). Excess dietary protein leads to an increase in the glomerular filtration rate (GFR) that is of little consequence in normal individuals. However, in patients with either microalbuminuria or overt albuminuria, a high-protein diet augments albuminuria and has been associated with a more rapid decline in GFR. Conversely, many studies have documented the fact that protein restriction reduces proteinuria, and because hyperfiltration and proteinuria are independent risk factors for the progression of renal disease, dietary protein restriction has been advocated as a potential renoprotective measure in CKD. On the basis of available data, it is reasonable to suggest that the benefit of protein restriction remains to be proven conclusively. If a low-protein diet is instituted (0.6 to 1 g/day) in patients with CKD, then it is important that 50% of the protein come from high biologic value sources and that the caloric intake be maintained at 35 kcal/kg/day to prevent the development of malnutrition. Growth retardation is a major problem in children with CKD, and protein restriction is generally not advocated. In patients with the nephrotic syndrome, an intake of 1 g/kg/day of protein is advised. Once ESRD has supervened, protein requirements rise. HD patients should receive 1 to 1.2 g/kg/day, whereas CAPD patients require a higher intake (1.2 to 1.3 g/kg) to allow for ongoing peritoneal losses.

Sodium

As CKD progresses, the ability to excrete the daily dietary sodium intake diminishes. Sodium retention occurs in most forms of CKD and contributes to the development of hypertension and hence progressive end-organ hypertensive injury. The typical Western diet is high in sodium (100 to 300 mmol/day) and the recommended sodium intake to limit hypertension and edema in patients with CKD is less than 100 mmol/day (43 mmol = 1 g). In dialysis patients excess sodium intake is associated with higher interdialytic weight gains and intradialytic hypotension as a result of the need for ultrafiltration of large fluid volumes over a relatively short time interval. The degree of sodium restriction in patients with ESRD depends on the residual urine output: in an anuric patient the intake should be less than 100 mmol/day, but this restriction can be safely increased by 50 mmol/500 mL of residual urine output. In patients with rare cases of salt-wasting nephropathy, sodium supplementation may be required to prevent intravascular volume depletion.

Potassium

The average U.S. diet contains 50 to 150 mmol (25 mmol = 1 g) of potassium/day. Hyperkalemia is usually uncommon until the GFR falls to less than 20 mL/min in the absence of distal tubular dysfunction (hyperkalemic distal renal tubular acidosis) or agents that block distal potassium secretion (e.g., angiotensin-converting enzyme inhibitors or nonsteroidal anti-inflammatory drugs). In general, dietary potassium restriction (<100 mmol/day) controls serum potassium levels in most patients with advanced CKD. In ESRD more intensive restriction is required, especially in anuric HD patients (50 to 75 mmol/day). CAPD and HD patients with significant residual urine output may require less intensive restriction. In patients with ESRD, the presence of inappropriate hypokalemia suggests poor dietary protein intake.

Calcium and Phosphorus

In early renal failure, serum calcitriol levels fall, and secondary hyperparathyroidism is nearly universal. As renal failure progresses, a reduction in parathyroid expression of vitamin D receptor as well as calcium receptor renders these glands resistant to both calcitriol and calcium. Dietary phosphorus further increases parathyroid hyperplasia in addition to parathyroid hormone synthesis and secretion. A normal individual typically ingests 1 to 1.5 g of phosphorus/day, mainly from dietary protein intake. As GFR falls, phosphate restriction (<600 to 800 mg/day) can be achieved by moderate protein restriction, in particular by limiting the intake of dairy products. However, as the GFR decreases to less than 20 to −5 mL/min, phosphate binders are usually required to maintain normal serum phosphate levels (< 5.5 mg/dL [1.8 mmol/L]). Calcium carbonate, calcium acetate, and sevelamer HCl are all effective in lowering serum phosphorus levels. Calcium-based binders are usually used as first-line agents. It is important to understand that if the primary goal is a reduction in phosphate absorption, then the binders should be administered with food. If hypocalcemia is the major concern, then they should be administered between meals to maximize systemic absorption. The total dose of elemental calcium provided by the calcium-based phosphate binders should not exceed 1.5 g/day, and the total intake of elemental calcium (including dietary calcium) should not exceed 2 g/day. Contraindications to the use of calcium binders include hypercalcemia and/or persistent "relative" hypo-parathyroidism (parathyroid hormone <150 pg/mL [<16.5 pmol/L] on two consecutive measurements). In such patients, sevelamer HCl may be used as a first-line agent. A more detailed discussion of metabolic bone disease in CKD/ESRD, including the indication for vitamin therapy, is found in Chapter 30, Renal Osteodystrophy.

Dietary Lipids

Cardiovascular disease is the leading cause of death in end-stage renal failure, and the expert opinion is that the management of dyslipidemia in patients with CKD should be equivalent to that in patients with known coronary heart disease. In addition, hyperlipidemia has been postulated to play a role in progression of renal disease. Whether progression can be slowed by dietary or pharmacologic modification of lipid levels is less clear. The safety and efficacy of a low-fat, low-cholesterol diet in patients with CKD has not been conclusively proven. Restriction of dietary fat should probably be avoided when there is evidence of PEM. In general, the dietary recommendations for fat intake mirror those given to the general population: 20% to 25% of caloric intake should come from fat. This should include less than 7% of calories as saturated fat, less than 10% of calories as polyunsaturated fat, and the remainder as monounsaturated fat. According to National Kidney Foundation Kidney Disease Outcomes Quality Initiative (K/DOQI) guidelines, complex carbohydrates should account for 50% to 60% of total calories.

Vitamins and Trace Elements in Uremia

Vitamin deficiencies may occur in renal failure. Dietary limitation, malabsorption, impaired cellular metabolism, circulating inhibitors, or increased losses (dialysis) jeopardize the intake of micronutrients. Because the symptoms of vitamin deficiency are often subtle in their manifestations and may be mistaken for symptoms of uremia, routine vitamin supplementation is widely practiced. Patients with advanced CKD, especially those consuming protein-, phosphate-, or potassium-restricted diets, should receive vitamin B complex and folate supplementation (1 mg/day). Once the patient is receiving dialysis, water-soluble vitamin losses may accelerate, particularly those of vitamin B_1 (thiamine). To circumvent this and other water-soluble vitamin deficiencies, a multivitamin specially formulated for patients with CKD/ESRD that contains the Recommended Daily Allowances (RDAs) of vitamin C, folate, niacin, thiamine, riboflavin, vitamin B_6, vitamin B_{12} 6 mcg and pantothenic acid is prescribed (e.g., Nephrocaps).

Importantly, special requirements for vitamin intake are imposed by dialysis. For example, HD patients given vitamin C in excess (>100 mg) may develop systemic oxalosis, and excessive pyridoxine supplementation has been reported to cause a peripheral neuropathy. Recently, extensive interest has arisen about the accumulation of homocysteine by patients with kidney disease; homocysteine levels are high in dialysis patients and could contribute to the development of arteriosclerosis in these patients. In theory, supplements of vitamin B_6 and folic acid could help reduce homocysteine levels, but a definite beneficial effect on cardiovascular outcomes remains to be demonstrated.

The requirements for fat-soluble vitamins are even more difficult to establish than the requirements for water-soluble vitamins. It has also been suggested that fat-soluble vitamins may participate in some of the complications of kidney failure. For these reasons, fat-soluble vitamins should be given only to patients with a well-defined indication, and supplements providing all vitamins should not be prescribed to avoid the dangers of toxicity.

In summary, evidence indicates that vitamin intake by reasonably nourished HD patients is often insufficient to meet the RDAs for normal subjects. In addition, there is evidence that the requirements for vitamin B_6 and folate may be increased in uremia, especially in patients receiving erythropoietin therapy. Thus, the practice of prescribing a water-soluble vitamin supplement for HD patients may be useful and probably does little harm. However, in view of the reports that peripheral neuropathy and hyperoxemia can occur with high doses of pyridoxine and vitamin C, respectively, "megavitamin" therapy should be avoided.

Recommendations for providing trace element supplements for uremic patients are controversial for several reasons: it is very difficult to determine whether body stores are sufficient, insufficient, or excessive, and it is difficult to prove that symptoms are reversed solely by the administration of trace elements. Based on postmortem studies, the distribution of trace elements in different tissues of uremic patients is abnormal, but it is not clear that these abnormalities are clinically important. Therefore, unless specific indications are present, supplemental trace elements should not be given. An exception would be patients receiving long-term parenteral or enteral nutrition.

Management of Malnutrition

Once the diagnosis of malnutrition is made, the initial evaluation should include attempts to identify reversible causes of diminished intake. These include dietary restrictions, drugs that interfere with taste, and depressive illness. In patients with gastroparesis (e.g., diabetic autonomic neuropathy) metoclopramide and erythromycin have been used with some success to improve gastric emptying. Uremia is a leading cause of anorexia and evidence of worsening malnutrition such as loss of lean body mass or a fall in serum albumin concentration are indications to commence renal replacement therapy in subjects with advanced CKD. In those patients receiving maintenance HD or PD, evidence of underdialysis should be specifically sought because suboptimal clearance rates can lead to anorexia and weight loss. This is best identified by assessing the patient's clearance as measured by the Kt/V (see Chapter 36, Hemodialysis, and Chapter 37, Peritoneal Dialysis). In the setting of malnutrition, the clinician should aim for a Kt/V value of at least 1.3 in HD patients and a weekly Kt/V of more than 2 in PD patients. Abdominal distension due to the instilled dialysate can occasionally interfere with appetite in PD patients. If abdominal distension is a persistent problem, then the patient should drain the abdomen before meals to minimize this complication.

Nutritional Supplements

If the preceding interventions do not yield an improvement in appetite and lean body mass, then nutritional supplementation should be considered. Oral supplementation is the preferred option and specially formulated supplements are available for patients with stage V CKD/ESRD. Specialty supplements typically have low potassium and phosphate contents and a high caloric content relative to their volume. In patients with severe malnutrition and persistent poor intake, consideration can be given to overnight nasogastric feeding. Intradialytic parenteral nutrition has been advocated as a treatment option in patients with severe malnutrition with or without gastroparesis; however, definitive outcome data are lacking. Given its substantial cost and the lack of compelling evidence of benefit, it should probably be reserved for patients unable to tolerate oral supplementation. The institution of total parenteral nutrition is reserved for those patients unable to consume more than 50% of their prescribed caloric intake by the enteral route. Specially formulated preparations are required in ESRD because most generic total parenteral nutrition solutions are high in potassium, phosphate, and magnesium. Close attention to electrolyte serum levels during total parenteral nutrition administration in ESRD is essential to prevent the development of life-threatening electrolyte disturbances.

Other Options

Malnutrition in the PD patient may respond to a dialysate containing amino acids rather than glucose as the osmotic agent. Intraperitoneal amino acid administration is postulated to enhance net nitrogen balance and overall nutritional status. A commercially available formulation is available (Nutrineal) in the United States and Europe, but definitive guidelines for its use are lacking at this time. A reasonable approach is to use an amino acid solution in 1 to 2 exchanges per day in malnourished patients who are resistant to or unable to tolerate oral supplementation. Serial biochemical and anthropometric measurement can be used to assess the response to therapy. A failure to respond within 3 to 4 months should be considered evidence of a lack of efficacy, and the agent should be discontinued. Control of metabolic acidosis (>25 mmol/L) with oral sodium bicarbonate has been demonstrated to improve nutritional parameters in one small clinical trial. Other treatment options include the administration of recombinant human growth hormone or the anabolic steroid nandrolone in selected patients.

Specific Pharmacologic Approaches to Clinical Renoprotection

32

SPECIFIC PHARMACOLOGIC INTERVENTION: A RISK FACTOR–BASED APPROACH

In many patients with chronic renal disease, progressive loss of renal function occurs despite the absence of any overt activity of the underlying renal disorder. The accepted hypothesis is that common mechanisms account for the progressive loss of renal function regardless of the underlying nature of the original disease. Systemic and glomerular hypertension, proteinuria, and metabolic abnormalities such as hyperlipidemia are assumed to be common mediators in the pathophysiology of focal glomerulosclerosis, the probable final common pathway of progressive renal damage. In many renal conditions, hypertension, proteinuria, and metabolic abnormalities are simultaneously present. This clustering of risk factors is presumably of prime importance for renal outcome because the interaction of these risk factors probably accelerates progressive renal damage. To prevent progressive loss of renal function, as a matter of clinical common sense, any prevailing primary damaging factors amenable to intervention should be eliminated. However, in many patients no disease-specific factors accessible to intervention can be identified and treatment strategies should be targeted to ameliorating common renal risk factors. Such interventions have been shown to effectively slow the rate of loss of renal function in diabetic as well as in nondiabetic patients. Importantly, clinical studies have consistently demonstrated the importance of proteinuria as a promoter of progressive renal damage. Therefore, reduction of proteinuria is the central element of any renoprotective regimen.

RISK FACTORS FOR LOSS OF RENAL FUNCTION AND RENOPROTECTIVE BENEFIT OF SPECIFIC INTERVENTION

Hypertension

Whereas malignant hypertension has for decades been recognized to lead to rapid loss of renal function, the role of less severe hypertension in progressive renal damage is less well defined. Epidemiologic data for patients entering dialysis programs suggest a substantial role for hypertension, with hypertensive nephrosclerosis being the second most common cause of end-stage renal failure, surpassed only by diabetes. Among patients with a diagnosis of hypertensive nephrosclerosis, however, only 6% had a history of malignant hypertension, a finding that strongly suggests a causal role for less severe hypertension in the development of end-stage renal failure. In addition, large epidemiologic screening investigations have found blood pressure, specifically diastolic blood pressure, to be a predictor of end-stage renal disease in the general population. Remarkably, in some studies the association with increased renal risk is already apparent with systolic and diastolic pressures well within the normotensive range. Although hypertension is very common, the development of renal failure is a rare event, suggesting that the impact of blood pressure on long-term renal function depends on the concomitant presence of either a specific susceptibility to hypertensive renal damage or the presence of other renal risk factors (or a combination thereof). Several predictors of loss of renal function have been identified in hypertensive populations, including racial factors, impaired glucose tolerance, increased uric acid levels, and elevated serum creatinine levels.

In patients with chronic kidney disease (CKD) hypertension is common, and its prevalence increases with deteriorating renal function. Hypertension is consistently associated with a poor renal outcome in patients with CKD. In diabetic patients, the development of hypertension is closely associated with the transition from normoalbuminuria to microalbuminuria, with subsequent progression to overt proteinuria, and with progressive loss of renal function. Likewise in nondiabetic renal disease, hypertension is associated with a poor long-term renal outcome across a spectrum of renal disorders.

Blood Pressure Reduction

Antihypertensive therapy has been the cornerstone of renoprotective intervention for decades. Reduced blood pressure is associated with a more favorable course of long-term renal function in diabetic as well as nondiabetic patients. Evidence for the renoprotective effect of a reduction in blood pressure is supported by several studies investigating the long-term renal effects of more aggressive blood pressure control. In patients with essential hypertension, more effective stabilization of renal function is obtained with a blood pressure level of 129/86 mm Hg than with a blood pressure level of 139/90 mm Hg. In diabetic nephropathy, the importance of aggressive blood pressure reduction for preservation of renal function has been extensively demonstrated in observational studies. Trials comparing angiotensin-converting enzyme (ACE) inhibitors with conventional antihypertensive agents in insulin-dependent diabetes mellitus (type 1 diabetes), as well as in non–insulin-dependent diabetes mellitus (type 2 diabetes), show that loss of renal function is ameliorated more effectively in the treatment groups with lower blood pressures, specifically those assigned to receive ACE inhibitors. Although non–blood pressure-related effects of ACE inhibitors are likely to be involved in renoprotection as well, the association between blood pressure reduction and the protection obtained against loss of renal function is strong.

Target Blood Pressure

The target blood pressure for renoprotection in nondiabetic renal disease depends on the severity of proteinuria. In patients with proteinuria of 1 to 3 g/day, a mean arterial pressure of 92 mm Hg (125/75 mm Hg) provides superior renoprotection compared with a mean arterial pressure of 98 mm Hg (corresponding to 135/80 mm Hg). This additional benefit is not observed in patients with protein loss of less than 1 g/day. Ethnic factors may also have an impact on the benefit of a given blood pressure level with proteinuric black patients appearing to receive more benefit from tighter blood pressure control then white subjects. Although the evidence from multiple trials is of an indirect nature, analysis appears to support a target blood pressure not exceeding 130/85 mm Hg in CKD. Stabilization of renal function may require a target mean arterial pressure of 95 mm Hg, which corresponds to approximately 120/80 mm Hg. For diabetic patients, even though no formal trials comparing different target levels have been performed, the recommendation is a target blood pressure less than 120 to 130 systolic and 80 to 85 mm Hg diastolic for microalbuminuric patients. From the clinical standpoint, efforts to achieve these target blood pressures often require the use of multiple antihypertensive agents.

Glomerular Hypertension

Experimental studies have shown that glomerular hypertension/hyperfiltration occurs as a renal adaptive response to loss of functional renal mass. This serves initially to maintain glomerular filtration rate (GFR), but ultimately it is maladaptive and accelerates the decline in renal function. Hyperfiltration is worsened by high protein intake, which may contribute to the accelerating effect of high protein intake on the progression of CKD. A reduction in elevated glomerular capillary pressure rather than a reduction in systemic blood pressure closely correlates with protection against the development of focal glomerulosclerosis in several experimental renal conditions. Indirect data suggest that a reduction in intraglomerular hydrostatic pressure may be relevant to the outcome of renoprotective interventions in humans as well. In nondiabetic and diabetic renal disease, the early renal hemodynamic response (but not the response of systemic blood pressure) to antihypertensive therapy has been shown to predict its long-term renoprotective efficacy. A slight drop in GFR at the onset of treatment, which may indicate a reduction in glomerular hydrostatic pressure, predicts a favorable long-term course of renal function, suggesting that a reduction in glomerular pressure may play a role in long-term renoprotection in humans.

Proteinuria

A pathogenetic role for proteinuria in progressive loss of renal function is suggested by many experimental and clinical studies. Proteinuria consistently predicts the rate of loss of renal function in CKD and is the best predictor of end-stage renal failure in patients with CKD. Remarkably, the association between proteinuria and the rate of progression is present not only in conditions in which proteinuria might reflect the severity or activity of a primary glomerular disorder but also in chronic pyelonephritis and vesicoureteral reflux in which the glomerulus is not the primary site of injury. This consistent relationship is the basis of the hypothesis that proteinuria is a key factor in a vicious circle of non–disease-specific factors that account for progressive renal function loss. However, it should be recognized that in many patients progression to end-stage renal failure without significant proteinuria suggests that its impact relative to disease-specific factors may vary among different populations.

Reduction of Proteinuria

Antihypertensive regimens associated with a better reduction in proteinuria typically provide better renoprotection in patients with CKD. The association between a reduction in proteinuria and renal prognosis applies not only to antihypertensive treatment but also to remission of proteinuria attained spontaneously or by treatment of the underlying renal disease (e.g., immunosuppressive treatment). The consistent relationship between residual proteinuria and long-term renal prognosis demonstrates first and foremost that a reduction in proteinuria is a prerequisite for renoprotection. In individual patients, the long-term renal prognosis correlates with the initial antiproteinuric response to therapy. For clinical purposes, it is important that the response be apparent early after the start of therapy to allow early distinction between patients who will benefit from the intervention and those in whom additional therapy may be required. Furthermore, in view of the consistent relationship between a reduction in proteinuria and renoprotection, attempts to maximally suppress proteinuria are likely to be a fruitful approach to improve renoprotection.

Hyperlipidemia

Dyslipidemia is common in renal disease, and lipid nephrotoxicity has been hypothesized to be involved in the progression of renal damage. This association may be particularly relevant in proteinuric renal disease, which is associated with hyperlipidemia. However, the common forms of primary hyperlipidemia do not appear to initiate overt renal disease in normal individuals. Nevertheless, several clinical studies have suggested that hyperlipidemia is associated with a faster rate of renal function loss in patients with CKD and in hypertensive individuals. A secondary analysis from the Modification of Diet in Renal Disease (MDRD) study identified high-density lipoprotein cholesterol as a predictor of the rate of decline in renal function, thereby supporting the relevance of the lipid profile. However, a causal association between hyperlipidemia and the rate of progression has not been conclusively proven and any effect may be reflective of the confounding effects of proteinuria.

Reduction of Lipids

In patients with CKD 3-hydroxy-3-methylglutaryl-coenzyme A (HMG-CoA) reductase inhibitors effectively reduce total cholesterol, low-density lipoprotein cholesterol, and apolipoprotein B but the effects on proteinuria levels have been varied. The results of meta-analysis studies support a tendency toward a reduction in proteinuria by reducing lipids. However, no study has demonstrated slowing of disease progression, but it should be noted that the power to detect such a change was low in most studies. In summary, more solid data are required, especially on the long-term outcome of renal function, to substantiate the possible renoprotective benefit in humans provided by HMG-CoA reductase inhibition.

Genetic Factors

Familial clustering of diabetic nephropathy and the association of several renal disorders (e.g., membranous glomerulopathy, immunoglobulin A nephropathy, and focal segmental sclerosis) with distinct human leukocyte antigen (HLA) patterns suggested that susceptibility to the development of these disorders was subject to genetic influences. A role for genetic factors in modifying the course of renal function loss is also suggested by interethnic differences in outcome and by the remarkably constant individual progression rate as opposed to the large interindividual differences in the rate of progression, even for subjects suffering from the same underlying disorder. To date, the most attention has focused on a common insertion (I)/deletion (D) polymorphism for the *ACE* gene. ACE levels in serum and renal tissue are higher in DD homozygotes and an association between the DD genotype and more rapid loss of renal function has been reported in a variety of renal disorders.

Miscellaneous

Morbid obesity has long been known to be associated with focal glomerulosclerosis. Less extreme obesity is now increasingly being recognized as a renal risk factor in CKD. The mechanism underlying the renal risk of obesity is not well characterized and may relate to its association with other renal risk factors such as hypertension, diabetes mellitus, and lipid abnormalities and possibly hyperfiltration.

Importantly, weight loss by ingestion of a hypocaloric diet can result in significant reductions in proteinuria in obese patients. An increasing body of evidence indicates that cigarette smoking is associated with an increased rate of loss of renal function. The effect appears to be particularly prominent in diabetic nephropathy, but it is also apparent in nondiabetic renal disease.

PHARMACOLOGIC APPROACHES

Antihypertensive Treatment

Reduction in blood pressure is of prime importance in the prevention of disease progression in CKD, and this can be achieved with all of the currently available classes of antihypertensive agents. Whether the choice of a particular antihypertensive agent matters for long-term renoprotection, independent of the reduction in blood pressure achieved, is a matter of active debate.

Recent meta-analyses of the effects of ACE inhibitors support a renoprotective effect of renin-angiotensin-aldosterone system (RAAS) blockade beyond blood pressure control in nondiabetic and diabetic patients, and this finding is supported by recent data on the renoprotective effects of angiotensin II type 1 (AT1) receptor blockade.

Angiotensin-Converting Enzyme Inhibitors

Comparative clinical studies have found more effective preservation of renal function by ACE inhibitors than by other antihypertensive agents. The benefit of ACE inhibitors appears to be most evident in those patients with the highest risk of progression to end stage renal disease based on their initial rate of loss of renal function or baseline proteinuria. Nevertheless, patients with less severe proteinuria also benefit from ACE inhibition. In diabetic patients with either microalbuminuria or overt nephropathy, ACE inhibition attenuates the long-term rate of renal function loss independent of its effects on blood pressure. The benefit of these drugs is found, in part, in their effects to facilitate efferent glomerular arteriolar dilation by antagonizing the effects of angiotensin II as they lower blood pressure. Thus, there is a more consistent reduction in both systemic and glomerular capillary pressure. Special attention should be paid to adequate dosing of these agents, because in many studies the renoprotective effect was observed at the higher end of the dosing range. The goals of therapy should be blood pressure less than 130/85 (<125/80 if proteinuria > 1 g is present), a reduction in proteinuria to less than 300 mg/24 hr, and a loss of GFR of less than 2 ml/yr. The dose of the individual ACE-inhibitor should be maximized until these goals are attained or side effects preclude further dose augmentation. Interestingly, ACE inhibition also appears to be able to induce regression toward normoalbuminuria in subjects with microalbuminuria and reduce not only the risk for nephropathy but also overall mortality and cardiovascular events in diabetic patients with high cardiovascular risk.

Angiotensin II Type 1 Receptor Blockers

In patients with essential hypertension, as well as in patients with CKD, angiotensin receptor blockers (ARBs) induce a gradual fall in blood pressure that is associated with renal hemodynamic changes and a reduction in proteinuria similar to that achieved by ACE inhibition. The renoprotective profile of this class was recently substantiated by a series of landmark studies, which demonstrated that AT1 blockade protected hypertensive patients with type 2 diabetes from progressing from the microalbuminuric state to overt nephropathy and slowed the loss of renal function in type 2 diabetics with overt nephropathy compared with conventional treatment. As with ACE inhibition, the renoprotective effect mediated by the ARBs appears to be linked to the reduction in proteinuria. Treatment goals are the same as those outlined earlier for ACE inhibition.

Calcium Channel Blockers

Calcium channel blockers (CCBs) are effective antihypertensive agents in patients with CKD. Their renoprotective effects, however, have been questioned because of the possible deleterious effects of increased glomerular pressure mediated by attenuation of glomerular afferent arteriolar tone. Most studies of the effects of calcium channel blockade in CKD have used RAAS blockade as the regimen for comparison. To date RAAS blockade–based regimens have been favored over CCB-based regimens in most diabetic and nondiabetic renal disease trials. This effect may be even more pronounced in African-American patients with hypertensive nephrosclerosis. A comparison of CCBs with a placebo—not usually warranted in renal disease populations—provides an additional perspective: in older subjects with systolic hypertension, active therapy with the CCB nitrendipine resulted in a reduction in proteinuria and serum creatinine compared with placebo. All in all, it would be reasonable to assume that the renoprotective properties of the CCBs are closely linked to their antihypertensive properties and that a renoprotective benefit can be expected only in patients in whom blood pressure is rigorously controlled. In most patients they should be considered as "add-on" therapy to RAAS blockade when the latter agents fail to adequately control blood pressure.

β-Blockers

In patients with CKD, β-blockers are generally effective in reducing blood pressure. However, no studies are available to support specific renoprotection by β-blocker–based antihypertensive treatment and β-blockers are less effective than ACE inhibitors for long-term renoprotection in nondiabetic patients, as well as in African-American patients with type 2 diabetes. However, other well-controlled studies have found a similar rate of loss of renal function with β-blockers and ACE inhibitors, suggesting that β-blockers are useful for long-term renoprotection, possibly because of their effects on blood pressure.

Diuretics

In many patients with CKD, diuretics are required for effective blood pressure control. Accordingly, diuretics are part of the therapeutic regimen in many studies. Nonetheless, their long-term renoprotective effect in humans has not been established. However, diuretics are indispensable in renoprotective intervention in view of the importance of control of volume status and blood pressure in patients with overt renal disease. Whether different diuretics are equivalent for renoprotection is unknown. The specific cardioprotective effects of aldosterone blockade by spironolactone suggest that this issue may be relevant to renal patients as well. Although spironolactone appears to have added antiproteinuric efficacy in addition to ACE inhibition, it is unclear whether this finding reflects specific aldosterone blockade or just its effect on volume control. Of note, in renal patients the combination of RAAS blockade and aldosterone blockade requires close consideration of safety issues in light of the risk of development of hyperkalemia.

RISK FACTOR PROFILE IN RENAL PATIENTS

Clustering of Renal Risk Factors and Concordance with Cardiovascular Risk Factors

Renal risk factors can be identified in most renal patients, and several risk factors are often simultaneously present. In light of the evidence for synergism between different renal risk factors, this simultaneous presence has considerable clinical impact. Proteinuria in particular appears to cluster with hypertension, as well as with metabolic risk factors.

The main clinical and demographic factors associated with increased renal risk are also well-established risk factors for cardiovascular morbidity and mortality. This concordance may reflect the similarity of the pathophysiologic pathways of progressive glomerulosclerosis and interstitial sclerosis with the process of atherosclerosis. Patients with CKD have a particularly high risk for cardiovascular morbidity and mortality. The increased risk is attributed in large part to risk factors, such as demographic factors, hypertension, hyperlipidemia, and smoking, which are also present in the population with nonrenal conditions.

Proteinuria is a consistent predictor of cardiovascular mortality in the CKD population. Remarkably, increased cardiovascular risk is present not only in overtly proteinuric individuals but also in microalbuminuric diabetic and nondiabetic subjects. The grim clinical consequences of the dual risk associated with this risk factor profile is reflected by the fivefold to sixfold increased risk for myocardial infarction in nephrotic patients as opposed to the normal population. Hyperlipidemia is usually proportional to the severity of the proteinuria, with a particularly atherogenic lipid profile including an elevation of the highly atherogenic lipoprotein (a).

CLINICAL MANAGEMENT

A Framework for Renoprotective Intervention

An overall framework for renoprotective intervention is required in patients with CKD. Most patients with a risk for loss of renal function will eventually die of cardiovascular causes. Treatment aims should therefore also explicitly include an overall reduction in cardiovascular risk. To achieve this goal, however, aggressive and costly therapy is required and must be continued for many years. A risk factor–based approach may serve to properly identify patients who are likely to benefit from such aggressive treatment while alleviating the burden of treatment in those at low risk.

Primary Prevention

PRIMARY PREVENTION OF RENAL FUNCTION LOSS IN HYPERTENSION   The main preventive measure is effective blood pressure reduction. At present, no data are available to substantiate a specific renal advantage with any particular class of antihypertensive agents for hypertensive patients in the absence of overt renal disease or proteinuria. The choice of a preferred drug for the individual patient can thus be guided by specific indications and contraindications as a result of comorbid conditions. A systolic blood pressure less than 140 mm Hg has been recommended to prevent loss of renal function in essential hypertension; however, the target goal should be lower in patients with microalbuminuria (< 130/85 mm Hg).

PRIMARY PREVENTION IN DIABETES MELLITUS   In both type 1 diabetes and type 2 diabetes, improved glycemic control and aggressive blood pressure control have clearly been shown to be effective in primary prevention of renal disease. Antihypertensive treatment with ACE inhibitors provides primary prevention of nephropathy while treatment with the ARB irbesartan dose dependently prevents progression from microalbuminuria to overt albuminuria. In the natural history of type 1 diabetes, the onset of microalbuminuria, defined as an excretion rate of 30 to 300 mg/day or 20 to 200 mg/min, is a strong predictor of subsequent progression to overt nephropathy. Therefore, the discovery of microalbuminuria should trigger the commencement and subsequent monitoring of renoprotective intervention therapy in diabetes mellitus. Accordingly, the first step in primary prevention of nephropathy in type 1 diabetes is screening for microalbuminuria on an annual basis 5 years after diagnosis. With type 2 diabetes, a larger proportion of patients may have microalbuminuria at the time of diagnosis or shortly thereafter; thus, screening of patients with type 2 diabetes should start at the time of diagnosis. In addition, blood pressure should be monitored at least annually in type 1 diabetes and type 2 diabetes and antihypertensive treatment should be instituted if required to achieve a target blood pressure less than 130/85 mm Hg. If microalbuminuria is discovered, then pharmacologic therapy should be instituted irrespective of blood pressure. Based on the evidence available, ACE inhibitors can be recommended as first-choice agents in type 1 diabetes and ARBs in type 2 diabetes. Monitoring of therapy should include monitoring of microalbuminuria as well as blood pressure, with a goal of stabilization and eventual reduction of microalbuminuria and a blood pressure less than 130/85 mm Hg. If the response to therapy is insufficient, a diuretic should be added.

Secondary Prevention

In patients with established renal disease, the primary causal factors for ongoing renal damage, if present, should first be eliminated. The benefit of rigorous blood pressure control is supported by many studies. Reduction of blood pressure to less than 130/80 mm Hg has been recommended for renal patients. For proteinuric patients, the target blood pressure should be even lower. In patients with proteinuria greater than 1 g/day, additional benefit is obtained by blood pressure reduction to 125/75 mm Hg.

Because of the importance of proteinuria as a renal risk factor, its presence should act as a guide for therapy. Even if blood pressure is in the so-called normotensive range, the presence of proteinuria should prompt the institution of antiproteinuric therapy. In light of the consistent predictive value of a reduction in proteinuria for subsequent renoprotection, not only a reduction in blood pressure but also a reduction in proteinuria should be main targets of renoprotective intervention. The proven renoprotective efficacy of ACE inhibitors renders them first-choice agents in patients at high risk for deterioration of renal function, such as nondiabetic patients with overt proteinuria and patients with diabetic nephropathy. In type 2 diabetes, the renoprotective efficacy of ARBs has now been established, and thus they are first-choice drugs. In patients without proteinuria, notably those with polycystic kidneys and tubulointerstitial disease, other classes of drugs, such as β-blockers and CCBs, may also be used as first-line drugs. In addition to dietary sodium restriction, adjunctive therapy in subjects with overt proteinuria should preferably include dietary protein restriction. Even though conflicting study outcomes have generated controversy about the benefit of protein restriction, meta-analysis supports the renoprotective benefit of protein restriction in nondiabetic as well as diabetic subjects (see also Chapter 31, Nutritional Therapy in Renal Disease).

Additional measures in renal patients should include control of prevalent cardiorenal risk factors. The main measures are discontinuation of smoking and control of hyperlipidemia. Specific antihyperlipidemic therapy is required in many renal patients. HMG-CoA reductase inhibitors are effective for this purpose and may be combined with fibric acid derivatives in patients with high triglyceride levels.

Monitoring of Renoprotective Therapy

Usually, chronic loss of renal function is a gradual process that takes years or decades to progress to end-stage renal failure. This gradual deterioration in renal function has implications for monitoring the efficacy of renoprotective interventions. A slight reduction in GFR at the onset of antihypertensive therapy predicts better long-term renoprotection. This drop presumably reflects functional hemodynamic changes, such as a drop in glomerular capillary pressure, that are favorable in the long run. However, when the drop in GFR is substantial or the clinical condition of the patient is compatible with renal artery stenosis, it is important to exclude renal artery stenosis, especially when the treatment includes ACE inhibition or an ARB.

In individual patients, even with sophisticated and frequent measurements, the rate of decline in GFR is usually too slow to monitor and, thus, renoprotective therapy cannot be titrated. Titration based on intermediate parameters that predict future loss of renal function provides a better alternative. Although blood pressure should obviously be monitored, proteinuria (or albuminuria) is the best predictor of future loss of renal function and thus reflects the renoprotective efficacy of the regimen. Proteinuria can therefore guide adjustment of therapy.

Optimizing Response to Therapy

Despite recent advances, chronic renal disease is still essentially a progressive condition. To achieve better prevention of end-stage renal failure strategies are needed to optimize renoprotective interventions by an integrated regimen of pharmacologic and nonpharmacologic measures.

Sodium Status

The disturbed sodium and volume homeostasis in most renal patients leads to expanded extracellular volume and hypertension, which is particularly prominent in proteinuric patients. In specific patient categories such as African Americans and microalbuminuric diabetic patients, blood pressure is often exquisitely sodium sensitive, and diuretic therapy is often required to obtain effective blood pressure control. This dependence of response on volume status applies particularly to ACE inhibitors and AT1 receptor blockers. The effect of sodium status on antiproteinuric efficacy may be partly related to its concomitant effects on blood pressure, but the intrarenal effects of sodium status may be important as well, as suggested by the prominent effect of sodium restriction on proteinuria in contrast to its relatively modest effect on blood pressure. Therefore, sodium restriction and diuretic therapy, if required, are essential components of an optimal renoprotective regimen.

Protein Intake

Dietary protein restriction can reduce proteinuria in patients with CKD; however, conclusive outcome data for prevention of end-stage renal disease are lacking. However, protein restriction can enhance the antiproteinuric effect of ACE inhibition. In severe proteinuria, institution of protein restriction during ACE inhibitor therapy can yield a reduction in proteinuria of up to 33%. Thus, the effects of ACE inhibition and dietary protein restriction appear to be additive for reduction in proteinuria, and if proteinuria persists despite blockade of the RAAS, then protein restriction should be considered.

Dose Titration for Proteinuria

In view of the importance of proteinuria, it may be surprising that few data are available on dose-response curves for proteinuria with the use of ACE inhibitors or ARBs. The dose-response curves for blood pressure and proteinuria are not necessarily similar. A progressive antiproteinuric effect from ACE inhibitors may occur at higher doses than those needed for maximal blood pressure reduction or for achieving the recommended target blood pressure values. For AT1 receptor blockade, the optimal antiproteinuric effect of losartan is obtained at a higher dose than that needed for the maximal blood pressure response in nondiabetic as well as diabetic nephropathy. Importantly, the responses of blood pressure and proteinuria are not always concordant, and a common trend across several studies seems to be that in subjects with normal blood pressure, an antiproteinuric effect can be obtained with doses that do not or only slightly affect blood pressure. For a balanced view of the renoprotective potential of supramaximal doses of ACE inhibitors or ARBs, further studies in different populations are needed, as well as research on the issue of tolerability. The benefits of high-dose ACE inhibitor or ARB monotherapy should also be weighed against those of dual blockade of the RAAS (see the next section). For the moment, controlled studies to support specific dose recommendations for long-term renoprotection are lacking. However, the treatment targets—blood pressure control *plus* optimal reduction of proteinuria (<300 mg/24 hr)—should guide titration of therapy. If proteinuria persists despite good blood pressure control, increasing the dose is worth a try, although it may not be invariably effective.

Combination Therapy

Combinations of drugs with different mechanisms of action can exert additive effects. For renal protection, several combinations are of specific interest as judged by their effect on intermediate renal parameters. First, as noted earlier, during ACE inhibition, cotreatment with diuretics can overcome the effects of high sodium intake on blood pressure and proteinuria. Thus, combination therapy provides a way to overcome resistance to antiproteinuric efficacy. In light of the different levels of RAAS blockade, a case may be made for combining ACE inhibitors with ARBs. In renal disease populations, several studies thus far have reported that combined therapy with an ACE inhibitor and an AT1 receptor blocker exerts a more effective antiproteinuric response than either does as monotherapy in diabetic as well as nondiabetic nephropathy.

However, dose considerations may be relevant. In studies reporting an added effect of dual blockade, the doses used were deliberately chosen to be submaximal—with the rationale of possibly inducing fewer side effects than with the drugs used separately. Thus, the efficacy of dual blockade could be due to more effective RAAS blockade as such; however, efficacy might also have been achieved with a higher dose of either drug. For the purpose of maximal reduction in proteinuria, it would also be relevant to assess whether dual blockade, at optimal doses of both drugs, would result in a further reduction in proteinuria. The available data suggest an enhanced potential of dual blockade over monotherapy, but this additive effect may not apply to all conditions. Optimal dosing schedules, also in relation to other optimizing measures such as volume control, will have to be developed further.

Time Course

In nondiabetic patients, it takes several weeks to achieve the maximum reduction in proteinuria, which should be taken into account when one titrates for optimal reduction of proteinuria. In microalbuminuric type 1 diabetes, on the other hand, the time course of reduction in albuminuria parallels the reduction in blood pressure, with maximal responses already occurring in the first week of treatment, which may reflect the greater renal impact of blood pressure in these patients. The lack of similar data for other antihypertensive agents or for diabetic patients with overt nephropathy precludes recommendation of a fixed schedule for the time course of titration at this time.

VI

Drugs and the Kidney

Diuretics

33

INDIVIDUAL CLASSES OF DIURETICS

Carbonic Anhydrase Inhibitors

Site of Action
Carbonic anhydrase inhibitors work in the proximal tubule.

Mechanism of Action
Carbonic anhydrase inhibitors work by inhibition of luminal and cellular carbonic anhydrase. The net result is impaired Na^+, Cl^-, and HCO_3^- absorption, leading to an alkaline diuresis. Diuretic efficacy is limited by distal Na^+ and HCO_3^- absorption and development of metabolic acidosis.

Pharmacokinetics
Acetazolamide (Diamox) is readily absorbed. Its $t_{1/2}$ (half-life) is 13 hours. Methazolamide (Neptazane) has less plasma protein binding, a longer $t_{1/2}$, and greater lipid solubility, all of which favor penetration into aqueous humor and cerebrospinal fluid. It has fewer renal effects and therefore is preferred for treatment of glaucoma.

Clinical Indications
Carbonic anhydrase inhibitors can be used with $NaHCO_3$ infusion to cause an alkaline diuresis that increases the excretion of weakly acidic drugs (e.g., salicylates and phenobarbital) or acidic metabolites (urate). Chloride-responsive metabolic alkalosis is best treated by administering Cl^- with K^+ or Na^+. However, if this produces unacceptable extracellular volume (ECV) expansion, acetazolamide (250 to 500 mg/day) and KCl can be used to increase HCO_3^- excretion. These agents are useful in glaucoma because they diminish the transport of HCO_3^- and Na^+ by the ciliary process, thereby reducing intraocular pressure. Acetazolamide is

also used in a dosage of 125 mg twice daily as prophylaxis against mountain sickness, probably through stimulation of respiration and diminishing of cerebral blood flow. In established mountain sickness, it improves oxygenation and pulmonary gas exchange. It can stimulate ventilation in patients with central sleep apnea.

Adverse Effects
Adverse effects include lethargy, abnormal taste, paresthesia, gastrointestinal distress, malaise, and decreased libido. These symptoms can be diminished by $NaHCO_3$, but this increases the risk of nephrocalcinosis and nephrolithiasis, which occur at a 10-fold higher rate in patients receiving acetazolamide. Symptomatic metabolic acidosis develops in 50%. Acidosis is more common in elderly patients, diabetic patients, and patients with chronic kidney disease (CKD). An alkaline urine favors partitioning of renal ammonia into blood rather than its elimination in urine and may precipitate encephalopathy in patients with liver failure.

Osmotic Diuretics

Site of Action
Osmotic diuretics act as osmotic particles in tubule fluid, rather than on a specific transport pathway.

Mechanism of Action
Mannitol is freely filtered but poorly reabsorbed. The osmotic gradient created results in the loss of fluid and Na^+, K^+, Cl^-, and HCO_3^-.

Pharmacokinetics and Dosage
Mannitol is distributed in the ECV and is filtered freely at the glomerulus. Consequently, the $t_{1/2}$ for plasma clearance depends on the glomerular filtration rate (GFR) and can be prolonged up to 36 hours in advanced renal failure. It can be infused intravenously in daily doses of 50 to 200 g as a 15% or 20% solution or 1.5 to 2 g/kg of a 20% solution over 30 to 60 minutes to treat raised intraocular or intracranial pressure.

Clinical Indications
Mannitol is used in the management of severe head injury for which it is more effective than loop diuretics or hypertonic saline in reducing brain water content. Mannitol can also prevent and/or reverse the dialysis disequilibrium syndrome. There is no clear evidence that mannitol or any diuretic is effective in prevention

or treatment of acute renal failure (ARF) and its routine application in this setting is discouraged.

Adverse Effects
The osmotic abstraction of cell water initially causes hyponatremia and hypochloremia. Later, when the excess extracellular fluid is excreted, the decrease in cell water concentrates K^+ and H^+ within cells, which increases the gradient for their diffusion into the extracellular fluid, leading to hyperkalemic acidosis. These electrolyte changes are normally rapidly corrected by the kidney, provided that renal function is adequate. Later, hypernatremic dehydration may develop if free water is not provided, because urinary concentrating ability is inhibited. Importantly, in patients with renal failure, hemodilution and hyperkalemic metabolic acidosis may occur after administration of mannitol and the consequent circulatory overload, central nervous system depression, and severe electrolyte disturbances can trigger the need for emergency hemodialysis.

Loop Diuretics

Site of Action
The site of action of loop diuretics is the luminal aspect of the thick ascending limb of the loop of Henle (TAL).

Mechanism of Action
They work by inhibition of the $Na^+/K^+/2Cl^-$ cotransporter termed *NKCC2*. These are potent diuretics (25% of Na^+ reabsorption occurs in the TAL). Other effects of loop diuretics include a reduction in the medullary concentrating gradient as a result of a reduction in solute reabsorption in the water-impermeable TAL. This impairs free water excretion during both water loading and dehydration. Loop diuretics increase the fractional excretion of Ca^{2+} by up to 30% by decreasing the lumen-positive transepithelial potential that promotes paracellular Ca^{2+} reabsorption from the lumen. The loop of Henle is the major nephron segment for reabsorption of Mg^{2+}, and loop diuretics increase fractional Mg^{2+} excretion by more than 60%, also by diminishing voltage-dependent paracellular transport. Furosemide also has a unique venodilatory action mediated by an endothelium-dependent hyperpolarizing action that can acutely lower central filling pressures in the setting of congestive heart failure (CHF).

Pharmacokinetics
Furosemide is well absorbed; its bioavailability averages 50%. It is more than 90% albumin bound, and the kidney is the primary

route of elimination. In contrast, bumetanide and torsemide have better oral bioavailability and are metabolized in the liver. The duration of action of torsemide is approximately twice as long, but clinically relevant differences in salt-depleting action are not evident. In patients with CKD, the elimination of furosemide, unlike bumetanide or torsemide, is greatly reduced because its metabolism to the inactive glucuronide occurs in the kidney. In patients with CKD due to differences in the elimination routes, there is therefore a tradeoff when a loop diuretic is selected in CKD: Furosemide can accumulate and cause ototoxicity at high doses, whereas bumetanide retains its metabolic inactivation but is therefore somewhat less potent. Renal clearance of the active form of loop diuretics falls in proportion to the creatinine clearance. In addition, metabolic acidosis impairs the luminal secretion of weak organic acids including loop diuretics. These two factors explain why diuretic secretion is often impaired in advanced CKD. Also, a low serum albumin concentration, as may occur in the nephrotic syndrome, may enhance furosemide metabolism leading to a loss of efficacy.

Clinical Indications
These are described under "Clinical Uses of Diuretics."

Adverse Effects
These are discussed under "Adverse Effects of Diuretics."

Thiazides

Site of Action
Thiazides work at the early distal convoluted tubule.

Mechanism of Action
Thiazide diuretics block the thiazide-sensitive Na^+/Cl^- cotransporter, which mediates 40% of coupled reabsorption of Na^+ and Cl^-. Thiazides impair maximal urinary dilution, but not maximal urinary concentration, thereby predisposing to hyponatremia particularly in elderly patients. Thiazides also decrease Ca^{2+} excretion by enhancing basolateral Na^+/Ca^{2+} exchange and stimulating proximal reabsorption of Ca^{2+} in response to ECV depletion.

Pharmacokinetics
Thiazides are readily absorbed and are extensively bound to plasma proteins. They are eliminated largely by secretion into the proximal tubule where they mediate their effects. The $t_{1/2}$ is prolonged in renal failure and in elderly patients; however, because the secreted component is clinically active, the prolonged

$t_{1/2}$ actually reduces their natriuretic efficacy. The more lipid-soluble drugs (e.g., bendroflumethiazide and polythiazide) are more potent, have a more prolonged action, and are more extensively metabolized. Chlorthalidone has a particularly prolonged action, whereas indapamide is sufficiently metabolized to limit accumulation in renal failure.

Clinical Indications
These are described under "Clinical Uses of Diuretics."

Adverse Effects
These are described under "Adverse Effects of Diuretics."

Distal Potassium-Sparing Diuretic Agents

Distal K^+-sparing diuretics comprise those that directly inhibit luminal Na^+ entry (e.g., amiloride and triamterene) and those that are competitive antagonists of aldosterone (e.g., spironolactone and eplerenone).

Site of Action
Their site of action is the principal cells in the late distal convoluted tubule and initial connecting tubule and the cortical collecting duct.

Mechanism of Action
These diuretics inhibit Na^+ uptake via the epitheal Na^+ channel (ENaC), resulting in a natriuresis and diminished electrochemical gradient for K^+ secretion. Trimethoprim and pentamidine have amiloride-like actions and can cause hyperkalemia. Spironolactone is a competitive inhibitor of aldosterone. The latter stimulates Na^+ resorption and K^+ secretion in the distal convoluted tubule by increasing the activity of ENaC. Distal K^+-sparing diuretics cause a modest natriuresis, and their more clinically relevant actions are to reduce the excretion of K^+.

Pharmacokinetics
Triamterene is well absorbed. The drug and its metabolites are secreted in the proximal tubule with half-lives of 3 to 5 hours. Triamterene and its active metabolites accumulate in patients with cirrhosis because of decreased biliary secretion and in elderly patients and in those with renal disease because of decreased renal excretion. Amiloride is incompletely absorbed, has a duration of action of approximately 18 hours. It accumulates in renal failure and may worsen renal function. Spironolactone is readily absorbed, has a $t_{1/2}$ of 20 hours and takes 10 to 48 hours to become maximally effective.

Clinical Indications
Distal K^+-sparing agents are used primarily as K^+-sparing agents in patients with hypokalemic alkalosis. Amiloride can prevent amphotericin-induced hypokalemia and hypomagnesemia.

Adverse Effects
The risk of hyperkalemia is dose-dependent and increases considerably in patients with renal failure or in those receiving K^+ supplements, angiotensin-converting enzyme (ACE) inhibitors, angiotensin receptor blockers (ARBs), nonsteroidal anti-inflammatory drugs, β-blockers, heparin, or ketoconazole. Impaired net acid excretion can cause metabolic acidosis, which worsens hyperkalemia. Amiloride and triamterene accumulate in renal failure and triamterene accumulates in cirrhosis. Therefore, these drugs should be avoided in these situations. Spironolactone can cause impotence, loss of libido, gynecomastia, or postmenopausal bleeding. A related drug, eplerenone, causes less gynecomastia.

Dopamine

In low doses (1 to 3 mcg/kg/min), dopamine is natriuretic, owing primarily to a modest increase in the GFR and a reduction in proximal reabsorption attributed to a cyclic adenosine monophosphate–induced inhibition of the Na^+/H^+ antiporter. "Renal dose dopamine" has little or no renal effect in critically ill patients or in patients with sepsis, and controlled trials have failed to detect an improved outcome in patients given dopamine. Renal-dose dopamine for the treatment of ARF lacks efficacy, is expensive, and can cause cardiac arrhythmias, and its use is actively discouraged.

ADAPTATION TO DIURETIC THERAPY: CLINICAL IMPLICATIONS

Diuretics entrain a set of homeostatic mechanisms that limit their fluid-depleting actions and contribute to diuretic resistance and adverse effects. The first dose of a diuretic normally produces a brisk diuresis. However, in subjects consuming a normal-salt diet, a new equilibrium is attained within one day when body weight stabilizes and daily fluid and electrolyte excretion no longer exceeds intake. This occurs because of a combination of post-diuretic salt retention, the development of a contraction alkalosis that inhibits the efficacy of loop diuretics, and diuretic tolerance (which is class specific). In contrast, during salt restriction the first dose of furosemide produces a blunted natriuresis, but Na$^+$ balance cannot be restored because of the low level of dietary Na$^+$ intake, and the patient continues to lose both Na$^+$ and body weight. There are several clinical implications from these findings. First, even in subjects receiving powerful loop diuretics, dietary salt intake must be restricted to obviate postdiuretic salt retention and to ensure the development of a negative NaCl balance. Second, during prolonged diuretic administration, subjects may be particularly responsive to another class of diuretic. Third, diuretic therapy should not be stopped abruptly unless dietary salt intake is effectively curtailed, because the adaptive mechanisms limiting salt excretion persist for days after diuretic use. Fourth, selection of a diuretic with a prolonged action or more frequent administration of the diuretic will enhance NaCl loss by limiting the time available for postdiuretic salt retention. Indeed, continuous infusion of a loop diuretic is more effective than the same dose given as a bolus injection in volunteers, in patients with cardiac disease, and in those with chronic renal failure despite a similar delivery of diuretic to the urine. Fifth, prevention or reversal of diuretic-induced metabolic alkalosis may enhance diuretic efficacy.

Diuretic Resistance

If diuretic resistance is seen, the first step is to select the appropriate target response (e.g., a specific body weight) and to ensure that the edema is due to inappropriate renal NaCl and fluid retention rather than to lymphatic or venous obstruction. The next step is to exclude noncompliance or concurrent use of nonsteroidal anti-inflammatory drugs. Thereafter, dietary NaCl intake should be quantitated (24-hour Na$^+$ excretion). For patients with mild edema or hypertension, a "no added salt" diet may be sufficient to reduce daily Na$^+$ intake to 100 to 120 mmol. For patients with diuretic resistance, the help of a dietitian is usually necessary to reduce daily Na$^+$ intake to 80 to 100 mmol. The next step is to double the dose of the diuretic or, better, to give two daily doses. Furosemide and bumetanide act for only 3 to 6 hours. Two divided doses, by interrupting postdiuretic salt retention, produce a greater response than the same total dose given once daily. Concurrent disease may impair the absorption of the diuretic. Thus, a more bioavailable diuretic, such as torsemide, may be preferable. Diuretic resistance is often accompanied by a pronounced metabolic alkalosis. This may be reversed by KCl or by adding a distal K$^+$-sparing diuretic. Adaptive changes in downstream nephron segments during prolonged diuretic therapy provide a rational basis for combining diuretics (see the next section).

If there is no response, consideration should be given to a trial of intravenous loop diuretic infusion or ultrafiltration.

Diuretic Combinations

Combination diuretic therapy using agents acting on separate natriuretic mechanisms can significantly augment the diuretic response.

Loop Diuretics and Thiazides

A loop diuretic and a thiazide (e.g., hydrochlorothiazide or metolazone) are synergistic in normal subjects and in those with edema or renal insufficiency. Metolazone is equivalent to bendrofluazide in enhancing NaCl and fluid losses in furosemide-resistant subjects with CHF or the nephrotic syndrome. Patients with advanced chronic renal failure (GFR < 30 mL/min) that is unresponsive to thiazide alone have a marked natriuresis when the thiazide is added to loop diuretic therapy, probably by blockade of enhanced distal tubular Na^+ reabsorption. However, close clinical surveillance is imperative when combination therapy is initiated because of a high incidence of hypokalemia, excessive ECV depletion, and azotemia.

Loop Diuretics or Thiazides and Distal Potassium-Sparing Diuretics

Amiloride or triamterene increases furosemide natriuresis only modestly but curtails the excretion of K^+ and net acid and preserved total body K^+. Distal K^+-sparing agents are generally contraindicated in renal failure because they may cause severe hyperkalemia and acidosis.

ADVERSE EFFECTS OF DIURETICS

Fluid and Electrolyte Abnormalities

Extracellular Volume Depletion and Azotemia

Diuretics normally do not decrease the GFR. However, renal failure can be precipitated by vigorous diuresis in patients with impaired renal function, severe edema, or cirrhosis and ascites. A rise in the ratio of blood urea nitrogen to creatinine (> 20:1) suggests ECV depletion.

Hyponatremia

Hyponatremia is usually described with thiazide therapy. The mechanisms include enhanced arginine vasopressin release in response to volume depletion and more importantly specific effects on the urinary concentrating capacity. This effect is relatively specific for thiazides, which inhibit urinary dilution, whereas loop diuretics inhibit both urinary concentration and dilution. Mild, asymptomatic hyponatremia can be treated by withdrawing diuretics, restricting the daily intake of free water to 1 to 1.5 L, restoring any K^+ and Mg^{2+} losses, and replenishing NaCl if the patient is clearly volume depleted. Severe, symptomatic hyponatremia complicated by seizures is an emergency requiring intensive treatment. The ideal management remains controversial but usually involves the controlled administration of hypertonic saline (see Chapter 7, Pathophysiology of Water Metabolism).

Hypokalemia

The serum K^+ concentration (S_K) of patients not receiving KCl supplements falls by an average of 0.3 mmol/L with furosemide and by 0.6 mmol/L with thiazides. Mild diuretic-induced hypokalemia (S_K 3 to 3.5 mmol/L) increases the frequency of ventricular ectopy, the clinical significance of which in otherwise healthy subjects is unknown. Severe hypokalemia (S_K <3 mmol/L) is associated with a doubling of serious ventricular dysrhythmias, muscular weakness, and rhabdomyolysis. Lesser degrees of hypokalemia can precipitate dysrhythmias in patients with known ischemic heart disease, subjects taking digoxin, or patients with a prolonged QT interval. Hypokalemia can be prevented by increasing intake of K^+ by 20 to 40 mmol daily. In the presence of alkalosis, hyperaldosteronism, or Mg^{2+} depletion, hypokalemia is quite unresponsive to dietary KCl. A more effective, convenient, and predictable strategy therefore is to prescribe combined therapy with a distal K^+-sparing agent such as amiloride or triamterene, which prevents diuretic-induced hypokalemia and alkalosis and provides further natriuresis and antihypertensive efficacy.

Hyperkalemia

Distal potassium-sparing diuretics decrease K^+ secretion and predispose to hyperkalemia. Recently, trimethoprim and pentamidine have been identified as amiloride-like agents that inhibit K^+ secretion in the collecting ducts.

Hypomagnesemia

During prolonged therapy with thiazides and loop diuretics, serum Mg^{2+} concentration (S_{Mg}) falls by 5% to 10% and diuretic-induced hyponatremia and hypokalemia cannot be reversed fully until any Mg^{2+} deficit is replaced. Symptoms of hypomagnesemia include depression, muscular weakness, and atrial fibrillation and can be corrected by administration of magnesium oxide or sulfate. Distal K^+-sparing agents and spironolactone diminish Mg^{2+} excretion.

Hypercalcemia

Thiazides increase the serum concentrations of total and ionized calcium (S_{Ca}). Persistent hypercalcemia should prompt a search for a specific cause, for example, an adenoma of the parathyroid glands. In contrast, loop diuretics and saline infusion are used in association with volume expansion to treat hypercalcemia.

Acid-Base Changes

Metabolic alkalosis induced by thiazides or loop diuretics is an important adverse factor in patients with hepatic cirrhosis and ascites, in whom the alkalosis may provoke hepatic coma by partitioning ammonia into the brain, and in those with underlying pulmonary insufficiency, in whom the alkalosis can impair ventilatory drive. Diuretic-induced metabolic alkalosis is best managed by administration of NaCl or KCl, but a distal K^+-sparing diuretic or occasionally a carbonic anhydrase inhibitor, should be considered. Spironolactone and distal K^+-sparing diuretics can cause hyperkalemic metabolic acidosis, especially in elderly patients, those with renal impairment or cirrhosis, and those receiving KCl supplements.

Metabolic Abnormalities

Hyperglycemia

Diuretic therapy, especially with thiazides, impairs carbohydrate tolerance and occasionally precipitates diabetes mellitus. The increase in blood glucose concentration is greatest during initiation of therapy and is reversed rapidly after discontinuation of diuretics even after many years of therapy. The effect can be corrected by reversal of hypokalemia or hypomagnesemia or administration of spironolactone. Care should be taken to monitor blood glucose after initiation of thiazide therapy, particularly in obese or diabetic patients. Measures to prevent this complication include coadministration of a distal, K^+-sparing diuretic, spironolactone, ACE inhibitor, or ARB, prescribing extra KCl, or reducing the thiazide dosage.

Hyperlipidemia

Administration of loop diuretics or thiazides increases the plasma concentrations of total cholesterol, triglycerides, and low-density lipoprotein cholesterol, but reduces concentration of high-density lipoprotein cholesterol. Therefore, it raises the low-density lipoprotein-to-high-density lipoprotein cholesterol ratio. Importantly, most studies have shown that serum cholesterol returns to baseline over 3 to 12 months of thiazide therapy and when combined with lifestyle management, 4 years of thiazide therapy for hypertension is associated with a modest improvement in the lipid profile.

Hyperuricemia
Prolonged thiazide therapy for hypertension increases the serum urate concentration by approximately 35%, and this can lead to gout.

Other Adverse Effects

Impotence
The incidence of impotence is much higher in patients receiving thiazides than in normal subjects.

Ototoxicity
Loop diuretics can cause deafness that may occasionally be permanent. The risk is greater with ethacrynic acid and when it is combined with another ototoxic drug (e.g., an aminoglycoside), during high-dose bolus intravenous therapy in patients with renal failure if plasma levels are increased, and in hypoalbuminemic subjects.

Hazards in Pregnancy and Newborns
The use of thiazides can be maintained during pregnancy in those whose hypertension has been controlled by them, and they can be used in pregnancy to treat pulmonary edema. Prolonged furosemide therapy in preterm infants can cause renal calcification. Diuretics can be transferred from the mother to the infant in breast milk.

Drug Allergy
A reversible photosensitivity dermatitis occurs rarely during thiazide or furosemide therapy. High-dose furosemide in renal failure can cause bullous dermatitis. Diuretics may cause a more generalized dermatitis, sometimes with eosinophilia, purpura, or blood dyscrasia. Occasionally, they cause a necrotizing vasculitis. Cross-sensitivity can occur with other sulfonamide drugs. Acute interstitial nephritis with fever, skin rash, and eosinophilia may develop abruptly some months after initiation of therapy with a thiazide or, less often, with furosemide.

Ethacrynic acid is chemically dissimilar from other loop diuretics and can be a substitute.

Adverse Drug Interactions
Hyperkalemia in patients receiving distal K^+-sparing diuretics can be precipitated by concurrent therapy with KCl, ACE inhibitors, ARBs, heparin, ketoconazole, trimethoprim, or pentamidine. Loop diuretics and aminoglycosides potentiate ototoxicity and nephrotoxicity. Diuretic-induced hypokalemia increases digitalis toxicity fourfold. Plasma lithium concentrations increase during thiazide therapy because of increased proximal lithium reabsorption. Nonsteroidal anti-inflammatory drugs may impair the diuretic, natriuretic, antihypertensive, and venodilating responses to diuretics and predispose to renal vasoconstriction and a fall in GFR. Used together, indomethacin and triamterene may precipitate acute urinary obstruction and renal failure.

CLINICAL USES OF DIURETICS

Edematous Conditions

Diuretic therapy for edema should be initiated with the lowest effective dose and only after treatment of the underlying etiology has been initiated. Dietary Na^+ intake should be monitored and restricted to 100 to 120 mmol/24 hr in patients with mild edema. Increasingly severe restrictions of dietary salt to 80 to 100 mmol/24 hr are required for patients with refractory edema.

Cardiac Failure
The therapeutic approach for cardiac failure depends on the cause of the left ventricular dysfunction.

Acute Ischemic Left Ventricular Failure
Intravenous furosemide for left ventricular failure complicating acute myocardial infarction can rapidly reduce the left ventricular filling pressure primarily by increasing venous capacitance, an effect that is an antecedent to any diuretic effect. The ensuing diuresis reduces left ventricular end-diastolic pressure further. However, ischemia can lead to diastolic dysfunction. In this setting, diuretic-induced volume losses can reduce cardiac output, occasionally to the point of hypotension and shock. Accordingly, intravenous diuretics should not be used in patients with cardiogenic shock and must be used carefully in those with acute left ventricular failure, especially when diastolic dysfunction is suspected.

Chronic Stable Congestive Heart Failure

Diuretics are extremely useful in the long-term management of chronic, stable CHF. Loop diuretic therapy can improve cardiac output and congestive symptoms. On the other hand, because the failing heart has a decreased capacity to regulate its contractility in response to changes in venous return, if diuretic therapy is overzealous, patients may suffer from a decreased effective blood volume (orthostatic hypotension, weakness, fatigue, decreased exercise ability, and prerenal azotemia). Therefore, salt-depleting therapy requires continual reassessment and judicious use of other measures (e.g., vasodilators, ACE inhibitors, or ARBs). Diuretics should be used cautiously in those with diastolic dysfunction. A recent study has shown that patients with CHF have an improved outcome if randomly assigned to receive spironolactone (25 to 50 mg/day), even if they are receiving concurrent ACE inhibitor therapy.

There is impaired diuretic responsiveness in patients with advanced CHF due to delayed absorption and diminished tubular secretion. Thus, resistance should be anticipated in patients with severe CHF, and the diuretic dosage should be increased accordingly. Mild CHF often responds to dietary Na^+ restriction (100 to 120 mmol/day) and low doses of a thiazide diuretic. As cardiac failure progresses, larger, more frequent doses of loop diuretics and tighter control of dietary salt intake (80 to 100 mmol/day) are required. For the patient with refractory CHF, the addition of a second diuretic acting at the proximal tubule (e.g., acetazolamide) or a downstream site (e.g., a thiazide) can produce a dramatic diuresis, even in individuals with impaired renal function. Many patients with advanced CHF and diuretic resistance have a satisfactory diuresis after addition of spironolactone (25 to 100 mg/day). In patients with diuretic resistance, admission to the hospital for an continuous intravenous infusion of furosemide may be required (20 to 160 mg/day as needed).

Right Ventricular Failure

The requirement for diuretic therapy in patients with pure right heart failure or cor pulmonale is not compelling. A decrease in venous return induced by vigorous diuresis may worsen right heart function, and the clinical emphasis should be on reversal of chronic hypoxemia.

Cirrhosis of the Liver

Patients with advanced cirrhosis of the liver are Na^+ avid but have a blunted response to furosemide because of hypoalbuminemia, leading to diminished tubular delivery. In relative terms, these patients have an enhanced natriuretic response to diuretics acting in the distal nephron. Thus, thiazides and, in particular, spironolactone are a rational choice for treating edema and ascites in the cirrhotic patient. Cirrhotic patients with peripheral edema may tolerate a diuresis of 1 to 3 kg/day. However, because the daily ascites drainage is limited to 300 to 900 mL, the maximum daily weight loss in nonedematous patients should not exceed 0.3 to 0.5 kg. Mild edema can be treated by dietary restriction of Na^+ (100 mmol/day) and free water (1.5 L/day) if the S_{Na} falls to less than 130 mmol/L. Patients with milder ascites require stricter reduction of salt and may respond to spironolactone (25 to 100 mg/day). More severe ascites may require bed rest and a combination of furosemide and spironolactone (40 to 160 mg of furosemide/100 to 400 mg of spironolactone). Patients with diuretic resistance may be considered for transjugular portosystemic shunting or repeated large volume paracentesis. The traditional belief that paracentesis is dangerous in such patients has been challenged by controlled trials showing that it is more effective than diuretic therapy in relieving ascites and reducing length of hospital stay but that it does not influence mortality rates. Even repeated, large-volume paracenteses (4 to 6 L/day) are safe if intravenous albumin (25 to 50 g with each procedure) is administered.

The most common problems with furosemide in cirrhosis are electrolyte disturbances and volume depletion. Hypokalemia is related to preexisting K^+ depletion and hyperaldosteronism. It can be countered by the use of spironolactone or distal K^+-sparing agents. However, patients with cirrhosis can develop hyperkalemic metabolic acidosis with spironolactone.

Nephrotic Syndrome

Diuretics are central to the management of the nephrotic syndrome. These patients typically have some degree of diuretic resistance; therefore, loop diuretics are the agents of first choice because of their more potent natriuretic effects. Decreased diuretic delivery into tubular fluid and diuretic binding to filtered albumin within the tubule lumen contribute to the observed diuretic resistance. The administration of albumin in combination with furosemide to enhance diuretic efficacy has long been practiced. Controlled trials suggest that any effect is modest at best. A more logical approach to diuretic resistance is to limit albuminuria with an ACE inhibitor or ARB or both, which also may combat the associated coagulopathy, dyslipidemia, edema, and progressive loss of renal function.

Idiopathic Edema

Idiopathic edema affects women predominantly. It causes fluctuating salt retention and edema, exacerbated by orthostasis. The effects of diuretic therapy in this setting are unclear, and patients are best treated by salt restriction.

Nonedematous Conditions

Acute Renal Failure

Diuretics can be used to treat edema or to convert ARF to nonoliguric ARF. Most patients with severe ARF show diuretic resistance, and the administration of high-dose diuretic therapy (>1 g/day) can provoke hearing loss and therefore cannot be recommended. Importantly, furosemide therapy for ARF does not reduce mortality but may reduce the need for dialysis by diminishing hyperkalemia, acidosis, or fluid overload. The use of bumetanide or torsemide, which are hepatically metabolized, may lead to less drug accumulation and less risk of ototoxicity.

Chronic Renal Insufficiency

Salt and water retention are almost invariable in chronic renal insufficiency and contribute to the development of hypertension. Dietary salt restriction should be the cornerstone of therapy; however, if this is not sufficient, then diuretic therapy is indicated. Thiazide diuretics are relatively ineffective in patients with a moderate to severe degree of chronic renal insufficiency (creatinine clearance <35 mL/min), although thiazide diuretics such as metolazone at high doses do retain some efficacy even in quite advanced chronic renal insufficiency, particularly when used in combination with a loop diuretic. Therefore, loop diuretics are preferred in this setting. The response to diuretics is limited by a reduction in the absolute rate of NaCl reabsorption in the kidney that is the target for the diuretic and by a reduction in diuretic delivery to the urine. However, the maximal increase in fractional excretion of Na^+ produced by furosemide is maintained quite well in CKD because there is a relative three- to fourfold increase per residual nephron in the expression of the $Na^+/K^+/2Cl^-$ cotransporter in the TAL. Torsemide has the greatest oral bioavailability in chronic renal failure. For patients with refractory conditions, a loop diuretic infusion (e.g., bumetanide, 1 mg/hr for 12 hours) produces a greater natriuresis than bolus injections. High plasma levels of furosemide can cause ototoxicity, and it is advisable to set a ceiling dose in patients with CKD.

Hypercalcemia

Ca^{2+} excretion is increased by osmotic or loop diuretics. Hypercalcemia activates a Ca^{2+}-sensing protein that inhibits fluid and NaCl reabsorption in the TAL and impairs renal concentration. The ensuing ECV depletion further limits Ca^{2+} excretion by reducing the GFR and enhancing proximal fluid and Ca^{2+} reabsorption. Therefore, the initial therapy for hypercalcemia is volume expansion with saline. Once volume expansion is achieved an infusion of a loop diuretic (e.g., 80 to 120 mg of furosemide every 1 to 2 hours) causes the loss of approximately 80 mg of Ca^{2+} per dose. Fluid and electrolytes should be replaced quantitatively.

Nephrolithiasis

Thiazides reduce stone formation in hypercalciuric and even normocalciuric patients by reducing excretion of Ca^{2+} and oxalate. Some patients continue to form stones and require additional citrate therapy. Ca^{2+} excretion can be enhanced by addition of amiloride or a low-salt diet. $KHCO_3$ produces a greater reduction in Ca^{2+} excretion than KCl when given with hydrochlorothiazide.

Diabetes Insipidus

Thiazides can reduce urine flow by about 50% in patients with central or nephrogenic diabetes insipidus. Antidiuresis is related to a decreased GFR, enhanced water reabsorption in the proximal and distal tubules, and an increase in papillary osmolarity.

Antihypertensive Drugs

34

INDIVIDUAL AGENTS

Angiotensin-Converting Enzyme Inhibitors

Class Mechanisms of Action

The angiotensin-converting enzyme (ACE) inhibitors inhibit the activity of ACE, which converts the angiotensin I (AI) to the potent hormone angiotensin II (AII). Because AII plays a crucial role in maintaining and regulating blood pressure by vasoconstriction and renal sodium and water retention, the ACE inhibitors are powerful tools for targeting multiple pathways that contribute to hypertension.

Class Members

There are currently more than 15 ACE inhibitors in clinical use. Each drug has a unique structure, but they all have remarkably similar clinical effects. The pharmacodynamic properties of the ACE inhibitors are outlined in Table 34–1.

Class Renal Effects

In patients with hypertension, ACE inhibitors restore the pressure-natriuresis relationship to normal, resulting in a natriuresis and lower arterial blood pressure. In the setting of restricted sodium intake, the response is exaggerated. The decrease in aldosterone results in decreased potassium excretion, particularly in patients with impaired renal function. The antikaliuretic effect is typically transient but can be exacerbated by concomitant administration of potassium-sparing diuretics, potassium supplements, and non-steroidal anti-inflammatory drugs and potassium levels should be monitored rigorously.

The reduction of proteinuria is a key therapeutic goal in management of chronic kidney disease. All ACE inhibitors decrease urinary protein excretion in normotensive and hypertensive patients with chronic renal disease of various origins. Individual response rates

Table 34–1: Pharmacodynamic Properties of the Common Angiotensin-Converting Enzyme Inhibitors

Generic (Trade) Name	Dose Range	Dosing Interval	Maximal Daily Dose
Captopril (Capoten)	12.5–50	bid/tid	150
Benazepril (Lotensin)	10–20	qd	40
Enalapril (Vasotec)	10–40	qd/bid	40
Quinapril (Accupril)	20–80	qd	80
Ramipril (Altace)	2.5–20	qd/bid	40
Trandolapril (Mavik)	2–4	qd	8
Fosinopril (Monopril)	5–40	qd/bid	40
Perindopril (Aceon)	4–8	qd	8
Lisinopril (Zestril, Prinivil)	20–40	qd	40

vary widely and are strongly influenced by drug dose and changes in dietary sodium. Notably the effect of ACE inhibitors on reduction of proteinuria is abolished with high salt intake. Many patients with impaired renal function exhibit a reversible fall in glomerular filtration rate (GFR) with ACE inhibitor therapy that is not detrimental. This fall in GFR occurs because of the hemodynamic changes, but the long-term reduction in perfusion pressure is renoprotective. Indeed, type 1 diabetic patients with the greatest initial decline in GFR have the slowest rate of loss of renal function over time. It should be emphasized that ACE inhibitors should not be withdrawn immediately if a modest increase in serum creatinine is noted; a 20% to 30% decline in GFR can be expected and close monitoring is warranted. The improvement in clinical outcome is not restricted to hypertensive patients. In normotensive diabetic patients, studies demonstrate that ACE inhibitors can normalize GFR, markedly reduce the progression of renal disease, and normalize microalbuminuria. The ACE inhibitors have superior antiproteinuric efficacy compared with other classes of antihypertensive agents, with the exception of angiotensin receptor blockers (ARBs). Clinical trials also demonstrate a superior renoprotective effect of ACE inhibitors in African Americans, a group once thought not to benefit from this class of drug. In the African American Study of Kidney Disease, hypertensive patients with proteinuria greater than 300 mg/day had a much slower rate of progression of kidney disease when treated with an ACE inhibitor than with a dihydropyridine calcium antagonist (CA).

Class Efficacy and Safety
ACE inhibitors are recommended for initial monotherapy in patients with mild, moderate, and severe hypertension regardless

of age, race, or sex. ACE inhibitors are indicated as first-line therapy in hypertensive patients with heart failure and systolic dysfunction, those with type 1 diabetes and proteinuria, patients after myocardial infarction with reduced systolic function, and patients with left ventricular dysfunction. Indeed, all hypertensive diabetic patients, even those with no evidence of nephropathy, should be given ACE inhibitors for cardiovascular risk reduction. African Americans have been found to respond less well to lower doses than Caucasians, but higher doses are as effective. ACE inhibitors elicit an adequate response in 40% to 60% of patients, and response rates are enhanced by salt restriction or the addition of low-dose hydrochlorothiazide (HCTZ).

ACE inhibitors are contraindicated in patients with known renovascular hypertension or hypersensitivity to ACE inhibitors. ACE inhibitors may cause fetal or neonatal injury or death when used during the second and third trimesters of pregnancy. Exposure to ACE inhibitors limited to the first trimester has not been associated with injury. If a patient becomes pregnant during treatment, the ACE inhibitor should be discontinued and alternative treatment found; termination of pregnancy is not warranted. Hyperkalemia rarely requires discontinuation of therapy and is more likely to develop in patients with renal insufficiency or diabetes or those taking potassium-sparing drugs. The most common side effect of ACE inhibitors is a dry, hacking, nonproductive, and often intolerable cough that is reported in up to 20% of patients. This is managed by switching to an ARB (see later). Angioedema is a rare but potentially life-threatening complication of ACE inhibitor therapy. It occurs in less than 0.2% of patients within hours of the first dose of ACE inhibitor or occasionally after prolonged use. First-dose hypotension occurs more commonly in volume-depleted states, patients with high-renin hypertension, and those with systolic heart failure. In high-risk patients, therapy should be initiated with lower doses and preferably after discontinuation of diuretics. Other complications include a metallic taste sensation, leukopenia, and anemia. Fatal agranulocytosis has been reported.

Angiotensin II Type I Receptor Antagonists

Class Mechanisms of Action
The ARBs selectively antagonize AII directly at the angiotensin II type 1 (AT1) receptor. Because AII plays a crucial multifactorial role in maintaining and regulating blood pressure, blockade

Table 34–2: Pharmacodynamic Properties of the Common Angiotensin Receptor Blockers

Generic (Trade) Name	Dose Range	Dosing Interval	Maximal Daily Dose
Eprosartan (Teveten)	200–400	qd/bid	400
Irbesartan (Avapro)	150–300	qd	300
Losartan (Cozaar)	50–100	qd/bid	100
Valsartan (Diovan)	80–160	qd	320
Candesartan (Atacand)	8–32	qd	32
Telmisartan (Micardis)	40–80	qd	80
Olmesartan (Benicar)	20–40	qd	40

of the AT1 receptor with ARBs is a powerful tool for targeting multiple pathways that contribute to hypertension.

Class Members
The ARB class is composed of peptide and nonpeptide analogs that vary in structure, mechanism of receptor inhibition, metabolism, and potency. There are currently seven drugs in clinical use. The pharmacodynamic properties of the ARBS are outlined in Table 34–2.

Class Renal Effects
Angiotensin receptor blockade significantly decreases urinary protein excretion in a manner broadly similar to that observed with ACE inhibition. Antiproteinuric effects have been described in diabetic and nondiabetic patients and with renal transplant recipients. The maximal antiproteinuric effect occurs at 3 to 4 weeks. In patients with diabetic nephropathy, ARBs reduce proteinuria by up to 30% and can reduce microalbuminuria to baseline in one third of patients. Long-term renoprotection with these agents substantially retards the progression of renal disease and reduces overall mortality in patients with type 2 diabetes independent of changes in blood pressure. Thus, the ARBs should be the foundation of therapy in patients with type 2 diabetes and nephropathy. Whether the antiproteinuric effects are equivalent to or better than those of ACE inhibitors remains to be determined. However, they do appear to have additive antiproteinuric effects. It is recommended that patients receiving ACE inhibitor therapy with persistent hypertension or proteinuria should be considered for combined treatment with angiotensin receptor antagonist therapy. A property unique to the losartan molecule is induction of uricosuria. This effect is not associated with an increased risk of nephrolithiasis nor

is it observed with ACE inhibitors or other ARBs, and it is not related to inhibition of the renin-angiotensin system. The decrease in serum uric acid may be beneficial, because it has been suggested that hyperuricemia is a risk factor for renal disease progression and coronary artery disease.

Class Efficacy and Safety

All AT1 receptor blockers have been demonstrated to lower blood pressure effectively and safely in patients with mild, moderate, and severe hypertension regardless of age, sex, or race. They are indicated as first-line monotherapy or add-on therapy for hypertension and are comparable in efficacy to ACE inhibitor therapy. They are safe and effective in patients with renal insufficiency, diabetes, heart failure, renal transplants, coronary artery disease, and left ventricular hypertrophy (LVH) and have been shown to protect against hypertensive end-organ disease, such as LVH, stroke, end-stage renal disease, and possibly diabetes. Although they may not be the most efficacious agents in terms of blood pressure reduction in blacks, they are equally or more efficacious in offering target organ protection and arresting disease progression than agents that do not inhibit the renin-angiotensin system.

The long onset of action of 4 to 6 weeks avoids the first-dose hypotension and rebound hypertension commonly seen with other drugs. The addition of thiazide diuretics potentiates the therapeutic effect and increases response rates to 70% to 80% and is more effective than increasing the dose of ARB. ARBs are contraindicated in patients with known renovascular hypertension and may cause fetal or neonatal death when used during the second and third trimesters of pregnancy. As with ACE inhibitors, an abrupt decline in GFR may be observed in the setting of renal hypoperfusion; this typically responds to withdrawal of the drug and/or optimization of renal perfusion. In clinical trials, hyperkalemia occurs in less than 1.5% of patients and is comparable to that observed with ACE inhibitor therapy. It is more likely to develop in patients with renal insufficiency or diabetes or those taking potassium-sparing drugs. ARBs have no effect on serum lipids in hypertensive patients but may improve the abnormal lipoprotein profile of patients with proteinuric renal disease. Clinically relevant side effects are not observed more often than in placebo-treated patients. Because ARBs do not interfere with kinin metabolism, cough is rare and the incidence of cough in patients with a history of ACE inhibitor–induced cough is no greater than in those receiving placebo. Similarly, the incidence of angioedema and facial swelling is no greater than with placebo.

β-Adrenergic Antagonists

Mechanisms of Action

β-Adrenergic blocking drugs exert their effects by attenuation of sympathetic stimulation through competitive antagonism of catecholamines at the β-adrenergic receptor. In addition to β-blockade properties, certain drugs have antihypertensive effects mediated through several different mechanisms including α_1-adrenergic blocking activity, β_2-adrenergic agonist activity, and perhaps effects on nitric oxide–dependent vasodilator action. Partial agonist activity is a property of certain β-adrenergic blockers that results in less slowing of the resting heart rate but the overall clinical significance remains unclear. β-Adrenergic receptor blockers may be nonspecific and block both β_1- and β_2-adrenergic receptors, or they may be relatively specific for β_1-adrenergic receptors. β_1-Receptors are found predominantly in heart, adipose, and brain tissue, whereas β_2-receptors predominate in the lung, liver, smooth muscle, and skeletal muscle. Many tissues, however, have both β_1- and β_2-receptors, including the heart, and it is important to realize that the concept of a cardioselective drug is only relative. The bioavailability of β-blockers varies greatly, and they are eliminated primarily by hepatic metabolism.

Class Members

The β-adrenergic antagonists are classified and reviewed on the basis of the following subclasses: nonselective β-adrenergic antagonism, nonselective β-adrenergic antagonism with partial agonist activity, and β_1-selective adrenergic antagonism. Their pharmacodynamic and pharmacokinetic properties are outlined in Table 34–3.

Table 34–3: Pharmacodynamic Properties of the Common β-Blockers

Generic (Trade) Name	Dose Range (mg)	Dosing Interval	Maximal Daily Dose (mg)
Nadolol	40–80	qd	320
Propranolol	80–320	bid	640
Timolol	20–40	bid	60
Pindolol	10–40	qd-bid	60
Atenolol	50–100	qd	200
Metoprolol	100–200	qd-bid	450
Bisoprolol	5–20	qd	40
Acebutolol	400–800	qd	1200

Renal Effects of β-Adrenergic Blockers

In general, the acute administration of a β-adrenergic blocker usually results in reduction of GFR.

The degree of reduction in GFR is typically modest and not of clinical significance in most patients. In patients with impaired kidney function, dosage adjustment of atenolol is necessary (Table 34–4).

Table 34–4: Antihypertensive Drugs Requiring Dose Modification* in Renal Insufficiency: Estimated Glomerular Filtration Rate (Creatinine Clearance)

Drug	10–15 mL/min	<10 mL/min	Dialysis
Angiotensin-converting enzyme inhibitors			
Benazepril	50%	25%	Negligible
Captopril	50%	25%	(H) 50%
Cilazapril	50%	25%	(H) 50%
Enalapril	50%	25%	(H) 50%
Fosinopril	No change	No change	75%
Lisinopril	50%	25%	(H) 50%
Perindopril	75%	50%	–
Quinapril	50%	25%	–
Ramipril	50%	25%	–
Trandolapril	50%	25%	–
Angiotensin receptor blockers			
Candesartan	No change	No change	Negligible
Eprosartan	No change	50%	Negligible
Irbesartan	No change	–	Negligible
Losartan	No change	No change	Negligible
Olmesartan	–	–	–
Telmisartan	No change	No change	Negligible
Valsartan	No change	No change	–
β-Adrenergic antagonists			
Nadolol	50%	25%	(H) 50%
Carteolol	50%	25%	–
Penbutolol	No change	50%	Negligible
Pindolol	No change	50%	Negligible
Atenolol	50%	25%	(H) 50%
Bisoprolol	50%	25%	Negligible
Acebutolol	50%	30%–50%	(H) 50%
Celiprolol	50%	Avoid	–
Nebivolol	50%	–	–

Continued

Table 34–4: (cont'd)

Drug	10–15 mL/min	<10 mL/min	Dialysis
Calcium antagonists			
No dose adjustment required in renal failure			
Central β₂-adrenergic or imidazole I1 agonists			
Methyldopa	No change	50%	(H) 50%
Clonidine	50%	25%	Negligible
Peripheral adrenergic-neuronal blocking agents			
Guanethidine	No change	50%	(avoid) —
Direct-acting vasodilators			
Hydralazine	No change	75%	‡Negligible
Minoxidil	50%	50%	(H and P) 50%

*Percent of total dose given.

‡Slow acetylators.

H, hemodialysis; P, peritoneal dialysis.

Efficacy and Safety of β-Adrenergic Antagonists

The Sixth Report of the Joint National Committee on Prevention, Detection, Evaluation, and Treatment of High Blood Pressure (JNC VI) recommended a β-blocker or diuretic as appropriate initial therapy for hypertension. This recommendation was based on numerous randomized clinical trials showing a reduction in mortality and morbidity with these agents. β-Adrenergic antagonists are effective therapy for patients in all age-groups. Patients older than 60 years of age have an antihypertensive response to atenolol that is comparable to that of patients treated with diltiazem, HCTZ, or captopril. The response is, however, less in elderly black patients, and some studies have suggested that β-adrenergic blockers may be less efficacious in black than in white patients compared with therapy with calcium channel blockers and thiazides. β-Blockers are suitable first-line therapy for elderly patients with hypertension in whom they are effective for primary prevention of stroke, myocardial infarction, and sudden death. At present, β-blockers appear to be effective for many hypertensive elderly patients, particularly those with comorbid conditions and tachycardia; however, they may be somewhat less effective than diuretics or CAs as first-line therapy. Other indications include a prior history of coronary artery disease or congestive heart failure where a mortality benefit has been convincingly demonstrated. β-Adrenergic blockers have been widely used to treat women with hypertension in the third trimester of pregnancy.

The main side effects associated with β-adrenergic blockade include central nervous system symptoms of lethargy, sedation, sleep disturbance, depression, and visual hallucinations; sexual dysfunction in males; constipation, diarrhea, nausea, or indigestion; hyperkalemia; and impaired glucose tolerance. β-Blockade can also blunt the effects of epinephrine secretion resulting from hypoglycemia, which may result in hypoglycemia unawareness. Patients with severe bronchospastic airway disease should not receive β-adrenergic blockers. In patients with mild to moderate disease, β_1-selective agents may be used cautiously. Symptoms of peripheral vascular disease may be exacerbated by β-blocker therapy. Abrupt withdrawal of β-adrenergic blockers may be associated with overshoot hypertension and worsening angina in patients with coronary artery disease, and myocardial infarction has been reported. These withdrawal symptoms may be due to increased sympathetic activity, which is a reflection of possible adrenergic receptor up-regulation during chronic sympathetic blockade. Gradual tapering of β-blockers decreases the risk of withdrawal.

Calcium Antagonists

Mechanisms of Action

CAs have emerged as an important therapeutic class of medications for a variety of cardiovascular disorders. Initially introduced in the 1970s as antianginal agents, they are now widely advocated as first-line therapy for hypertension. Each class of CA is quantitatively and qualitatively unique, possessing differential sensitivity and selectivity for binding pharmacologic receptors as well as the slow calcium channel in various vascular tissues. This differential selectivity of action has important clinical implications for the use of these drugs and explains why the CAs vary considerably in their effects on regional circulatory beds, sinus and atrioventricular (AV) nodal function, and myocardial contractility. It further explains the diversity of indications for clinical use, ancillary effects, and side effects. CAs uniformly lower peripheral vascular resistance in patients regardless of race, salt sensitivity, age, or comorbid conditions. Interestingly the maximal vasodilatory response to the CAs is inversely related to the patient's plasma renin activity. Thus, it is possible that these agents are of specific benefit in patients with low-renin hypertension, such as blacks.

Class Members

CAs are a very heterogeneous group of compounds and differ with respect to pharmacologic profile, pharmacokinetic profile, clinical indications, and side effect profile (Table 34–5). The two primary subtypes are the dihydropyridines (nifedipine, felodipine, amlodipine, nicardipine, isradipine, and nisoldipine) and nondihydropyridines. The nondihydropyridines are further divided into two classes: benzothiazepines (diltiazem) and diphenylalkylamines (verapamil). Although all CAs vasodilate coronary and peripheral arteries, the dihydropyridines are the most potent. Their potent vasodilatory action prompts a rapid compensatory increase in sympathetic nervous activity, mediated by baroreceptor reflexes. Longer-acting dihydropyridines, however, do not appear to activate the sympathetic nervous system. In contrast, the nondihydropyridines are moderately potent arterial vasodilators but directly decrease AV nodal conduction and have negative inotropic and chronotropic effects, not abrogated by the reflex increase in sympathetic tone. Because of their negative inotropic action, they are contraindicated in patients with systolic heart failure. Short-acting agents are no longer recommended for the treatment of hypertension because the powerful stimulation of the sympathetic nervous system by the vasodilation may predispose patients to angina, myocardial infarction, and stroke.

Table 34–5: Pharmacodynamic Properties of the Common Calcium Channel Blockers

Generic (Trade) Name	Dose Range (mg)	Dosing Interval	Maximal Daily Dose (mg)
Diltiazem	60–120	qd	480
Diltiazem SR	120–240	bid	480
Amlodipine	5–10	qd	10
Felodipine	5–10	qd	10
Isradipine	2.5–10	bid	20
Nicardipine	20–120	tid	120
Nifedipine	10–30	qid	120
Nifedipine SR	30–60	bid	120
Verapamil	80–120	qid	480
Verapamil SR	90–240	bid	480

SR, slow release formulation.

Class Renal Effects

Acute administration of CAs results in little change or augmentation of the GFR and renal plasma flow, no change in the filtration fraction, and reduction of renal vascular resistance. The long-term effects of CAs on renal function are controversial and variable. Some hypertensive patients exhibit an exaggerated increase in GFR and renal plasma flow in response to the dihydropyridines, and this may lead to an increase in protein excretion of up to 40%. In contrast, felodipine, diltiazem, and verapamil do not appear to have this effect and may lower protein excretion, possibly by also decreasing efferent arteriolar tone and glomerular pressure. The clinical implications remain to be determined. In blacks with hypertension and mild to moderate renal insufficiency with proteinuria greater than 1 g/day, renoprotection with an ACE inhibitor far exceeds any effect of the dihydropyridine calcium channel blocker amlodipine, with which renal function may deteriorate. Hypertensive patients with diabetic nephropathy also fare considerably worse with amlodipine therapy than with an ARB both in terms or renoprotection and overall mortality. However, coadministration of amlodipine with an ARB does not abrogate the protective effect on kidney function. It is postulated that selective dilation of the afferent arteriole favors an increase in glomerular capillary pressure that perpetuates renal disease progression. CAs represent an important treatment option for renal transplant recipients. Administration of CAs may help preserve long-term renal function by protecting against cyclosporine nephrotoxicity and, possibly, by contributing to immunomodulation.

Class Efficacy and Safety

Approximately 70% to 80% of hypertensive patients in stage I and II respond to monotherapy. In contrast to other vasodilators, the CAs attenuate the reflex increase of neurohormonal activity that accompanies reduction in blood pressure, and in the long term they inhibit or do not change sympathetic activity. The CAs are effective in young, middle-aged, and elderly patients with all ranges of hypertension. CAs are equally efficacious in patients with high or low plasma renin activity regardless of dietary salt intake or race. They are effective and safe in patients with hypertension and coronary artery disease and end-stage renal disease. The long-acting agents produce sustained systolic and diastolic blood pressure reductions of 16 to 28 and 14 to 17 mm Hg, respectively, with no appreciable development of tolerance.

Among the different classes, the dihydropyridines appear to be the most powerful for reducing blood pressure but may also be associated with greater activation of baroreceptor reflexes. Verapamil and to a lesser extent diltiazem exert greater effects on the heart and less vasoselectivity. They typically reduce heart rate, slow AV conduction, and depress contractility. CAs are contraindicated in patients with severely depressed left ventricular function (except perhaps amlodipine), hypotension, sick sinus syndrome (unless a pacemaker is in place), second- or third-degree heart block, and atrial arrhythmias associated with an accessory pathway. They should not be used as first-line antihypertensive agents in patients with heart failure, patients after myocardial infarction, those with unstable angina, or blacks with proteinuria greater than 300 mg/day. Conversely, CAs are indicated and may be preferred in patients with metabolic disorders such as diabetes, peripheral vascular disease, and stable ischemic heart disease. They may also be ideal agents for elderly hypertensive patients because they tend to lower the risk of stroke more than other classes of agents.

The CAs are generally well tolerated and are not associated with significant perturbations of glycemic balance, lipemic control, or sexual dysfunction. Orthostatic changes do not occur because venoconstriction remains intact. The most common side effect of the dihydropyridines is peripheral edema. It is a result of uncompensated precapillary vasodilation and is not responsive to diuretics but may improve with the addition of an ACE inhibitor, which preferentially vasodilates postcapillary beds. Other side effects related to vasodilation include headache, nausea, dizziness, and flushing. The nondihydropyridines verapamil and isradipine more commonly cause constipation and nausea. Another common side effect of the dihydropyridines is gingival hyperplasia.

Properties beyond their antihypertensive actions make the CAs particularly useful in certain clinical situations. CAs not only lower arterial pressure but increase coronary blood flow. With the exception of the short-acting dihydropyridines, most CAs reduce heart rate, improve myocardial oxygen demand, improve ventricular filling, and conserve contractility, making them ideal for patients with angina or diastolic dysfunction. Verapamil may also be used for secondary cardioprotection to reduce reinfarction rates in patients intolerant of β-blockers unless they have concomitant heart failure. In general, the antihypertensive effects of CAs are enhanced more in combination with β-blockers or ACE inhibitors than with diuretics. Concomitant therapy with β-blockers and nondihydropyridine CAs, however, is potentially dangerous because they may have additive effects on suppressing heart rate, AV node conduction, and cardiac contractility, especially in patients with end-stage renal disease.

Drug interactions are not uncommon. Concurrent use of a CA and amiodarone exacerbates sick sinus syndrome and AV block. Diltiazem, verapamil, and nicardipine have been shown to increase cyclosporine, tacrolimus, and sirolimus levels by 25% to 100% by inhibiting the cytochrome P-450$_{3A4}$ isoenzyme, which metabolizes the calcineurin inhibitors. Concomitant administration of nifedipine, diltiazem, nicardipine, and verapamil with the digitalis glycosides results in up to a 50% increase in serum digoxin concentrations.

CAs may be associated with an increased risk of gastrointestinal hemorrhage, particularly in elderly persons. The safety of CAs in treating cardiovascular diseases remains controversial. There is clear evidence that CAs reduce cardiovascular mortality and morbidity, particularly with stroke; however, short-acting agents such as nifedipine have been associated with a small increased risk for myocardial infarction in meta-analyses compared with other agents. Currently, there is no evidence to prove the existence of either additional beneficial or detrimental effects of CAs on coronary disease events, including fatal or nonfatal myocardial infarctions and other deaths from coronary heart disease. Because of a potential risk, however, as well as simplicity and improved compliance, longer-acting agents should be considered over short-acting CAs for the treatment of hypertension.

Central Adrenergic Agonists

Mechanisms of Action

Central adrenergic agonists act by crossing the blood-brain barrier and have a direct effect on α_2-adrenergic and imidazole (I_1 subtype) receptors located in the midbrain and brainstem. In addition to decreasing total sympathetic outflow, binding to these receptors results in increases in vagal activity. Clonidine is a stimulant of both α-adrenergic receptors and imidazole receptors whereas α-methyldopa acts on the former. More selective imidazole receptor stimulants such as moxonidine and rilmenidine activate the I_1 receptors. The classical α_2-receptor agonists such as clonidine and α-methyldopa trigger vasodilatation in resistance vessels and hence a reduction in peripheral vascular resistance and blood pressure. Despite the vasodilator action, reflex tachycardia generally does not occur as a result of peripheral sympathetic inhibition. The selective I_1 receptor agonists moxonidine and rilmenidine are predominantly arterial vasodilators. The effects of these drugs are mediated by inhibition of the sympathetic outflow, and moxonidine use is also associated with the reduction in plasma renin activity.

Renal Effects of Central α₂-Adrenergic Agonists

Central α_2-agonists and imidazole I_1 agonists have little, if any, clinically important effect on renal plasma flow or GFR in hypertensive patients. Some dosage adjustment is required for patients with renal disease (Table 34–4).

Antihypertensive Efficacy and Safety

These agents have been shown to be effective monotherapy for hypertension in all age and racial groups. There are no significant effects on carbohydrate tolerance and the central α_2-adrenergic agonists appear to be neutral with respect to lipid metabolism. These agents may also be of benefit in patients with congestive heart failure, in whom they may abrogate the activation of deleterious neurohumoral and neuroendocrine compensatory mechanisms.

Stimulation of α_2-adrenergic receptors in the central nervous system induces several side effects of these drugs including sedation and drowsiness. The most common side effect related to α_2-adrenergic activation is dry mouth due to a centrally mediated inhibition of cholinergic transmission. Clonidine in high doses may precipitate a paradoxical hypertensive response related to stimulation of postsynaptic vascular α_2-adrenergic receptors. Methyldopa has been associated with a positive results on a direct Coombs test with or without hemolytic anemia. The α_2-adrenergic agonists are associated with sexual dysfunction and may produce gynecomastia in men and galactorrhea in both men and women. Abrupt cessation of α_2-adrenergic blockers may result in rebound hypertension tachycardia, tremor, anxiety, headache, nausea, and vomiting within 18 to 36 hours.

Central and Peripheral Adrenergic Neuronal Blocking Agents

Mechanisms of Action and Class Member

Reserpine reduces blood pressure by lowering the activity of central and peripheral noradrenergic neurons, resulting in a rapid reduction in cardiac output, heart rate, and peripheral vascular resistance. The half-life is 50 to 100 hours. Extensive hepatic metabolism occurs; 1% is recovered as unchanged compound in the urine. The maximal clinical effect is observed 2 to 3 weeks after initiation of therapy. No dosage adjustment is necessary for patients with renal insufficiency.

Renal Effects

GFR and renal plasma flow are not affected by reserpine therapy.

Efficacy and Safety
Reserpine has been shown to be effective as a single agent or in combination with HCTZ. Reserpine used in combination with a diuretic has shown efficacy comparable to that of combinations of β-blockers and diuretics. The most common side effect of reserpine is nasal congestion, which is reported in up to 20% of patients. Inability to concentrate, sedation, sleep disturbance, and depression have been reported, possibly as a result of depletion of central dopaminergic and serotoninergic neuronal stores.

Direct-Acting Vasodilators

Mechanisms of Action
The direct-acting vasodilators reduce systolic and diastolic blood pressure by decreasing peripheral vascular resistance. Decreases in arterial pressure are associated with a fall in peripheral resistance and a reflex increase in cardiac output. Sodium and water retention is promoted due to the stimulation of renin release.

Class Members
Hydralazine is a direct-acting arteriole vasodilator. Initial oral doses in hypertension should be 10 mg four times daily, increasing to 50 mg four times daily over several weeks. Patients may require doses of up to 300 mg/day. Dosing can be changed to twice daily for maintenance. The drug may also be used as an intravenous bolus injection or as a continuous infusion. Oral absorption is 50% to 90% of the dose and the drug is up to 90% protein bound. Patients with mild to moderate renal insufficiency should have the dosing interval increased to every 8 hours. In severe renal failure, the dose interval should increase to every 8 to 24 hours.

Minoxidil is a direct vasodilator. It is more potent than hydralazine and induces a more marked activation of adrenergic drive. For severe hypertension the initial recommended dose is 5 mg as a single daily dose, increasing to 10 to 20 or 40 mg in single or divided doses. Minoxidil is usually used in conjunction with salt restriction and diuretics to prevent sodium retention. Concomitant therapy with a β-adrenergic blocking agent is often required for increases in heart rate. Renal excretion is 90%. Dosage adjustments may be required in patients with renal failure (see Table 34–4).

Renal Effects of Direct-Acting Vasodilators
Hydralazine and minoxidil both increase the secretion of renin and therefore cause elevations of AII and aldosterone. Retention of salt and water may be due to direct drug effects on the proximal convoluted tubule. GFR and renal plasma flow are unaffected.

Efficacy and Safety

Minoxidil is commonly reserved for severe or intractable hypertension. When added to a diuretic and a β-blocker, minoxidil is generally well tolerated. Hypertrichosis is common. Pericarditis and pericardial infusions have been observed. An increase in left ventricular mass has been reported, possibly due to adrenergic hyperactivity. Chronic treatment with hydralazine has been associated with the development of systemic lupus erythematosus (6% to 10%). Generally, the syndrome occurs early in therapy, but it can occur after many years of treatment. A positive antinuclear antibody titer is used to confirm a clinical diagnosis of lupus. It occurs primarily in slow acetylators. The syndrome is reversible when hydralazine is discontinued, but it may require months for complete clearing of symptoms.

Moderately Selective Peripheral α$_1$-Adrenergic Antagonists

Mechanisms of Action

The nonselective agents phentolamine and phenoxybenzamine have an occasional role in hypertension management. Phentolamine is used parenterally, and the longer acting agent phenoxybenzamine has been used orally for the management of hypertension associated with pheochromocytoma.

Class Members

Phenoxybenzamine irreversibly binds to α-receptors and lowers peripheral resistance. The usual oral dose of phenoxybenzamine for pheochromocytoma is 10 mg twice daily, gradually increasing every other day to doses ranging between 20 and 40 mg two or three times a day. A β-blocker may be administered if tachycardia becomes excessive during therapy; however, the pressor effects of a pheochromocytoma must be controlled by α-blockade before β-blockers are given. With oral use of phenoxybenzamine, pheochromocytoma symptoms decrease after several days. Administration of phenoxybenzamine to patients with renal impairment should be done cautiously. Specific dosage recommendations are not available.

Phentolamine is an α-adrenergic blocking agent that produces peripheral vasodilatation in cardiac stimulation with a resulting fall in blood pressure in most patients. The drug is used parenterally. The usual dose is 5 mg repeated as needed. The onset of activity with intravenous dosing is immediate. The drug is metabolized by the liver with 10% excreted in the urine as unchanged drug.

Renal Effects
Phenoxybenzamine has no clear effect on the renin-angiotensin-aldosterone axis. Salt and water retention does not occur. GFR and effective renal plasma flow would be expected to increase in proportion to the degree of blockade of α-adrenergic receptors.

Efficacy and Safety
Tachycardia may result from α-adrenergic blockade, which unmasks the β-adrenergic effects of epinephrine-secreting tumors. This may be controlled with concurrent use of a β-adrenergic antagonist. α-Adrenergic blockade must be initiated before β-adrenergic blockade to avoid paradoxical hypertension. Side effects of phenoxybenzamine are sedation, weakness, nasal congestion, hypertension, and tachycardia.

Peripheral α_1-Adrenergic Antagonists

Mechanisms of Action
Drugs of this class (doxazosin and prazosin) are selective for the postsynaptic α_1-adrenergic receptor. Because of the selective α_1 action, the reflex tachycardia associated with blockade of the presynaptic α_2-receptor is decreased substantially.

Renal Effects
GFR and renal blood flow are maintained during long-term treatment with these agents. No dosage adjustment is necessary in patients with renal disease (see Table 34–4).

Efficacy and Safety
Patients receiving doxazosin as their initial antihypertensive drug have been found to have poorer blood pressure control compared with those receiving a chlorthalidone-based treatment. In clinical studies, patients receiving doxazosin had no difference in the incidence of fatal coronary heart disease or nonfatal myocardial infarction but did have higher rates of stroke and congestive heart failure compared with those receiving diuretic-based regimens. α_1-Blockers potentially have beneficial effects on lipid metabolism. These drugs have been consistently shown to result in a modest reduction in total and low-density lipoprotein cholesterol and a small increase in high-density lipoprotein cholesterol.

Use of α-blockers has been associated with regression of LVH. Whether this is a result of effective blood pressure reduction or a specific pharmacologic property of these drugs remains to be established. The most important side effect of α_1-adrenergic receptor blockers is the first-dose effect. This is a result of orthostatic hypotension and causes lightheadedness, palpitations, and occasionally syncope. It can be minimized by initiating therapy with a small dose taken at bedtime. This effect can be exacerbated in patients with underlying autonomic insufficiency. α_1-Adrenergic antagonists are also used for symptomatic treatment of prostatic hypertrophy.

Selective Aldosterone Receptor Antagonists

Class Mechanism and Class Member

Eplerenone is a selective aldosterone receptor antagonist that may have antihypertensive effects distinct from its diuretic properties. Although it is a much less potent mineralocorticoid receptor blocker than spironolactone, it is much more specific and has little agonist activity for estrogen and progesterone receptors. Therefore, it is associated with a lower incidence of gynecomastia, breast pain, and impotence in men and diminished libido and menstrual irregularities in women.

Class Renal Effects

Selective aldosterone receptor antagonism may have benefits for the kidney independent of its effects on blood pressure. Both experimental and clinical studies have demonstrated that AII may be associated with progression of renal disease. Despite having no observable effects on glomerular hemodynamics, selective aldosterone receptor antagonism therapy may provide an incremental opportunity to protect the kidney in combination with ACE inhibitor or AII receptor blocker therapy by inhibiting the effects of aldosterone that persist despite therapy with these drugs.

Class Efficacy and Safety

Eplerenone lowers blood pressure when administered at doses of 25, 50, or 200 mg twice daily in a dose-dependent fashion. Clinical trials also demonstrated that eplerenone has antihypertensive activity that is additive with that of either an ACE inhibitor or AII receptor blocker. In diabetic hypertensive patients with microalbuminuria, adding eplerenone to ACE inhibitor therapy reduces proteinuria more than the ACE inhibitor alone independent of effects on blood pressure. The advantage of eplerenone over spironolactone in clinical practice is probably related to fewer endocrine side effects because of more selective aldosterone receptor antagonism.

Vasopeptidase Inhibitors

Omapatrilat (BMS-186716) is the first of the new class of agents termed vasopeptidase inhibitors. Omapatrilat is an orally active, long-acting selective competitive inhibitor of neutral endopeptidase and ACE. As a result of this combined activity, omapatrilat potentiates multiple endogenous vasodilatory peptides, including the natriuretic peptides, bradykinin, and adrenomedullin, while also inhibiting generation of the vasoconstrictive peptide AII. The drug is metabolized in the liver and its half-life is 14 to 19 hours. Most metabolites are excreted in the urine with less than 1% as unchanged drug. Cytochrome P-450 enzymes are not involved in the metabolism of omapatrilat, nor does this chemical affect P-450 isoenzymes. Omapatrilat has no known interaction with other medications.

Class Renal Effects
Vasopeptidase inhibitors that combine the dual effects of ACE and neutral endopeptidase inhibition offer substantial promise for renal protection in that they provide an excellent strategy not only for reducing blood pressure but also for reducing glomerular capillary pressure and proteinuria.

Class Efficacy and Safety
Clinical trials with omapatrilat have demonstrated a dose-dependent efficacy in reduction of systolic and diastolic blood pressure (10 to 80 mg). Reductions in systolic blood pressure are more substantial with fully titrated omapatrilat (20 to 80 mg daily) than with fully titrated lisinopril or amlodipine. Moreover, in diabetic patients receiving omapatrilat monotherapy (20 to 80 mg) blood pressure lowers by the same degree as amlodipine (2.5 to 10 mg); however, omapatrilat also yields statistically significant reductions in proteinuria not observed with amlodipine monotherapy. Omapatrilat may also have promise as a new treatment strategy in congestive heart failure. Despite the marked potential for omapatrilat for the treatment of both hypertension and congestive heart failure, a higher incidence of angioedema (2% to 3% of patients) thought to be related to increased bradykinin concentration has delayed its clinical approval.

SELECTION OF ANTIHYPERTENSIVE DRUG THERAPY

Blood pressure is only one of many surrogate markers of risk contributing to cardiovascular disease, and the optimal goal blood pressure for different patients may be somewhat different, depending on coexistent cardiovascular risk factors. Therefore, the treatment of high blood pressure and the estimation of goal blood pressure requirements need to be carefully individualized for each patient.

Choosing Appropriate Agents

The choice of initial therapy in hypertension depends on a variety of factors including patient age, sex, race, obesity, and coexistent cardiovascular or renal disease. The chief considerations for initial therapy in older patients should include the major pathophysiologic problem, which is an increase in peripheral vascular resistance. Systolic hypertension, a wide pulse pressure, diastolic dysfunction, and a propensity for orthostasis are characteristic. Ideal therapeutic strategies for these patients include a low dose of HCTZ, 12.5 to 25 mg/day. Thiazide diuretics function primarily as vasodilators and are particularly effective in controlling systolic blood pressure. Thiazide diuretics also facilitate vasodilation with other therapeutic classes, particularly those that block the renin-angiotensin-aldosterone axis, and they can be used together as fixed-dose combinations. Calcium channel blockers are also useful vasodilators in older patients. They are much better tolerated in the lower half of their dosing range. α-Blockers may be useful in older men with benign prostatic hypertrophy. β-Blockers may impair baroreceptor responses in older patients and worsen orthostasis and should be used with caution. Treatment of isolated systolic hypertension in older patients often requires multiple drugs. Regardless of the agents that are used, a slow careful titration approach is recommended, preferably with doses increasing no more often than every 3 months.

Sex differences may be important in the selection of antihypertensive therapy. The use of ACE inhibitors and AII receptor blockers should be avoided in pregnant women because of their possible teratogenic effects. Optimal therapy in a pregnant woman includes α-methyldopa, hydralazine, or β-blockers because they have a proven safety record with minimal risk of teratogenic effects. In women with osteoporosis, thiazide diuretics are ideal agents because they antagonize calciuria and facilitate bone mineralization. Women experience more cough with ACE inhibitors and more pedal edema with calcium channel blockers than men do. Race may play a role in choice of antihypertensive agents. Blacks typically present with hypertension at an earlier age, have more substantial elevations in blood pressure, and have earlier development of target organ damage than their demographically similar matched white counterparts. In addition, significant racial differences in the response to antihypertensive medications exists possibly because of higher sensitivity to salt in black patients. In general, thiazide diuretics and calcium channel blockers have more robust antihypertensive properties at lower doses in blacks than other commonly used therapeutic classes. Higher doses of ACE inhibitors or ARBs are often required to achieve the same level of blood pressure reduction as seen in other racial groups. It is not uncommon for multiple drugs to be required to reach the target blood pressure. Consequently, fixed-dose combinations may prove to be most useful in this population group as part of the strategy to simplify the approach. Hispanic and Asian Americans do not appear to have different hypertensive responses to commonly used drugs than white Americans.

Obese hypertensive patients often have other medical problems that complicate management of hypertension. β-Blockers may be helpful in diminishing sympathoadrenal drive. Vasodilators, such as HCTZ and ACE inhibitors, ARBs, and calcium channel blockers, are useful for reducing peripheral vascular resistance. Combinations of these drugs may also be helpful. With the tendency for expanded plasma volume, thiazide diuretics can be helpful because they provide both an opportunity to cause vasodilation and mild volume reduction. Often, these patients require multiple drugs to achieve goal blood pressure, and simplification strategies are important. Because of the increased occurrence of cardiovascular risk clustering phenomena in these patients, drug therapies that are metabolically neutral are ideal.

In patients with coronary artery disease, it is important to remember that most coronary artery perfusion occurs during diastole. Hence, pharmacotherapy should be targeted to slowing heart rate to enhance perfusion during diastole. β-Blockers and heart rate-lowering calcium channel blockers, such as nondihydropyridines, are ideal for this purpose. Agents that block the renin-angiotensin-aldosterone axis are the most effective in reducing LVH. If patients have dyspnea, it is important to use an echocardiogram to distinguish between diastolic and systolic dysfunction. The treatment of diastolic dysfunction should include therapies that facilitate ventricular relaxation and reduce heart rate (β-blockers and calcium channel blockers). With systolic dysfunction, drugs that block the renin-angiotensin-aldosterone axis are more suitable for providing both preload and afterload reduction.

For the specific requirement of patients with established renal disease see Chapter 24, Essential Hypertension.

Refractory Hypertension

Refractory hypertension is a term used to characterize hypertension that fails to respond to what the clinician considers to be an adequate antihypertensive regimen. True refractory hypertension is unusual, and a methodologic approach should be taken to help facilitate blood pressure control in these patients because lack of control puts them at greater risk for cardiovascular complications. A variety of factors interfere with the ability to normalize blood pressure, the most important of which is noncompliance. This problem derives from many factors, including inadequate education, a poor clinician-patient relationship, lack of understanding about side effects, and the complexity of multidrug regimens. Pseudohypertension is commonly observed in older hypertensive patients who have hardened atherosclerotic arteries, which are not easily compressible. This condition interferes with auscultatory measurements of blood pressure and greater apparent pressure is required to compress the sclerotic vessel than the intra-arterial blood pressure requires. Another common cause of pseudohypertension is improper measurement. This occurs when the blood pressure is taken with an inappropriately small cuff in people with large arm circumference. Because of the substantial proportion of hypertensive patients who are obese, it is critical to have the appropriate cuff size for determining auscultatory pressure.

Some clinicians may view "white coat hypertension" as a cause of refractory hypertension. This is an area of contentious debate in that elevated office readings despite lower home readings still provide important predictive value for the development of cardiovascular events. Some clinical studies indicate that patients with so-called white coat hypertension also have LVH and may not have an appropriate nocturnal dip in blood pressure.

Volume overload is an important and common cause of refractory hypertension. It may be related to excessive salt intake or the inability of the kidney to excrete an appropriate salt and water load because of either endocrine abnormalities or intrinsic renal disease. Salt sensitivity is particularly common in patients of African-American descent. A careful clinical examination coupled with judicious use of either thiazide or loop diuretics is critical in achieving ideal blood volume to restore the antihypertensive efficacy of most classes of drugs. It is also appropriate to consider educating the patient about avoiding foods that are rich in salt content, such as processed foods.

Drug-related causes of refractory hypertension are common and need to be carefully assessed in each patient. Perhaps the most common drugs that cause refractory hypertension are over-the-counter preparations of sympathomimetics such as nasal decongestants, appetite suppressants, and nonsteroidal anti-inflammatory drugs. Unfortunately, patients may not always recognize over-the-counter preparations as a medication. Therefore, careful questioning with a specific focus on these types of medications should be a routine procedure during the evaluation for refractory hypertension. In addition, oral contraceptives, ethanol, cigarettes, and cocaine can be complicating factors that interfere with the ability of medications to lower blood pressure.

Obesity is an often overlooked cause of refractory hypertension because it is commonly associated with obstructive sleep apnea. Secondary causes of hypertension might also be considered as a cause of refractory hypertension. Chronic kidney disease and renal vascular disease are not uncommon and are easily recognized. Additional endocrine abnormalities include hyperaldosteronism, pheochromocytoma, or hypo- or hyperthyroidism and hyperparathyroidism; rarely, aortic coarctation can be a cause of refractory hypertension.

Strategies to control blood pressure in patients with refractory hypertension should first deal with issues related to compliance, simplifying the medical regimen, and being sure that side effects are not playing a role. Subsequently, one can evaluate medications and try to choose those that work well with one another to facilitate a nearly additive antihypertensive response. Most drugs reduce systolic blood pressure by approximately 8 to 10 mm Hg. Consequently, it is not unusual for patients whose systolic blood pressure is 40 or 50 mm Hg from the goal to require four or five medications or possibly even more. One should also ensure that volume excess is controlled and that there are no drug-drug interactions or clinical situations that would promote diuretic resistance such as excessive salt intake.

DRUG TREATMENT OF HYPERTENSIVE URGENCIES AND EMERGENCIES

The terms *hypertensive urgency* and *hypertensive emergency* are used loosely in clinical practice with a great deal of overlap. The distinction between the two is important because the management approach is substantially different. A hypertensive emergency is a clinical syndrome in which severe hypertension results in ongoing target organ damage manifested by encephalopathy, retinal hemorrhage, papilledema, acute myocardial infarction, stroke, or acute renal dysfunction. Any delay in control of blood pressure may lead to irreversible sequelae, including death. Hypertensive emergencies are unusual but require immediate hospitalization in an intensive care unit, with careful and judicious use of intravenous vasodilators to lower systolic and diastolic blood pressure cautiously to approximately 140/90 mm Hg (see Table 34–6). In contrast, hypertensive urgencies are clinical situations in which a patient has a marked elevation in blood pressure (greater than 200/130 mm Hg) but no evidence of ongoing target organ damage. These patients do not require emergency therapy and can be managed cautiously on an outpatient basis (Table 34–7).

Parenteral Drugs, Direct-Acting Vasodilators

Diazoxide is a pure arterial dilator that is used primarily in the treatment of acute hypertensive emergencies. The "minibolus" (1 mg/kg administered at intervals of 5 to 15 minutes) and the continuous infusion of diazoxide have become the preferred methods of administration to avoid excessive reduction in blood pressure. Diazoxide acts rapidly, and the blood pressure effect persists for up to 12 hours. It has a plasma half-life of 17 to 31 hours. In renal disease, the plasma half-life is prolonged, and dose reduction is required. Concurrent administration of a β-adrenergic antagonist can control reflex tachycardia. Transient hyperglycemia occurs in most patients and the blood glucose level should be monitored. Hydralazine is a direct-acting vasodilator and may be given intramuscularly as a rapid intravenous bolus injection. It acts rapidly, and the blood pressure effect persists for up to 6 hours. It is less potent that diazoxide, and the blood pressure response is less predictable.

Sodium nitroprusside is the most potent of the parenteral vasodilators, and it dilates both arteriolar resistance and venous capacitance vessels. It has the advantages of being immediately effective when given as an infusion and of having an extremely short duration of action, which permits minute-to-minute adjustments in blood pressure control. The disadvantages of nitroprusside therapy include the need for intra-arterial blood pressure monitoring, the need to protect the solution from light during infusion, and the potential for toxic effects from metabolic side products. Nitroprusside is rapidly metabolized to cyanide and then to thiocyanate. Thiocyanate is excreted largely in the urine; it has a plasma half-life of 1 week in normal subjects and accumulates if renal insufficiency is present. Toxic concentrations of cyanide or thiocyanate may occur if nitroprusside infusions are given for

Table 34-6: Parenteral Drugs Used in the Treatment of Hypertensive Emergencies

Drug	Dose (Maximal)	Onset of Action	Peak Effect	Duration of Action
Direct-acting vasodilators				
Diazoxide	7.5–30 mg/min infusion or 1 mg/kg bolus q5–15 min (300 mg)	1–5 min	30 min	4–12 hr
Hydralazine	0.5–1.0 mg/min infusion or 10–50 mg intramuscularly	1–5 min	10–80 min	3–6 hr
Nitroglycerin	5–100 mcg/min infusion	1–2 min	2–5 min	3–5 min
Nitroprusside	0.25–10 mcg/kg/min infusion	Immediate	1–2 min	2–5 min
β₁-Adrenergic antagonist				
Esmolol	250–500 mcg/min ×1 (loading dose), then 50–100 mcg/kg/min ×4 (maintenance); maintenance dose may be increased to maximum 300 mg/kg/min	1–2 min	5 min	10–30 min
α₁- and β-Adrenergic antagonist				
Labetalol	2 mg/min infusion or 0.25 mg/kg	5 min	10 min	3–6 hr
Ganglionic blockers	Trimethaphan 0.5–10 mg/min infusion bolus over 2 min (300 mg)	Immediate	1–2 min	5–10 min
Angiotensin-converting enzyme inhibitor				
Enalaprilat	0.625–5.0 mg bolus over 5 min q6hr	5–15 min	1–4 hr	6 hr
Peripheral α-Adrenergic Antagonist				
Phentolamine	0.5–1.0 mg/min infusion or 2.5–5.0 mg bolus	Immediate	3–5 min	10–15 min
Calcium antagonist				
Nicardipine	5–15 mg/hr	5–10 min	45 min	50 hr
Dopamine D₁-like receptor agent				
Fenoldopam	0.01–1.6 mcg/min constant infusion	5–15 min	30 min	5–10 min

Table 34–7: Rapid-Acting Oral Drugs Used in the Treatment of Hypertensive Emergencies

Drug	Dosage (Maximal)	Onset of Action	Peak Effect	Duration of Action
Labetalol	100–400 mg q12h (2400 mg)	1–2 hr	2–4 hr	8–12 hr
Clonidine	0.2 mg initially, then 0.1 mg/hr (0.8 mg)	30–60 min	2–4 hr	6–8 hr
Diltiazem	30–120 mg q8h (480 mg)	< 15 min	2–3 hr	8 hr
Enalapril	2.5–10 mg q6h (40 mg)	< 60 min	4–8 hr	12–24 hr
Captopril	12.5–25 mg qh (150 mg)	< 15 min	1 hr	6–12 hr
Enalapril	2.5–10 mg q6h (40 mg)	< 60 min	4–8 hr	12–24 hr
Prazosin	1–5 mg q2h (20 mg)	< 60 min	2–4 hr	6–12 hr

more than 48 hours or at infusion rates greater than 2 mg/kg/min; the maximal dose rate of 10 mg/kg/min should not last more than 10 minutes. Toxic manifestations include air hunger, hyperreflexia, confusion, and seizures. Lactic acidosis and venous hyperoxemia are laboratory indicators of cyanide intoxication. The drug should be promptly discontinued and levels of cyanide measured.

Intravenous nitroglycerin produces, in a dose-related manner, dilation of both arterial and venous beds. At lower doses, its primary effect is on preload; at higher infusion rates, afterload is reduced. Nitroglycerin may also dilate both epicardial coronary vessels and their collaterals, increasing blood supply to ischemic regions. Effective coronary perfusion is maintained, provided that blood pressure does not fall excessively or heart rate does not increase significantly. Nitroglycerin has an immediate onset of action but is rapidly metabolized to dinitrates and mononitrates. Patients with normal or low left ventricular filing pressure or pulmonary wedge pressure may be hypersensitive to the effects of nitroglycerin. Therefore, continuous monitoring of blood pressure, heart rate, and pulmonary capillary wedge pressure must be performed to assess the correct dose. Intravenous nitroglycerin may be the drug of choice in the treatment of the patient with moderate hypertension associated with coronary ischemia. The principal side effects are headache, nausea, and vomiting. Tolerance may develop with prolonged use.

β₁-Selective Adrenergic Antagonist

Esmolol hydrochloride is a short-acting β₁-selective adrenergic antagonist used in the management of hypertensive emergencies (see Table 34–6). Efficacy should be assessed after the 1-minute loading dose and 4 minutes of a maintenance infusion. If an adequate therapeutic effect is observed, the maintenance infusion should be maintained. If an adequate therapeutic effect is not observed, the same loading dose can be repeated for 1 minute followed by an increased maintenance rate of infusion. Extravasation of esmolol hydrochloride may cause serious local irritation and skin necrosis. Esmolol shares all of the toxic potential of the β₁-adrenergic antagonists previously discussed. It may be particularly useful for the treatment of postoperative hypertension and hypertension associated with coronary insufficiency. Esmolol is hydrolyzed rapidly in blood, and negligible concentrations are present 30 minutes after discontinuance. Because the kidneys eliminate the deesterified metabolite of esmolol, the drug should be used cautiously in patients with renal insufficiency.

Labetalol

The α₁- and β-adrenergic antagonist labetalol may be given by either repeated intravenous injection or slow continuous infusion (see Table 34–6). The maximal blood pressure–lowering effect occurs within 5 minutes of the first injection. Patients should be in the supine position for administration of the drug to avoid symptomatic postural hypotension. It has been proved to be safe and useful in hypertensive urgencies and emergencies in pregnant women.

Ganglionic Blocking Agent

Trimethaphan camsylate blocks transmission of impulses at both sympathetic and parasympathetic ganglia and is used exclusively for the treatment of hypertensive emergencies. It has an immediate onset of action when administered as a continuous infusion (see Table 34–6). The resulting dramatic reduction of blood pressure requires intra-arterial monitoring. The main disadvantage is patients should be supine for administration of the drug to avoid profound postural hypotension. It has been shown to be useful for acute blood pressure reduction in patients with acute aortic dissection. Other disadvantages include the potential for tachyphylaxis after sustained infusion (48 hours) and the appearance of side effects associated with parasympathetic and sympathetic blockade and histamine release.

α-Adrenergic Antagonist

Phentolamine mesylate is a nonselective α-adrenergic antagonist used primarily in the treatment of hypertension associated with pheochromocytoma. It has a rapid onset of action when administered intravenously as either a bolus or a continuous infusion (see Table 34–6). The duration of action is 10 to 15 minutes. It has a plasma half-life of 19 minutes; approximately 13% of a single dose appears in the urine as unchanged drug. Adverse effects include those associated with nonselective α-adrenergic blockade, as discussed earlier.

Calcium Antagonists

Nicardipine hydrochloride, a dihydropyridine CA, is administered by slow continuous infusion, resulting in a dose-dependent decrease in blood pressure. Onset of action is within minutes; 50% of the ultimate decrease occurs in 45 minutes, but a final steady state does not occur for about 50 hours (see Table 34–6). Discontinuation of infusion is followed by a 50% offset of action in 30 minutes, but gradually decreasing antihypertensive effects exist for about 50 hours. It has been shown to be safe and effective in pediatric hypertensive emergencies.

Dopamine D_1-Like Receptor Agonist

Fenoldopam mesylate, a dopamine D_1-like receptor agonist, is used for acute hypertensive treatment. Its elimination half-life is 5 minutes, and steady-state concentrations are reached within 20 minutes. Clearance of the active compound is not altered by end-stage renal disease or hepatic disease. Side effects include a reflex increase in heart rate, an increase in intraocular pressure, headache, flushing, nausea, and hypotension.

Hypertensive Urgency

A more gradual, progressive reduction in systemic blood pressure may be achieved after the oral administration of drugs having rapid absorption in hypertensive urgencies. These include (1) the α_1- and β-adrenergic antagonist labetalol, (2) the central α_2-adrenergic agonist clonidine, (3) the CAs diltiazem and verapamil, (4) the ACE inhibitors captopril and enalapril, (5) the postsynaptic α_1-adrenergic antagonist prazosin, and (6) a combination of oral therapies. The doses and pharmacodynamic effects of rapid-acting oral drugs used commonly in the treatment of hypertensive emergencies are given in Table 34–7. Note that rapid-acting oral dihydropyridine CAs such as sublingual nifedipine are no longer recommended because they may cause large and unpredictable reductions in blood pressure with resultant ischemic events.

Clinical Considerations in the Acute Reduction of Blood Pressure

Acute reduction of blood pressure carries the risk of impairing the blood supply to vital structures such as the brain and the heart. Consequently, every effort should be made to avoid excessive reduction of blood pressure. Short-term, rapid reduction of blood pressure may decrease cerebral blood flow sufficiently to precipitate ischemia and infarction in patients with chronic hypertension. This may be a risk in patients with atherosclerotic disease of the cerebral blood vessels in whom there may be areas of uneven cerebral perfusion. Sudden drops in blood pressure can also interfere with coronary perfusion during diastole and result in myocardial ischemia, infarction, or arrhythmia. In addition, rapid reduction of blood pressure may result in a reflex increase in heart rate, which would also interfere with coronary perfusion during diastole. For these reasons, careful, cautious, and controlled reduction in blood pressure is necessary in these patients. For most hypertensive emergencies, a parenteral drug such as sodium nitroprusside is ideal. However, if the patient has coronary disease, the use of intravenous nitroglycerin or esmolol or both is a useful approach because they can induce coronary dilation or slow heart rate, respectively. Intravenous nicardipine could also be used because it facilitates coronary vasodilation. Patients with acute aortic dissection are best treated with a β-adrenergic antagonist plus nitroprusside or a ganglionic blocker such as trimethaphan. Patients with hypertensive encephalopathy or central nervous system hemorrhage may be best treated with drugs that do not cause cerebral vasodilation such as a hydralazine, nitroprusside, nicardipine, or fenoldopam. Fenoldopam may be helpful in patients with kidney diseases, because it maintains renal blood flow.

Prescribing Drugs in Renal Disease

35

INITIAL PATIENT ASSESSMENT FOR DRUG DOSING

Patients with chronic kidney disease require multiple medications, and special care is needed to avoid drug-related toxicity. Clinical evaluation always begins with a careful history and physical examination with specific regard to the patient's volume status and muscle mass. Reviewing the possibility of drug interactions before choosing a drug regimen is essential, and drug therapy should be individualized to take advantage of the fact that one drug can be used to treat several conditions. Individualization of the drug regimen requires measurements of body height and weight and estimation of the volume of distribution. Many clinicians use the average of the measured body weight and the ideal body weight as the value on which to base drug doses. A loading dose equivalent to the dose given to a patient with normal renal function should always be given to patients with renal impairment if the physical examination suggests a normal extracellular fluid volume. The maintenance dose adjustment thereafter depends on the measured or estimated glomerular filtration rate.

DRUG REMOVAL BY DIALYSIS

Factors Affecting Clearance

Drug removal by conventional hemodialysis occurs primarily by the process of drug diffusion across the dialysis membrane. Drug removal by conventional hemodialysis is most effective for drugs that have a molecular weight of less than 500 D and that are less than 90% protein bound with a small volume of distribution. Removal of low-molecular-weight drugs is enhanced by increasing the blood and dialysate flow rates and by using large surface area dialyzers.

The hemodialysis clearance of a drug can be estimated from the following relationship:

$$Cl_{HD} = Cl_{urea} \times (60/MW_{drug}),$$

where Cl_{HD} is drug clearance by hemodialysis, Cl_{urea} is urea clearance by the dialyzer (typically 150 to 200 mL/min), and MW_{drug} is the molecular weight of the drug.

The use of porous dialysis membranes during high-flux dialysis improves the clearance of drugs with a higher molecular weight. The removal of drugs during high-flux dialysis depends more on treatment time, blood and dialysate flow rates, distribution volume, and binding of the drug to serum proteins. Typically much more drug of a high molecular weight is removed during high-flux dialysis than during conventional hemodialysis.

Peritoneal dialysis is much less efficient for removal of drugs than hemodialysis. As with conventional hemodialysis, clearance is most effective for low-molecular-weight drugs with a small volume of distribution. In contrast, many drugs are well absorbed when placed in the peritoneal dialysate. Higher-molecular-weight drugs may be somewhat more removed by peritoneal dialysis because of secretion into peritoneal lymphatic fluid.

Molecular weight, membrane characteristics, blood flow rate, and the addition of dialysate determine the rate and extent of drug removal during continuous renal replacement therapy (CRRT). Because of the large pore size of membranes used for CRRT and the fact that most drugs are smaller than 1500 D, drug removal by CRRT does not depend greatly on molecular weight. The volume of distribution of a drug is the most important factor determining removal by CRRT. A volume of distribution greater than 0.7 L/kg substantially decreases drug removal by CRRT. In addition, protein binding of more than 80% provides a substantial barrier to drug removal by convection or diffusion. The addition of continuous dialysis to continuous hemofiltration increases drug clearance, depending on blood and dialysate flow rates. As during high flux dialysis, drug removal parallels the removal of urea and creatinine. The simplest method for estimating drug removal during CRRT is to estimate urea or creatinine clearance during the procedure.

Recommendations for dosing selected drugs in patients with impaired renal function are given in Table 35–1. These recommendations are meant only as a guide and do not imply efficacy

Table 35–1: Drug Doses in Renal Failure

Drug	Dose Method	GFR >50 (mL/min)	GFR 10–50 (mL/min)	GFR <10 (mL/min)	Supplemental Dose after Hemodialysis	CAPD	CRRT
Acarbose	D	50% to 100%	Avoid	Avoid	Unknown	Unknown	Avoid
Acebutolol	D	100%	50%	30% to 50%	None	None	Dose for GFR 10–50
Acetazolamide	I	q6h	q12h	Avoid	No data	No data	Avoid
Acetohexamide	I	Avoid	Avoid	Avoid	Unknown	Unknown	Avoid
Acetohydroxamic acid	D	100%	100%	q8h	Unknown	Unknown	Unknown
Acetominophen	I	q4h	q6h	q8h	Dose after dialysis	None	Dose for GFR 10–50
Acetylsalicylic acid	I	q4h	q4–6h	Avoid	Dose after dialysis	None	Dose for GFR 10–50
Acrivastine		Unknown	Unknown	Unknown	Unknown	Unknown	Unknown
Acyclovir	D, I	5 mg/kg q8h	5 mg/kg q12–24h	2.5 mg/kg q24h	Dose after dialysis	Dose for GFR <10	3.5 mg/kg/day
Adenosine	D	100%	100%	100%	None	None	Dose for GFR 10–50
Albuterol	D	100%	75%	50%	Unknown	Unknown	Dose for GFR 10–50
Alcuronium	D	Avoid	Avoid	Avoid	Unknown	Unknown	Avoid
Alfentanil	D	100%	100%	100%	Unknown	Unknown	Dose for GFR 10–50
Allopurinol	D	75%	50%	25%	1/2 dose	Unknown	Dose for GFR 10–50
Alprazolam	D	100%	100%	100%	None	Unknown	Dose for GFR 10–50
Altretamine	D	Unknown	Unknown	Unknown	No data	No data	NA
Amantadine	I	q24–48h	q48–72h	q7d	Unknown	None	Unknown
Amikacin	D, I	60% to 90% q12h	30% to 70% q12–18h	20% to 30% q24–48h	2/3 normal dose	15–20 mg/L/day	Dose for GFR 10–50
Amiloride	D	100%	50%	Avoid	NA	NA	NA
Amiodarone	D	100%	100%	100%	None	None	Dose for GFR 10–50
Amitriptyline	D	100%	100%	100%	None	Unknown	NA
Amlodipine	D	100%	100%	100%	None	None	Dose for GFR 10–50
Amoxapine	D	100%	100%	100%	None	None	NA
Amoxicillin	I	q8h	q8–12h	q24h	Dose after dialysis	250 mg q12h	NA

Continued

Table 35-1: (cont'd)

Drug	Dose Method	GFR > 50 (mL/min)	GFR 10–50 (mL/min)	GFR < 10 (mL/min)	Supplemental Dose after Hemodialysis	CAPD	CRRT
Amphotericin	I	q24h	q24h	q24–36h	None	Dose for GFR < 10	Dose for GFR 10–50
Amphotericin B colloidal	I	q24h	q24h	q24–36h	None	Dose for GFR < 10	Dose for GFR 10–50
Amphotericin B lipid	I	q24h	q24h	q24–36h	None	Dose for GFR < 10	Dose for GFR 10–50
Ampicillin	I	q6h	q6–12h	q12–24h	Dose after dialysis	250 mg q 12h	Dose for GFR 10–50
Amrinone	D	100%	100%	50% to 75%	No data	No data	Dose for GFR 10–50
Anistreplase	D	100%	100%	100%	Unknown	Unknown	Dose for GFR 10–50
Astemizole	D	100%	100%	100%	Unknown	Unknown	NA
Atenolol	D, I	100% q24h	50% q48h	30% to 50% q96h	25–50 mg	None	Dose for GFR 10–50
Atovaquone	D	100%	100%	100%	None	None	Dose for GFR 10–50
Atracurium	D	100%	100%	100%	Unknown	Unknown	Dose for GFR 10–50
Auranofin	D	50%	75%	Avoid	None	None	None
Azathioprine	D	100%	Avoid	50%	Yes	Unknown	None
Azithromycin	D	100%	100%	100%	None	None	None
Azlocillin	I	q4–6h	q6–8h	q8h	Dose after dialysis	Dose for GFR < 10	Dose for GFR 10–50
Aztreonam	D	100%	50% to 75%	25%	0.5 g after dialysis	Dose for GFR < 10	Dose for GFR 10–50
Benazepril	D	100%	50% to 75%	25% to 50%	None	None	Dose for GFR 10–50
Bepridil		Unknown	Unknown	Unknown	None	None	No data
Bctamethasone	D	100%	100%	100%	Unknown	Unknown	Dose for GFR 10–50
Betaxolol	D	100%	100%	50%	None	None	Dose for GFR 10–50
Bezafibrate	D	70%	50%	25%	Unknown	Unknown	Dose for GFR 10–50
Bisoprolol	D	100%	75%	50%	Unknown	Unknown	Dose for GFR 10–50
Bleomycin	D	100%	100%	50%	None	None	Dose for GFR 10–50
Bopindolol	D	100%	100%	100%	None	None	Dose for GFR 10–50

Bretylium	D	100%	25% to 50%		None	None	Dose for GFR 10-50
Bromocriptine	D	100%	100%		Unknown	Unknown	Unknown
Brompheniramine	D	100%	100%		Unknown	Unknown	NA
Budesonide	D	100%	100%		Unknown	Unknown	Dose for GFR 10-50
Bumetanide	D	100%	100%		None	None	NA
Bupropion	D	100%	100%		Unknown	Unknown	NA
Buspirone	D	100%	100%		Unknown	Unknown	NA
Busulfan	D	100%	100%		None	Unknown	Dose for GFR 10-50
Butorphanol	D	100%	75%		Unknown	Unknown	NA
Capreomycin	I	q24h	q24h		Unknown	None	Dose for GFR 10-50
Captopril	D, I	100% / q8h–12h	75% / q12–18h	50% / q24h	Give dose after HD only	25% to 30%	Dose for GFR 10-50
Carbamazepine	D	100%	100%		None	None	None
Carbidopa	D	100%	100%		Unknown	Unknown	Unknown
Carboplatin	D	100%	50%	25%	1/2 dose	Unknown	Dose for GFR 10-50
Carmustine	D	Unknown	Unknown		Unknown	Unknown	Unknown
Carteolol	D	100%	50%	25%	Unknown	Unknown	Dose for GFR 10-50
Carvedilol	D	100%	100%		None	None	Dose for GFR 10-50
Cefaclor	D	100%	100%	50%	250 mg after dialysis	250 mg q8–12h	Dose for GFR 10-50
Cefadroxil	I	q12h	q12–24h	q24–48h	0.5–1.0 g after dialysis	0.5 g/day	Dose for GFR 10-50
Cefamandole	I	q6h	q6–8h	q12h	0.5–1.0 g after dialysis	0.5–1.0 g q12h	Dose for GFR 10-50
Cefazolin	I	q8h	q12h	q24–48h	0.5–1.0 g after dialysis	0.5 g q12h	Dose for GFR 10-50
Cefepime	I	q12h	q16–24h	q24–48h	1.0 g after dialysis	Dose for GFR < 10	Not recommended
Cefixime	D	100%	75%	50%	300 mg after dialysis	200 mg/day	Not recommended
Cefmenoxime	D, I	1.0 g q8h	0.75 g q8h	0.75 g q12h	0.75 g after dialysis	0.75 g q12h	Dose for GFR 10-50
Cefmetazole	I	q16h	q24h	q48h	Dose after dialysis	Dose for GFR < 10	Dose for GFR 10-50
Cefonicid	D, I	0.5 g/d	0.1 g–05 g/day	0.1 g/day	None	None	None
Cefoperazone	D	100%	100%		1 g after dialysis	None	None
Ceforanide	I	q12h	q12–24h	q24–48h	0.5–1.0 g after dialysis	None	1.0 g/day

Continued

Table 35–1: (cont'd)

Drug	Dose Method	GFR > 50 (mL/min)	GFR 10–50 (mL/min)	GFR < 10 (mL/min)	Supplemental Dose after Hemodialysis	CAPD	CRRT
Cefotaxime	I	q6h	q8–12h	q24h	1 g after dialysis	1 g/day	1 g q12h
Cefotetan	D	100%	50%	25%	1 g after dialysis	1 g/day	750 mg q12h
Cefoxitin	I	q8h	q8–12h	q24–48h	1 g after dialysis	1 g/day	Dose for GFR 10–50
Cefpodoxime	I	q12h	q16h	q24–48h	200 mg after dialysis	Dose for GFR < 10	NA
Cefprozil	D, I	250 mg q12h	250 mg q12–16h	250 mg q24h	250 mg after dialysis	Dose for GFR < 10	Dose for GFR < 10
Ceftazidime	I	q8–12h	q24–48h	q48h	1 g after dialysis	0.5 g/day	Dose for GFR 10–50
Ceftibuten	D	100%	50%	25%	300 mg after dialysis	Dose for GFR < 10	Dose for GFR 10–50
Ceftizoxime	I	q8–12h	q12–24h	q24h	1 g after dialysis	0.5–1.0 g/day	Dose for GFR 10–50
Ceftriaxone	D	100%	100%	100%	Dose after dialysis	750 mg q12h	Dose for GFR 10–50
Cefuroxime axetil	D	100%	100%	100%	Dose after dialysis	Dose for GFR < 10	NA
Celiprolol	D	100%	100%	75%	Unknown	None	Dose for GFR 10–50
Cephalexin	I	q8h	q12h	q12h	Dose after dialysis	Dose for GFR < 10	NA
Cephalothin	I	q6h	q6–8h	q12h	Dose after dialysis	1 g q12h	1 g q8h
Cephapirin	I	q6h	q6–8h	q12h	Dose after dialysis	1 g q12h	1 g q8h
Cephradine	D	100%	50%	25%	Dose after dialysis	Dose for GFR < 10	NA
Cetirizine	D	100%	100%	30%	None	Unknown	NA
Chloralhydrate	D	100%	Avoid	Avoid	None	Unknown	NA
Chlorambucil	D	Unknown	Unknown	Unknown	Unknown	Unknown	Unknown
Chloramphenicol	D	100%	100%	100%	None	Unknown	None
Chlorazepate	D	100%	100%	100%	Unknown	None	NA
Chlordiazepoxide	D	100%	100%	50%	None	Unknown	Dose for GFR 10–50
Chloroquine	D	100%	100%	50%	None	None	None

Chlorpheniramine	D	100%	100%	100%	None	Unknown	NA
Chlorpromazine	D	100%	100%	100%	None	None	Dose for GFR 10-50
Chlorpropamide	D	50%	Avoid	Avoid	Unknown	None	Avoid
Chlorthalidone	D	q24h	q24h	Avoid	NA	NA	NA
Cholestyramine	D	100%	100%	100%	None	None	Dose for GFR 10-50
Cidofovir	D, I	100% q12h	100% q12h	66% q24h	No data	None	Dose for GFR 10-50
Cilastatin	D	50% to 100%	Avoid	Avoid	Avoid	No data	Avoid
Cilazapril	D, I	100%	50%	10% to 25% q72h	None	Avoid	Avoid
Cimetidine	D, I	75% q24h	50% q24-48h	25%	None	None	Dose for GFR 10-50
Cinoxacin	D	100%	50%	Avoid	None	None	Dose for GFR 10-50
Ciprofloxacin	D	100%	50% to 75%	50%	Avoid	Avoid	Avoid
Cisapride	D	100%	100%	50%	250 mg q12h	250 mg q8h	200 mg IV q12h
Cisplatin	D	100%	100%	50%	Unknown	Unknown	50% to 100%
Cladribine	D	75%	75%	50%	Yes	Unknown	Unknown
Clarithromycin	D	Unknown	Unknown	Unknown	Dose after dialysis	Unknown	Unknown
Clavulanic acid	D	100%	100%	50% to 75%	Dose after dialysis	Dose for GFR < 10	Dose for GFR 10-50
Clindamycin	D	100%	100%	100%	None	None	None
Clodronate	D	Unknown	Unknown	Avoid	Unknown	Unknown	Unknown
Clofaziamine		100%	100%	100%	None	None	No data
Clofibrate	I	q6-12h	q12-18h	Avoid	None	Unknown	Dose for GFR 10-50
Clomipramine	D	Unknown	Unknown	Unknown	Unknown	Unknown	NA
Clonazepam	D	100%	100%	100%	None	None	NA
Clonidine	D	100%	100%	100%	None	Unknown	Dose for GFR 10-50
Codeine	D	75%	75%	50%	None	Unknown	Dose for GFR 10-50
Colchicine	D	100%	100%	50%	None	Unknown	Dose for GFR 10-50
Colestipol	D	100%	100%	100%	None	None	Dose for GFR 10-50
Cortisone	D	100%	100%	100%	None	Unknown	Dose for GFR 10-50
Cyclophosphamide	D	100%	100%	75%	1/2 dose	Unknown	Dose for GFR 10-50
Cycloserine	I	q12h	q12-24h	q24h	None	None	Dose for GFR 10-50

Continued

Table 35-1: (cont'd)

Drug	Dose Method	GFR > 50 (mL/min)	GFR 10-50 (mL/min)	GFR < 10 (mL/min)	Supplemental Dose after Hemodialysis	CAPD	CRRT
Cyclosporine	D	100%	100%	100%	None	None	100%
Cytarabine	D	100%	100%	100%	Unknown	Unknown	Dose for GFR 10-50
Dapsone	D	100%	No data	No data	None	Dose for GFR < 10	No data
Daunorubicin	D	100%	100%	100%	Unknown	Unknown	Unknown
Delavirdine		100%	100%	100%	None	No data	Dose for GFR 10-50
Desferoxamine	D	100%	100%	100%	Unknown	Unknown	Dose for GFR 10-50
Desipramine	D	100%	100%	100%	None	None	NA
Dexamethasone	D	100%	100%	100%	Unknown	Unknown	Dose for GFR 10-50
Diazepam	D	100%	100%	100%	None	Unknown	100%
Diazoxide	D	100%	100%	100%	None	None	Dose for GFR 10-50
Diclofenac	D	100%	100%	100%	None	None	Dose for GFR 10-50
Dicloxacillin	D	100%	100%	100%	None	None	NA
Didanosine	I	q12h	q24h	q24-48h	Dose after dialysis	Dose for GFR <10	Dose for GFR <10
Diflunisal	D	100%	50%	50%	None	None	Dose for GFR 10-50
Digitoxin	D	100%	100%	50% to 75%	None	None	Dose for GFR 10-50
Digoxin	D, I	100% q24h	25% to 75% q36h	10% to 25% q48h	None	None	Dose for GFR 10-50
Dilevalol	D	100%	100%	100%	None	None	Unknown
Diltiazem	D	100%	100%	100%	None	None	None
Diphenhydramine	D	100%	100%	100%	None	None	NA
Dipyridamole	D	100%	100%	100%	Unknown	Unknown	Dose for GFR 10-50
Dirithromycin		100%	100%	100%	None	None	Dose for GFR 10-50
Disopyramide	I	q8h	q12-24h	q24-40h	None	None	Dose for GFR 10-50
Dobutamine	D	100%	100%	100%	No data	No data	Dose for GFR 10-50
Doxacurium	D	100%	50%	50%	Unknown	Unknown	Dose for GFR 10-50
Doxazosin	D	100%	100%	100%	None	None	Dose for GFR 10-50
Doxepin	D	100%	100%	100%	None	None	Dose for GFR 10-50

Doxorubicin	D	100%	100%	100%	None	Unknown	Dose for GFR 10–50
Doxycycline	D	100%	100%	100%	None	None	Dose for GFR 10–50
Dyphylline	D	75%	50%	25%	1/3 dose	Unknown	Dose for GFR 10–50
Enalapril	D	100%	75% to 100%	50%	20% to 25%	None	Dose for GFR 10–50
Epirubicin	D	100%	100%	100%	Unknown	Unknown	Dose for GFR 10–50
Erbastine	D	100%	50%	50%	Unknown	Unknown	Dose for GFR 10–50
Erythromycin	D	100%	100%	50% to 75%	None	None	None
Estazolam	D	100%	100%	100%	Unknown	Unknown	NA
Ethacrynic acid	I	q8–12h	q8–12h	Avoid	None	None	NA
Ethambutol	I	q24h	q24–36h	q48h	Dose after dialysis	Dose for GFR < 10	Dose for GFR 10–50
Ethchlorvynol	D	100%	Avoid	Avoid	None	None	NA
Ethionamide	D	100%	100%	50%	None	None	None
Ethosuximide	D	100%	100%	100%	None	Unknown	Unknown
Etodolac	D	100%	100%	100%	None	None	Dose for GFR 10–50
Etomidate	D	100%	100%	100%	Unknown	Unknown	Dose for GFR 10–50
Etoposide	D	100%	75%	50%	None	Unknown	Dose for GFR 10–50
Famciclovir	I	100%	q12–48h	50% q48h	Dose after dialysis	No data	Dose for GFR 10–50
Famotidine	D	50%	25%	10%	None	None	Dose for GFR 10–50
Fazadinium	D	100%	100%	100%	Unknown	Unknown	Dose for GFR 10–50
Felodipine	D	100%	100%	100%	None	None	Dose for GFR 10–50
Fenoprofen	D	100%	100%	100%	None	None	Dose for GFR 10–50
Fentanyl	D	100%	75%	50%	NA	NA	NA
Fexofenadine	I	q12h	q12–24h	q24h	Unknown	Unknown	Dose for GFR 10–50
Flecainide	D	100%	100%	50% to 75%	None	None	Dose for GFR 10–50
Fleroxacin	D	100%	50% to 75%	50%	400 mg after dialysis	400 mg/day	NA
Fluconazole	D	100%	100%	100%	200 mg after dialysis	Dose for GFR < 10	Dose for GFR 10–50
Flucytosine	I	q12h	q16h	q24h	Dose after dialysis	0.5–1.0 g/day	Dose for GFR 10–50
Fludarabine	D	100%	75%	50%	Unknown	Unknown	Dose for GFR 10–50
Flumazenil	D	100%	100%	100%	None	Unknown	NA

Continued

Table 35-1: (cont'd)

Drug	Dose Method	GFR > 50 (mL/min)	GFR 10-50 (mL/min)	GFR < 10 (mL/min)	Supplemental Dose after Hemodialysis	CAPD	CRRT
Flunarizine	D	100%	100%	100%	None	None	None
Fluorouracil	D	100%	100%	100%	Yes	Unknown	Dose for GFR 10–50
Fluoxetine	D	100%	100%	100%	Unknown	Unknown	NA
Flurazepam	D	100%	100%	100%	None	Unknown	NA
Flurbiprofen	D	100%	100%	100%	None	None	Dose for GFR 10–50
Flutamide	D	100%	100%	100%	Unknown	Unknown	Unknown
Fluvastatin	D	100%	100%	100%	Unknown	Unknown	Dose for GFR 10–50
Fluvoxamine	D	100%	100%	100%	None	Unknown	NA
Foscarnet	D	28 mg/kg	15 mg/kg	6 mg/kg	Dose after dialysis	Dose for GFR < 10	Dose for GFR 10–50
Fosinopril	D	100%	100%	75% to 100%	None	None	Dose for GFR 10–50
Furosemide	D	100%	100%	100%	None	None	NA
Gabapentin	D, I	400 mg tid	300 mg q12–24h	300 mg qd	300 mg load, then 200–300 mg		Dose for GFR 10–50
Gallamine	D	75%	Avoid	Avoid	NA	NA	Dose for GFR 10–50
Ganciclovir	I	q12h	q24–48h	q48–96h	Dose after dialysis	Dose for GFR < 10	2.5 mg/kg/day
Gemfibrozil	D	100%	100%	100%	None	Unknown	Dose for GFR 10–50
Gentamicin	D, I	60% to 90% q8–12h	30% to 70% q12h	20% to 30% q24–48h	2/3 normal dose	3–4 mg/L/day	Dose for GFR 10–50
Glibornuride	D	Unknown	Unknown	Unknown	Unknown	Unknown	Avoid
Gliclazide	D	Unknown	Unknown	Unknown	Unknown	Unknown	Avoid
Glipizide	D	100%	100%	100%	Unknown	Unknown	Avoid
Glyburide	D	Unknown	Avoid	Avoid	None	None	Avoid
Gold sodium thiomalate	D	50%	Avoid	Avoid	None	None	Avoid
Griseofulvin	D	100%	100%	100%	None	None	None
Guanabenz	D	100%	100%	100%	Unknown	Unknown	Dose for GFR 10–50
Guanadrel	I	q12h	q12–24h	q24–48h	Unknown	Unknown	Dose for GFR 10–50

Guanethidine	I	q24h	q24h	q24-36h	Unknown	Unknown	Avoid
Guanfacine	D	100%	100%	100%	None	None	Dose for GFR 10-50
Haloperidol	D	100%	100%	100%	None	None	Dose for GFR 10-50
Heparin	D	100%	100%	100%	None	None	Dose for GFR 10-50
Hexobarbital	I	q8h	q8h	q8-16h	None	Unknown	NA
Hydralazine	D	100%	100%	100%	None	None	Dose for GFR 10-50
Hydrocortisone	D	100%	50%	20%	Unknown	Unknown	Dose for GFR 10-50
Hydroxyurea	D	Unknown	Unknown	Unknown	Unknown	Unknown	Dose for GFR 10-50
Hydroxyzine	D	100%	100%	100%	100%	100%	100%
Ibuprofen	D	Unknown	Unknown	Unknown	None	None	Dose for GFR 10-50
Idarubicin	D	100%	100%	Unknown	Unknown	Unknown	Unknown
Ifosfamide	D	100%	100%	75%	Unknown	Unknown	Dose for GFR 10-50
Iloprost	D	100%	100%	50%	Unknown	Unknown	Dose for GFR 10-50
Imipenem	D	100%	50%	25%	Dose after dialysis	Dose for GFR < 10	Dose for GFR 10-50
Imipramine	D	100%	100%	100%	None	None	NA
Indapamide	D	100%	100%	Avoid	None	None	NA
Indinavir	D	100%	100%	100%	None	Dose for GFR < 10	Nos data
Indobufen	D	50%	25%	25%	Unknown	Unknown	NA
Indomethacin	D	100%	100%	100%	None	None	Dose for GFR 10-50
Insulin	D	75%	50%	50%	None	None	Dose for GFR 10-50
Ipratropium	D	100%	100%	100%	None	None	Dose for GFR 10-50
Isoniazid	D	100%	100%	50%	Dose after dialysis	Dose for GFR < 10	Dose for GFR < 10
Isosorbide	D	100%	100%	100%	10-20 mg	None	Dose for GFR 10-50
Isradipine	D	100%	100%	100%	None	None	Dose for GFR 10-50
Itraconazole	D	100%	100%	50%	100 mg q12-24h	100 mg q12-24h	100 mg q12-24h
Kanamycin	D, I	60% to 90% q8-12h	30% to 70% q12h	20% to 30% q24-48h	2/3 normal dose	15-20 mg/L/day	Dose for GFR 10-50

Continued

623

Table 35–1: (cont'd)

Drug	Dose Method	GFR > 50 (mL/min)	GFR 10–50 (mL/min)	GFR < 10 (mL/min)	Supplemental Dose after Hemodialysis	CAPD	CRRT
Ketamine	D	100%	100%	100%	Unknown	Unknown	Dose for GFR 10–50
Ketanserin	D	100%	100%	100%	None	None	Dose for GFR 10–50
Ketoconazole	D	100%	100%	100%	None	None	None
Ketoprofen	D	100%	100%	100%	None	None	Dose for GFR 10–50
Ketorolac	D	100%	50%	50%	None	None	Dose for GFR 10–50
Labetolol	D	100%	100%	100%	None	None	Dose for GFR 10–50
Lamivudine	D, I	100%	50–150 mg qd	25 mg qd	Dose after dialysis	Dose for GFR < 10	Dose for GFR 10–50
Lamotrigine	D	100%	100%	100%	Unknown	Unknown	Dose for GFR 10–50
Lansoprazole	D	100%	100%	100%	Unknown	Unknown	Unknown
Levodopa	D	100%	100%	100%	Unknown	Unknown	Dose for GFR 10–50
Levofloxacin	D	100%	50%	25% to 50%	Dose for GFR < 10	Dose for GFR < 10	Dose for GFR 10–50
Lidocaine	D	100%	100%	100%	None	None	Dose for GFR 10–50
Lincomycin	I	q6h	q6–12h	q12–24h	None	None	NA
Lisinopril	D	100%	50% to 75%	25% to 50%	20%	None	Dose for GFR 10–60
Lispro Insulin	D	100%	75%	50%	None	None	None
Lithium carbonate	D	100%	50% to 75%	25% to 50%	Dose after dialysis	None	Dose for GFR 10–50
Lomefloxacin	D	100%	50% to 75%	50%	Dose for GFR < 10	Dose for GFR < 10	NA
Loracarbef	I	q12h	q24h	q3–5 d	Dose after dialysis	Dose for GFR < 10	Dose for GFR 10–50
Lorazepam	D	100%	100%	100%	None	Unknown	Dose for GFR 10–50
Losartan	D	100%	100%	100%	Unknown	Unknown	Dose for GFR 10–50
Lovastatin	D	100%	100%	100%	Unknown	Unknown	Dose for GFR 10–50
Low–molecular–weight heparin	D	100%	100%	50%	Unknown	Unknown	Dose for GFR 10–50
Maprotiline	D	100%	100%	100%	Unknown	Unknown	NA

Meclofenamic acid	D	100%	100%	100%	None	None	Dose for GFR 10-50
Mefenamic acid	D	100%	100%	100%	None	None	Dose for GFR 10-50
Mefloquine		100%	100%	100%	None	None	Dose for GFR 10-50
Melphalan	D	100%	75%	50%	Unknown	Unknown	Dose for GFR 10-50
Meperidine	D	100%	75%	50%	Avoid	Unknown	Avoid
Meprobamate	I	q6h	q9-12h	q12-18h	None	None	NA
Meropenem	D, I	500 mg q6h	250-500 mg q12h	250-500 mg q24h	Dose after dialysis	Dose for GFR < 10	Dose for GFR 10-50
Metaproterenol	D	100%	100%	100%	Unknown	Unknown	Dose for GFR 10-50
Metformin	D	50%	25%	Avoid	Unknown	Unknown	Avoid
Methadone	D	100%	100%	50% to 75%	None	None	NA
Methenamine mandelate	D	100%	Avoid	Avoid	NA	NA	NA
Methicillin	I	q4-6h	q6-8h	q8-12h	None	None	Dose for GFR 10-50
Methimazole	D	100%	100%	100%	Unknown	Unknown	Dose for GFR 10-50
Methotrexate	D	100%	50%	Avoid	Yes	None	Dose for GFR 10-50
Methyldopa	I	q8h	q8-12h	q12-24h	250 mg	None	Dose for GFR 10-50
Methylprednisolone	D	100%	100%	100%	Yes	Unknown	Dose for GFR 10-50
Metoclopramide	D	100%	75%	50%	None	Unknown	50% to 75%
Metocurine	D	75%	50%	50%	Unknown	Unknown	Dose for GFR 10-50
Metolazone	D	100%	100%	100%	None	None	NA
Metoprolol	D	100%	100%	100%	50 mg	None	Dose for GFR 10-50
Metronidazole	D	100%	100%	50%	Dose after dialysis	Dose for GFR < 10	Dose for GFR 10-50
Mexiletine	D	100%	100%	50% to 75%	None	None	None
Mezlocillin	I	q4-6h	q6-8h	q8h	None	None	Dose for GFR 10-50
Miconazole	D	100%	100%	100%	None	None	None
Midazolam	D	100%	100%	50%	NA	NA	NA
Midodrine		5-10 mg q8h	5-10 mg q8h	5 mg q8h	5 mg q8h	No data	Dose for GFR 10-50
Miglitol	D	50%	Avoid	Avoid	Unknown	Unknown	Avoid

Continued

Table 35–1: (cont'd)

Drug	Dose Method	GFR > 50 (mL/min)	GFR 10–50 (mL/min)	GFR < 10 (mL/min)	Supplemental Dose after Hemodialysis	CAPD	CRRT
Milrinone	D	100%	100%	50 to 75%	No data	No data	Dose for GFR 10–50
Minocycline	D	100%	100%	100%	None	None	Dose for GFR 10–50
Minoxidil	D	100%	100%	100%	None	None	Dose for GFR 10–50
Mitomycin C	D	100%	100%	75%	Unknown	Unknown	Unknown
Mitoxantrone	D	100%	100%	100%	Unknown	Unknown	Dose for GFR 10–50
Mivacurium	D	100%	50%	50%	Unknown	Unknown	Unknown
Moricizine	D	100%	100%	100%	None	None	Dose for GFR 10–50
Morphine	D	100%	75%	50%	None	Unknown	Dose for GFR 10–50
Moxalactam	I	q8–12h	q12–24h	q24–48h	Dose after dialysis	Dose for GFR < 10	Dose for GFR 10–50
Nabumetone	D	100%	100%	100%	None	None	Dose for GFR 10–50
N-Acetylcysteine	D	100%	100%	75%	Unknown	Unknown	100%
Nadolol	D	100%	50%	25%	40 mg	None	Dose for GFR 10–50
Nafcillin	D	100%	100%	100%	None	None	Dose for GFR 10–50
Nalidixic acid	D	100%	Avoid	Avoid	Avoid	Avoid	NA
Naloxone	D	100%	100%	100%	NA	NA	Dose for GFR 10–50
Naproxen	D	100%	100%	100%	None	None	Dose for GFR 10–50
Nefazodone	D	100%	100%	100%	Unknown	Unknown	NA
Nelfinavir	D	No data	No data	No data	No data	No data	No data
Neostigmine	D, I	100%	50%	25%	Unknown	Unknown	Dose for GFR 10–50
Netilmicin	D, I	50% to 90% q8–12h	20% to 60% q12h	10% to 20% q24–48h	2/3 normal dose	3–4 mg/L/day	Dose for GFR 10–50
Nevirapine	D	100%	100%	100%	None	Dose for GFR < 10	Dose for GFR 10–50
Nicardipine	D	100%	100%	100%	None	None	Dose for GFR 10–50
Nicotinic acid	D	100%	50%	25%	Unknown	Unknown	Dose for GFR 10–50
Nifedipine	D	100%	100%	100%	None	None	Dose for GFR 10–50
Nimodipine	D	100%	100%	100%	None	None	Dose for GFR 10–50

Drug		GFR >50	GFR 10–50	GFR <10	Hemodialysis	CAPD	CVVH
Nisoldipine	D	100%	100%	100%	None	None	Dose for GFR 10–50
Nitrazepam	D	100%	100%	100%	Unknown	Unknown	NA
Nitrofurantoin	D	Avoid	Avoid	Avoid	NA	NA	NA
Nitroglycerine	D	100%	100%	100%	No data	No data	Dose for GFR 10–50
Nitroprusside	D	100%	100%	100%	None	None	Dose for GFR 10–50
Nitrosoureas	D	75%	75%	25% to 50%	None	Unknown	Unknown
Nizatidine	D	50%	50%	25%	Unknown	Unknown	Dose for GFR 10–50
Norfloxacin	I	q12–24h	q12–24h	Avoid	NA	NA	NA
Nortriptyline	D	100%	100%	100%	None	None	NA
Ofloxacin	D	50%	50%	25% to 50%	100 mg bid	Dose for GFR <10	300 mg/day
Omeprazole	D	100%	100%	100%	Unknown	Unknown	Unknown
Ondansetron	D	100%	100%	100%	Unknown	Unknown	Dose for GFR 10–50
Orphanadrine	D	100%	100%	100%	Unknown	Unknown	NA
Ouabain	I	q24–36h	q24–36h	q36–48h	None	None	Dose for GFR 10–50
Oxaproxin	D	100%	100%	100%	None	None	Dose for GFR 10–50
Oxatomide	D	100%	100%	100%	None	None	NA
Oxazepam	D	100%	100%	100%	None	Unknown	Dose for GFR 10–50
Oxcarbazepine	D	100%	100%	100%	Unknown	Unknown	Unknown
Paclitaxel	D	100%	100%	100%	Unknown	Unknown	Dose for GFR 10–50
Pancuronium	D	50%	50%	Avoid	Unknown	Unknown	Dose for GFR 10–50
Paroxetine	D	50% to 75%	50% to 75%	50%	Unknown	Unknown	NA
PAS	D	50% to 75%	50% to 75%	50%	Dose after dialysis	Dose for GFR <10	Dose for GFR 10–50
Penbutolol	D	100%	100%	100%	None	None	Dose for GFR 10–50
Penicillamine	D	Avoid	Avoid	Avoid	1/3 dose	Unknown	Dose for GFR 10–50
Penicillin G	D	75%	75%	20% to 50%	Dose after dialysis	Dose for GFR <10	Dose for GFR 10–50
Penicillin VK	D	100%	100%	100%	Dose after dialysis	Dose for GFR <10	NA
Pentamidine	I	q24–36h	q24–36h	q48h	None	None	None

Continued

Table 35-1: (cont'd)

Drug	Dose Method	GFR > 50 (mL/min)	GFR 10–50 (mL/min)	GFR < 10 (mL/min)	Supplemental Dose after Hemodialysis	CAPD	CRRT
Pentazocine	D	75%	75%	50%	None	Unknown	Dose for GFR 10–50
Pentobarbital	D	100%	100%	100%	None	Unknown	Dose for GFR 10–50
Pentopril	D	50% to 75%	50% to 75%	50%	Unknown	Unknown	Dose for GFR 10–50
Pentoxifylline	D	100%	100%	100%	Unknown	Unknown	100%
Perfloxacin	D	100%	100%	100%	None	None	Dose for GFR 10–50
Perindopril	D	100%	75%	50%	25% to 50%	Unknown	Dose for GFR 10–50
Phenelzine	D	100%	100%	100	Unknown	Unknown	NA
Phenobarbital	I	q8–12h	q8–12h	q12–16h	Dose after dialysis	1/2 normal dose	Dose for GFR 10–50
Phenylbutazone	D	100%	100%	100%	None	None	Dose for GFR 10–50
Phenytoin	D	100%	100%	100%	None	None	None
Pindolol	D	100%	100%	100%	None	None	Dose for GFR 10–50
Pipecuronium	D	100%	50%	25%	Unknown	Unknown	Dose for GFR 10–50
Piperacillin	I	q4–6h	q4–6h	q8h	Dose after dialysis	Dose for GFR < 10	Dose for GFR 10–50
Piretanide	D	100%	100%	100%	None	None	NA
Piroxicam	D	100%	100%	100%	None	None	Dose for GFR 10–50
Plicamycin	D	100%	75%	50%	Unknown	Unknown	Unknown
Pravastatin	D	100%	100%	100%	Unknown	Unknown	Dose for GFR 10–50
Prazepam	D	100%	100%	100%	Unknown	Unknown	NA
Prazosin	D	100%	100%	100%	None	None	Dose for GFR 10–50
Prednisolone	D	100%	100%	100%	Yes	Unknown	Dose forGFR 10–50
Prednisolone	D	100%	100%	100%	Yes	Unknown	Dose for GFR 10–50
Prednisone	D	100%	100%	100%	None	Unknown	Dose for GFR 10–50
Primaquine	D	100%	100%	100%	None	None	Dose for GFR 10–50
Primidone	I	q8h	q8–12h	q12–24h	1/3 dose	Unknown	Unknown
Probenecid	D	100%	Avoid	Avoid	Avoid	Unknown	Avoid
Probucol	D	100%	100%	100%	Unknown	Unknown	Dose for GFR 10–50
Procainamide	I	q4h	q6–12h	q8–24h	200 mg	None	Dose for GFR 10–50

Drug		GFR >50	GFR 10–50	GFR <10	Hemodialysis	CAPD	CRRT
Promethazine	D	100%	100%	100%	Unknown	Unknown	Dose for GFR 10–50
Promethazine	D	100%	100%	100%	None	None	100%
Propafenone	D	100%	100%	100%	None	None	Dose for GFR 10–50
Propofol	D	100%	100%	100%	Unknown	Unknown	Dose for GFR 10–50
Propoxyphene	D	100%	Avoid	Avoid	None	None	NA
Propranolol	D	100%	100%	100%	None	None	Dose for GFR 10–50
Propylthiouracil	D	100%	100%	100%	Unknown	Unknown	Dose for GFR 10–50
Protryptyline	D	100%	100%	100%	None	None	NA
Pyrazinimide	D	Avoid	Avoid	Avoid	Avoid	Avoid	Avoid
Pyridostigmine	D	50%	35%	20%	Unknown	Unknown	Dose for GFR 10–50
Pyrimethamine	D	100%	100%	100%	None	None	None
Quazepam	D	Unknown	Unknown	Unknown	Unknown	Unknown	NA
Quinapril	D	75% to 100%	75% to 100%	75%	25%	None	Dose for GFR 10–50
Quinidine	D	100%	100%	75%	100–200 mg	None	Dose for GFR 10–50
Quinine	I	q8h	q8–12h	q24h	Dose after dialysis	Dose for GFR < 10	Dose for GFR 10–50
Ramipril	D	100%	50% to 75%	25% to 50%	20%	None	Dose for GFR 10–50
Ranitidine	D	75%	50%	25%	1/2 dose	None	Dose for GFR 10–50
Reserpine	D	100%	100%	Avoid	None	Dose for GFR < 10	Dose for GFR 10–50
Ribavirin	D	100%	100%	50%	Dose after dialysis	Dose for GFR < 10	Dose for GFR <10
Rifabutin	D	100%	100%	100%	None	None	Dose for GFR 10–50
Rifampin	D	100%	50% to 100%	50% to 100%	None	Dose for GFR < 10	Dose for GFR < 10
Ritonavir	D	100%	100%	100%	None	Dose for GFR < 10	Dose for GFR 10–50
Saquinavir	D	100%	100%	100%	None	Dose for GFR < 10	Dose for GFR 10–50
Secobarbital	D	100%	100%	100%	None	none	NA
Sertraline	D	100%	100%	100%	Unknown	Unknown	NA
Simvastatin	D	100%	100%	100%	Unknown	Unknown	Dose for GFR 10–50

Continued

Table 35-1: (cont'd)

Drug	Dose Method	GFR >50 (mL/min)	GFR 10-50 (mL/min)	GFR <10 (mL/min)	Supplemental Dose after Hemodialysis	CAPD	CRRT
Sodium valproate	D	100%	100%	100%	None	None	None
Sotalol	D	100%	30%	15% to 30%	80 mg	None	Dose for GFR 10-50
Sparfloxacin	D, I	100%	50% to 75%	50% q48h	Dose for GFR <10	No data	Dose for GFR 10-50
Spectinomycin	D	100%	100%	100%	None	None	None
Spironolactone	I	q6-12h	q12-24h	Avoid	NA	NA	Avoid
Stavudine	D, I	100%	50% q12-q24h	50% q24h	Dose after dialysis	No data	Dose for GFR 10-50
Streptokinase	D	100%	100%	100%	NA	NA	Dose for GFR 10-50
Streptomycin	I	q24h	q24-72h	q72-96h	1/2 normal dose	20-40 mg/L/day	Dose for GFR 10-50
Streptozotocin	D	100%	75%	50%	Unknown	Unknown	Unknown
Succinylcholine	D	100%	100%	100%	Unknown	Unknown	Dose for GFR 10-50
Sufentanil	D	100%	100%	100%	Unknown	Unknown	Dose for GFR 10-50
Sulbactam	I	q6-8h	q12-24h	q24-48h	Dose after dialysis	0.75-1.5 g/day	750 mg q12h
Sulfamethoxazole	I	q12h	q18h	q24h	1 g after dialysis	1 g/day	Dose for GFR 10-50
Sulfinpyrazone	D	100%	100%	Avoid	None	None	Dose for GFR 10-50
Sulfisoxazole	I	q6h	q8-12h	q12-24h	2 g after dialysis	3 g/day	Not applicable
Sulindac	D	100%	100%	100%	None	None	Dose for GFR 10-50
Sulotroban	D	50%	30%	10%	Unknown	Unknown	Unknown
Tamoxifen	D	100%	100%	100%	Unknown	Unknown	Dose for GFR 10-50
Tazobactam	D	100%	75%	50%	1/3 dose	Dose for GFR <10	Dose for GFR 10-50
Teicoplanin	I	q24h	q48h	q72h	Dose for GFR <10	Dose for GFR <10	Dose for GFR 10-50
Temazepam	D	100%	100%	100%	None	None	NA
Teniposide	D	100%	100%	100%	None	None	Dose for GFR 10-50
Terazosin	D	100%	100%	100%	Unknown	Unknown	Dose for GFR 10-50
Terbutaline	D	100%	50%	Avoid	Unknown	Unknown	Dose for GFR 10-50
Terfenadine	D	100%	100%	100%	None	None	NA
Tetracycline	I	q8-12h	q12-24h	q24h	None	None	Dose for GFR 10-50

Drug	Method	GFR >50	GFR 10–50	GFR <10			
Theophylline	D	100%	100%	Unknown	1/2 dose	Unknown	Dose for GFR 10–50
Thiazides	D	100%	100%	Avoid	NA	NA	NA
Thiopental	D	100%	100%	75%	NA	NA	NA
Ticarcillin	D, I	1–2 g q4h	1–2 g q8h	1–2 g q12h	3 g after dialysis	Dose for GFR < 10	Dose for GFR 10–50
Ticlopidine	D	100%	100%	100%	Unknown	Unknown	Dose for GFR 10–50
Timolol	D, I	100%	100%	100%	None	None	Dose for GFR 10–50
Tobramycin	D, I	60% to 90% q8–12h	30% to 70% q12h	20% to 30% q24–48h	2/3 normal dose	3–4 mg/L/day	Dose for GFR 10–50
Tocainide	D	100%	100%	50%	200 mg	None	Dose for GFR 10–50
Tolazamide	D	100%	100%	100%	Unknown	Unknown	Avoid
Tolbutamide	D	100%	100%	100%	None	None	Avoid
Tolmetin	D	100%	100%	100%	None	None	Dose for GFR 10–50
Topiramate	D	100%	50%	25%	Unknown	Unknown	Dose for GFR 10–50
Topotecan	D	75%	50%	25%	Unknown	Unknown	Dose for GFR 10–50
Torsemide	D	100%	100%	100%	None	None	NA
Tranexamic acid	D	50%	25%	10%	Unknown	Unknown	Unknown
Tranylcypromine	D	Unknown	Unknown	Unknown	Unknown	Unknown	NA
Trazodone	D	100%	Unknown	Unknown	Unknown	Unknown	NA
Triamcinolone	D	100%	100%	100%	Unknown	Unknown	Dose for GFR 10–50
Triamterene	I	q12h	q12h	Avoid	NA	NA	Avoid
Triazolam	D	100%	100%	100%	None	NA	NA
Trihexyphenidyl	D	Unknown	Unknown	Unknown	Unknown	None	Unknown
Trimethadione	I	q8h	q8–12h	q12–24h	Unknown	Unknown	Dose for GFR 10–50
Trimethoprim	I	q12h	q18h	q24h	Dose after dialysis	q24h	q18h
Trimetrexate	D	100%	50% to 100%	Avoid	No data	No data	No data
Trimipramine	D	100%	100%	100%	None	None	NA
Tripelennamine	D	Unknown	Unknown	Unknown	Unknown	Unknown	NA
Triprolidine	D	Unknown	Unknown	Unknown	Unknown	Unknown	NA
Tubocurarine	D	75%	50%	Avoid	Unknown	Unknown	Dose for GFR 10–50
Urokinase	D	Unknown	Unknown	Unknown	Unknown	Unknown	Dose for GFR 10–50

Continued

Table 35–1: (cont'd)

Drug	Dose Method	GFR > 50 (mL/min)	GFR 10–50 (mL/min)	GFR < 10 (mL/min)	Supplemental Dose after Hemodialysis	CAPD	CRRT
Vancomycin	D, I	500 mg q6–12h	500 mg q24–48h	500 mg q48–96h	Dose for GFR < 10	Dose for GFR < 10	Dose for GFR 10–50
Vecuronium	D	100%	100%	100%	Unknown	Unknown	Dose for GFR 10–50
Venlafaxine	D	75%	50%	50%	None	Unknown	NA
Verapamil	D	100%	100%	100%	None	None	Dose for GFR 10–50
Vidarabine	D	100%	100%	75%	Infuse after dialysis	Dose for GFR < 10	Dose for GFR 10–50
Vigabatrin	D	100%	50%	25%	Unknown	Unknown	Dose for GFR 10–50
Vinblastine	D	100%	100%	100%	Unknown	Unknown	Dose for GFR 10–50
Vincristine	D	100%	100%	100%	Unknown	Unknown	Dose for GFR 10–50
Vinorelbine	D	100%	100%	100%	Unknown	Unknown	Dose for GFR 10–50
Warfarin	D	100%	100%	100%	None	None	None
Zafirlukast	I	100%	100%	100%	Unknown	Unknown	Dose for GFR 10–50
Zalcitabine	D	100%	q12h	q24h	Dose after dialysis	No data	Dose for GFR 10–50
Zidovudine (AZT)	D, I	200 mg q8h	200 mg q8h	100 mg q8h	Dose for GFR < 10	Dose for GFR < 10	100 mg q8h
Zileuton		100%	100%	100%	None	Unknown	Dose for GFR 10–50

CAPD, chronic ambulatory peritoneal dialysis; CRRT, continuous renal replacement therapies; D, decreasing individual doses; GFR, glomerular filtration rate; HD, hemodialysis; I, increasing individual doses; NA, not applicable.

or safety of a recommended dose in an individual patient. A loading dose equivalent to the usual dose in patients with normal renal function should be considered for drugs with a particularly long half-life. The table indicates potential methods for adjusting the dose by decreasing the individual doses or increasing the dose interval. In the table, when the dose method (D) is suggested, the percentage of the dose for normal renal function is given. When the interval method (I) is suggested, the actual dose interval is provided. When the dose interval can safely be lengthened beyond 24 hours, extended parenteral therapy may be completed without prolonging hospitalization. In patients requiring chronic hemodialysis, many drugs need to be given only at the end of the dialysis treatment, improving compliance.

The effect of the standard clinical treatment on drug removal is shown for hemodialysis, chronic ambulatory peritoneal dialysis, and CRRT. Most of these recommendations were established before very-high-efficiency hemodialysis treatments were practical, continuous cycling nocturnal peritoneal dialysis was common, and diffusion was added to hemofiltration in CRRTs. Some drugs that have high dialysis clearance rates do not require supplemental doses after dialysis if the amount of the drug removed is not sufficient, as is the case if the volume of distribution is large. To ensure efficacy when information about dialysis loss is not available and to simplify dosimetry, maintenance doses of most drugs should be given after dialysis. Peritonitis is a major complication of peritoneal dialysis, and the treatment of choice is the intraperitoneal administration of antibiotics. In general, there is excellent drug absorption after intraperitoneal administration of common antibiotics.

Dosing Considerations for Specific Drug Categories

Analgesics
Most analgesics are eliminated by hepatic biotransformation. However, the accumulation of active metabolites can result in central nervous system toxicity and seizures. The use of morphine, meperidine, and dextropropoxyphene in patients with impaired renal function should be avoided. Hydromorphone is suitable for patients with severe pain. Prolonged narcosis is associated with codeine and dihydrocodeine, whereas the use of fentanyl may lead to prolonged sedation.

Anticonvulsants
Generalized major motor seizures occur in patients with uremia, and phenytoin is one of the most commonly used drugs for

such seizures. For any given total serum phenytoin level, the concentration of active, free drug is higher in uremic patients than in patients with normal renal function, increasing the risk of toxicity. Dose increments of phenytoin should be small, sufficient time should be allowed for the drug to reach steady-state levels, and measurement of free serum phenytoin concentration should be done often in uremic patients who are not showing a response to therapy.

Antihypertensive and Cardiovascular Agents

Antihypertensive and cardiovascular agents are the most commonly prescribed drugs for patients with renal disease. Many cardiovascular drugs or their metabolites have prolonged half-lives and can accumulate in patients with renal insufficiency. Adverse effects are typically related to the pharmacologic effect of the drugs, and adverse events can be avoided by careful dose titration to clinical effect especially with newer, longer-acting formulations. Angiotensin-converting enzyme inhibitors and angiotensin receptor antagonists are widely used in the management of progressive renal disease and hypertension. The initial doses of angiotensin-converting enzyme inhibitors and angiotensin receptor antagonists should be low and carefully titrated, and renal function and serum potassium levels should be monitored for evidence of hyperkalemia.

The use of antiarrhythmic agents requires particular care and frequent monitoring for electrocardiographic evidence of toxicity, such as a prolonged QT interval or widening of the QRS complex on an electrocardiogram.

Diuretics are widely used in patients with chronic renal failure to control volume overload and aid in the management of hypertension. Diuretic-induced hypovolemia can result in a further decrease in renal function and volume status should be carefully evaluated during diuretic therapy. Potassium-sparing diuretics (i.e., amiloride, spironolactone, and triamterene) must be avoided in patients with creatinine clearance less than 30 mL/min because of the risks associated with hyperkalemia. As renal function decreases, tubular secretion of loop diuretics falls and larger doses are required to effect a diuresis. Thiazides lose their diuretic efficacy when the glomerular filtration rate falls below about 30 mL/min; however, the combination of a thiazide and loop diuretic can prove more effective than a higher dose of either agent alone.

Antimicrobial Agents

Inappropriate loading dose reduction that results in ineffectively low plasma concentration is a significant danger in patients with renal impairment. A single loading dose of antibiotic, equivalent to the usual maintenance dose for patients with normal renal function should almost always be given to patients with impaired renal function. Subsequent doses and dose intervals can be individualized on the basis of the relative importance of maintaining therapeutic peak or trough concentrations (see earlier). Uremia may mask the clinical presentation of infection and the signs of antibiotic-toxicity in patients with renal failure. Adverse reactions to antimicrobial treatment in patients with impaired renal function are usually caused by the accumulation of drugs or their metabolites to toxic levels with repeated doses and may affect any organ system. Drug toxicity should be considered in antibiotic-treated patients with renal insufficiency who develop new symptoms and therapeutic drug monitoring is essential in all patients with renal impairment to avoid toxicity to the kidney and other organs. Specific care should be taken with the use of aminoglycosides because nephrotoxicity can occur even if serum levels are "normal."

Hypoglycemic Drugs

Diabetic nephropathy is the leading cause of end-stage renal disease in the United States. Careful selection of hypoglycemic drugs and consideration of dosage is important for patients with impaired renal function. The kidney accounts for almost 30% of the elimination of insulin from the body and as renal function decreases, insulin clearance also falls. Hypoglycemia is more common in diabetic patients with impaired renal function. Patients with impaired renal function have an increased risk of hypoglycemia when they are treated with insulin or oral hypoglycemic drugs, and doses should be adjusted accordingly. In patients with renal failure, the use of long-acting sulfonylureas (e.g., glyburide) is accompanied by an enhanced risk of hypoglycemia, and the use of metformin is associated with a higher risk of lactic acidosis. Therefore, the use of these drugs is discouraged.

Nonsteroidal Anti-inflammatory Drugs

Nonsteroidal anti-inflammatory drugs (NSAIDs) are potent inhibitors of renal prostaglandin synthesis, and their use typically results in a decreased glomerular filtration rate in patients with chronic renal failure. NSAIDs also cause salt and water retention and trigger hyperkalemia in patients with even modest renal impairment. NSAIDs should be used cautiously in patients with decreased renal function and avoided in those with congestive heart failure, volume contraction, or liver failure. There is no advantage in the use of selective inhibitors of cyclooxygenase-2 over nonselective NSAIDs. The development of acute interstitial nephritis, occasionally in association with a minimal change–like glomerular lesion, is a well recognized complication of both NSAID and cyclooxygenase-2 use.

Sedatives, Hypnotics, and Drugs Used in Psychiatry

Anxiety and depression are often clinical correlates of renal failure. Excessive sedation is the most common complication of centrally acting agents in renal failure and is often inappropriately ascribed to the effects of uremia. The short-term administration of benzodiazepines is safe; however, care must be taken to avoid long-acting agents and those with active metabolites such as diazepam, chlordiazepoxide, and flurazepam. Phenothiazines and tricyclic antidepressants can produce confusion, orthostatic hypotension, and excessive sedation. Lithium carbonate, used in the management of bipolar disorder, is excreted by the kidney and has a narrow therapeutic range. Dose reduction and plasma lithium level monitoring is required in all patients with impaired or unstable renal function. Life-threatening lithium toxicity may be managed by dialysis. Repeated treatments are often required to deal with the rebound in serum levels often observed after dialysis.

VII

Renal Replacement Therapy

Hemodialysis

36

THE HEMODIALYSIS POPULATION

Demographics

More than 300,000 patients in the United States with end-stage renal disease (ESRD) are receiving hemodialysis. The annual incidence of patients entering hemodialysis programs is approximately 250 per 1 million people, representing more than 70,000 new patients per year. Notably, the prevalence rate for African-American patients with ESRD is approximately 4 times that of the general population and 6.5-fold that of the Caucasian population.

Morbidity and Mortality of Hemodialysis Patients

As access to hemodialysis has expanded, the number of comorbid diseases in patients at initiation of therapy has increased. Hemodialysis patients typically have high coincident rates of diabetes mellitus, cardiovascular disease, cerebral vascular disease, and chronic lung disease. These conditions result in frequent hospitalizations, particularly in older patients. Specific risk factors for hospital admission include receiving hemodialysis for less than 1 year, a hematocrit less than 30%, and an inadequate dialysis dose (urea reduction ratio < 60%). The annual mortality rate for the population with ESRD in the United States is approximately 182 per 1000 patient-years with cardiovascular disease and infections accounting for most deaths. The striking mortality rates associated with hemodialysis are reflected in the finding that at age 60 the life expectancy of a hemodialysis patient is only 5 years compared with 20 years for a healthy individual.

TRANSITION FROM CHRONIC KIDNEY DISEASE TO HEMODIALYSIS

Reducing Comorbidity

Optimal pre-ESRD management includes treatment strategies focused on the following clinical issues:

- Strict blood pressure and glycemic control
- Blockade of the renin-angiotensin-aldosterone system
- Management of anemia
- Avoidance of nephrotoxins (e.g., radiocontrast material and nonsteroidal anti-inflammatory drugs)
- Prevention of renal osteodystrophy
- Dietary intervention to minimize malnutrition while moderating protein intake
- Patient education regarding treatment options in ESRD
- Appropriate placement of vascular or peritoneal access
- Evaluation for renal transplantation (including preemptive transplantation)

Comorbid conditions must also be treated with particular emphasis placed on the management of cardiovascular risk factors including the treatment of anemia with erythropoietin. The key to optimal management of the patient with chronic kidney disease is early input from a nephrologist (glomerular filtration rate < 60 mL/min). Early management has been shown to reduce morbidity and mortality rates among patients entering renal replacement programs.

Starting Hemodialysis

Common indications for initiation of hemodialysis in patients with acute renal failure include uncontrolled hypertension, pulmonary edema, acidosis, hyperkalemia, pericarditis, and encephalopathy. These indications should never be reasons for initiating chronic maintenance hemodialysis because the goal for patients is a smooth transition from chronic kidney disease to ESRD. Although there is no agreed on absolute level at which hemodialysis should be initiated, therapy should be started at a level of residual renal function above which the major symptoms of uremia supervene. Among the criteria for initiating dialysis are residual creatinine clearances of 15 and 10 mL/min, which roughly correspond to serum creatinine concentrations of 6 and 8 mg/dL for diabetic and nondiabetic patients, respectively. These are general guidelines, and it may be necessary to initiate hemodialysis in patients even earlier in the course of their disease if they have otherwise uncorrectable symptoms or signs of renal failure such as nausea and vomiting, weight loss, intractable congestive heart failure, or hyperkalemia. The restless leg syndrome, asterixis, and a reversal of the sleep-wake cycle are early neurologic manifestations of uremia. If alternative explanations for these symptoms and signs cannot be discerned, they should be indications for initiating dialysis.

VASCULAR ACCESS

Arteriovenous Fistula

A native vein fistula is the vascular access of choice in hemodialysis patients. The most commonly used site is at the wrist, where the cephalic vein is connected to the radial artery. A significant percentage of radial-cephalic fistulas fail to mature or thrombose (25% to 35%) especially in female, diabetic, and older hemodialysis patients. An alternative to the radial-cephalic fistula is a brachiocephalic fistula or a brachiobasilic fistula. Because the basilic vein in the upper arm lies under deep fascia, the vein must be dissected and transposed into a more convenient subcutaneous position ("basilic vein transposition"). Compared with brachiocephalic fistulas, transposed brachiobasilic fistulas are more likely to mature, but have a higher long-term thrombosis rate. Better patency has been reported for upper arm fistulas compared with lower arm fistulas or arteriovenous grafts, supporting the trend toward creation of upper arm arteriovenous fistulas as the access of choice in patients with poor forearm venous anatomy. Preoperative ultrasonographic imaging can increase the success rate for the surgical placement of arteriovenous fistulas. The chosen vein should be at least 2.5 mm in diameter at the point of anastomosis to increase the fistula success rate. Another successful strategy for increasing the usage of arteriovenous fistulas involves ligation of tributary veins when the fistula fails to mature promptly. The average time to first use of a fistula is more than 8 weeks and because commencement of hemodialysis with an arteriovenous-fistula is associated with better long-term patient outcomes, timely insertion is essential.

Arteriovenous Grafts

Dialysis arteriovenous grafts made of expanded polytetrafluoroethylene have the advantage of low early thrombosis rates, ease of surgical placement, and a relatively short time between access creation and successful cannulation. However, these short-term advantages are more than outweighed by the long-term increased risk for infection and thrombosis compared with native vein fistulas. The 1- and 2-year primary patency rates for expanded polytetrafluoroethylene grafts are only 50% and 25%, respectively. Graft thrombosis accounts for 80% of all vascular access dysfunction, and in more than 90% of thrombosed grafts, venous stenosis at or distal to the graft vein anastomosis is detected. This can be managed by either surgical revision or balloon angioplasty. Infection in the graft should be suspected when fever is accompanied by pain over the graft or evidence of new-onset graft dysfunction. Graft infection should be treated as a matter of clinical urgency and requires removal of the infected graft combined with systemic antibiotic therapy for at least 3 weeks. There are no compelling clinical trial data suggesting a benefit from either antiplatelet or anticoagulant strategies in the prevention of arteriovenous graft or fistula thrombosis.

Vascular Access Monitoring and Surveillance

Physiologic monitoring of access function may improve clinical outcomes by helping to identify patients with a risk of arteriovenous graft failure and facilitating elective correction of venous stenotic lesions. Approaches include physical examination, static and dynamic venous pressure monitoring, vascular access blood flow monitoring, vascular access imaging by Doppler ultrasound, and measurement of access recirculation. Although fistulography remains the gold standard for assessing access patency, it is not suitable for routine surveillance studies. Indications for fistulography with or without angioplasty include the following clinical findings suggestive of early venous outflow stenosis:

- Prolonged bleeding from needle puncture sites
- Elevated venous pressures on hemodialysis (> 100 mm Hg)
- Edema of the arm
- Evidence of recirculation (> 10%)
- Arterio-venous graft flow less than 600 mL or reduced by 25% from baseline

Although venous stenoses develop less often and at a slower rate in patients with native arteriovenous fistulas compared with arteriovenous grafts, it has been suggested that vascular access blood flow monitoring has utility in this patient population as well.

Venous Catheters

Cuffed, tunneled dialysis catheters have the advantage of immediate usability and relatively easy placement. However, they are associated with strikingly high rates of patient morbidity. They should only be used as a bridge to use of an arteriovenous access or as a permanent vascular access in patients for whom all other peripheral access options have been exhausted. Tunneled catheters are, not unsurprisingly, associated with a high rate of local exit site infections, bacteremia/septicemia ("line sepsis"), and thrombotic complications. The importance of line sepsis as a cause of mortality in ESRD patients cannot be overemphasized. There is up to a 300-fold higher mortality from sepsis in all dialysis patients compared with the general population, and the incidence of catheter-associated bloodstream infection is at least 2 to 4 episodes per 1000 patient-catheter days. The clinician needs to be ever vigilant in the care of the patient with a tunneled line. Clinical findings suggestive of a catheter infection include a fever, tenderness over the tunnel or exit site, and rigors during dialysis. If infection is suspected then intravenous vancomycin and gentamicin should be administered pending the results of blood cultures. The coverage can be adjusted when the results of bacteriologic evaluation are available. If infection is confirmed, then the treatment of catheter-related bacteremia is as follows:

- Removal of the catheter with delayed replacement until defervescence in patients with severe clinical symptoms
- Catheter exchange by guidewire in patients with minimal symptoms and normal-appearing tunnel and exit site
- Catheter replacement by guidewire with creation of a new tunnel in patients with exit site or tunnel infection only

In all cases, patients should be treated with at least 3 weeks of systemic antibiotic therapy. However, even using these conservative strategies, 15% to 20% of patients with catheter-related bacteremias experience complicated infections, including osteomyelitis, discitis, endocarditis, and septic arthritis. Catheter-related bacteremia due to *Staphylococcus aureus* is particularly associated with metastatic infection. The use of mupirocin ointment at the catheter exit site may decrease the incidence of *S aureus*–associated bacteremias. Attempting to treat catheter-related bacteremia with antibiotics without catheter removal is unsuccessful in most patients. Venous catheters are also subject to frequent episodes of thrombosis, requiring thrombolytic therapy or replacement of the catheter. The long-term use of cuffed venous catheters also leads to the development of central venous stenosis and right atrial thrombi. Because subclavian vein stenosis may preclude the subsequent successful placement of ipsilateral arteriovenous fistulas or grafts, the use of subclavian venous catheters is generally contraindicated in dialysis patients except as a last resort.

ARTIFICIAL PHYSIOLOGY: GENERAL PRINCIPLES OF HEMODIALYSIS

Dialysis relies on the mass transfer across semipermeable membranes. The hemodialysis membrane separates the blood and dialysate compartments. Diffusion, convection, and ultrafiltration across the membrane are properties that are integral to the dialysis procedure.

- *Diffusion:* The movement of solutes from one compartment to another across a semipermeable membrane, relying on a concentration gradient between the two compartments.
- *Ultrafiltration:* Fluid movement across a semipermeable membrane driven by a hydrostatic pressure gradient.
- *Convection:* Movement of solutes by bulk flow in association with fluid removal. It is not dependent on concentration gradients and the magnitude of its contribution to clearance is directly related to the ultrafiltration rate.

Diffusion is the principal mechanism for toxin removal during hemodialysis, although convective clearance does contribute if ultrafiltration also takes place. Convective clearance is the mechanism of toxin removal by the depurative process known as hemofiltration, which is commonly used in the setting of continuous renal replacement therapy in critically ill patients.

Clearance

The clearance of a substance is the amount removed from plasma, divided by the average plasma concentration over the time of measurement. Clearance is expressed in moles or weight of the substance per volume per time and can be thought of as the volume of plasma that can be completely cleared of the substance in a unit of time. The goals of dialysis are straightforward: to remove accumulated fluid and toxins. With respect to toxins, the goal is to maintain their concentrations below the levels at which they produce uremic symptoms. However, the toxic levels of retained substances are not used as performance measures for dialysis because their identities are unknown. Instead, the efficacy of dialysis is primarily judged by the clearance of urea. Several variables affect clearance by the dialyzer, including blood and dialysate flow rates, dialyzer surface area, dialytic time, and the inherent transport characteristics of the membrane for high- and low-molecular-weight substances, respectively.

Hemodialysis Membranes: Effects and Characteristics

The surface area, surface charge, and pore size are properties of the membrane that directly govern the molecules which can diffuse from blood to the dialysate. Virtually all of the commercial dialyzers available in the United States are configured as large cylinders packed with hollow fibers, known as *hollow-fiber dialyzers*. Blood flows within the hollow fibers, and dialysate flows outside and around these fibers, generally in a countercurrent fashion whereby dialysate flow is in the opposite direction to blood flow. Dialyzer membranes are one of three basic types based on the structural compound used in the synthesis of the membrane:

- *Cellulose:* These are polysaccharide-based membranes manufactured from cotton fibers. They are low flux and are considered "bioincompatible" (see later).
- *Semisynthetic:* These are cellulosic membranes modified by the addition of a synthetic material to increase biocompatibility.
- *Synthetic:* Synthetic membranes are composed of one of the following: polyacrylonitrile, polysulfone, polymethylmethacrylate or polyamide. They are generally more biocompatible than cellulose-based membranes and have higher permeability and flux characteristics.

During hemodialysis, patients may experience a number of reactions that are a direct consequence of establishing the extracorporeal circuit. The number and severity of these reactions define the degree of dialysis biocompatibility. The clinical manifestations of bioincompatibilty include chest and back pain, dyspnea, nausea, vomiting, and hypotension. Fortunately, more severe anaphylactic reactions are rare and usually reflect contamination with bacterial peptides. Complement activation through the alternative pathway, with generation of the anaphylatoxins C3a and C5a, mediates most of the effects of bioincompatibility.

THE DIALYSIS PRESCRIPTION

The goal of hemodialysis in patients with ESRD is to restore the body's intracellular and extracellular fluid environment toward that of healthy individuals with functioning kidneys to the greatest extent possible. The prescription for an individual hemodialysis session must take into account an examination and physiologic assessment of individual patient needs to achieve these goals. The variables in the hemodialysis procedure that may be manipulated by the physician on the basis of clinical assessment include the following:

1. Choosing the type of dialyzer
2. Establishing blood and dialysate flows
3. Prescribing the time for the dialysis procedure
4. Prescribing the dialysate composition
5. Determining the frequency of the dialysis procedure
6. Determining the intensity of anticoagulation of the extra-corporeal circuit

Dialyzer Choice

The three most critical determinants in making a decision about the choice of dialyzer are its solute clearance capacity, ultrafiltration capacity, and biocompatibility. The ideal hemodialysis membrane would have a high clearance of low- and middle-molecular-weight uremic toxins, negligible loss of vital solutes, and adequate ultra-filtration capacity in an effort to maximize efficiency and reduce adverse metabolic effects from the hemodialysis procedure. Additional characteristics of the ideal dialyzer would be a low blood volume compartment, beneficial biocompatibility effects, high reliability, and low cost. The capacity for fluid removal by a dialyzer is described by its ultrafiltration coefficient, which corre-lates directly with its permeability. A low ultrafiltration coefficient implies a low permeability to water and vice versa.

Anticoagulation for Hemodialysis

The most widely used anticoagulant for dialysis is heparin. For most patients, heparin is administered systemically during the dialysis procedure as a single bolus or incrementally during the dialysis treatment. In routine hemodialysis practice, the intensity of anticoagulation is not measured, but in some circumstances, the activated clotting time is used. A simple method of heparin administration is the systemic administration of 50 to 100 units/kg of heparin at the initiation of dialysis, often followed by a bolus of 100 units/hr. When activated clotting time is being measured, the target activated clotting time is approximately 50% above base-line values. In fractional anticoagulation, a smaller initial bolus of heparin is administered (10 to 50 units/kg), followed by an infusion of 500 to 1000 units/hr. Fractional heparinization can be used to achieve less intensive anticoagulation for which the tar-get activated clotting time is maintained at 25% (fractional) or 15% (tight fractional) above the baseline value. These approaches are generally reserved for patients with a higher risk for bleeding complications (see later). For patients with a high risk for bleeding, heparin is occasionally administered as regional anticoagulation, in which only the extracorporeal dialyzer circuit is anticoagulated by administering heparin into the arterial line and protamine into the venous line. As an alternative to regional anticoagulation for patients at high risk for bleeding, dialysis may be performed without any anticoagulation. By using the saline flush technique, hemodialysis is initiated at a high blood flow rate to reduce thrombogenicity, and the dialyzer is flushed every 15 to 60 minutes with 50 mL of saline. This technique is not likely to be successful when high blood flow rates are not attainable and when a high ultrafiltration rate is required. For patients with a high risk for serious adverse events from hemorrhage, the following guidelines are recommended.

Heparin-free dialysis (including regional anticoagulation):

- Significant bleeding risk
- Within 7 days of major operative procedure (14 days if intracranial)
- Within 72 hours of visceral organ biopsy
- Pericarditis
- A major surgical procedure anticipated within 8 hours after dialysis

Fractional anticoagulation:

- More than 7 days after major surgery
- More than 72 hours after visceral organ biopsy
- Dialysis within 8 hours before a surgical procedure

Blood and Dialysate Flow

Blood and dialysate flow rates are critical elements of the dialysis prescription that can be altered to modify solute clearance. Blood and dialysate flow rates typically range from 300 to 500 and 500 to 800 mL/min, respectively. Studies have demonstrated that the practical upper limit of effective dialysate flow is twice the blood flow rate, beyond which the gain in solute removal is minimal. In clinical practice, the efficacy of angioaccess may affect solute clearance obtained at a given prescribed blood flow rate. Should venous outflow be restricted, there is an increased likelihood of backflow (called *recirculation*) from the venous to the arterial side of the access so that "dialyzed" blood reenters the dialytic circuit, thereby decreasing the efficiency of solute clearance.

The fractional recirculation (R) is calculated using the formula:

$$R = Cs - Ca/Cs - Cv$$

In this equation, *Cs*, *Ca*, and *Cv* are the concentrations (C) of the measured solute in systemic (*s*), arterial line (*a*), and venous (*v*) blood. Recirculation is measured as follows: after arterial line and venous line samples are obtained during dialysis, the blood flow is abruptly reduced to 50 mL/min, with the dialysate flow off and a peripheral sample is obtained from the arterial line after 150% of the volume from the needle to the sample point has been cleared (usually between 20 and 30 seconds). A recirculation rate of more than 10% is considered significant and mandates evaluation of the vascular access.

Dialysis Time

The clearance of any of a solute, such as urea, can be increased by lengthening the dialysis treatment. Because the typical dialysis prescription emphasizes optimal blood and dialysate flows and the selection of dialyzers with large mass transfer coefficient characteristics, the duration of dialysis is often the sole variable that can be used to augment solute clearance during an individual dialysis session. However, because diffusive solute clearance depends on solute concentration on the blood side, the efficiency of solute removal declines over the course of the dialysis procedure. A longer duration of the dialysis procedure also allows for a lower net ultrafiltration rate per hour for a given targeted ultrafiltration goal over the course of the procedure. This may result in fewer intradialytic symptoms such as hypotension and cramping.

Dialysate Composition

Sodium

The sodium concentration of the dialysate plays a crucial role in determining cardiovascular stability during hemodialysis. Historically, the dialysate sodium concentration was maintained at hyponatremic levels (130 to 135 mEq/L) to favor diffusive sodium loss during the dialysis procedure. However, this favored fluid shifts from the extracellular to the intracellular space, thereby exacerbating the plasma volume–depleting effects of hemodialysis. In addition, the osmolar changes and fluid shifts resulted in a high incidence of dialysis disequilibrium, characterized by headaches, nausea, vomiting, and, in severe cases, seizures. As a consequence, the use of hyponatremic dialysate has largely been abandoned. The current standard is to have a dialysate sodium concentration close to that of plasma. The prescription of high sodium dialysate has become a common practice in an attempt to reduce intradialytic hypotension. Unfortunately, this approach may lead to polydipsia, increased interdialytic weight gain, and increased interdialytic hypertension, thereby offsetting the beneficial effects of increased intradialytic hemodynamic stability. Therefore, strategies have evolved that involve varying the dialysate sodium concentration over the course of a dialysis session, referred to as *sodium modeling*. Sodium modeling is often performed in a stepwise fashion, in which the initial dialysate sodium concentration is greater than or equal to 145 mEq/L and, during the second half of the dialysis session, is abruptly reduced, or it may be reduced gradually over the course of the dialysis session ("linear sodium modeling"). Although sodium modeling can reduce the frequency of hypotension during dialysis, it is unclear whether this technique offers any advantage over a fixed dialysate sodium concentration of 140 to 145 mEq/L.

Potassium

The fractional decline in the plasma potassium concentration during hemodialysis is proportionately greater when there is a higher predialysis potassium concentration. However, the flux of potassium from the intracellular compartment to the extracellular space lags behind the transfer of potassium across the dialysis membrane. Hence, after the hemodialysis session, there is an increase in the plasma potassium concentration of approximately 30% over 4 to 5 hours due to movement of potassium from the intracellular to the extracellular space. Most of the cardiac arrhythmias that arise from the fall in the serum potassium concentration occur during the first half of the dialysis session. It is important to realize that it is the rapidity of the fall in plasma potassium concentration rather than the absolute plasma potassium level that determines the risk for interdialytic cardiac arrhythmias. The selection of a dialysate potassium concentration is empirical and is guided by patient-specific factors. Generally, a dialysate potassium concentration of 1 to 3 mEq/L is used in most patients. Patients who have excessive potassium loads from diet, medications, hemolysis, tissue breakdown, or gastrointestinal bleeding may require a lower dialysate potassium concentration. Low dialysate potassium concentrations should be used with caution, however, because an analysis has found an association between low dialysate potassium concentrations and sudden cardiac death in outpatient hemodialysis patients.

Calcium

Given the use of calcium-based phosphate binders and the aggressive use of vitamin D analogs, a standard dialysate calcium concentration of 2.5 to 3 mEq/L is preferred to prevent interdialytic hypercalcemia and elevations in the calcium-phosphate product, which are associated with vascular calcification.

Buffers

Hemodialysis therapy cannot remove large quantities of free hydrogen ions because of their low concentration in the blood. As a result, correction of the acidosis is largely achieved by using a dialysate with a higher concentration of bicarbonate than is present in the blood (30 to 40 mmol/L), promoting flux of base from the dialysate into the blood. Higher dialysate bicarbonate concentrations are sometimes used to fully correct metabolic acidosis due to the adverse effects of metabolic acidosis on protein catabolism and nutritional status in maintenance hemodialysis patients. Acetate-based dialysates are no longer in routine use.

Glucose

In general, an optimal dialysate glucose concentration is 100 to 200 mg/dL for most patients. However, in diabetic patients, insulin doses may require adjustment to account for this dialysis-imposed "glucose clamp," in which levels of plasma glucose may be kept constant during dialysis owing to the concentration in the dialysate.

Dialysate Temperature

Dialysate temperature is generally maintained between 36.5 and 38°C at the inlet of the dialyzer. Under normal circumstances there is an increase in body temperature during dialysis owing to ultrafiltration-induced volume contraction during hemodialysis that results in peripheral vasoconstriction, which in turn limits peripheral heat loss. Eventually, there is a reflex dilatation of peripheral blood vessels, which allows heat escape but reduces peripheral vascular resistance, resulting in an intradialytic fall in blood pressure. This led to the suggestion that lowering dialysate solution temperature might permit increased hemodynamic stability in hypotension-prone dialysis patients. Clinical trials have demonstrated that the provision of low temperature dialysis (35°C) improves cardiovascular stability during hemodialysis.

Ultrafiltration Rate

Modern dialysis machines possess ultrafiltration control systems that allow remarkably precise titration of the ultrafiltration prescription. Prescription of the ultrafiltration rate in maintenance hemodialysis patients is generally based on an assessment of estimated dry weight. *Dry weight* is defined as the lowest weight a patient can tolerate without the development of signs or symptoms of intravascular hypovolemia. Tolerance of the ultrafiltration rate during hemodialysis is largely determined by the rate of vascular refilling from the interstitium. Efforts to minimize intradialytic volume depletion include online hematocrit monitoring, which estimates blood volume changes during dialysis to allow appropriate adjustment of ultrafiltration rates before the development of overt hypotension. An additional approach involves the use of variable ultrafiltration rates during the hemodialysis procedure, known as ultrafiltration modeling. Studies suggest that combining sodium and ultrafiltration profiling may significantly reduce hemodialysis-related symptoms.

HEMODIALYSIS ADEQUACY

Multiple lines of evidence implicate inadequate dialysis prescriptions and underdelivery of the prescribed dose of dialysis as central factors responsible for the high mortality seen in ESRD. Monitoring the delivered dose of dialysis has therefore become a central facet of the management of patients with ESRD. However, the task of assessing treatment adequacy by indexing the dose of dialysis to a simple plasma level of urea or creatinine is unhelpful. In the first instance they are not the major uremic toxins and, in addition, the plasma levels reflect not only dialysis clearance but also nutritional intake and muscle mass, respectively. Therefore, clinicians have related the measured clearance of urea to outcome using one of two well-accepted methods (urea kinetic modeling):

- Kt/V_{urea}
- Urea reduction ratio

Kt/V is the fractional clearance of urea (Kt) as a function of its volume of distribution (V) where K equals the dialyzer clearance of urea (a function of the K_0A urea and the blood and dialysate flows), and t is the time on dialysis. The Kt/V is related to the pre- and postdialysis urea levels. Both urea generation and fluid removal during dialysis increase the postdialysis blood urea nitrogen (BUN). As a result, models that ignore urea generation and volume changes yield a lower value for Kt/V, because it appears that dialysis has been less efficient. The more complex models take into account urea generation rates during dialysis, dialysis-induced changes in total body water, and urea rebound postdialysis. A useful formula for calculating the Kt/V is

$$Kt/V = -\ln (R - 0.008 \times t) \div (4 - 3.5 \times R) \times UF/W$$

where ln is the natural logarithm; R is the post-predialysis urea ratio; t is the dialysis session length in hours; UF is ultrafiltration volume in 1 hour; and W is postdialysis weight in kilograms.

Great care should be taken in measuring the postdialysis urea level because this is central to the accurate estimation of Kt/V.

Both cardiopulmonary and access recirculation can significantly affect the BUN level measured from the arterial inflow port. To avoid this potential source of error, the blood flow pump should be slowed to 50 mL/min for 1 to 2 minutes before the sample is drawn from the "arterial" inflow access port at the end of dialysis. The value obtained from the formula above is known as the single-pool, unequilibrated Kt/V. A postdialysis urea level from blood drawn 30 to 60 minutes after dialysis will be higher owing to the equilibration of intracellular and blood urea levels. A value derived from this figure is known as a double-pool, equilibrated Kt/V. The difference between these two values is usually greater with shorter dialysis treatment times and averages 0.2. Despite the apparent significance of the figure, clinical studies evaluating the importance of Kt/V have used the single-pool, unequilibrated approach.

The simpler method for quantifying of the delivered dose of hemodialysis is the urea reduction ratio (URR) (i.e., predialysis BUN – postdialysis BUN/predialysis BUN). The URR depends exclusively on the changes that occur in urea levels during intermittent hemodialysis. Although URR has been shown to correlate with survival in a fashion similar to Kt/V and is recognized by National Kidney Foundation's Disease Outcomes Quality Initiative (K/DOQI) guidelines as a valid index of hemodialysis adequacy, Kt/V is a more precise index of small molecule clearance.

Clinical Importance of Kt/V and URR

Evidence supporting the importance of measuring the clearance of urea derives from the National Cooperative Dialysis Study (NCDS). The NCDS suggested that removal of urea strongly predicted morbidity and that urea kinetic modeling could be used to guide the dosing of hemodialysis in individual patients. Although the primary results of the NCDS were not expressed in terms of Kt/V subsequent retrospective analysis suggested that a Kt/V of less than 0.8 or a URR of less than 0.5 were associated with a significant rise in all-cause patient mortality. Whereas the NCDS was able to define a dose of dialysis below which an unacceptable number of complications occur, it was not designed to define an optimal level of dialysis beyond which no further improvement was realized. To address the question of what the optimal dialysis dose is, the National Institutes of Health initiated a multicenter, prospective, randomized trial to assess the impact of the dialysis prescription on morbidity and mortality of hemodialysis patients—The HEMO Study. An equilibrated Kt/V of 1.05 was compared with an equilibrated

Kt/V of 1.45, comparable, on average, to single-pool *Kt/V* values of 1.25 and 1.65, respectively. The effect on mortality and morbidity of high-flux versus low-flux dialyzers was also compared. All-cause mortality was the primary outcome and morbidity assessed from hospitalization, time to hospitalization for cardiovascular and infectious causes, and time to a decline in serum albumin concentration were secondary outcome measures. The primary outcome, death from any cause, was not influenced by the dialysis dose or the dialyzer flux assignment. The main secondary outcomes, including first hospitalization for cardiac causes or infection or all-cause mortality, declines in albumin or all-cause mortality, and all hospitalization not related to vascular access problems, also did not differ between the dose and the flux groups. Subgroup analysis suggested that females randomly assigned to the high-dose hemodialysis group had a lower risk of mortality. Subjects who had received hemodialysis for a longer time *at entry into the study* also had a lower mortality rate if they were allocated to the high-flux arm of the study.

Based on the earlier data current K/DOQI guidelines mandate a single-pool *Kt/V* of at least 1.2 for both adult and pediatric hemodialysis patients (or an average URR of > 65%). However, it is would appear prudent to provide a margin above the minimal dose to protect the patient from receiving less dialysis than intended due to factors that result in lower than intended clearance including suboptimal blood flows, poor blood pump calibration, poor access function, or premature treatment termination. Of note, the HEMO Study should not be used as a justification to reduce hemodialysis time nor is it possible to conclude from the HEMO Study that minimizing time while maintaining an "acceptable" *Kt/V* is justified.

ALTERNATIVE CHRONIC HEMODIALYSIS PRESCRIPTIONS

The results of the HEMO Study can only be applied to three times weekly hemodialysis, as is practiced in the United States. Worldwide there is increasing interest in different treatments times and frequencies designed to improve the clearance of larger substances with a view to improving mortality and morbidity rates. The removal of high-molecular-weight substances depends on membrane porosity and on the length of the dialysis treatment. It is possible to argue that, for the full benefit of high flux membranes to be realized, longer treatment times than those used in the HEMO Study are required. Alternative approaches include the following:

Short, daily hemodialysis. This involves five to seven treatments per week, each lasting 1.5 to 2.5 hours and the use of high-flux biocompatible membranes at blood flow rates higher than 400 mL/min and dialysate flow rates of 500 to 800 mL/min. This form of therapy has been associated with significant improvement in serum albumin levels, calcium-phosphate levels, and volume control in small scale studies. No mortality data are available.

Nocturnal hemodialysis. This is also performed five to seven times per week, with each treatment lasting 6 to 8 hours, and the use of biocompatible membranes at blood flow rate of 200 to 300 mL/min and dialysate flows of 200 to 300 mL/min. Although the number of patients studied has been rather limited, multiple lines of evidence suggest that significant improvements in nitrogen intake, caloric intake, and serum albumin level result. Once again convincing outcome data are lacking; however, one report described the use of nocturnal hemodialysis in children with growth retardation and failure to thrive with peritoneal dialysis. Treatment with nocturnal hemodialysis was well tolerated and resulted in improved nutritional status and quality of life and catch-up growth.

Slow, long hemodialysis. This is given three times weekly, with blood flow rates of 200 to 250 mL/min and a dialysis time of 6 to 8 hours. The single-pool Kt/V is typically 1.6 to 1.8. This procedure is practiced in Tassin in France and has been associated with improvements in blood pressure control and better overall nutritional status.

MANAGEMENT OF THE MAINTENANCE HEMODIALYSIS PATIENT

Infection and Immunity

Infection is the second leading cause of death in hemodialysis (10% to 20%) after cardiovascular diseases, with septicemia accounting for more than 75% of these infectious deaths. Risk factors for septicemia in hemodialysis patients include older age, diabetes mellitus, hypoalbuminemia, temporary vascular access, and the reprocessing of dialyzers. Clinical data demonstrate that central venous catheters are a major source of bacterial colonization and infection in hemodialysis patients compared with patients using arteriovenous grafts or arteriovenous fistulas.

Most infections in hemodialysis patients are caused by common catalase-producing bacteria such as *Staphylococcus* species, rather than opportunistic infections. There is increasing concern about the development of antibiotic resistance in hemodialysis patients. The common occurrence of methicillin-resistant *S aureus* infections over time has led to the frequent use of vancomycin to treat suspected and proven septicemia. This in turn has led to the emergence of vancomycin-resistant *Enterococcus* infections in many dialysis units.

Viral infections are also common in hemodialysis patients. The frequency of hepatitis B infection has fallen as a result of the introduction of recombinant erythropoietin coupled with the availability of the hepatitis B vaccine; however, infections still occur. Hemodialysis patients may acquire hepatitis B infection from community sources, from transmission in hemodialysis centers due to inadequate infection control precautions, or from accidental breaks in infection control technique. The hepatitis C virus (HCV) has become the most important cause of liver disease among hemodialysis patients and is also a major concern for hemodialysis staff. The prevalence of anti-HCV antibody positivity in hemodialysis units varies from 5% to 40%. The clinical course of HCV infection in hemodialysis patients tends to be chronic and indolent with a characteristic fluctuating course and multiple peaks and troughs in alanine aminotransferase levels. Current recommendations are that hemodialysis patients should be considered a high-risk population for HCV infection and should undergo periodic screening. Isolation of HCV carriers within the hemodialysis unit is not recommended beyond the use of standard universal precautions. Although most hemodialysis patients with HCV infection remain asymptomatic over a long period, identified patients should be instructed to avoid additional hepatic toxins, including alcohol consumption and potentially hepatotoxic medications. Antiviral therapy with interferon-α is recommended for selected categories of HCV-infected hemodialysis patients.

Human immunodeficiency virus infection appears to be increasing in incidence in hemodialysis patients. According to the Centers for Disease Control and Prevention, in 2000, 1.5% of hemodialysis patients had human immunodeficiency virus infection and 0.4% had acquired immunodeficiency syndrome. There is no contraindication to highly active antiretroviral therapy in the population receiving dialysis.

All hemodialysis patients should receive hepatitis B, pneumococcal, and influenza vaccines. Patients with chronic kidney disease should receive three doses of recombinant hepatitis B vaccine as early in the course of renal disease as possible because only 50% to 75% of dialysis patients develop protective antibody levels against hepatitis B surface antigen compared with more than 90% of healthy adults. Revaccination with up to three additional doses is recommended for those hemodialysis patients who do not develop protective antibody levels. Anti-hepatitis B surface antigen testing is recommended 1 to 2 months after vaccination of hemodialysis patients to demonstrate protective antibody levels. Additional postvaccination testing is recommended annually. A booster dose is recommended if the anti-hepatitis B surface antigen titer falls to less than 10 mUnits/mL. A single dose of the 23-valent pneumococcal polysaccharide vaccine is recommended intramuscularly or subcutaneously for all dialysis patients older than 2 years of age. Revaccination is recommended 3 years after the previous dose for children and after at least 5 years in adults. Influenza vaccination is recommended annually for hemodialysis patients because of an increased risk for influenza-related mortality. Household members and health care workers in contact with hemodialysis patients should also be vaccinated annually to decrease influenza transmission rates. The influenza vaccine is also recommended for children receiving hemodialysis.

Vaccines routinely administered in childhood (i.e., measles, mumps, and rubella vaccines; varicella vaccine; inactivated polio virus vaccine; diphtheria, tetanus, and pertussis vaccine; and *Haemophilus* influenza type B conjugate vaccine) are generally recommended for children receiving hemodialysis. Oral polio virus vaccine, which is no longer available in the United States, is not recommended because of a theoretical risk of producing paralytic polio.

The pathogenesis and management of anemia, cardiovascular disease, calciphylaxis, and nutrition in the dialysis population are discussed in detail in Chapter 27, Hematologic Consequences of Renal Failure; Chapter 28, Cardiovascular Aspects of Chronic Kidney Disease; Chapter 30, Renal Osteodystrophy; and Chapter 31, Nutritional Therapy in Renal Disease.

COMPLICATIONS OF HEMODIALYSIS

Hemodialysis is a relatively safe procedure, with an estimated 1 death in 75,000 treatments as a result of technical error. The age of the patient; the presence of underlying medical conditions such as diabetes mellitus, coronary artery disease, or congestive heart failure; and the patient's degree of compliance with a complex medical regimen necessary in end-stage disease influence the frequency and severity of adverse events.

Hypotension

Hypotension is the most common acute complication of hemodialysis (Table 36–1). The incidence of hypotension in the dialysis population ranges between 15% and 30%. During ultrafiltration, a protein-free ultrafiltrate of plasma is removed from the intravascular space. The resultant rise in plasma oncotic pressure causes fluid to move from the interstitial and intracellular spaces to replenish plasma volume. Hypotension results when the rate of intravascular volume depletion exceeds the rate of refilling of this space, especially if total peripheral resistance and cardiac output cannot compensate for the loss of intravascular volume. Very large interdialytic weight gains cannot easily be removed during a typical treatment (usually lasting between 3.5 and 4 hours), even in the presence of volume overload, because the refilling of

---

Table 36–1: Causes of Intradialytic Hypotension

Common
- High ultrafiltration rate (> 1 L/hr)
  - Excessive interdialytic weight gain
- Inappropriately low "dry weight"
- Rapid reduction in plasma osmolality
- Autonomic neuropathy
  - Diabetes mellitus
  - Amyloidosis
- Underlying cardiac dysfunction
  - Diastolic dysfunction
  - Systolic dysfunction
  - Arrhythmia
- Medications
  - β-Blockers/α-blockers/nitrates/calcium channel blockers
- Food ingestion during dialysis (splanchnic vasodilation)

Uncommon
- Septicemia
- Myocardial infarction
- Pericardial tamponade
- Dialyzer reaction
- Occult hemorrhage
- Adenosine release due tissue ischemia
- Acetate-based dialysate

---

intravascular space is time dependent. Hypotension is probable with ultrafiltration rates in excess of 1.5 L/hr. Hypotension can also occur when the weight of the patient is at or below his or her estimated dry weight and volume shifts no longer are able to compensate for intravascular depletion and maintain blood pressure. As mentioned earlier, the estimated dry weight of a patient is defined as that weight below which the patient develops symptomatic hypotension, *in the absence of edema and excessive interdialytic weight gains.*

The composition of the dialysate can influence blood pressure in several ways. Sodium and calcium concentrations and the temperature of the dialysis fluid are among the factors that influence the frequency of hypotension during dialysis. The process of diffusion also leads to a decline in plasma osmolality because of removal of solutes. The magnitude of the fall in effective plasma osmolality ranges between 10 and 25 mOsm/kg. The fall in plasma osmolality creates an osmotic gradient between the plasma and the interstitial and intracellular spaces. Fluid moves from the plasma into cells and the interstitium, resulting in a reduction in plasma volume. This intravascular volume loss is superimposed on volume removed by ultrafiltration, and its magnitude can be as much as 1 to 1.5 L during the treatment. This shift is opposed by an increase in oncotic pressure induced by ultrafiltration. Increases in the concentration of sodium, the principal osmotic agent in the dialysate, reduce this osmotic gradient. The frequency of hypotension reported at a dialysate sodium concentration of 140 mEq/L is substantially lower than the frequency at 130 mEq/L. An increase in interdialytic hypertension has not been a major problem at the higher sodium concentration and the use of dialysate with a sodium concentration of 140 mEq/L is common. The calcium concentration of the dialysate has also been shown to affect myocardial contractility. Higher calcium concentrations in the dialysate, up to a concentration of 3.5 mEq/L, have been associated with improved contractility, independent of the nature of other factors in the dialysate. However, with the increasing use of calcium salts to prevent hyperphosphatemia, hypercalcemia is seen more often when the calcium concentration of dialysate is this high. Dialysate temperature has been shown to affect blood pressure during hemodialysis. Dialysate cooled to 35°C reduces the frequency of hypotensive episodes because vasoconstriction is potentiated at this temperature.

Patients undergoing hemodialysis are often receiving antihypertensive agents or other medications that can interfere with the normal hemodynamic response to ultrafiltration and loss of blood volume into the dialytic circuit. β-Adrenergic receptor blockers reduce myocardial contractility and prevent a compensatory increase in the heart rate, thus interfering with a major defense mechanism supporting blood pressure during dialysis. Verapamil can be expected to exert a similar effect. Vasodilators can prevent vasoconstriction in response to ultrafiltration. The development of several antihypertensive agents formulated to be administered orally as a single daily dose or by a transdermal delivery system (nifedipine and clonidine, respectively) has reduced the incidence of drug-induced hypotension. These agents are generally well tolerated and may often be used on the same day as dialysis because high peak levels are avoided. Nitroglycerin ointment can often aggravate the propensity for hypotension by inducing peripheral vasodilatation.

Management of Hypotension

The immediate management of hypotension is achieved by placing the patient in the Trendelenburg position, administering a 100- to 200-mL normal saline bolus, and reducing the ultrafiltration rate, at least temporarily. Alternatives to saline are occasional mannitol and albumin administration. Supplemental oxygen also may be useful to improve hypoxemia and cardiac contractility in some patients. The next step is to evaluate the cause of hypotension. This involves determining whether hypotension occurs early or late in the treatment period. In a previously stable patient who is free of edema and signs of congestive heart failure and in whom hypotension occurs late in the treatment, the most common cause is underestimation of the patient's dry weight. Reducing the amount of ultrafiltration during hemodialysis, which effectively raises postdialysis dry weight, corrects the hypotension. In contrast, the patient with excessive intradialytic weight gains may become hypotensive before the dry weight is achieved because the rate at which fluid can be mobilized to refill the intravascular space is limited. In this instance, dialysis time or frequency may need to be increased for removal of all necessary fluid at a tolerable rate. Whenever possible, doses of short-acting antihypertensive medication should not be administered at least 4 hours before the hemodialysis treatment. Many of the long-acting blood pressure medications can be taken at bedtime to avoid peak concentrations during dialysis. In patients with frequent hypotension early into the treatment, pericarditis with tamponade must be suspected.

A multifaceted approach often can prevent hypotension. Sodium and ultrafiltration modeling can be applied to the treatment. The newer dialysis machines have programs that permit the dialysate sodium or the ultrafiltration rate, or both, to be automatically changed during the treatment. The dialysate sodium level can be gradually altered during the treatment from an initial concentration of 150 mEq/L to 140 mEq/L, allowing easier mobilization of fluid during the treatment. Most dialysis machines allow dialysate temperature to be easily lowered to 35°C. At this dialysate temperature, thermal energy is transferred from the patient to the dialysate, and the resultant vasoconstriction raises blood pressure. For patients with persistent hypotension or autonomic insufficiency, the oral α_1-adrenergic agonist midodrine can be prescribed. A dose of 5 to 10 mg given 30 to 60 minutes before hemodialysis has been proved to be effective in reducing the incidence of hypotension in small-scale studies.

Cramps

Muscle cramps occur with as many as 20% of dialysis treatments. Although their pathogenesis is uncertain, cramps are associated with high ultrafiltration rates and low dialysate sodium concentrations, indicating that they are caused by acute extracellular volume contraction. Cramps are managed by reducing the ultrafiltration rate and administering normal saline (200 mL) or small volumes (5 mL) of 23% hypertonic saline or 50% dextrose in water. In nondiabetic patients 50% dextrose in water is especially useful, particularly near the conclusion of the dialysis treatment, because as glucose is metabolized, hyperosmolality and intravascular volume expansion in the postdialysis period are avoided. The pain resulting from very severe cramps may be alleviated by administration of agents such as diazepam but at the risk of increased hypotension. Quinine sulfate, an agent that increases the refractory period and excitability of skeletal muscle, is effective in preventing cramping if administered 1 to 2 hours before dialysis commences. Patients using quinine must be observed for the development of thrombocytopenia. In patients with excessive weight gain, dialysis time must be increased to prevent cramps during attempts to achieve the patient's dry weight.

Dialysis Disequilibrium Syndrome

Dialysis disequilibrium refers to a constellation of symptoms including nausea and vomiting, restlessness, headaches, and fatigue during hemodialysis or in the immediate postdialysis period. Severe disequilibrium may result in life-threatening emergencies, including seizures, coma, and arrhythmias. These symptoms are believed to arise from rapid rates of change in solute concentration and pH in the central nervous system.

Dialysis disequilibrium is most commonly seen in situations in which the initial solute concentrations are very high and the rate at which they decline is rapid as may occur during the first few hemodialysis sessions in a uremic patient. Milder symptoms may occur in patients in chronic maintenance hemodialysis, particularly if noncompliant behavior has resulted in missed or shortened treatments. In particular, the shorter treatment times that are possible because of dialyzers of high clearance (high-efficiency and high-flux dialyzers) may lead to symptoms in smaller individuals who have low urea volumes.

During the initiation of hemodialysis in a new patient, measures that reduce the rate of osmolar change are helpful. The use of smaller surface area dialyzers and reduced rates of blood flow and maintenance of the direction of flow of dialysate in the same direction as blood flow (rather than the customary countercurrent configuration) are measures that can be used to lower solute clearance rates and reduce symptoms. Daily dialysis for 3 to 4 days with gradual increases in dialysis time and blood flow often prevents symptoms and signs of disequilibrium. The aim for dialysis should be a URR of less than 40%. Patients with a particularly high risk for disequilibrium (BUN > 150 mg/dL [50 mmol/L]) can receive prophylactic mannitol (12.5 g of hypertonic mannitol) at the start of the hemodialysis session and hourly thereafter until the end of the treatment. A high dialysate sodium level (e.g., 145 mg/L) may also be helpful. For severe headache, seizures, or obtundation, the dialysis procedure should be immediately terminated and the airway secured. Intravenous administration of diazepam is useful for treating seizures caused by disequilibrium and this may be followed by intravenous mannitol to raise the plasma osmolality.

Arrhythmias and Angina

Patients with ESRD often have several predisposing factors for arrhythmias, including a high prevalence of ischemic heart disease, left ventricular hypertrophy, valvular sclerosis, and calcific deposits within the conducting system. Superimposed on these organic problems are the rapid changes in electrolyte concentrations inherent in efficient hemodialysis. Ventricular ectopic activity, including nonsustained ventricular tachycardia, is seen most often in patients who are taking digoxin, particularly when the dialysate potassium concentration is less than 2 mEq/L. Supraventricular tachycardiac and atrial fibrillation also can be precipitated by hypotension and coronary ischemia.

The physician must attempt to obtain a balance between the need to remove potassium that accumulates during the interdialytic period and the need to avoid low serum potassium levels that produce arrhythmias. In patients taking digoxin or those who have myocardial dysfunction, the use of a dialysate with a potassium concentration of 3 mEq/L may reduce the frequency of arrhythmias. The acute therapy for arrhythmias during hemodialysis is similar to that for patients with normal renal function, but appropriate dose adjustments must be made for those drugs normally removed by the kidney. A reassessment of the need for digoxin should also be considered. Digoxin is often started before dialysis is started, in an attempt to improve cardiac contractility and lessen congestive heart failure. After initiation of dialysis, patients' vascular volume status can often be well controlled by adjustments to this estimated dry weight, and digoxin therapy can be discontinued.

Occasional episodes of atrial fibrillation after dialysis also occur in some patients at the end of dialysis. In many patients, these are self-limited episodes that last 1 to 2 hours, which controlled ventricular rate and no signs or symptoms of ischemia. Neither digoxin nor anticoagulation is definitely indicated in these patients because the risk of subsequent more serious arrhythmias with concomitant digoxin and hypokalemia may be greater.

Angina often occurs during dialysis. Coronary artery disease is common in patients receiving dialysis. The anemia associated with chronic renal failure adds to the risk of episodes of angina. Increases in heart rate often accompany ultrafiltration during diffusive clearance, making angina a likely event in patients with coronary artery disease. There is often a need to withhold β-blockers immediately before the hemodialysis treatment. Tachyarrhythmias and hypotension can also precipitate angina. Supplemental oxygen should be administered if angina occurs, the blood flow should be slowed, and hypotension should be treated if present. If hypotension is not present, sublingual nitroglycerin may be given, but the patient should be in the recumbent position.

Hypoglycemia

Carbohydrate metabolism is quite abnormal in patients with chronic renal failure. Although there is a peripheral resistance to the effects of insulin in uremia, the half-life of insulin is significantly prolonged when the glomerular filtration rate is less than 20 mL/min. The effect of a given dose of insulin is enhanced after dialysis is instituted because an improvement in peripheral responsiveness to insulin. The implication of the foregoing is that a diabetic patient who takes a usual dose of insulin may experience hypoglycemia when undergoing dialysis against a bath with a fixed glucose concentration (i.e., glucose clamp) that is too low for the amount of insulin being administered. It is often necessary to decrease the dose of insulin on the same day as dialysis to prevent hypoglycemic episodes. Diabetic patients should not receive dialysis against a bath that has a glucose concentration of less than 100 mg/dL.

Hemorrhage

The uremic environment produces impaired platelet functioning, changes in capillary permeability, and anemia, all of which can impair hemostasis. Increased blood loss from the gastrointestinal tract may also be present because of gastritis or angiodysplasia, lesions associated with renal failure. The initiation of hemodialysis is reported to partially correct the defects responsible for the platelet dysfunction and capillary permeability that occur in uremia. However, patients undergoing hemodialysis still have a higher risk of hemorrhagic events because of repeated exposure to heparin.

Acute bleeding episodes can occur at many sites; gastrointestinal blood loss, subdural and retroperitoneal hematomas, and the development of a hemopericardium may be life threatening. Patients with acute inflammatory pericarditis, those who have had trauma or who have had recent surgery, or those who have an underlying coagulopathy or thrombocytopenia have a particular risk for development of hemorrhagic complications during hemodialysis. In addition to acute bleeding episodes, patients undergoing hemodialysis are exposed to chronic, low-grade episodes of blood loss with each dialysis treatment. Between 5 and 10 mL of residual blood remains in the artificial kidney and tubing even after thorough rinsing. There may be blood loss as needles are inserted and removed and as repeated blood tests are performed. Blood loss has been estimated to be between 5 and 50 mL per dialysis treatment.

Prevention of bleeding episodes requires identification of patients who have an increased risk. In hospitalized patients, regional anticoagulation may be a useful alternative to heparin (see earlier). If the patient is closely supervised, the use of heparin-free dialysate may also be useful. In this case, blood coagulation of the extracorporeal circuit is prevented by maintenance of high blood flows (> 300 mL/min) and frequent flushes of saline into the extracorporeal circuit. There is a suggestion that a low hematocrit in itself predisposes to bleeding. The use of erythropoietin to increase hematocrit may lessen the risk of bleeding. Attention to iron stores and iron supplementation is therefore important in these patients. The use of low-molecular-weight heparin compounds should be avoided in patients with ESRD. Massive hemorrhage has been described with repeated use of these compounds in dialysis patients.

First-Use Syndrome or Blood-Membrane Interaction

The membrane interposed between the blood and dialysate should not be considered an inert material. Numerous reactions, involving the activation of the complement pathway and the coagulation cascade, as well as the formed elements of blood, occur during contact of the blood with the dialysis membrane.

First-Use Syndrome

The first-use syndrome refers to a symptom complex encountered when a new dialyzer made of cuprophane, a cellulosic material, is used. The symptoms associated with the first use of a dialyzer appear early, usually within the first half hour after commencement of treatment. One group of symptoms resembles an anaphylactic reaction, with urticaria, angioedema, and wheezing. A severe reaction is associated with profound hypotension and cardiac arrest.

Many patients who have had this reaction have elevated levels of immunoglobulin E directed against serum proteins that have interacted with ethylene oxide, a sterilizing agent used in the manufacture of dialyzers. Complement activation also has been implicated in some of these reactions. Noncellulosic membranes, such as those made from polyacrylonitrile, polysulfone, or polymethyl methacrylate, do not cause large amounts of complement to be released into the circulation, and they appear to be better tolerated as well. Anaphylactoid reactions have been reported when patients taking angiotensin-converting enzyme inhibitors undergo hemodialysis using polyacrylonitrile (AN69) membranes or other reused membranes of various kinds. These reactions occur despite the fact that the biocompatibility profile of these membranes, at least with respect to complement activation, is superior to that of new cuprophane membranes. Evidence indicates that AN69, because of its negative surface charge, is capable of generating bradykinin by activation of Hageman factor and the kallikrein-kininogen pathway. ACE is a potent kinase responsible for degrading bradykinin. Angiotensin-converting enzyme inhibition may lead to higher bradykinin levels and to the unopposed action of this substance. Bradykinin-induced hypotension and bronchoconstriction result. Treatment of mild forms of this syndrome is symptomatic, but anaphylactoid reactions need to be treated with epinephrine and steroids. Blood in the extracorporeal circuit should not be returned to the patient.

Peritoneal Dialysis | *37*

Less than 10% of patients receiving dialysis in the United States undergo peritoneal dialysis (PD) either in the form of continuous ambulatory peritoneal dialysis (CAPD) or continuous cycler peritoneal dialysis (CCPD). This is in stark contrast to the situation in other countries such as Canada, the United Kingdom, and Australia, where a much higher percentage of patients are managed using this technique. Although PD does not yield a survival advantage over intermittent hemodialysis (HD), in properly selected patients it offers a simple and effective form of renal replacement therapy without a need for angioaccess and allows patients to manage their condition in the comfort of their own home or work surroundings.

COMPONENTS OF THE PERITONEAL DIALYSIS SYSTEM

Renal replacement therapy with PD requires three key components:

- The PD catheter
- The PD solution
- The peritoneal membrane and its associated vascular supply

Catheters

Access to the peritoneal cavity with a permanent indwelling catheter is at present one of the key factors determining the long-term success of PD. One of the early catheter designs was introduced by Tenckhoff, and the term *Tenckhoff catheter* has become a commonly used term for all chronic PD catheters. Since the introduction of the original designs, modifications have been targeted to improving subcutaneous anchorage of the catheter, preventing catheter migration, and decreasing infectious complications related to the catheter.

Catheter Design and Insertion

ACUTE USE CATHETERS   Acute PD catheters are straight, relatively rigid conduits about 3 mm in diameter and 25 to 30 mm in length that can be placed at the bedside. With prolonged use, this catheter design, with bedside placement, is associated with a significant risk of peritonitis, malfunction, and bowel perforation. Therefore, in current practice, often because of the acuity and severity of illness in a patient with acute renal failure, most patients are treated with some form of HD or hemofiltration.

CHRONIC USE CATHETERS   Standard chronic indwelling peritoneal catheters are constructed of either silicone rubber or polyurethane. The intraperitoneal portion of long-term catheters usually contains many 1-mm side holes for the passage of fluid, but it may also have modifications to facilitate fluid movement, alleviate symptoms associated with inflow or drainage, decrease catheter migration, and prevent trapping by omentum. Most modern catheters have a "swan-neck" configuration. This catheter design has a lateral or downward external exit site and a permanent bend in the subcutaneous portion of the catheter. This bend produces an arcuate tunnel that is convex upward so that both the internal (peritoneal) and external (skin) exits point downward. This prevents catheter migration and cuff extrusion and decreases the likelihood of exit site infection.

The technique of PD catheter implantation has a significant influence on long-term catheter outcome. Catheters should be inserted under strictly sterile conditions according to five established standards: (1) the deep cuff should be in the anterior abdominal musculature, (2) the subcutaneous cuff should be near the skin surface and not less than 2 cm from the exit site to allow for drainage and provide a firm anchorage that prevents piston-like movements of the catheter; (3) the catheter exit should be positioned laterally; (4) the exit site should be directed downward or laterally; and (5) the intra-abdominal portion of the catheter should be placed between the visceral and parietal peritoneum and in the middle of loops of bowel. After catheter insertion, it is normal to flush the peritoneal cavity with 500 to 1500 mL of dialysis fluid until clear immediately after placement. Heparin (500 to 1000 units/L) can be added when fibrin is present. Optimally, PD should not be initiated until 10 to 14 days after catheter placement to allow wound healing and cuff maturation and minimize the risk of leakage or infection. If PD must be started immediately after implantation or before the optimal catheter break-in period, it is recommended that intermittent dialysis with low dialysate volumes (i.e., < 1500 mL) with the patient in the supine position be used. After catheter implantation, the exit site should be covered with sterile gauze and a nonocclusive dressing. The dressing should not be changed for several days unless excessive bleeding is evident. To ensure optimal tissue healing during this period, the catheter should be immobilized to prevent trauma to the exit site, and exit site sutures should be avoided. In addition, patients should avoid submerging the exit site in water during this period. Transfer from PD to HD is thought to be directly due to catheter-related problems in about 20% of patients—usually a catheter-related infection but, occasionally, catheter migration and dialysate leaks. Catheter survival rates are more than 90% at 1 year and range from 60% to 80% at 3 years.

Dialysis Solutions

Electrolytes

SODIUM   The concentration of Na^+ in the ultrafiltrate early in the course of a dwell is lower than that of serum. This occurs as a result of aquaporin-mediated transcellular movement of water across the peritoneal membrane that is sodium free, a process called sodium sieving. It is most pronounced in patients who are slow transporters (see later) and when hypertonic dialysis fluids are used. During long dwell periods, after transcellular water movement ceases, sodium moves from blood to the dialysate down its concentration gradient, and dialysate sodium concentrations increase. To avoid hypernatremia, most commercially available dialysis fluids now have a Na^+ concentration of 132 mEq/L. Also to circumvent the development of hypernatremia, it may be prudent to avoid repeated short dwell periods of exclusively hypertonic dialysis fluid unless the Na^+ concentration in the dialysis fluid is decreased.

POTASSIUM K^+ is not usually added to chronic PD fluid. In typical CAPD exchanges using dialysis fluid with no added K^+, dialysate K^+ approaches equilibrium toward the end of the exchange. Losses of about 35 mEq/day in the dialysate while a serum K^+ concentration of approximately 4 mEq/L is maintained are typical. With rapid cycling, K^+ losses are augmented, but maximal rates are about 8 mEq/hr. If needed, K^+ removal can be slowed by adding K^+ to the dialysate.

CALCIUM   Control of Ca^{2+} and phosphate balance in end-stage renal disease is important to prevent the long-term complications of renal osteodystrophy. Unfortunately, phosphorus is only poorly removed by standard PD. It was common practice in the past to treat hypocalcemia by using a relatively high dialysis

Ca^{2+} concentration (3.5 mEq/L). However, in the current era most patients receive Ca^{2+} salts as their primary phosphate binder. Therefore, the standard Ca^{2+} concentration is now 2.5 mEq/L.

Buffers

Current standard PD fluids use lactate as the buffer. A bicarbonate-based buffer system would be preferable for dialysis fluids, but precipitation of Ca^{2+} and Mg^{2+} carbonates and caramelization of glucose at physiologic pH during sterilization preclude its use. One significant drawback of lactate-based solutions is that the fluids have an unphysiologically low pH (5.5) which can lead to abdominal pain on instillation.

Osmotic Agents

Ultrafiltration in PD is driven by an osmotic gradient across the peritoneal membrane. The osmotic gradient is achieved by adding osmotically active agents to the dialysis solution, the most common of which is glucose.

GLUCOSE Glucose is the osmotic agent in standard dialysis solutions. Glucose is safe, effective, readily metabolized, and inexpensive. However, rapid absorption, the potential for metabolic derangements (e.g., hyperglycemia, hyperinsulinemia, hyperlipidemia, and obesity) are significant clinical drawbacks. Most standard PD fluids contain one of three concentrations of glucose: 1.5%, 2.5%, or 4.25%. At present, glucose remains the standard osmotic agent, but other osmotic agents (e.g., polyglucose and amino acids) are also used in clinical practice.

GLUCOSE POLYMERS The commercially prepared glucose polymer icodextrin is currently in clinical use. The ultrafiltration profiles of glucose polymers differ substantially from those of glucose. Ultrafiltration with glucose is rapid, occurs early in the dwell period, and decreases with time as glucose is absorbed. In contrast, polyglucose is not absorbed across the peritoneal membrane and its lymphatic absorption is slow. Therefore, ultrafiltration increases linearly with time as the polyglucose solution maintains a slow, but sustained, colloid osmotic force. This is ideal for producing sustained ultrafiltration over long dwell periods of up to 18 hours. Initial studies have shown that these solutions are safe and well tolerated, with ultrafiltration rates similar to those of 2.5% dextrose and markedly better than those of 1.5% dextrose during overnight dwell. Complications include rash and sterile peritonitis. Indications for the use of polyglucose include the long dwell times associated with CAPD (overnight) and CCPD (daytime), patients with loss of ultrafiltration capacity, episodes of peritonitis, and patients with diabetes mellitus (to decrease the glucose load).

AMINO ACIDS Protein malnutrition is a significant risk factor for morbidity and mortality in dialysis patients. In PD there is an obligatory daily loss of protein and amino acids into the peritoneal effluent. In this setting a potential advantage of amino acid–containing fluids is that the amino acids would contribute to protein synthesis without the concomitant phosphorus load associated with oral protein sources. The nutritional outcomes of initial clinical studies were disappointing. However, subsequent studies using a 1.1% mixture of essential and nonessential amino acid solutions performed in Europe have suggested a clinical benefit in patients with adverse nutritional parameters, who had the best sustained response to intraperitoneal amino acids. Ultrafiltration rates for 1.1% amino acid solutions are similar to those for 1.5% dextrose solutions. Complications of amino acid–containing solutions include the development of metabolic acidosis and increased levels of serum urea nitrogen.

Peritoneal Membrane

Anatomy
The peritoneal membrane is the primary interface between blood and the dialysate compartments. It is across this membrane that water and solute must be transported. The total surface area of the peritoneal membrane (parietal and visceral) is thought to approximate the body surface area in most adults (i.e., 1 to 2 m²). Children have a disproportionately larger peritoneal surface area than most adults do. The peritoneal cavity generally contains about 100 mL or less of fluid, but a normal-sized adult can usually tolerate 2 L or more without discomfort or compromise of pulmonary function.

CLINICAL USE OF PERITONEAL DIALYSIS

Choice of Dialysis Modality

A key factor in facilitating a smooth transition from chronic kidney disease to renal replacement therapy is early patient education on the different dialysis modalities that should commence when the glomerular filtration rate is less than 30 mL/min (stage IV chronic kidney disease). Late referral increases the need for acute HD and substantially reduces the take-on rate for PD. In choosing PD as a potential dialysis modality, the nephrologist should first determine whether the individual patient has any potential contraindications (Table 37–1).

Table 37–1: Contraindications to Peritoneal Dialysis

Absolute contraindications
    Extensive abdominal adhesions
    Loss of ultrafiltration capacity
    Large surgically irreparable hernias
    Diaphragmatic hernia
    Bladder exstrophy, gastroschisis, or omphalocele
Relative contraindications
    Anuria (especially if weight > 100 kg)
    Morbid obesity
    Diverticulitis or inflammatory bowel disease
    (The presence of an ileostomy or colostomy is not considered
    a contraindication)

Peritoneal Dialysis Modalities

CONTINUOUS AMBULATORY PERITONEAL DIALYSIS   CAPD is the
basic form of PD and is still in widespread use. Patients typically
undergo four manual exchanges per day: three daytime exchanges
of about 5 hours each and one overnight exchange of about 8 or
9 hours. By adjusting the dwell volume appropriately (see the later
section on adjusting the PD prescription), most CAPD patients
can achieve an adequate dose of dialysis.

CYCLER DIALYSIS   In cycler PD an automated cycler machine is
programmed to deliver three or more fluid exchanges, typically
during a 7- to 12-hour period overnight. Most patients will also
carry dialysate in the peritoneum for part or all of the day; these
patients are considered to have a "wet day" or, alternatively, are
described as performing CCPD. In some cases, the patient will
perform one or more manual exchanges during the day in addition to the last bag fill exchange. Few patients will perform
cycler dialysis overnight and not perform a last bag fill. These
patients are considered to have a "dry day" or, alternatively, are
described as performing nightly intermittent peritoneal dialysis
(NIPD).

TIDAL PERITONEAL DIALYSIS   Tidal PD consists of the repeated
instillation of small tidal volumes of dialysis fluid with the use
of an automated cycler. Variables requiring a choice include
reserve volume, tidal outflow volume, tidal replacement volume,
flow rates, and frequency of exchanges. Theoretically, maintaining an intraperitoneal reservoir by not attempting to
completely drain the peritoneal cavity after each dwell results in
more continuous contact of the dialysate with the peritoneal
membrane. There is little evidence to suggest that tidal PD can

provide clearance superior to that provided by cycler dialysis. However, it may decrease abdominal discomfort during inflow and outflow.

Choice of Peritoneal Dialysis Modality

The patient's peritoneal membrane transport characteristics must be known to optimize the PD prescription. These characteristics are determined by using the peritoneal equilibration test (PET). The PET is a semiquantitative measure of peritoneal solute transport. It is performed as follows:

1. After an overnight dwell, 2 L of 2.5% dextrose dialysis fluid is instilled into the peritoneum. The patient is rolled side-to-side with every 400 mL to ensure proper fluid distribution.
2. The dialysate is allowed to dwell for 4 hours.
3. Dialysate urea, creatinine, glucose, and Na^+ concentrations are measured at time 0 and after 2 and 4 hours of dwell time.
4. Serum values are determined after 2 hours.
5. The 4-hour drain volume is also obtained.

For each for these dwell times, dialysate/plasma (D/P) ratios are obtained for urea and creatinine (Cr). The ratio of glucose at the time of draining to the initial glucose concentration in dialysis fluid (D/D_0) is also obtained. The results of the PET categorize patients into one of four transport categories by using the D/P Cr ratio at 4 hours: high (D/P Cr ratio > 0.81), high-average (D/P Cr ratio between 0.81 and 0.65), low-average (D/P Cr ratio between 0.65 and 0.50), or low (D/P Cr ratio < 0.50). Based on these results, the PD prescription that would best match the patient's transport characteristics can be chosen (Table 37–2). Most patients are either high-average or low-average transporters and can usually perform either CAPD or CCPD and achieve both an adequate dose of dialysis and ultrafiltration. Patients who are low transporters have a slow increase in the D/P Cr ratio and therefore benefit from a longer dwell time. Thus, these patients are more likely to achieve adequate dialysis with evenly spaced, long dwell periods (CAPD or CCPD with a last bag fill and midday exchange). Patients who are high transporters have a rapid increase in the D/P ratio in the first 1 to 2 hours of dwell time, followed by a decline in the D/P value. These patients are more likely to achieve adequate dialysis when receiving cycler dialysis. If these patients require daytime dwell periods to achieve adequate dialysis, they are most likely to benefit from dwell times less than 3 hours; they will derive little benefit from one daytime dwell that lasts the entire day.

Table 37–2: Baseline Peritoneal Equilibrium Test Prognostic Value

Solute Transport Modality	Ultrafiltration	Predicted Ccr	Preferred PD
High	Poor	Adequate	NPD, DAPD*
High-average	Adequate	Adequate	Standard-volume PD†
Low-average	Good	Adequate	High-volume PD‡
Low	Excellent	Inadequate	High-volume PD‡

*May need to do a midday exchange or a daytime polyglucose dwell to maintain ultrafiltration.

†CAPD with 8 to 10 L or CCPD with a dialysis solution inflow of 6 to 8 L overnight and 2 L in the daytime for clearance, but may need a dry day, polyglucose, or midday exchange to maintain ultrafiltration.

‡CAPD with greater than 9 L/day, CAPD with a nightly exchange device, or CCPD with inflow greater than 8 L overnight and/or 2 L daytime and possible midday exchange.

CAPD, circulating ambulatory peritoneal dialysis; CCPD, continuous cycling peritoneal dialysis; CCr, creatinine clearance; DAPD, daytime ambulatory peritoneal dialysis; NPD, nightly peritoneal dialysis; PD, peritoneal dialysis.

From Twardowski ZJ: Nightly peritoneal dialysis. Why? Who? How? And when? *ASAIO Trans* 36:8–16, 1990.

ADEQUACY OF PERITONEAL DIALYSIS

When patients initiate PD, a good proportion of their total solute clearance is provided by residual renal function. Over a period of 24 to 36 months, this residual renal function will decline to zero and this loss may be associated with a failure to achieve clearance targets. Thus, PD adequacy must be measured often and on a regular basis to ensure that the patient is receiving adequate dialysis. The National Kidney Foundation Dialysis Outcomes Quality Initiative (K/DOQI) guidelines recommend that total solute clearance (Kt/V_{urea} and weekly creatinine clearance) be measured 2 to 4 weeks after PD is started and again before 6 months. Clearance should be measured every 4 months thereafter.

$$\text{Weekly } Kt/V_{urea} = (\text{24-hour volume} \times \text{D/P urea}) + (\text{24 hour urine volume} \times \text{U/P urea}) \times 7$$

$$\text{Weekly creatinine clearance} = (\text{24-hour volume} \times \text{D/P creatinine}) + ([\text{UCr} \times \text{24-hour urine volume}] \div \text{PCr}) \times 7$$

These figures may be adjusted to ideal body weight.

The K/DOQI clinical practice guidelines provide evidence-based guidelines for the provision of adequate PD including recommendations for an adequate dose of dialysis.

Based on many clinical studies the guidelines recommend the following in adult patients:

- CAPD
  - $Kt/V_{urea} > 2$
  - Creatinine clearance 60 L/wk/1.73 m^2 (high or high-average transporters) or 50 L/wk/1.73 m^2 (low or low-average transporters)
- Cycler dialysis
  - NIPD: $Kt/V_{urea} > 2.2$ and creatinine clearance > 66 L/wk/1.73 m^2
  - CCPD: $Kt/V_{urea} > 2.1$ and creatinine clearance > 63 L/1.73 m^2

In malnourished patients, the estimate of body surface area should be adjusted according to the patient's ideal body weight. Clinical studies have convincingly demonstrated that loss of residual renal function is a predictor of mortality in the PD population. Therefore, measures to preserve residual renal function (angiotensin-converting enzyme inhibition, hypertension control, and avoidance of nephrotoxins) are extremely important in the PD patient.

WRITING THE DIALYSIS PRESCRIPTION

Initial Prescription

Ideally, PD should not be started until the peritoneal catheter has been in place for at least 14 days to minimize the risk of leakage around the catheter site and peritonitis. PD is typically prescribed empirically by using data based on the patient's weight, residual renal function, and any lifestyle constraints that may be present. The guidelines in Table 37–3 are modified from the K/DOQI clinical practice guidelines. Patients should be monitored closely during the training period to ensure that the 4-hour drain volumes are those expected for the percent dextrose PD solution that is being used and that no drainage is observed around the catheter exit site.

Adjustments to the Initial Dialysis Prescription

Two to four weeks after initiation of PD, 24-hour collections of urine and dialysate should be performed, along with serum

Table 37–3: Recommended Prescriptions for Patients Starting CAPD or CCPD

	Estimated GFR of > 2 mL/min	*Estimated GFR of ≤ 2 mL/min*
CAPD		
BSA < 1.7 m²	4 × 2-L exchanges/day	4 × 2.5-L exchanges/day
BSA 1.7–2 m²	4 × 2.5-L exchanges/day	4 × 3-L exchanges/day
BSA ≥ 2 m²	4 × 3-L exchanges/day	4 × 3-L exchanges/day
CCPD		
BSA < 1.7 m²	4 × 2 L (9 hr/night) + 2 L/day	4 × 2.5 L (9 hr/night) + 2 L/day
BSA 1.7–2 m²	4 × 2.5 L (9 hr/night) + 2 L/day	4 × 3 L (9 hr/night) +2 L/day
BSA ≥ 2 m²	4 × 3 L (9 hr/night) + 3 L/day	4 × 3 L (9 hr/night) +3 L/day

BSA, body surface area; CAPD, continuous ambulatory peritoneal dialysis; CCPD, continuous cycling peritoneal dialysis; GFR, glomerular filtration rate. Modified from Burkart JM, Schreiber M, Korbet SM, et al: Solute clearance approach to adequacy of peritoneal dialysis. *Perit Dial Int* 16:457–470, 1996.

chemistry panels and a complete blood count to calculate the weekly Kt/V urea and creatinine clearance. The initial PET should be performed approximately 1 month after the initiation of dialysis. This test is performed to rule out unexpected problems and also to identify patients who are either high or low transporters. High transporters will need short dwell prescriptions and may begin to have ultrafiltration problems as residual kidney function fails. Low transporters usually require high-volume CAPD or CCPD to maintain adequate dialysis as residual kidney function falls. If clearance values are below target, the prescription should be modified and adequacy testing repeated.

Further Adjustments to the Dialysis Prescription

For CAPD patients, two methods can be used to increase dialysis adequacy. The most common approach is to increase the dwell volume in 500-mL increments. Accordingly, a patient receiving four 2-L exchanges per day would have the prescription increased to four 2.5-L exchanges per day. Alternatively, a nocturnal exchange device is available that supplies an extra exchange overnight, thus providing the patient with a total of five exchanges per day.

For cycler dialysis patients, several methods are available for improving adequacy. These methods include increasing the dwell volume of an individual exchange, increasing the time spent overnight on the cycler, increasing the number of exchanges on the cycler, or increasing the number of daytime dwell periods. Sometimes a combination of these measures is used in an individual patient.

For high transporters, both clearance and ultrafiltration can be optimized by the use of rapid-cycle, short-dwell exchanges. In patients who are low or low-average transporters, however, higher clearances will probably be achieved with the equally spaced dwell of CAPD than with classic cycler therapy. Anuric patients who are either low transporters or with transport values greater than 100 kg will probably require a combination of CAPD and CCPD for adequate dialysis.

PERITONEAL DIALYSIS IN SPECIAL POPULATIONS

Rapid Transporters

Approximately 10% to 15% of CAPD patients are high transporters. The key characteristics of this patient sub-group are the following:

- Rapid equilibration of small solute concentration between the dialysate and that of the blood
- Higher rates of transperitoneal protein loss
- Rapid absorption of dialysate glucose, leading to an early fall in ultrafiltration rates which can lead to volume expansion

Patients who are high transporters have been shown to have an increased risk for mortality and hypoalbuminemia and increased incidence of weakness, fatigue, and hospitalization.

This increased rate of mortality and morbidity in high transporters has several possible etiologies. First, these patients have a higher rate of hypoalbuminemia, which is associated with a higher mortality in all patients with end-stage renal disease. Second, increased glucose absorption can lead to a variety of pathologic processes, including hyperlipidemia, hyperinsulinemia, and obesity. Third, and perhaps most importantly, loss of intraperitoneal osmotic pressure because of glucose absorption leads to reduced ultrafiltration, volume overload, and hypertension. Approaches to the management of the high transporter include the use of cycler dialysis with rapid exchanges to prevent glucose equilibrium and allow for preservation of ultrafiltration capacity. Second, the use of icodextrin can reduce glucose absorption by more than one third and thereby result in improved fluid control.

Elderly Patients

Elderly patients may have a substantial number of comorbid medical conditions that may limit their ability to perform their own PD therapy. It is estimated that about 60% of patients older than 80 years need assistance with dialysis exchanges, exit site care, and medications. If family support is not available, assistance can be provided by nursing home staff, daily care centers, or home care nurses. Not surprisingly, patients who are bedridden have a higher rate of peritonitis, perhaps because of an increased frequency of diverticulitis and bladder incontinence. Exit site infections, however, appear to be less common in older patients than in younger patients, probably because of the decreased activity level of the older group. Elderly patients are more likely to have problems related to constipation, which can be a cause of mechanical dysfunction of the Tenckhoff catheter. Thus, constipation must be assessed in all PD patients and treated appropriately.

Patients with Diabetes Mellitus

Potential advantages of PD in diabetes mellitus include the following:

1. Lack of anticoagulation and its possible benefit on diabetic retinopathy
2. Increased removal of middle molecules, which may help prevent or minimize the complications of diabetic neuropathy

Potential disadvantages of PD include the following:

1. Constant exposure to a hyperglycemic environment
2. Increased risk of peritonitis because of immunosuppression in diabetic patients

There is no difference in the natural history of diabetic complications (retinopathy or neuropathy) among patients receiving PD compared with those receiving HD. Most, but not all, studies have shown no difference in the rates and severity of peritonitis among diabetic and nondiabetic patients. Although intraperitoneal administration of insulin has been advocated as a potential benefit of PD in patients with diabetes mellitus, it has been associated with a higher rate of peritonitis, erratic glycemic control, subcapsular liver steatosis, and malignant omentum syndrome and is therefore not advised.

Pediatric Patients

PD is widely considered to be the treatment of choice for renal failure in infants and young children when transplantation is not an immediate option. PD therapy allows children of all ages to receive dialysis in their homes with no or minimal dietary restrictions. Importantly, studies have demonstrated that significantly more PD patients attend school full-time than do HD patients both at initiation of dialysis and at 6, 12, and 24 months of follow-up. An additional benefit of PD over HD is the well-documented increase in quality of life for both pediatric patients and their parents.

The most common cause of treatment failure is recurrent peritonitis and ultrafiltration failure. K/DOQI guidelines state that the target dose of PD in children should meet or exceed the adult standard but note that morbidity and mortality data for dose and outcomes are lacking. Strategies to improve clearance include the use of continuous therapies and maximizing drain volume, especially by optimizing the exchange volume or by using either hypertonic dextrose solutions or icodextrin.

PERITONEAL DIALYSIS IN A NONCHRONIC SETTING

Acute Renal Failure

See Chapter 9, Acute Renal Failure.

Nonuremic Uses of Peritoneal Dialysis

Congestive Heart Failure
Numerous case reports have described the use of PD to treat patients with congestive heart failure. Potential benefits of this modality for congestive heart failure include improvements in functional status, ejection fraction, and quality of life and a decrease in hospitalization rates. Patients have resolution of volume overload, including lower extremity edema and ascites.

Hypothermia
Patients who are severely hypothermic can be treated with heated (42 to 46°C) humidified oxygen, intravenous fluids warmed to 43°C, and PD with dialysate warmed to 43°C.

Liver Disease
Patients with liver disease and ascites can be successfully treated with PD. In patients transferred for hemodynamic instability

while receiving HD, stabilization of blood pressure can be achieved with PD. Peritoneal losses of protein have been shown to decrease substantially over time, from greater than 30 g/day to less than 10 g/day.

COMPLICATIONS OF PERITONEAL DIALYSIS

Malnutrition

Malnutrition affects between 40% to 75% of all PD patients and is a significant risk factor for mortality and hospitalization in chronic PD patients. Malnutrition may reflect underdialysis as residual renal function declines or excessive protein loss in the dialysate, or inflammation as indicated by a high C-reactive protein level may also contribute. Hypoalbuminemia, a marker of malnutrition, in PD patients is associated with older age, diabetes mellitus, female sex, the D/P Cr ratio, PET results, and a longer duration of dialysis. The K/DOQI guidelines recently recommended dietary protein intake of 1.2 to 1.3 g/kg/day for chronic PD patients. Consideration also needs to be given to peritoneal protein losses, however, because these losses average 5 to 15 g/day but can be considerably higher with episodes of peritonitis. Patients undergoing chronic PD should have a total daily energy intake of 35 kcal/kg if younger than 60 years and 30 kcal/kg if 60 years or older. This intake includes both dietary intake and the energy intake derived from glucose absorbed from the peritoneal dialysate.

Cardiovascular Disease

Multifactorial atherosclerotic risk factors in PD patients include not only the traditional risk factors but also coronary calcification, hypoalbuminemia, hyperhomocysteinemia, and elevated levels of C-reactive protein and lipoprotein(a). Medical therapy, including aspirin, β-blockers, angiotensin-converting enzyme inhibitors, and lipid-lowering agents should be initiated if indications exist. Revascularization can be performed with either percutaneous transluminal coronary angioplasty or coronary artery bypass grafting, with the latter procedure preferred in patients with multivessel disease, impaired left ventricular function, severe symptoms, or ischemia.

Hypertension

Hypertension occurs in 50% to 90% of PD patients and may, in some cases, reflect fluid retention as a result of impaired ultrafiltration. Treatment of volume overload and hypertension in PD patients includes the prescription of loop diuretics, preservation of residual renal function, reduction of dietary salt intake, and prevention and treatment of peritoneal ultrafiltration failure.

Hyperlipidemia

PD is associated with an increased prevailing serum glucose concentration because of constant absorption from the peritoneal cavity. As a result, PD patients are susceptible to the development of hyperglycemia and hyperinsulinemia. In addition, dialysate protein loss of 5 to 15 g/day results in the loss of all lipoproteins, with preferential loss of small molecules such as high-density lipoprotein. Therefore, it is not surprising that PD patients have a more atherogenic profile than HD patients. Dietary modification is typically unsuccessful and may compromise nutritional intake; therefore, most PD patients require pharmacologic therapy for treatment of dyslipidemia. Guidelines developed by the International Society for Peritoneal Dialysis recommend that low-density lipoprotein cholesterol levels be less than 100 mg/dL and that 3-hydroxy-3-methylglutaryl-coenzyme A reductase inhibitors be used as first-line therapy.

Homocysteine

Most PD patients have elevated homocysteine. Although homocysteine is removed by PD, the removal rate is not high enough to allow for the correction of hyperhomocysteinemia. Folic acid supplementation can decrease homocysteine levels in PD patients, but no randomized clinical trials have been conducted to investigate the effect of folate supplementation on rates of cardiovascular events in PD patients with elevated homocysteine levels.

Comparison of Hemodialysis and Peritoneal Dialysis

The mortality and hospitalization rates for HD and PD have been compared in many studies. The results of these analyses have been contradictory, with some studies showing a survival advantage for HD, other studies showing a survival advantage for PD, and still other studies showing no difference in mortality rates. The differing results probably reflect selection bias, the use of different variables in multivariate models, variations in the dose of dialysis delivered and inadequate sample sizes. Based on the available data, it is reasonable to assume broadly similar outcomes for PD and HD, with the exception of morbidly obese and elderly diabetic patients. Notably, patient satisfaction is often higher for patients receiving PD than those receiving HD, but once again this result may reflect selection bias.

Indications for Switching from Peritoneal Dialysis to Hemodialysis

In some situations a patient may not be able to continue PD and may need to switch to HD. First, despite adjustment of the PD prescription, the patient may not be able to achieve adequate dialysis. A complete assessment of the possible causes for the inadequate dialysis should be undertaken, including patient noncompliance with the dialysis prescription and sampling and collection errors. Noncompliance with some part of the dialysis prescription is fairly common in PD patients. Inadequate ultrafiltration can be seen either in patients who are high transporters or in patients who have a mechanical defect that impairs adequate outflow of dialysate from the peritoneal cavity. High transporters also have a risk for excessive protein loss in the dialysate, which can lead to a significant decline in serum albumin levels. If malnutrition develops and cannot be rectified by aggressive nutritional supplementation and correction of underlying comorbid medical conditions, treatment should be switched to HD. Finally, patients who have frequent episodes of peritonitis, peritoneal access failure that cannot be readily corrected, or severe hypertriglyceridemia are also poor candidates for continuation of PD.

Noninfectious Complications

Mechanical Complications

INFLOW PAIN　Inflow pain is typically due to positioning of the catheter tip adjacent to tissue that cannot move during fluid infusion. This type of pain is minimized when curled-tip catheters with multiple outflow pores are used but may require catheter repositioning. Pain may also be related to the dialysate composition. An abnormally low dialysate pH may transiently cause pain in some patients. If low pH is the cause of the pain, it can be mitigated by adding 4 to 5 mEq/L of $NaHCO_3$ to the dialysis solution before infusion.

OUTFLOW FAILURE　Outflow failure is detected when the drained volume is substantially less than the instilled volume. If both outflow failure and inflow failure are present, they are probably due to either a kink in the catheter or catheter obstruction by fibrin or clots. If obstruction is suspected, the catheter can often be opened with an injection of urokinase or tissue plasminogen activator. Catheter kinking is usually treated by catheter replacement. Other causes of outflow failure include catheter migration (subdiaphragmatic), omental wrapping, and adherence of bowel (as seen with constipation). In such cases, the clinician should rule out constipation and then obtain a plain radiograph to determine the position of the catheter. If the catheter tip has migrated, repositioning can be attempted with a malleable metal rod under fluoroscopic guidance, with guidewires, with channel cleaning brushes, and, as a last resort, via peritoneoscopy. Catheters with a swan-neck configuration between the two cuffs also have a much lower rate of catheter migration than do catheters without the swan-neck configuration.

CATHETER DAMAGE PD catheters can be damaged by exposure to antibacterial agents that are strong oxidants (alcohol and iodine), by accidental injury from sharp objects, and simply by wear from long-term use. Repair of damaged catheters by splicing the old catheter with extension tubing is often successful but should not usually be attempted if the breakage is less than 2 cm from the exit site.

Complications Related to Increased Intra-abdominal Pressure

HERNIAS A retrospective study of hernias over a 15-year period determined that the risk of hernia formation was 5% in cycler dialysis patients and 13% in CAPD patients with up to 15% of these hernias progressing to incarceration or strangulation. There does not appear to be a relationship between exchange volume and the rate of hernia formation. The most common hernias are umbilical, inguinal, or pericatheter or located at a previous surgical site. Risk factors for hernia formation include previous abdominal surgery and patient weight less than 60 kg. Because of the potential risk of serious complications, surgical repair should be strongly considered in all cases. PD can be restarted several days after surgery, initially at a volume of 1 to 1.5 L and then with gradual reinstatement of the patient's original peritoneal prescription over the next 2 to 4 weeks.

DIALYSATE LEAKS, INCLUDING HYDROTHORAX Dialysate leaks are seen in about 5% to 10% of CAPD patients. Leaks that occur within 30 days of PD catheter placement are called early leaks, and they are usually pericatheter leaks. Risk factors for early dialysate leaks include initiation of PD immediately after catheter placement and the use of nonstandard techniques for PD catheter insertion. Leaks that occur well after the initiation of dialysis are abdominal wall, genital, or pleural leaks. These leaks usually have a more subtle manifestation, which can include weight gain, peripheral or genital edema, subcutaneous swelling, edema, and apparent ultrafiltration failure, and for pleural leaks, shortness of breath. Hydrothorax probably occurs when peritoneal dialysate traverses the diaphragm through lymphatics or through defects in the diaphragm itself, most often through tendinous defects or diaphragmatic blebs. The clinical manifestations of hydrothorax can vary from an asymptomatic finding on routine chest radiography to severe respiratory compromise.

Genital edema can be caused by leakage of dialysate from a defect in the abdominal wall, an inguinal hernia, or a patent processus vaginalis. A pleural peritoneal leak can also be diagnosed by the presence of a high glucose concentration in pleural fluid. Treatment of dialysate leakage is initially conservative and entails withholding PD treatments for 1 to 2 weeks with HD support. If the leak recurs, pleurodesis can be attempted although there is a paucity of supportive data. Surgical repair of the pleuroperitoneal defect requires open thoracotomy, and many clinicians favor a switch to HD rather than subjecting the patient to the operative risk.

ALTERATIONS IN RESPIRATORY FUNCTION In seated patients, infusion of 2 L of dialysate results in a decrease in the partial pressure of oxygen (PO_2) and functional reserve, as well as a decrease in vital capacity of about 10% to 20%. Despite these findings, most patients with obstructive airway disease are able to tolerate CAPD without difficulty, perhaps because the "stretch" that the diaphragm undergoes with increased intra-abdominal volume improves the efficiency of its contractions. Patients with restrictive lung disease, however, are likely to be symptomatic when receiving PD, with the most severe symptoms occurring while they are supine. An instillation test can be used to assess the potential for respiratory compromise in patients with severe pulmonary disease.

BACK PAIN Increased intra-abdominal pressure and volume tend to pull the lumbar vertebrae into a more lordotic position. The net effect is increased stress on the spine. Many patients with end-stage renal disease already have degenerative disk disease, osteoporosis, or facet disease at initiation of dialysis, and their therapy may be complicated by the onset of renal osteodystrophy, which also has a predilection for symptomatology in this area. The addition of dialysate may lead to new onset or worsening of back pain in these patients. Treatment is targeted to reducing intra-abdominal pressure, which may be achieved in some patients by decreasing instilled volumes or switching to cycler dialysis therapy.

Ultrafiltration Failure
Ultrafiltration failure may be defined clinically by the presence of fluid overload despite restriction of fluid intake and the use of three or more hypertonic (4.25% dextrose) exchanges per day.

Membrane failure is often not the cause of volume overload (noncompliance with dietary sodium restriction, loss of residual urine output, and dialysate leaks are other common causes). After exclusion of other issues, a comparison of the baseline with current PET results (including D/P ratios and dialysate sodium concentrations) is recommended. Most authorities now prefer a modified PET in which 4.25% dextrose (3.86% glucose) is used to maximize the osmotic gradient and sodium profiling. With this equilibration test, the definition of true membrane failure is ultrafiltration of less than 400 mL after a 4-hour dwell period. The prevalence and frequency of ultrafiltration failure are uncertain but are approximately 2.5% after 1 year of dialysis, 9.5% at 3 years, and 30.9% after 6 years.

ULTRAFILTRATION FAILURE IN A PATIENT WITH HIGH SOLUTE TRANSPORT Patients with loss of ultrafiltration and current 4-hour PET results showing D/D_0 glucose less than 0.3 and D/P Cr greater than 0.81 are characterized as high solute transporters. These patients tend to have poor ultrafiltration because of rapid glucose absorption and dissipation of the osmotic gradient. Some patients have these transport characteristics at baseline, and if their dwell times are mismatched for their membrane transport characteristics, they often appear to have ultrafiltration failure as they lose residual renal function and no longer have urine flow as a supplement to net daily fluid losses. In other patients, loss of ultrafiltration is due to a change in membrane transport from baseline. When permanent loss of ultrafiltration develops, it is most commonly due to an increase in solute transport (historically called type I ultrafiltration failure). Because peritonitis leads to a similar, but transient, increase in transport, this diagnosis cannot be made in patients with a recent episode of peritonitis. Clinically, most of these patients can be managed by introducing glucose polymers and shortening dwell times, which will usually improve net ultrafiltration while maintaining total solute clearance.

ULTRAFILTRATION FAILURE AND NO CHANGE/AVERAGE SOLUTE TRANSPORT Loss of ultrafiltration in patients with no change or average transport characteristics tends to be due to catheter malfunction, fluid leaks, excessive lymphatic reabsorption, and a decrease in intracellular water transport.

DIALYSATE LEAKS Leak of dialysate from the peritoneal cavity into extra-abdominal tissue, such as the abdominal wall, results in decreased drain volume because of leakage of fluid and increased lymphatic absorption from abdominal tissues. This condition has no effect on diffusive or convective transport and tends to be associated with a normal decrease in dialysate Na^+ and unchanged PET values.

CATHETER MALPOSITION Mechanical problems such as migration of the catheter from the pelvic space to a subdiaphragmatic position can result in an inability to drain, an increase in residual volume, and a decrease in drain volume. Again, no change in D/P Cr values or an abnormal decrease in dialysate Na^+ is observed. Catheter position can easily be determined from a plane film radiograph. Occasionally extensive intra-abdominal adhesions resulting from recurrent or severe peritonitis may limit dialysate flow throughout the abdomen. This results in fluid trapping and can decrease the amount of peritoneal membrane surface area that is in contact with dialysate.

SCLEROSING ENCAPSULATING PERITONITIS Patients with this syndrome present with anorexia, weight loss, nausea, vomiting, intermittent bowel obstruction, ascites, bloody dialysate, malnutrition, and decreased peritoneal transport of solute and water. At laparotomy, patients are found to have a thick-walled, membranous cocoon entrapping loops of bowel. The cause is uncertain; however, chemical irritants have been implicated. The overall incidence is uncertain, but the condition is believed to occur in 0.5% to 0.9% of the overall PD population, with the risk increasing with time receiving PD such that it affects 15% to 20% of the subpopulation of PD patients receiving therapy for longer than 8 years. Surgical intervention has been disappointing; therefore, prevention is the key. The use of lactate-containing dialysis solutions, avoidance of intraperitoneal infusion of chemical irritants such as chlorhexidine, and prevention of severe prolonged episodes of peritonitis by early diagnosis, aggressive treatment, and early catheter removal when indicated may reduce the frequency of encapsulating peritonitis.

Infectious Complications

Peritonitis and exit site infections are the major complications of PD and are a leading cause of hospitalization of PD patients. When compared with surgical peritonitis, PD-related bacterial peritonitis is usually due to a single pathogen, and the infection is generally confined within the peritoneum and is seldom associated with positive blood cultures or abscess formation. Typically, many of these patients can be treated on an outpatient basis.

Prevention of Peritonitis
Presumed sources of bacterial peritonitis are as follows:

* Intraluminal (touch contamination during the spike procedure)
* Periluminal (related to catheter infection)
* Transvisceral migration (diverticulitis)

- Hematogenous
- Vaginal leak

Since the introduction of PD, several modifications to the components of the PD system have led to significant falls in infection rates.

Y SYSTEMS The first modification of the standard technique to result in a consistent reduction in peritonitis rates was the introduction of the Y set. This system incorporates "flush-before-fill" technology, with any possible contamination of the spike being flushed away from the peritoneum by draining after introduction of the spike. A further modification includes a preattached bag of dialysate to eliminate the need to "spike" the bag of dialysate, which further reduces peritonitis rates. These technologies are associated with peritonitis rates ranging from 0.7 to 1.7 episodes per year.

STAPHYLOCOCCUS NASAL CARRIAGE The annual probability of *Staphylococcus aureus* peritonitis developing is about 15%. The probability that a CAPD patient will have a peritoneal catheter removed because of this infection is 3% to 7.5% (20% to 50% for each infection). The primary reservoir for *S aureus* is within the anterior nares, and carriers have an increased risk for the development of *S aureus* exit site infections and peritonitis. Intranasal mupirocin twice a day for 5 days reduces the incidence of *S aureus* catheter infections, but not *S aureus* peritonitis or catheter loss. Use of topical daily mupirocin at the exit site has also been shown to reduce overall exit site infections and, at times, the incidence of *S aureus* peritonitis. Most clinicians advise the use of mupirocin ointment as part of routine exit site care or in the nares of carriers to prevent infections.

CATHETER-RELATED PERITONITIS Peritonitis is often related to concomitant catheter infections. Therefore, prevention of peritonitis requires optimal catheter implantation and exit site care (see earlier).

Peritonitis

DIAGNOSIS Peritonitis is often easily diagnosed on clinical grounds. Most patients present with the some or all of the following symptoms:

- Abdominal pain
- Cloudy dialysate fluid
- Fever (> 37.5°C)
- Nausea

Patients rarely have other systemic signs and symptoms and are seldom hypotensive. Findings on physical examination are typical of those from any cause of peritonitis and include abdominal tenderness, decreased bowel sounds, guarding, and occasionally, rebound tenderness. Because of the increased incidence of hernias in PD patients, the possibility of peritonitis as a result of ischemic bowel from an incarcerated hernia must always be considered; therefore, ventral, incisional, and inguinal hernias must be looked for, and other intra-abdominal disease must be ruled out.

Standard laboratory investigation for the diagnosis of peritonitis includes peritoneal fluid cell counts with differential, Gram stain, and culture. Findings suggestive of peritonitis include a peritoneal fluid white blood cell count greater than 100 cells/mm^3, most of which are polymorphonuclear white blood cells. Gram stains of peritoneal fluid are seldom helpful, but if the response is positive, they are predictive of culture results 85% of the time. Blood cultures are rarely positive. Cultures of the dialysate should be obtained immediately, but the availability of culture results should not delay the onset of therapy. If proper culture technique is followed, peritoneal cultures should be positive for approximately 90% of patients with peritonitis. If peritoneal fluid cultures are repeatedly sterile and peritoneal fluid white blood cell counts continue to be elevated, other diagnoses must be considered, including eosinophilic peritonitis, tuberculosis, or icodextrin use.

Occasionally, the dialysis effluent is bloody; however, this does not always imply a peritoneal pathologic condition. Bloody effluent commonly occurs after Tenckhoff catheter placement. Gynecologic causes (e.g., reverse menstruation, ovarian cyst rupture, or endometriosis) are the next most common findings. Sclerosing peritonitis should be considered in patients with an associated loss of ultrafiltration capacity. Free intraperitoneal air can occasionally be seen in patients treated by PD, but this finding on an acute abdominal series is not pathognomonic of a perforated viscus in these patients. However, the finding of free air should lead to consideration of perforation in the presence of peritonitis, especially with gram-negative rod or polymicrobial infections.

INFECTIOUS CAUSES OF PERITONITIS

Gram-Positive Peritonitis. Staphylococcus epidermidis was originally the most common causative agent of peritonitis, presumably as a result of touch contamination or pericatheter routes of infection. *S epidermidis* typically causes mild cases of peritonitis that tend to respond rapidly to therapy. *S aureus,* in contrast, is a much more virulent pathogen, and infection with this organism is more likely to be more resistant to therapy and be associated with progressive membrane damage.

Gram-Negative Peritonitis. Gram-negative peritonitis typically responds to appropriate antibiotic therapy, but *Pseudomonas* infections are particularly difficult to eradicate. The bowel, skin, urinary tract, contaminated water, and animal contact have been implicated as sources of gram-negative peritonitis. Peritonitis associated with severe diarrhea has been caused by *Campylobacter* infection.

Pseudomonas Peritonitis. *Pseudomonas* peritonitis deserves special consideration. Although most pseudomonal infections respond to combination antibiotic therapy, in up to 25% of patients catheter removal is required. If *Pseudomonas* peritonitis is related to an exit site or catheter infection, the response rate falls below 35%, and catheter removal is commonly required.

Fungal Peritonitis. The initial signs and symptoms in patients with fungal peritonitis tend to be no different from those in patients with bacterial peritonitis and are most often due to *Candida* species. Fungal peritonitis is often preceded by a recent history of bacterial peritonitis and previous antibiotic therapy. The standard of antifungal therapy has been to treat with intravenous amphotericin B. Other antifungal agents have been used and include fluorocytosine, ketoconazole, miconazole, and econazole. Once-a-day oral fluconazole has been used to treat *Candida* peritonitis, but usually the catheter has to be removed. Given the practical difficulties involved in catheter removal and the available clinical evidence, a reasonable therapeutic plan in hemodynamically stable patients with *Candida* peritonitis involves initiation of appropriate antifungal therapy with close monitoring of the patient. If significant clinical improvement is not seen by 48 hours, then the catheter should be removed. Therapy should be continued for a period of at least 10 days after catheter removal. Fluconazole has no activity against filamentous fungi, for which intravenous amphotericin B is the antifungal agent of choice. Fungal peritonitis from other causes typically requires use of antifungal agents and catheter removal. *Aspergillus* peritonitis has been treated with catheter removal and antifungal therapy.

Tuberculosis. Except for its more insidious onset, tuberculous peritonitis is similar to other forms of peritonitis in clinical manifestations. In general, it represents reactivation of a latent peritoneal focus rather than a primary infection. Tuberculous peritonitis is usually accompanied by a predominance of lymphocytes in the effluent, but this is not always the case. The diagnosis is often delayed and may require peritoneal biopsy. Management involves removal of the catheter and triple antitubercular therapy (isoniazid, rifampin, and pyrazinamide).

TREATMENT OF PERITONITIS   After appropriate investigations have been performed, it may be helpful to perform a few rapid exchanges initially if the patient is in pain or if the patient has sepsis to remove the endotoxin load and reduce inflammation. Empirical antimicrobial treatment should be commenced immediately thereafter without waiting for microbial culture results, and therapy can be tailored at a later point when these become available (Tables 37–4 and 37–5). Occurrences in most patients can be managed on an outpatient basis; indications for admission would include hypotension, severe pain, or evidence of an underlying abdominal pathologic condition. Recommendations are to start therapy with cefazolin or cephalothin (to cover gram-positive bacteria) and ceftazidime or an aminoglycoside (to cover gram-negative bacteria) in most patients unless clinical conditions mandate another approach. In general, empirical vancomycin use is not recommended. The recommended duration of therapy for *S aureus* is a total of 21 days. If *S aureus* is identified and no clinical improvement is seen by 3 or 4 days, rifampin is added. For other gram-positive organisms, the final antibiotic therapy is guided by culture results, and the duration of therapy should be a total of 14 days.

After empirical therapy is initiated, if a gram-negative infection is identified, treatment should be directed by culture and sensitivity testing results. Continuation of an aminoglycoside or ceftazidime is recommended. Systemic levels do not need to be achieved, which should reduce the risk of ototoxicity. For single

Table 37–4: Empiric Initial Therapy for Peritoneal Dialysis–Related Peritonitis, Stratified for Residual Renal Function

| | Residual Urine Volume | |
Antibiotic	< 100 mL/day	> 100 mcL/day
Cefazolin or cephalothin	1 g/bag qd *or* 15 mg/kg/bag qd	20 mg/kg /bag qd
And one of the following:		
Ceftazidime	1 g/bag qd	20 mg/kg/bag qd
Gentamicin, tobramycin, netilmicin	0.6 mg/kg/bag qd	Not recommended
Amikacin	2.0 mg/kg/bag qd	Not recommended

This dosing regimen is for intermittent dosing and is given once during the first day for at least a 6-hour dwell.

Modified from Keane WF, Bailie GR, Boeschoton E, et al: Adult peritoneal dialysis–related peritonitis treatment recommendations: 2000 update. *Perit Dial Int* 20:396–411, 2000.

Table 37–5: Treatment Strategies after the Causative Agent Is Known

Gram-positive	
Enterococcus	Stop cephalosporins
	Start ampicillin, 125 mg/L/each bag
	Consider adding an aminoglycoside
	Duration of therapy, 14 days
Staphylococcus aureus	Stop ceftazidime or aminoglycoside
	Continue cephalosporin
	Consider adding rifampin, 600 mg/day PO
	If MRSA, change to vancomycin or clindamycin
Other gram-positive bacteria	Stop ceftazidime or aminoglycoside
	Continue cephalosporin
	If MRSE, consider vancomycin or clindamycin
Gram-negative	
Single gram-negative species	Adjust antibiotics to sensitivity:
	If < 100 mL/day of urine, aminoglycoside
	If > 100 mL/day of urine, ceftazidime
Pseudomonas	Continue ceftazidime and add:
	If < 100 mL urine, aminoglycoside
	If > 100 mL/day of urine, ciprofloxacin, 500 mg PO bid, *or* piperacillin, 4 g IV q12hr, *or* aztreonam, load 1 g/L; maintenance, 250 mg/L IP/bag
Multiple gram-negative species	Continue cefazolin and ceftazidime
	Add metronidazole, 500 mg q8hr IV
	Consider surgical evaluation

IV, intravenous; IP, intraperitoneal; MRSA, methicillin-resistant *Staphylococcus aureus*; PO, oral.
Modified from Keane WF, Bailie GR, Boeschoton E, et al: Adult peritoneal dialysis–related peritonitis treatment recommendations: 2000 update. *Perit Dial Int* 20:396–411, 2000.

gram-negative infections, the length of therapy should be 14 days. If *Pseudomonas aeruginosa* or *Xanthomonas* is identified, therapy should be extended for a total of 21 to 28 days, catheter removal is often required, and therapy with two antibiotics to which the organism is sensitive is recommended. For multiple gram-negative bacteria species or anaerobes (or for both), surgical evaluation should be considered, the initial empirical antibiotic treatment should be continued with adjustments pending culture and sensitivity results, and metronidazole should be added. For fungal peritonitis, a trial of antifungal agents may be warranted but if no obvious improvement is noted after 4 to 5 days, the catheter should be removed. It was thought that successful therapy should be continued for 4 to 6 weeks.

RELAPSING PERITONITIS Relapsing peritonitis is arbitrarily defined as another episode of peritonitis caused by the same organism associated with the preceding episode of peritonitis within 4 weeks of completion of the antibiotic course. In this situation, the clinician should first review the culture and sensitivity results, and noncompliance should be considered. If *S aureus* is cultured, because of the possibility of intracellular sequestration of bacteria, it is recommended that rifampin and another antibiotic, as guided by sensitivity results, be used for a total of 4 weeks. Consideration should also be given to catheter infection or intra-abdominal abscess. Tunnel infections may contribute to relapsing peritonitis. An ultrasound or computed tomography scan of the tunnel should be considered. Catheter removal is often necessary (in up to 80% of episodes of peritonitis associated with tunnel infections). The risk of tunnel infection seems to be greater early in the course of PD and in women with diabetes.

INDICATIONS FOR CATHETER REMOVAL Catheter removal is indicated for mechanical failure that does not respond to other maneuvers. Other indications for catheter removal include refractory peritonitis, peritonitis associated with tunnel infections, some cases of chronic exit site or tunnel infection, *Pseudomonas* peritonitis unresponsive to appropriate antibiotic therapy, slowly improving fungal peritonitis, fecal peritonitis, significant intra-abdominal disease, and continually relapsing peritonitis with no obvious cause.

EOSINOPHILIC PERITONITIS This complication is usually observed early after catheter placement and is typically associated with sterile peritoneal cultures. Associated peripheral eosinophilia may or may not be present and is assumed to be due to chemical stimuli leached from the catheter. Fungal peritonitis and peritonitis resulting from other causes must be carefully excluded. Most cases of eosinophilic peritonitis resolve spontaneously after 2 to 3 weeks.

Catheter Infections (Exit Site and Tunnel)

Exit site infection may be defined as the presence of marked peri-catheter redness and wetness or exudate in the sinus tract, with or without a positive culture. The formation of crust around the exit may not indicate infection. Positive cultures from the exit site in the absence of inflammation are indicative of colonization and not infection. Catheter infections may be confined to the exit site or may involve only the tunnel. Tunnel infections are often unsuspected and are only diagnosed with ultrasound or computed tomography scans, but they should always be suspected in patients with relapsing peritonitis. A tunnel infection can occur independently of an obvious exit infection and is thus defined as erythema, edema, or tenderness of the subcutaneous tunnel, with or without discharge from the exit or a positive culture.

EXIT SITE INFECTIONS Almost all healed exit sites are colonized by bacteria. Bacterial virulence is also important; the virulent pathogens *S aureus* and *P aeruginosa* are most likely to induce infection. Although *Pseudomonas* infections are relatively rare, the severity of these infections, the difficulty in eradicating them, and the negative impact that they have on catheter survival warrant careful monitoring of this pathogen. Prevention of exit site infections involves strict hygiene and reducing trauma at the exit site by catheter immobilization, especially in the immediate postoperative period.

TUNNEL INFECTIONS Actual tunnel infections are rare. More commonly, they represent infection of the deep cuff. Although exit site infections can be treated successfully by antibiotics, deep cuff infections are rarely cured by antibiotics alone and usually require catheter removal.

PREVENTION OF CATHETER INFECTIONS The primary means of preventing catheter infections is to have a dedicated, knowledgeable catheter implantation team. Administration of prophylactic antibiotics before catheter placement has been documented to prevent subsequent infection. Postoperatively, it is important to immobilize the catheter and minimize handling. The exit should be covered with a sterile gauze dressing, which is not changed for several days unless excessive bleeding occurs. No clear consensus has emerged on when the patient should start daily exit site care. Recommendations vary from 2 to 8 weeks after placement. Swan-neck catheters, disconnect Y systems, and eradication of *S aureus* nasal carriage (discussed earlier) may prevent exit site infections. At present, no consensus has been reached on recommendations for the standard chronic care of the exit site. Some clinicians favor use of simple soap and water and others favor use of povidone-iodine.

TREATMENT OF EXIT SITE INFECTIONS Few data are available on the therapeutic efficacy of the current methods for treatment of exit site or tunnel infections. Treatment recommendations include the use of hypertonic saline (3%), Na^+ hypochlorite, diluted hydrogen peroxide, or povidone-iodine to treat equivocal or mild exit site infections. Acutely inflamed, traumatized exits, or chronic exit site infections require use of topical and parenteral antibiotics. Topical antibiotics include chlorhexidine, dilute hydrogen peroxide, and gentamicin eyedrops. Because of the high incidence of resistance, gram-positive infections may need to be treated parenterally with vancomycin. Oral cephalosporins or a penicillinase-resistant antibiotic can also be used if the organism is not resistant to these agents. Persistent infections can be treated with a combination of vancomycin and rifampin. For gram-negative infections, ciprofloxacin is usually appropriate, although some *Pseudomonas* infections may require other antipseudomonal agents. The recommended duration of therapy is 2 to 4 weeks. Occasionally, deroofing of the tunnel or exteriorizing of the cuff may be helpful. Shaving the superficial cuff is also beneficial in about 50% of refractory exit infections.

Intensive Care Nephrology

38

Renal failure is a common complication in the critically ill patient. An understanding of the pathophysiology of respiratory failure, shock, and management of mechanical ventilation is essential for nephrologists who are active in the care of these patients.

ACUTE RESPIRATORY FAILURE

Acute respiratory failure can be defined as the inability of the respiratory system to meet the oxygenation, ventilation, or metabolic requirements of the patient. Respiratory failure can be divided into two main types: hypoxemic respiratory failure, which is failure to maintain adequate oxygenation, and hypercapnic respiratory failure, which is inadequate ventilation with CO_2 retention. Because nephrologists are often asked to assist with the acid-base management of these patients, it is important that they have an understanding of mechanical ventilation and the newer treatment strategies for acute respiratory distress syndrome. Several modes of mechanical ventilation, which differ in their indications, are now available:

Continuous positive airway pressure (CPAP). This is not a true form of mechanical ventilation, but it provides a supply of fresh gas at a constant, specified pressure. It is most commonly used in weaning trials or in patients without respiratory failure who require an endotracheal tube to maintain an airway.

Synchronized intermittent mandatory ventilation (SIMV). In this modality, the physician orders a set number of breaths, delivered every minute at a certain tidal volume, which is given in synchrony with inspiratory effort if the patient is able to generate inspiration. Any breaths beyond the set number must be generated by the patient.

Assist control mode or continuous mandatory ventilation (CMV). In this modality the ventilator delivers a breath every time the patient generates a negative inspiratory force, or at a set rate, whichever is the higher frequency. CMV minimizes the work of breathing done by the patient and therefore should be used in the presence of myocardial ischemia or profound hypoxemia. CMV can lead to dynamic hyperinflation (breath stacking or "auto-PEEP" [positive end-expiratory pressure]) in tachypneic patients or those with obstructive lung disease if there is inadequate time to exhale the full tidal volume.

Pressure control ventilation (PCV). This setting differs from SIMV and CMV in that the physician sets an inspiratory pressure, not a tidal volume. The tidal volume can vary from breath to breath, and thus the minute volume is variable.

Pressure support ventilation (PSV). This is a patient-triggered mode of ventilation in which a preset pressure is maintained throughout inspiration. When inspiratory flow falls below a certain level, inspiration is terminated. PSV is commonly used in patients who require minimal support or to assist the spontaneous breaths during SIMV.

Airway pressure release ventilation (APRV). This mode is used in a spontaneously breathing patient who is using CPAP. At the end of each ventilator cycle, the lungs are allowed to briefly deflate to ambient pressure, facilitating CO_2 elimination, and then are rapidly reinflated to the baseline pressure (CPAP) with the next breath.

In addition to the mode of ventilation, the physician prescribes the oxygen concentration to be delivered, the level of PEEP, the tidal volume, and the respiratory rate. When initially intubated, patients are typically given a high oxygen concentration, which is then tapered down as quickly as possible because of the postulated risks associated with "oxygen toxicity," including worsening lung compliance and interstitial edema. PEEP provides a continuous airway pressure above atmospheric, preventing collapse of alveoli and small airways at end-expiration, thus improving functional residual capacity and oxygenation. PEEP is most commonly set between 5 and 20 cm H_2O and titrated until adequate oxygenation is achieved. The level of PEEP directly increases airway pressures; thus, high levels of PEEP can result in barotrauma. Tidal volumes traditionally range from 10 to 15 mL/kg per breath, but, as will be discussed in the next section on adult respiratory distress syndrome, recent studies support the use of lower tidal volumes in patients with lung injuries.

ACUTE RESPIRATORY DISTRESS SYNDROME

Adult respiratory distress syndrome is characterized clinically by hypoxia that is refractory to oxygen therapy, decreased lung compliance, and diffuse infiltrates on chest tomography. Two categories of acute respiratory distress syndrome have been defined:

- Acute lung injury (ALI)
- Acute respiratory distress syndrome (ARDS)

Both are characterized by acute onset of hypoxemic respiratory failure with bilateral infiltrates on chest computed tomography scans and a pulmonary artery wedge pressure of less than 18 mm Hg or no clinical evidence of left atrial hypertension. ALI is present when the preceding criteria are present with an arterial O_2 tension-to-fraction of inspired O_2 (PaO_2/FIO_2) ratio of less than 300, and ARDS is present when the PaO_2/FIO_2 is less than 200.

Clinical Features

The acute stage of ARDS/ALI is characterized by the onset of acute respiratory failure, refractory hypoxemia, and radiographic evidence of bilateral infiltrates on a chest x-ray, typically in the dependent zones. Patients often require mechanical support as the work of breathing increases. Mechanically ventilated patients with ARDS often have very high airway pressures, a result of the reduction of ventilated alveoli and reduced compliance. This often necessitates a high minute ventilation to maintain an acceptable CO_2 tension (PCO_2). After the acute phase, many patients recover completely, yet some develop a fibrotic phase characterized by fibrosing alveolitis, persistent hypoxemia, and right ventricular failure.

Risk Factors and Pathophysiology

ALI and ARDS can develop in association with several clinical conditions, not all of which directly involve the pulmonary system. The most common condition associated with ARDS is sepsis. Other common risk factors include shock, the systemic inflammatory response syndrome (SIRS), pneumonia, multiple transfusions, near drowning, aspiration, trauma, pancreatitis, burns, coronary artery bypass grafting, and disseminated intravascular coagulation (DIC).

Treatment

Supportive mechanical ventilation is the primary treatment of ARDS. The goal should be to provide adequate oxygenation while avoiding further barotrauma to the lung that can worsen existing injury. Traditionally, tidal volumes used during mechanical ventilation were in the range of 12 to 15 mL/kg; however, it is now felt that the resulting barotrauma may exacerbate pulmonary dysfunction. In the ARDSNet trial, conventional mechanical ventilation (12 mL/kg ideal body weight) was compared with a lower tidal volume goal starting at 6 mL/kg ideal body weight. In each group, the tidal volume was decreased in increments of 1 mL/kg to maintain plateau pressures of less than 50 mm Hg for the traditional ventilation group and less than 30 mm Hg for the lower tidal volume group. The mortality rate was significantly better in the lower tidal volume group albeit at the expense of a higher $PaCO_2$ ("permissive hypercapnia") and a lower arterial pH. Permissive hypercapnia may result in significant acidosis in a patient with renal failure and may require a higher bicarbonate bath during hemodialysis or continuous renal replacement therapy (RRT), because increasing the minute volume to improve acid-base control is often not an option. In patients with severe ARDS not yet receiving RRT, large infusions of bicarbonate may not improve acidosis because the injured lung may not be able to expel the CO_2 produced. Tris(hydroxymethyl) aminomethane (THAM) is a buffer that accepts one proton per molecule, generating HCO_3^- but not CO_2. It has been shown to control arterial pH without increasing CO_2 in the presence of refractory respiratory acidosis. However, THAM is excreted by the kidneys, so its use is not recommended in renal failure.

Volume management in the patient with ALI or ARDS is controversial. Substantial data from animal experiments indicate that fluid restriction, the achievement of a net negative fluid balance, and reductions in pulmonary capillary wedge pressure improve outcomes. However, fluid restriction can reduce cardiac output and other data suggest that patients with ALI or ARDS may do better with a strategy that increases oxygen delivery, which usually requires volume expansion. On balance, maintaining euvolemia (wedge pressure, 10 to 14 mm Hg, central venous pressure 6 to 12 mm Hg) in patients with ARDS or ALI with use of fluids as guided by evidence of organ perfusion would be the most reasonable approach at this time. Other therapeutic strategies in the management of ARDS include systemic glucocorticoids, prone positioning during ventilation, aerosolized surfactant and inhaled nitric oxide. Although improvement in gas exchange and oxygenation has been observed with these approaches, they have not been found to lower mortality.

Effects on Renal Function

Renal dysfunction is a common occurrence in patients with ARDS or ALI. Whereas this may primarily reflect the effects of sepsis or hemodynamic instability, mechanical ventilation itself has been found to be a predictor of the need for dialysis. Positive intrathoracic pressure from mechanical ventilation reduces cardiac output by impairing venous return and raising right ventricular afterload. This is particularly true in the presence of high PEEP, as is often needed in ARDS.

HYPOVOLEMIC SHOCK

Hypovolemic shock is defined as a reduction in the effective circulating blood volume, which leads to an oxygen deficit in the tissues, because oxygen supply is not able to meet oxygen demand. The most common causes of hypovolemic shock are listed in Table 38–1.

Table 38–1: Etiology of Hypovolemic Shock

Blood loss
External
Trauma
Gastrointestinal bleeding
Internal
Aortic dissection/abdominal aortic aneurysm rupture
Trauma
Splenic laceration/rupture
Hepatic laceration/rupture
Pelvis/long bone fracture
Ruptured ectopic pregnancy
Fluid loss
Diabetic ketoacidosis
Adrenal crisis
Burns
Diarrhea
Vomiting
Lack of volume replacement
Debilitation
Coma/found down

Pathogenesis

Once 10% of circulating volume has been lost, compensatory mechanisms are activated to maintain cardiac output, including adrenal catecholamine release, activation of the sympathetic nervous system, generation of angiotensin II via activation of the renin-angiotensin-aldosterone system, and vasopressin released by the pituitary gland. Once the loss of volume exceeds approximately 40%, these compensatory mechanisms are overwhelmed, and overt hypotension and shock ensue. This results in tissue ischemia accompanied by lactate generation as a result of anaerobic metabolism. In the early stages this process is reversible, but if left untreated, irreversible shock ensues. This state is characterized by capillary pooling of blood and volume- and pressor-resistant hypotension. Although restoration of flow to an ischemic organ is critical for restoration of function, reperfusion itself may contribute to organ damage. Reperfusion injury can manifest as myocardial stunning, reperfusion arrhythmias, breakdown of the gut mucosal barrier, acute renal failure (ARF), hepatic failure, or multiorgan dysfunction syndrome.

Clinical Manifestations

Early in the course of hypovolemia, tachycardia, tachypnea, and orthostatic hypotension are observed. Orthostasis is a particularly reliable clinical sign. Once volume losses become profound, overt hypotension, oliguria, and peripheral cyanosis as a result of diminished perfusion ensue. Hypovolemic shock due to trauma or bleeding is usually apparent, but internal bleeding or the other causes listed in Table 38–1 may not be as obvious. Acidosis can occur, often from hypoperfusion of tissues, which results in lactate production. DIC can also occur during hypovolemic shock, resulting in microvascular thrombi formation, and may contribute to the multiple organ dysfunction often seen after traumatic or hypovolemic shock.

Diagnosis

In most patients with hypovolemic shock, it is readily apparent that trauma or blood loss is the primary cause, but care must be taken not to overlook septic, cardiogenic, or anaphylactic shock. Initial resuscitation should begin during the evaluation. For external blood loss, crossmatching of blood should be done while fluids are infused for resuscitation. Gastrointestinal bleeding can be evaluated and potentially treated with upper or lower endoscopic procedures once the patient's condition is stabilized or with angiographic techniques. In the event of trauma, chest radiography should be performed to rule out tension pneumothorax or hemothorax. If abdominal trauma has occurred, peritoneal lavage can be performed to assess for hemorrhage, most commonly from splenic or hepatic lacerations. If the patient's condition is stabilized, computed tomography or ultrasound can also be used to assess for the presence of intra-abdominal hemorrhage or organ injury. Laboratory tests should include a complete blood count; a chemistry panel, including electrolyte, creatinine, and glucose levels, and liver function tests; arterial blood gas measurements; arterial lactate level; blood type and crossmatch; and urinalysis. In the event of trauma or bleeding, coagulation studies should include a platelet count, prothrombin time, and partial thromboplastin time. If the cause of shock is not readily apparent, an electrocardiogram should be performed to rule out myocardial infarction (MI).

Management

Diagnostic procedures should not delay the resuscitation of the patient in shock. The primary goal in the treatment of hypovolemic shock is to return circulating volume to normal. Care must be taken when a transfusion is given, because a higher hematocrit can actually worsen oxygen balance by increasing viscosity and reducing capillary flow. Although elderly patients with MIs may benefit from transfusion to a hematocrit of 30%, large transfusions of blood have been associated with multiple organ dysfunction, and a liberal transfusion policy to a hemoglobin concentration of 10 to 12 g/dL has been associated with increased mortality. Measurement of oxygen delivery and consumption also require pulmonary artery catheter placement, which may be an independent risk factor for mortality; thus, many physicians use improvement in blood pressure, metabolic acidosis, and serial lactate levels as markers that oxygen delivery and consumption are adequate. Further treatment depends on the cause of shock. Traumatic shock often requires surgical exploration to treat the source of bleeding. Upper gastrointestinal bleeding due to ulcers can be treated medically with intravenous proton pump inhibitors or endoscopically by electrocautery, laser coagulation, or injection therapy. Esophageal varices can be treated with an infusion of somatostatin or with an interventional procedure such as injection sclerotherapy or placement of a Sengstaken-Blakemore tube. Lower gastrointestinal bleeding can be treated with endoscopic therapies. Surgery is an option for recurrent bleeding.

Fluid Resuscitation

Fluid resuscitation is the initial therapy in hypovolemic shock, because it helps to restore circulating volume and oxygen delivery.

The types of fluids used are quite varied (Table 38–2), and controversy exists as to which agent is the most efficacious. Isotonic crystalloid solutions have traditionally been used as the primary fluid for volume expansion. Normal saline (0.9%) and lactated Ringer's solution are both commonly used, although large volumes of lactated Ringer's solution should be avoided in patients with renal failure, because they can result in hyperkalemia. Approximately 75% of the crystalloid volume infused enters the interstitial space, whereas 25% remains in the intravascular space. This distribution has led to the use of colloid solutions, which are retained in the intravascular space to a much greater extent than isotonic crystalloids (see Table 38–2).

Crystalloid versus Colloid for Resuscitation

The most appropriate fluid for resuscitation of the patient in shock is controversial. Colloids offer the theoretical advantage of expanding the intravascular space with less volume. One liter of dextran 70 increases intravascular volume by 800 mL, 1 L of hetastarch by 750 mL, 1 L of 5% albumin by 500 mL, and 1 L of saline by 180 mL. Colloids increase blood pressure more rapidly than crystalloids and may be associated with a lower incidence of pulmonary edema. However, in the presence of sepsis, in which there is significant capillary leak, these factors may not be relevant. There is also evidence that colloids inhibit the coagulation system, cause anaphylactoid reactions, and increase the risk of ARF (hetastarch). Several meta-analyses have shown a trend toward increased mortality in heterogeneous groups of critically ill patients resuscitated with colloids that is a concern; the Cochrane Injuries Group Albumin Reviewers found that the risk of death was significantly increased in critically ill patients who received albumin, suggesting that it should no longer be used in critically ill patients outside of randomized, controlled trials. However, in a recent large randomized trial comparing fluid resuscitation in intensive care unit patients treated with 0.9% NaCl or 4% albumin showed that efficacy and safety were equal in both groups. Given the available data, and the potential risks of colloids, crystalloids still remain the cornerstone of volume resuscitation treatment, although patients with profound volume deficits may benefit from colloids in addition to crystalloids to hasten restoration of circulating volume.

Vasopressors

The use of vasopressors in patients with hypovolemic shock should be reserved for those in whom adequate fluid infusion has not improved hypotension. In this setting, a pulmonary artery catheter can help guide therapy, because persistent shock

Table 38-2: Fluids Used for Resuscitation

	Sodium Chloride (0.9%)	Ringer's Lactate	Sodium Chloride (3%)	Albumin (5%)	Hetastarch (6%)	Dextran 70 + Sodium Chloride	Urea-Gelatin
Sodium (mEq/L)	154	130	513	130–160	154	154	145
Chloride (mEq/L)	154	109	513	130–160	154	154	145
Potassium (mEq/L)	0	4	0		0	0	5.1
Osmolarity (mOsm/L)	308	275	1025	310	310	310	391
Oncotic pressure (mm Hg)	0	0	0	20	30	60	26–30
Lactate (mEq/L)	0	28	0	0	0	0	0
Maximum dose (mL/kg/24 hr)	None	None	Limited by serum Na+	None	20	20	20
Cost (L)	$1.26	$1.44	$1.28	$100	$27.50	$35.08	–

703

can be caused by either peripheral vasodilation or myocardial dysfunction. A wedge pressure of 12 to 16 mm Hg is indicative of adequate volume expansion. Early studies suggest that vasopressin can reverse shock unresponsive to fluids and catecholamines and can improve survival after cardiac arrest in hypovolemic shock.

Treatment of Acidosis

In patients with intractable shock, metabolic acidosis may persist despite volume expansion and improved oxygen delivery. Intravenous bicarbonate is often used in this setting in an attempt to improve cardiac function. However, decreased cardiac contractility in the presence of lactic acidosis may be partially due to hypoxemia, hypoperfusion, or sepsis, and establishing direct deleterious effects of the low pH is difficult. Furthermore, bicarbonate infusion has been theorized to cause worsening intracellular acidosis, because the CO_2 produced when bicarbonate reacts with acids can diffuse rapidly across the cell membrane, whereas bicarbonate cannot. Because the treatment of lactic acidosis with sodium bicarbonate has not been shown to be beneficial in clinical studies and the potential for adverse effects appears real, the routine administration of sodium bicarbonate in this setting should be discouraged unless further compelling evidence becomes available.

Effects of Shock on Renal Function

ARF is a common finding in a patient with shock. In the presence of shock compensatory mechanisms maintaining renal perfusion (prostaglandin/nitric oxide release and efferent arteriolar vasoconstriction) are overwhelmed, and ischemic renal injury supervenes. Other factors, including DIC with resultant microvascular thrombi, can aggravate the renal ischemic injury.

SEPSIS

Sepsis and septic shock are common causes of ARF. The nephrologist is often involved in the care of this disease, and complete understanding of the pathophysiology and newer therapeutic approaches for sepsis is critical in the management of this patient population.

Definition

The American College of Chest Physicians/Society of Critical Care Medicine Consensus Conference in 1991 led to a uniform definition of the systemic inflammatory response syndrome (SIRS),

Table 38–3: Definition of Systemic Inflammatory Response
Syndrome (SIRS), Sepsis, Severe Sepsis, and Septic Shock

SIRS	Presence of two or more of the following:
	  Temperature > 38°C or < 36°C
	  Heart rate > 90 beats/min
	  Respiratory rate > 20 breaths/min
	  White blood cell count > 20,000/mm³,
	  < 4,000/mm³, or < 10% immature neutrophils

Sepsis	SIRS in the presence of documented infection
Severe sepsis	Sepsis with hypotension, hypoperfusion, or organ dysfunction
Septic shock	Sepsis with hypotension despite volume resuscitation and evidence of organ dysfunction or hypoperfusion

sepsis, severe sepsis, and septic shock (Table 38–3). The mortality rate for patients with SIRS increases as more criteria are fulfilled, and the condition advances along the spectrum. The approximate mortality rate for patients with two SIRS criteria is 7%, with three SIRS criteria it is 10%, with four SIRS criteria it is 17%, with sepsis it is 16%, with severe sepsis it is 20%, and with septic shock it is 46%.

Source of Infection and Microbiology

In the 1960s and 1970s, gram-negative organisms were the most common causes of septic shock, but gram-positive organisms have now increased in prevalence. The most common primary sites of infection in sepsis are the respiratory tract (50%), intra-abdominal and pelvic sites (20%), the urinary tract (10%), skin (5%), and intravascular catheters (5%). Risk factors for the development of sepsis include immunocompromise (human immunodeficiency virus infection or cytotoxic/immunosuppressive therapy), malnutrition, alcoholism, malignancy, diabetes mellitus, advanced age, and chronic renal failure.

Pathophysiology

It had been hypothesized that the manifestations of sepsis result from an excessive inflammatory response to bacterial organisms; however, strategies targeted at modulating an "overactive" immune response (e.g., corticosteroids, tumor necrosis factor antagonists, or antiendotoxin antibodies) have been singularly unsuccessful. Emerging evidence suggests that sepsis is actually associated with a state of immunosuppression as characterized by lymphocyte apoptosis, abnormal neutrophil activity, loss of delayed type hypersensitivity responses, and an increased susceptibility to nosocomial infection. The coagulation system also plays a role in the manifestation of sepsis. Levels of protein C are decreased, and its conversion to activated protein C, which inhibits thrombosis, is down-regulated during sepsis. Levels of antithrombin III and tissue factor pathway inhibitor, both inhibitors of the coagulation pathway, are reduced in the presence of sepsis. These factors contribute to the widespread microvascular thrombosis that occurs during sepsis, a result of which is a reduction in perfusion to various tissues, which may lead to the multiorgan dysfunction syndrome seen in many patients with sepsis.

Clinical Features

Common clinical manifestations include changes in body temperature (fever or hypothermia), tachycardia, tachypnea, and leukocytosis or leukopenia. Hypotension is due to a combination of persistent vasodilatation (low systemic vascular resistance) and a decreased effective circulating volume (increased microvascular permeability and increased insensible losses). Impaired organ perfusion is suggested by confusion, restlessness, oliguria, and lactic acid accumulation. Once patients with septic shock have received fluid and volume resuscitation, most have an elevated cardiac output and decreased systemic vascular resistance. However, despite these findings, the heart may not be as hyperdynamic as it should be, given the clinical setting, possibly due to a myocardial depressant effect of sepsis. ARDS complicates sepsis in up to 40% of patients and is often the initial manifestation of the multiorgan dysfunction syndrome. Adrenal insufficiency is a common finding in septic shock, with a reported incidence of 25% to 40%. The threshold for diagnosing adrenal insufficiency should be a cortisol level of 25 to 30 mcg/mL, instead of the usual 18 to 20 mcg/mL in response to a low-dose (1 to 2 mcg) adrenocorticotropic hormone stimulation test. In addition, in a patient who is hypotensive and requires pressors, a baseline cortisol level of less than 25 mcg/mL should be considered diagnostic of adrenal insufficiency.

DIC is often seen in sepsis and is characterized by enhanced activation of coagulation with intravascular fibrin deposition and platelet consumption. The resulting microvascular thrombi can reduce organ blood flow contributing to the onset of multiorgan dysfunction syndrome. Laboratory studies in DIC typically show thrombocytopenia, with an elevation of the prothrombin time and activated partial thromboplastin time, as well as elevated D dimer levels. Critical illness polyneuropathy is a common occurrence in the presence of sepsis and is caused by axonal degeneration. It is characterized by hyporeflexia, distal weakness, and normal or slightly elevated creatine kinase levels and may complicate ventilator weaning. Recovery from muscle weakness can take up to 6 months. Renal dysfunction is found in up to 40% of patients with sepsis, and the mortality rate in these patients is greater than 50%.

Management

The management of sepsis is based primarily on eradication of the infection and support of the patient's hemodynamics and other organ systems.

Antibiotics

Identifying and treating the source should be the primary goals in the management of sepsis. The initial choice of antibiotic often depends on the suspected site of infection. When this is not known, initial antibiotic therapy is usually broad-spectrum coverage, and if culture results later identify a source, coverage can be narrowed. If no organism is isolated, initial broad-spectrum antibiotics can be continued as long as the patient's condition is improving. Immediate institution of antibiotic therapy is critical, because there is a 10% to 15% higher mortality in patients not treated promptly.

Hemodynamic Support

Intravascular volume depletion, peripheral vasodilation, and increased microvascular permeability all contribute to the hypotension seen in severe sepsis and septic shock, and aggressive volume resuscitation should be the primary initial therapy. The requirements for fluid resuscitation are very large, and up to 10 L of crystalloids are often required in the first 24 hours. Boluses of fluid should be given until blood pressure, heart rate, or evidence of end-organ perfusion such as urine output has improved. Early therapy is crucial, and a recent study showed that early, goal-directed therapy, using central venous pressure, mean arterial pressure, hematocrit, and central venous oxygen saturation as end points, lowered mortality (Fig. 38–1).

Despite adequate fluid resuscitation, many patients require vasopressor agents. Dopamine is recommended as the agent of first choice. However, tachycardia and arrhythmias may limit its use. Norepinephrine is as effective for raising blood pressure

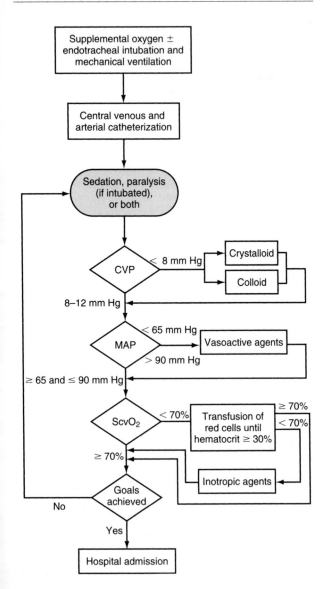

Figure 38–1. Protocol for early goal-directed therapy in sepsis. The protocol was as follows. A 500-mL bolus of crystalloid solution was given every 30 minutes to achieve a central venous pressure (CVP) of 8 to 12 mm Hg. If the mean arterial pressure (MAP) was less than 65 mm Hg, vasopressors were given to maintain a mean arterial pressure of at least 65 mm Hg. If the mean arterial pressure was greater than 90 mm Hg, vasodilators were given until it was 90 mm Hg or below. If the central venous oxygen saturation (Scvo2) was less than 70%, red cells were transfused to achieve a hematocrit of at least 30%. After the central venous pressure, mean arterial pressure, and hematocrit were thus optimized, if the central venous oxygen saturation was less than 70%, dobutamine administration was started at a dose of 2.5 mcg/kg of body weight/min, a dose that was increased by 2.5 mcg/kg/min every 30 minutes until the central venous oxygen saturation was 70% or higher or until a maximal dose of 20 mcg/kg/min was given. Dobutamine was decreased in dosage or discontinued if the mean arterial pressure was less than 65 mm Hg or if the heart rate was more than 120 beats/min. To decrease oxygen consumption, patients in whom hemodynamic optimization could not be achieved received mechanical ventilation and sedatives. From Rivers E, Nguyen B, Havstad S, et al: Early goal-directed therapy in the treatment of severe sepsis and septic shock. *N Engl J Med* 345:1368, 2001.

as dopamine but does not raise cardiac output as much as dopamine. Phenylephrine has purely α-adrenergic effects and fewer risks of tachyarrhythmias, but experience with it in septic shock is limited. Epinephrine can be used for refractory hypotension, but it has been shown to cause a rise in serum lactate levels. Dobutamine has been used in patients with sepsis to improve oxygen delivery, but it can potentiate hypotension due to β_2-adrenergic–mediated vasodilation. Dobutamine is recommended for patients with a low cardiac index (< 2.5 L/min/m²) after volume resuscitation, but if profound hypotension is present (systolic blood pressure < 80 mm Hg), it should be used in conjunction with an agent with more peripheral vasoconstrictor effects such as norepinephrine or phenylephrine. Emerging options include the use of vasopressin if other agents prove to be ineffective.

Treatment of the Coagulation Cascade

Treatment of the underlying condition will accelerate resolution of DIC. No specific therapy is recommended for DIC unless severe or life-threatening hemorrhage occurs, at which time replacement with platelets, fresh-frozen plasma, and possibly cryoprecipitate is indicated. In patients with severe sepsis (Acute Physiology and Chronic Health Evaluation [APACHE II] score of 25), the administration of activated protein C results in a significant reduction in overall mortality rates. Activated protein C acts as an anticoagulant, and, therefore, it should be used with caution in patients with an international normalized ratio greater than 3 or platelet count less than 30,000/mm³. Administration of activated protein C should be considered in all patients with a high risk of death from sepsis: three SIRS criteria and at least single organ dysfunction.

Nutrition and Glycemic Control
Nutritional support is a key component of the management of the critically ill patient. It is essential for maintaining optimal immune function and appears to decrease the susceptibility of critically ill patients to infection. The enteral route of nutrition is preferred because it is associated with a lower incidence of catheter-related bloodstream infection and may support the integrity of the intestinal mucosal barrier. Care must also be taken to maintain the blood glucose level at 80 to 110 mg/dL (4.4 to 6.1 mmol/L), with insulin if necessary, because this has been shown to significantly lower morbidity and mortality rates among critically ill patients.

Corticosteroids
Corticosteroids have long been the subject of studies in sepsis, the rationale being that minimization of the inflammatory cascade could improve outcome. Clinical studies of glucocorticoids in patients with sepsis have failed to demonstrate a beneficial effect; therefore, in the absence of evidence of adrenal insufficiency (see earlier), routine steroid therapy is not recommended.

Hemofiltration
The role of cytokines in sepsis and septic shock has led to the theory that removing them by hemofiltration may improve outcomes. However, most studies have shown no reduction in mortality rates. Therefore, in the absence of renal failure requiring RRT, there is no evidence to support the routine use of hemofiltration for sepsis.

CARDIOGENIC SHOCK

Cardiogenic shock is a state of decreased cardiac output in the presence of adequate intravascular volume, resulting in inadequate tissue perfusion. The diagnosis can be made clinically by the findings of poor tissue perfusion, such as oliguria or cool extremities, along with the hemodynamic criteria of sustained hypotension (systolic blood pressure < 90 mm Hg), reduced cardiac index (< 2.2 L/min/m^2), and congestion (pulmonary capillary wedge pressure > 18 mm Hg). The most common cause of cardiogenic shock is a massive myocardial infarct; other causes include smaller infarctions in patients with reduced left ventricular function, acute mitral regurgitation, rupture of the interventricular septum, myocarditis, end-stage cardiomyopathy, valvular heart disease, or hypertrophic cardiomyopathy.

Pathophysiology

Cardiogenic shock may occur once 40% of the myocardium is lost acutely. The resultant clinical sequelae of hypotension and tachycardia can potentiate the myocardial damage. The elevated wall stress resulting from left ventricular dilation and pump failure increases myocardial oxygen requirements, which also worsens ischemia.

Clinical Features

Hypotension is universal in cardiogenic shock. Tachycardia, arrhythmias, jugular venous distention, pulmonary rales, and a third heart sound may be observed. Signs of tissue hypoperfusion include confusion, mottling of the skin, and oliguria. ARF occurs in approximately one third of patients and is associated with a sharp increase in mortality as high as 90%. Multiple organ failure and lactic acidosis develop in many patients, primarily owing to ischemia from decreased cardiac output.

Evaluation

MI with reduced left ventricular systolic function is the most common cause; however, other causes of shock, such as sepsis, hypovolemia, and pulmonary embolism, need to be considered and excluded. An electrocardiogram should be performed, and if an inferior MI is suspected, a right-sided electrocardiogram should be performed to assess right-sided involvement. Routine blood tests, including measurement of cardiac enzymes, should be performed, a Foley catheter should be placed to monitor urine output, and a chest radiograph should be obtained. Echocardiography is a valuable tool to confirm the diagnosis of cardiogenic shock and can be used to identify potential mechanical causes that require surgical intervention.

Management

General Measures

Airway management and maintenance of adequate oxygenation should be the first concern during resuscitation. Intubation and mechanical ventilation may be required if adequate oxygenation cannot be maintained with supplemental oxygen or noninvasive ventilation with minimal work of breathing.

β-Blockers, angiotensin-converting enzyme inhibitors, and nitrates should be discontinued because they may worsen the patient's clinical state. If there is no evidence of pulmonary edema, an empirical fluid bolus (250 mL of 0.9% NaCl) can be administered. Significantly higher fluid requirements may be seen in patients with a right ventricular infarction to maintain left ventricular filling pressures. As in septic shock, tight glycemic control improves outcomes.

Inotropic Support

If hypotension persists despite optimization of filling pressures, then administration of inotropic agents should begin. Dobutamine improves myocardial contractility and cardiac output and is the drug of first choice when the systolic blood pressure is greater than 80 mm Hg. At lower systolic blood pressure, its vasodilatatory effects may worsen hypotension, and it should only be used in conjunction with another vasopressor. Dopamine (15 mcg/kg/min) is a reasonable choice in that setting, although it can precipitate tachycardia and arrhythmias at higher doses. Norepinephrine is a pure α-adrenergic agonist and can be used when there is an inadequate response to dopamine.

Milrinone and amrinone are phosphodiesterase inhibitors that improve cardiac output; however, they cause peripheral vasodilation and should not be used in patients with marginal blood pressures. Once the blood pressure has been stabilized, the treatment of pulmonary edema with diuretics and optimization of preload and afterload with direct vasodilator therapy can be considered. Emerging therapies include the use of recombinant human b-type natriuretic peptide, nesiritide, which can reduce pulmonary capillary wedge pressure and systemic vascular resistance and improve the urine output in diuretic-resistant patients.

Intra-Aortic Balloon Pumping

Intra-aortic balloon pumping can improve diastolic blood pressure and coronary perfusion and increase cardiac output in the presence of cardiogenic shock. Clinical studies have suggested that intra-aortic balloon pump placement improves survival, particularly in patients who have received thrombolytic therapy, probably owing to increased coronary blood flow. Intra-aortic balloon pumping has a complication rate of up to 15% (e.g., bleeding, limb ischemia, and bloodstream infection).

Coronary Reperfusion

The outcome of cardiogenic shock in the presence of MI is directly related to the patency of the coronary arteries involved. Therefore, interventions to open occluded arteries are crucial. Thrombolytics reduce the incidence of shock when given for acute MI, but once shock is established, the benefit is less clear. Emerging clinical evidence suggests that a more aggressive approach involving early revascularization (percutaneous procedures/coronary artery bypass grafting) results in improved outcomes in cardiogenic shock complicating acute MI. Ventricular assist devices have been used in patients with peri-infarction cardiogenic shock, acute myocarditis, and postcardiotomy shock as a bridge to either recovery of adequate myocardial function or transplantation.

Ultrafiltration

Ultrafiltration by continuous RRT has also been proposed as a treatment for severe refractory heart failure in patients who do not have uremia. In patients who are diuretic resistant, ultrafiltration, either by continuous or intermittent methods, can improve systemic hemodynamics; however, compelling outcome data are lacking. Although hemofiltration may improve congestive heart failure in some patients, removal of intravascular volume may not be tolerated by all patients and may lead to permanent renal dysfunction.

FULMINANT HEPATIC FAILURE

Definition

- *Fulminant hepatic failure* (FHF) is defined as severe acute liver failure in a patient with no preexisting liver disease, with encephalopathy developing within 2 weeks of the first manifestation of liver disease.
- *Subfulminant hepatic failure* (SFHF) is defined as liver failure that is complicated by encephalopathy between 3 and 12 weeks after the onset of jaundice.

Because the rate of onset of this disease process is an indicator of prognosis, with patients having the most rapid onset of encephalopathy also having the best chance of recovery, a newer definition has been proposed to classify FHF and SFHF. Hyperacute, acute, and subacute liver failure are defined by the time between the onset of jaundice and the development of encephalopathy (0 to 7 days, 8 to 28 days, and 29 days to 12 weeks, respectively). The survival rate of patients with hyperacute liver failure is 36%; for acute liver failure the survival rate is 7%, and for subacute liver failure it is 14%. The most common cause of hyperacute liver failure is acetaminophen overdose, although hepatitis A and B can also result in this condition. Acute liver failure is predominantly caused by viral hepatitis and drug reactions; subacute liver failure is most often caused by a hepatitis for which no viral cause can be found. A thorough history is critical for diagnosing drug-related FHF, which can be difficult in a profoundly encephalopathic patient. Conditions that can present as FHF are listed in Table 38–4.

Clinical Features

FHF presents with a variety of symptoms including nausea, vomiting, malaise, and jaundice. Hypoglycemia results from impaired gluconeogenesis, high insulin levels, and an inability to utilize stored glycogen. Metabolic acidosis is a consequence of poor tissue perfusion and an inability to clear lactate. Hypokalemia and hyponatremia also occur often. By definition, FHF requires that encephalopathy be present, the etiology of which is felt to be multifactorial. Hepatic encephalopathy is graded on a scale of 1 to 4 as listed in Table 38–5. Strong consideration should be given to intubation for airway protection as encephalopathy progresses through stage 3. Cerebral edema has been found in 40% of patients with FHF and advanced encephalopathy and leads to increased intracranial pressure (ICP) and decreased cerebral perfusion. This is manifested clinically by abnormal pupillary reflexes, systemic hypertension, and bradycardia. Invasive ICP monitoring for all patients with

Table 38–4: Causes of Fulminant Hepatic Failure

Viral hepatitis	Drug toxicity
Mushroom poisoning	Wilson disease
Autoimmune hepatitis	Metastatic tumor
Acute fatty liver of pregnancy	Budd-Chiari syndrome
HELLP syndrome	Portal vein thrombosis
Reye syndrome	Right-sided heart failure
Malignant hyperthermia	Acute rejection of liver transplant

Table 38–5: Stages of Hepatic Encephalopathy

Stage 1	Euphoria, anxiety, disruption of sleep, shortened attention span, mild confusion, slight asterixis
Stage 2	Slurred speech, lethargy, inappropriate behavior, asterixis, hypoactive reflexes, loss of continence
Stage 3	Marked confusion, incoherent speech, hyperactive reflexes, somnolent but arousable
Stage 4	Coma, unresponsive to pain, lacking asterixis

grade 3 and 4 encephalopathy has been shown to improve the outcome of liver transplantation by excluding those patients with low cerebral perfusion pressure (cerebral perfusion pressure = mean arterial pressure – ICP) who are likely to have permanent neurologic damage.

Coagulopathy and thrombocytopenia are common findings in FHF. Although hemorrhage is uncommon, the gastrointestinal tract is the most common site of bleeding, and intracranial hemorrhage may rarely occur spontaneously. Bacterial infections occur in up to 80% of patients with acute liver failure. Fungal infections are also common, the predominant organisms being *Candida albicans* or *Candida glabrata* and *Aspergillus*. There may be an absence of clinical signs of infection in FHF, so a high index of suspicion must be maintained, particularly when a patient's clinical condition undergoes a sudden deterioration. Renal dysfunction is present in up to 55% of all patients with FHF. Direct toxicity can be a result of acetaminophen overdose, radiocontrast material, or antibiotic use. The circulatory changes seen in FHF predispose patients to renal dysfunction (low systemic vascular resistance, hypotension, or renal vasoconstriction). Hepatorenal syndrome is a well-recognized occurrence and is discussed in Chapter 9, Acute Renal Failure. If RRT is required then continuous RRT should be considered first-line therapy in FHF, even in hemodynamically stable patients because intermittent RRT has been associated with a significant increase in ICP.

Evaluation

Initial laboratory tests should include chemistry profiles, coagulation studies, a complete blood count, a toxicology screen, viral serologic tests, ceruloplasmin (in patients younger than 40 years of age) and creatinine kinase levels, and urinalysis. Transaminase levels can be strikingly high, but the levels do not predict outcome. Increases in bilirubin and prothrombin levels and a reduction in the factor V level have prognostic value and should be followed closely. Signs of cardiac or renal failure should prompt consideration of Swan-Ganz catheter placement because the intravascular volume status can be difficult to determine otherwise in FHF. Sepsis must be looked for, including a search for fungal infections. Use of intravenous H_2 blockers is considered routine to prevent gastric bleeding with coagulopathy. A liver biopsy is needed for diagnosis in a minority of patients, because the etiology is usually evident. Transjugular biopsy has become the favored method with coagulopathy because the risk of bleeding is less than that with the percutaneous approach.

Management

Acetaminophen toxicity should be treated with *N*-acetylcysteine, which is effective up to 36 hours after an overdose of acetaminophen. Therefore, *N*-acetylcysteine should be given when acetaminophen overdose is suspected, even if levels are undetectable. The oral dose is 140 mg/kg initially, followed by 70 mg/kg every 4 hours for 17 doses. When given intravenously, the dose is a 150 mg/kg bolus followed by 70 mg/kg intravenously every 4 hours for 12 doses. Acyclovir should be used for herpes simplex infection and lamivudine has been proved to be of some benefit for hepatitis B infection. Acute fatty liver of pregnancy and the HELLP (*h*emolysis, *e*levated *l*iver enzymes, and *l*ow *p*latelets) syndrome require immediate delivery of the fetus. *Amanita* poisoning should be treated with high-dose penicillin (300,000 to 1 million units/kg/day), which has an antagonistic effect on the mushroom toxin amatoxin, and silybin (20 to 48 mg/kg/day), which blocks the hepatocellular uptake of amatoxin.

In most patients, therapy for FHF is supportive. Fluid resuscitation is often required in the acute setting because there is hypotension from decreased systemic vascular resistance, as well as redistributive losses. FFP continues to be used as a first-line agent for volume resuscitation, although there are no studies to support its use over that of normal saline. The use of albumin is controversial, given its association with poor outcomes in critical illness in general. Once volume resuscitation is complete, dextrose with 0.45% normal saline should be used for maintenance fluids, with careful monitoring of serum electrolytes. Hypotension that persists after fluid resuscitation is adequate, as evidenced by a wedge pressure of 12 to 14 mm Hg, requires vasopressors. Norepinephrine is most commonly used for its preferential effect on peripheral α-adrenergic receptors.

The treatment of hepatic encephalopathy is targeted to limiting the production of ammonia. Hypokalemia increases renal ammonia synthesis and should be aggressively treated. Lactulose reduces the gut absorption of ammonia and is the mainstay of therapy. Oral antibiotics (metronidazole and neomycin) have been used but do not offer any additional benefit over lactulose and should be reserved for lactulose-intolerant patients. Flumazenil may offer a short-term improvement in encephalopathy but does not appear to alter mortality rates.

Cerebral edema is a common cause of death in patients with FHF and should be treated aggressively. When ICP monitoring is performed, the cerebral perfusion pressure should be maintained above at least 50 mm Hg. Strategies to lower the ICP include raising the head of the bed to 20 to 30 degrees, measures to reduce fever, hyperventilation to a PCO_2 of 26 to 30 mm Hg and mannitol administration. Mannitol (0.5 to 1 g/kg) is effective in reducing ICP in patients with normal renal function. A diuresis of twice the volume of mannitol given should be expected in 1 hour. This dose can be repeated, but the serum osmolality must be monitored and mannitol stopped when the osmolality reaches 320 mOsm/kg. Complications of mannitol use include hypernatremia and volume depletion leading to ARF or, if renal excretion is impaired, volume overload and hyponatremia. In the setting of renal failure, mannitol can be coupled with hemofiltration to maintain the osmotic effect. Twice the volume of mannitol administered should be removed by ultrafiltration to ensure a beneficial effect.

Most patients with FHF develop coagulopathy, but spontaneous hemorrhage is uncommon. Parenteral vitamin K should be given for 3 days if coagulopathy develops, and fresh-frozen plasma should only be given for bleeding or in advance of invasive procedures. Other therapies, including insulin and glucagon, corticosteroids, and exchange transfusion, have not been shown to be beneficial. Emerging therapies for the treatment of FHF include liver dialysis units, bioartificial liver units, and the molecular adsorbent recirculating system. These are considered experimental treatments and are currently available only for investigational use in the United States.

RENAL REPLACEMENT THERAPY IN THE INTENSIVE CARE UNIT

For a complete discussion of dialytic modalities in ARF, see Chapter 9, Acute Renal Failure.

Extracorporeal Management of Poisoning

39

Extracorporeal treatment of poisoning is only required in a small minority of poisonings and only then when specific indications are met. Understanding the physiologic basis for these indications allows the clinician to effectively guide treatment of a drug overdose.

GENERAL MANAGEMENT OF POISONING AND DRUG OVERDOSE

Clinical History

The diagnosis of a toxic ingestion can often be established by the history, physical examination, and routine information from the toxicology laboratory. However, the overdose patient commonly presents to a health care facility in an obtunded state, making a thorough history difficult to obtain. For patients who are unable to give a history, questions about habits, hobbies, prescription medications, behavioral changes, and antecedent events should be directed to the family and friends. Discussions with emergency personnel also may reveal pertinent information. After initial airway and circulatory management, the clinician must gather data by means of physical examination and laboratory assessment to determine the cause of the toxic ingestion. The physician then must develop a treatment plan targeted to limiting the accumulation of toxin in the body.

Physical Examination

The physical examination findings of the poisoned patient are quite variable and often depend on the particular toxin ingested.

Patients require close monitoring because their conditions may deteriorate rapidly after the initial assessment. Frequent reevaluation of vital signs, cardiopulmonary condition, and neurologic status are essential for proper management. Specific clinical manifestations and physical findings pertaining to individual toxins are described in later sections of this chapter.

Laboratory Assessment

Laboratory assessment should include a complete blood cell count, comprehensive metabolic panel, serum osmolality, arterial blood gas determinations, urinalysis, urine drug screen, and serum acetaminophen and salicylate levels. An electrocardiogram is also indicated, because conduction disturbances within the myocardium are common in patients presenting with toxic ingestions. Two key laboratory features that assist in determining the type of toxin ingested are the anion gap and osmolal gap. A *high–anion gap metabolic acidosis* is characteristic of salicylate, methanol, and ethylene glycol toxicity or lactic acidosis due to hypotension/hypoxia. A low anion gap is observed with lithium, nitrate, iodine, and bromide poisoning. Ketosis may be present with acetone, isopropanol (i.e., isopropyl alcohol), and salicylate ingestion. The *osmolal gap* is the difference between the measured serum osmolality and the calculated osmolality.

The calculated osmolality is determined by the following formula:

$$Osm_{calculated}\ (mOsm/kg) = 2[Na]$$
$$= glucose/18 + blood\ urea\ nitrogen/2.8$$

The osmolal gap indicates the presence of an unmeasured solute and is considered to be elevated if the value is more than 10 to 12 mOsm/kg of H_2O. An elevated osmolal gap is most commonly seen with ethanol, ethylene glycol, isopropanol, and methanol toxicity. The concept of the osmolal gap is discussed in detail in a later section (see the section on diagnosis and laboratory data under "Ethylene Glycol").

DECONTAMINATION AND FACILITATED REMOVAL

Techniques That Prevent Further Absorption

Whole-Bowel Irrigation

Whole-bowel irrigation is performed with a solution containing electrolytes and iso-osmotic polyethylene glycol. The irrigating

Table 39–1: Clinical Uses of Multiple-Dose Activated Charcoal	
Agents effectively adsorbed	
Carbamazepine	Digoxin
Phenytoin	Dapsone
Phenobarbital	Salicylates
Theophylline	Quinine
Agents ineffectively adsorbed	
Aminoglycosides	
Heavy metals (e.g., arsenic, lead)	Phenothiazines
Tricyclic antidepressants	Calcium channel blockers
	Lithium

solution is given orally or through a nasogastric tube at a rate of 1 to 2 L/hr for adults until the rectal effluent is clear. Whole-body irrigation is indicated for toxins that are not well absorbed by activated charcoal (Table 39–1) and for overdoses with sustained-release medications. Contraindications include gastrointestinal bleeding or bowel obstruction or perforation.

Adsorbents

The most commonly used absorbent is activated charcoal, and it is a mainstay in the treatment of poisoning in the emergency room. The recommended dose of activated charcoal is 1 g/kg or a dose of 25 to 100 g. Multiple doses can be given every 4 hours, and the doses may be repeated for up to 24 hours or until serum drug levels are reduced to nontoxic concentrations. The efficacy of activated charcoal is greatest within 1 hour of ingestion, but its use should be considered for all poisonings, unless the specific agent binds poorly to the adsorbent or there are contraindications to its use. Activated charcoal is contraindicated in patients with altered levels of consciousness, at least until airway protection is established. Other contraindications include bowel obstruction or perforation. Other absorbents less commonly used include *sodium polystyrene sulfonate* (Kayexalate), which can, in high doses, limit lithium adsorption, and *cholestyramine,* which enhances the elimination of the organochlorines (e.g., chlordecone and lindane) and digoxin.

Ipecac

The clinical use of ipecac has declined dramatically over the past 20 years. Emetine acts locally in the gastrointestinal tract and systemically in the central nervous system (CNS) and successfully induces emesis in more than 90% of patients. Although data on the role and efficacy of ipecac have been controversial, no study has convincingly demonstrated that the clinical outcome of poisoned patients improved with the use of ipecac, and administration of this powerful emetic agent is not routinely advised. Absolute contraindications for the use of ipecac include altered mental status, ingestion of corrosive agents, and loss of protective airway reflexes.

Gastric Lavage

As with most methods of gastrointestinal decontamination, prompt administration of gastric lavage yields the highest efficacy. Gastric lavage can decrease the absorption of poisons by 10% to 25% if given within 30 to 60 minutes of the ingestion. However, it is a tedious and time-consuming procedure to perform and may actually facilitate adsorption by propelling tablets into the small intestine. Indications for gastric lavage include presentation to a health care facility within 1 hour of toxin ingestion or poisoning with a substance that is poorly absorbed by activated charcoal. Contraindications to gastric lavage include ingestion of a corrosive agent and a history of esophageal or gastric pathologic condition or surgery. Complications associated with gastric lavage include problems with placement of the orogastric tube into the trachea, esophageal perforation, aspiration, hypothermia, bleeding, cardiac arrhythmias, and hypoxia.

Techniques That Enhance Elimination

Urinary Alkalinization and Acidification

For a toxic ingestion, urinary alkalinization and acidification are two processes that can enhance renal clearance of a drug or toxin. The goal of altering the urinary pH is to shift the drug to its ionized form, thus inhibiting passive reabsorption in the tubule.

Before initiating alkaline diuresis, a basic metabolic panel, urinary pH, arterial pH, and serum concentration of the ingested toxin should be obtained to establish baseline parameters. Urinary alkalinization can be achieved by using intravenous 5% dextrose in water or 0.45% saline with one to three ampules of sodium bicarbonate (i.e., 50 to 150 mEq) added to each liter. The rate of infusion should initially be based on the volume status of the patient. After volume expansion, the rate of fluid replacement should match the urine output, with a goal of 2 to 3 mL/kg/hr and a urinary pH greater than 7.5. In patients with altered sensorium, a urinary catheter may be placed for accurate monitoring of urinary output. Serum electrolytes and urinary pH must be closely monitored every 2 to 3 hours during alkaline diuresis. The target range of urinary alkalinization is a pH value between 7.5 and 8.5. Urinary alkalinization effectively increases elimination of drugs such as phenobarbital, barbital, and salicylates. Complications of urinary alkalinization include hypokalemia, fluid overload, pulmonary edema, cerebral edema, hypernatremia (if free water restricted), and alkalemia. Alkalemia is a special concern in patients with renal dysfunction who are unable to excrete the bicarbonate load. Relative contraindications are congestive heart failure, renal failure, pulmonary edema, and cerebral edema.

Acid diuresis is effective in the elimination of amphetamines, fenfluramine, phencyclidine, and quinine. To achieve an acid diuresis, intravenous arginine (10 g) or lysine hydrochloride (10 g) is administered intravenously over 30 minutes, followed by oral ammonium chloride (4 g) every 2 hours. The goal of acid diuresis is a urinary pH of 5.5 to 6.5. However, acid diuresis has fallen out of favor due to its serious side effects including rhabdomyolysis and acute renal failure.

Antidotes
The management of certain poisonings requires the use of specific antidotes (Table 39–2). Although the use of antidotes may markedly diminish the mortality rate associated with certain

Table 39–2: Toxic Ingestions Treated with Specific Antidotes

Poison	Antidote
Acetaminophen	N-Acetylcysteine
β-Blocking agents	Glucagon, atropine, isoproterenol
Carbon monoxide	Oxygen
Cyanide	Sodium nitrite, sodium thiosulfate, oxygen
Digoxin	Digoxin-specific Fab antibody fragment
Ethylene glycol, methanol	Fomepizole and ethanol
Isoniazid	Pyridoxine
Metallic poisons	
Arsenic	Dimercaprol
Iron	Deferoxamine
Lead	Dimercaprol, edetate disodium calcium, penicillamine
Mercury	Dimercaprol, penicillamine
Nitrates, nitrites, phenacetin	Methylene blue
Opioids	Naloxone
Organophosphates	Atropine, pralidoxime
Benzodiazepines	Flumazenil

toxic exposures, no specific antidote is available for most toxic ingestions.

PRINCIPLES GOVERNING DRUG REMOVAL BY EXTRACORPOREAL TECHNIQUES

The clearance of a drug or toxin by extracorporeal therapy is determined by the pharmacokinetic and pharmacodynamic properties of the drug and by factors related to the extracorporeal technique itself. The factors that favor extracorporeal removal are outlined in Table 39–3.

EXTRACORPOREAL TECHNIQUES FOR DRUG REMOVAL

The indications for extracorporeal therapy in poisoning include the following:

- Clinical deterioration despite aggressive supportive therapy
- Ingestion of a dose that can cause toxicity or death if the agent can be removed at a rate that exceeds endogenous clearance
- Ingestion of a dose that can cause toxicity or death for which supportive therapy is ineffective

For any given drug, there is no absolute drug level that indicates when dialysis must be initiated; instead, the decision is based on the patient's clinical status and drug-related and dialysis-associated factors.

Table 39–3: Factors That Enhance Drug Removal by Extracorporeal Therapy

Drug-Related Factors	Dialysis-Related Factors
Low molecular weight (< 500 D)	Large surface area of dialysis membrane
Low protein binding (< 80%)	High-flux dialyzer
Low volume of distribution (< 1 L/kg)	High blood and dialysate flow
Water soluble	Increased ultrafiltration rate
Fast redistribution from peripheral compartments into blood	Increased time receiving dialysis

Hemodialysis

Characteristics of an ingested drug that make hemodialysis effective in toxin removal are the following:

- Low molecular weight (< 500 D)
- Small volume of distribution (< 1 L/kg)
- Low degree of protein binding
- High degree of water solubility

Choosing a dialyzer with a large surface area and increasing the blood flow and dialysate flow rates increase the clearance of low-molecular-weight toxins. High-flux dialyzers have more permeable membranes and can remove high-molecular-weight substances with greater efficiency. Drugs and chemicals that are removed by dialysis and hemoperfusion are listed in Table 39–4. After dialysis drug level rebound may occur as the drug redistributes from tissues into the plasma after its removal from the plasma compartment. It is important to check drug concentration levels and provide continued renal replacement therapy or repeated dialysis sessions if required. Acute hemodialysis requires cannulation, and a femoral approach is usually favored. A blood flow of more than 300 mL/min should be considered a minimum rate for efficient drug removal. The duration of the therapy is usually 4 to 8 hours but should be governed by the clinical response and serum drug concentrations. An additional benefit of hemodialysis is that it corrects any toxin-associated morbidities such as acute renal failure, pulmonary edema, and electrolyte disturbance.

Hemoperfusion

Hemoperfusion is a procedure that involves the passage of blood through an extracorporeal circuit with a disposable, sorbent-containing cartridge, typically activated charcoal or an exchange resin. Hemoperfusion is preferred when the toxin is lipid soluble

Table 39–4: Common Poisonings for Which Extracorporeal Therapy May Be Required

Hemodialysis	Hemoperfusion
Lithium	Theophylline
Ethylene glycol	Barbiturates
Methanol	Valproic acid
Isopropanol	
Salicylates	
Theophylline	
Valproic acid	

See text for specific indications.

or highly protein bound. The administration of hemoperfusion requires temporary vascular access through a double-lumen dialysis catheter and systemic anticoagulation. The blood flow rate should be maintained at more than 300 mL/min. Patients receiving hemoperfusion therapy must be monitored carefully for the following potential complications:

- Thrombocytopenia (typically a < 30% fall in platelet count; if the fall is higher, consider prostacyclin infusion)
- Transient leukopenia due to complement activation
- Hypofibrinogenemia
- Hypothermia
- Hypoglycemia

Many of these problems were associated with the type of cartridges used previously and have been overcome by coating of the charcoal with albumin cellulose nitrate. The principal disadvantage of hemoperfusion is the saturation of the adsorbent cartridge that occurs after 4 to 8 hours owing to clotting and adherence of cellular debris and plasma proteins to the adsorbent. The concurrent use of hemodialysis and hemoperfusion (hemoperfusion cartridge upstream of the dialyzer) is theoretically the optimal treatment in acute poisoning because it effectively removes toxin by adsorption and diffusion. However, hemodialysis-hemoperfusion is an expensive procedure, and the data on clinical outcomes are lacking.

Hemofiltration

Hemofiltration is a process in which solutes are removed by convection. Given the porosity of the membrane used, hemofiltration efficiently eliminates unbound high-molecular-weight toxins (40,000 D). Most poisons, however, are smaller, with a molecular size of less than 1000 D and thus hemofiltration does not offer much advantage over hemodialysis.

Continuous Renal Replacement Therapy/Peritoneal Dialysis/Plasma Exchange

Continuous renal replacement therapy is rarely used in patients with acute intoxication because of its low efficiency. However, continuous renal replacement therapy is advantageous when the ingested drug has a large volume of distribution and slow rate of redistribution from the peripheral tissue and has been used successfully to treat life-threatening lithium intoxication for which extended treatment time and gradual removal of intracellular lithium prevents postdialysis rebound. There is little role for peritoneal dialysis in acute poisoning, and it should only be considered when access to hemodialysis is not possible or contraindicated. The role of plasma exchange in acute poisoning is not well defined, but it may be considered for toxins that are highly protein bound (> 80%) and have low volumes of distribution (< 0.2 L/kg of body weight). One indication for plasma exchange is in the management of sodium chlorate poisoning, which causes hemolytic anemia. Plasma exchange removes sodium chlorate and eliminates red cell fragments and free hemoglobin.

INTOXICATIONS RESPONSIVE TO EXTRACORPOREAL THERAPY

Alcohols: Ethylene Glycol, Methanol, and Isopropanol

Intoxications with ethylene glycol, methanol, or isopropanol are associated with significant morbidity and mortality. These substances and their metabolites share several characteristics that make them ideal for removal by hemodialysis: low molecular weight, small volume of distribution, water solubility, and low levels of protein binding.

Ethylene Glycol

PHARMACOLOGY Ethylene glycol is a colorless, odorless, sweet-tasting substance most commonly found in antifreeze, solvents, hydraulic brake fluid, deicing solutions, detergents, lacquers, and polishes. It is rapidly absorbed by the gastrointestinal system, reaches a peak serum concentration 1 to 4 hours after ingestion, and has an elimination half-life of 3 hours. The accepted minimum lethal dose of ethylene glycol for an adult is 1 to 1.5 mL/kg.

METABOLISM Ethylene glycol itself is not toxic; instead, it is the accumulation of its metabolites that is responsible for its severe toxicity. Ethylene glycol is oxidized to glycoaldehyde by alcohol dehydrogenase. Aldehyde dehydrogenase then rapidly converts glycoaldehyde to glycolic acid, followed by the slow conversion of glycolic acid to glyoxylic acid; the final end products include oxalic acid, glycine, oxalomalic acid, and formic acid.

PATHOPHYSIOLOGY The underlying mechanisms of ethylene glycol toxicity are tissue destruction from calcium oxalate deposition and profound acidosis due to the accumulation of its metabolites (e.g., glycoaldehyde, glycolic acid, and lactate). In the kidney, reversible acute renal failure often develops.

CLINICAL PRESENTATION   The clinical course of ethylene glycol toxicity occurs in three phases:

Phase 1 is the neurologic phase, occurring 0.5 to 12 hours after ingestion and is characterized by inebriation without the odor of alcohol on the patient's breath. Nausea, vomiting, and hematemesis due to gastrointestinal irritation may be noted. As ethylene glycol undergoes metabolism to glycoaldehyde and glycolic acid (4 to 12 hours after ingestion), symptoms of CNS depression predominate. Altered consciousness may progress to coma and seizures in severe poisonings.

Phase 2 is the cardiopulmonary phase, occurring 12 to 24 hours after ingestion. During the second phase of ethylene glycol intoxication, calcium oxalate crystals deposit in the vasculature, myocardium, and lungs. Patients may develop tachycardia, mild hypertension, congestive heart failure, acute respiratory distress syndrome, severe metabolic acidosis, and multiorgan failure. Most deaths occur during this phase.

Phase 3 is the renal phase, occurring 24 to 72 hours after ingestion. In this final stage, calcium oxalate precipitates in the kidney, resulting in flank pain, acute tubular necrosis, hypocalcemia, microscopic hematuria, and oliguric acute renal failure.

With appropriate early medical intervention, ethylene glycol toxicity tends to resolve completely although permanent renal, CNS, and cranial nerve damage has been described.

DIAGNOSIS AND LABORATORY DATA   The diagnosis of ethylene glycol toxicity should be suspected in patients who present with the following features:

- Inebriation without the smell of alcohol
- Altered mental status
- High–anion gap metabolic acidosis/osmolal gap
- Hypocalcemia
- Calcium oxalate crystals in the urine (50% of patients, typically within 4 to 8 hours).

The osmolal gap is an extremely useful diagnostic tool in various alcohol intoxications. Because ethylene glycol is an osmotically active compound, it creates an osmolal gap. The osmolal gap is the difference between the measured osmolality, as determined by the freezing point depression method, and the calculated osmolality:

$$\Delta \, Osm_{gap} = Osm_{measured} - Osm_{calculated}$$

If coingestion of ethanol is suspected, the contribution of ethanol should be corrected for in the calculated osmolality as follows:

$$Osm_{calculated} \, (mOsm/kg) = 2[Na] + [glucose]/18 \\ + [blood \; urea \; nitrogen]/2.8 \\ + [ethanol]/4.6$$

The measured osmolality normally ranges between 270 and 290 mOsm/kg, and the normal osmolal gap is less than 10 to 12 mOsm/kg H_2O. An elevated osmolal gap suggests the presence of ethylene glycol, methanol, ethanol, isopropanol, propylene glycol, or acetone. It is important to recognize that, although an elevated osmolal gap is a significant clinical finding, a normal osmolal gap does not exclude the diagnosis of ethylene glycol or methanol poisoning. In the case of ethylene glycol toxicity, glycolic acid does not contribute to the osmolal gap, and patients who present later in the course of ethylene glycol intoxication may have a normal osmolal gap as the ethylene glycol is metabolized to glycolic acid.

TREATMENT The management of ethylene glycol intoxication includes aggressive fluid resuscitation to maintain urine output, correct dehydration, and prevent circulatory shock. Intravenous sodium bicarbonate should be administered if the serum bicarbonate concentration is less than 15 mEq/L or the arterial pH is less than 7.35. Seizures, which may be caused by hypocalcemia, should be controlled with standard anticonvulsant therapy. Asymptomatic hypocalcemia is not routinely used because it may exacerbate calcium oxalate crystal deposition. If seizures persist despite adequate anticonvulsant therapy, 10 to 20 mL of 10% calcium gluconate (0.2 to 0.3 mL/kg) can be infused slowly. The antidotes for ethylene glycol toxicity are ethanol and fomepizole. Indications for use of an antidote in ethylene glycol toxicity are (1) a plasma ethylene glycol concentration of more than 20 mg/dL, (2) documented recent ingestion of toxic amounts of ethylene glycol and an osmolal gap of more than 10 mOsm/L, or (3) a history or strong clinical suspicion of ethylene glycol poisoning and at least two of the following: arterial pH less than 7.3, serum bicarbonate level of less than 20 mEq/L, osmolal gap of more than 10 mOsm/L, or the presence of oxalate crystals in the urine. Ethanol can be given intravenously as 10% ethanol diluted in 5% dextrose in water. The loading dose of ethanol is 0.6 to 0.7 g of ethanol/kg (7.6 mL of 10% ethanol/kg), and the maintenance dose is 66 mg of ethanol/kg/hr (0.83 mL of 10% ethanol/kg/hr) for nondrinkers and 154 mg of ethanol/kg/hr (1.96 mL of 10% ethanol/kg/hr) for alcoholics. Serum ethanol concentrations should be monitored every 1 to 2 hours to ensure that blood levels remain therapeutic at 100 to 150 mg of ethanol/dL. Adverse effects of ethanol are hypoglycemia, inebriation, and CNS depression, which may mask the signs and symptoms of ethylene glycol toxicity.

Fomepizole (4-MP, 4-methylpyrazole) is a newer antidote that is a potent competitive inhibitor of alcohol dehydrogenase. Its use has largely replaced that of ethanol owing to its predictable pharmacokinetics and relatively few adverse effects. Adverse effects include headache, nausea, dizziness, eosinophilia, rash, tachycardia or bradycardia, and mild but transient elevation of the hepatic transaminases. Fomepizole is administered intravenously over 30 minutes. The loading dose of fomepizole is 15 mg/kg, followed by 10 mg/kg every 12 hours for four doses. After 48 hours, fomepizole is continued at 15 mg/kg every 12 hours until the ethylene glycol concentration is undetectable or less than 20 mg/dL and the patient is asymptomatic and has a normal arterial pH. During hemodialysis, the dosing interval must be changed to every 4 hours, or a constant infusion of 1 to 1.5 mg/kg/hr can be used to maintain adequate therapeutic levels of fomepizole.

Hemodialysis is an extremely effective method for the removal of ethylene glycol and its toxic metabolite, glycolic acid. The elimination half-life of ethylene glycol in patients receiving hemodialysis is 2.5 to 3.5 hours. Indications for hemodialysis are as follows: deteriorating clinical status despite supportive therapy, metabolic acidosis (arterial pH < 7.3), renal failure, or electrolyte abnormalities unresponsive to standard treatment.

Hemodialysis should be continued until the ethylene glycol level is undetectable or until it is less than 20 mg/dL, no metabolic acidosis is present, and no evidence of systemic toxicity persists. Rebound distribution of ethylene glycol may occur within 12 hours; therefore, serum osmolality and electrolytes should be monitored every 2 to 4 hours and treatment with ethanol or fomepizole continued for 24 hours after withdrawal of hemodialysis.

Methanol
PHARMACOLOGY   Methanol is a clear, colorless liquid used as a solvent, as an intermediate of chemical synthesis during various manufacturing processes, or as an octane booster in gasoline. Methanol is rapidly absorbed and distributed, with a mean absorption half-life of 5 minutes and mean distribution half-life of 8 minutes. Peak serum concentrations of methanol are reached within 30 to 60 minutes after ingestion, and the elimination

half-life (untreated) is 12 to 20 hours. The estimated minimum lethal dose is 10 mL, although this is highly variable.

METABOLISM Methanol is oxidized by alcohol dehydrogenase to formaldehyde, which is in turn rapidly metabolized to formic acid, the primary substance responsible for the toxicity of methanol poisoning.

CLINICAL PRESENTATION The *early stage* of methanol ingestion is characterized by CNS depression in which the patient appears inebriated and drowsy. This phase is mild and transient and is followed by a *latent interval* lasting 6 to 30 hours corresponding to the metabolism of methanol and the gradual accumulation of formic acid. There is no altered mental status during the latent interval, and the only presenting symptom may be blurred vision. In the *delayed stage* formic acid accumulates and systemic toxicity develops. The visual changes associated with methanol poisoning tend to occur rapidly and may include blurred vision, central scotoma, an impaired pupillary response to light, decreased visual acuity, photophobia, visual field defects, or progression to complete blindness. The visual abnormalities do not resolve in 25% to 33% of patients. The CNS effects of mild to moderate methanol toxicity are headache, vertigo, delirium, lethargy, restlessness, and confusion and coma and seizures in severe cases. Other symptoms during the delayed phase include nausea, vomiting, diarrhea, and abdominal pain from acute pancreatitis. Rarely, myoglobinuric acute renal failure may develop. Poor prognostic signs include severe metabolic acidosis, elevated formic acid levels, bradycardia, cardiovascular shock, anuria, and seizures or coma at presentation.

DIAGNOSIS AND LABORATORY DATA A methanol overdose should be considered in patients who present with visual changes, abdominal pain, high–anion gap metabolic acidosis, and an elevated osmolal gap. An osmolal gap is apparent during the early and latent phases of intoxication. During the delayed stage, as methanol is metabolized to formic acid, the osmolal gap may return to normal because formic acid is not osmotically active and a normal osmolal gap does not exclude the diagnosis of methanol poisoning. Other laboratory abnormalities include increased serum amylase levels due to parotitis or pancreatitis.

TREATMENT Once supportive care is initiated, treatment focuses on prevention of ocular toxicity, seizures, and coma due to the accumulation of the toxic metabolites formic acid and formaldehyde. Metabolic acidosis (pH < 7.3) is treated aggressively with sodium bicarbonate therapy, because the severity of intoxication and clinical outcome correlate with the degree of acidosis.

The rate-limiting step of methanol metabolism is mediated by 10-formyl tetrahydrofolate synthetase, which is folic acid dependent and administration of folic acid (50 mg given intravenously every 4 hours for five doses and then once daily) may increase the metabolism of formic acid to carbon dioxide and water. Other measures include aggressive intravenous fluid support to maintain adequate urine output, and control of seizures with standard anticonvulsants. As in the treatment of ethylene glycol poisoning, inhibitors of alcohol dehydrogenase, ethanol and fomepizole, are used in methanol intoxication, and treatment should be initiated without delay. The indications for the use of antidotes in methanol overdose are plasma methanol concentration greater than 20 mg/dL, documented recent ingestion of toxic amounts of methanol and osmolal gap of more than 10 mOsm/kg of H_2O, or a history or strong clinical suspicion of methanol poisoning and at least two of the following: arterial pH less than 7.3, a serum bicarbonate level less than 20 mEq/L (mmol/L), or an osmolal gap more than 10 mOsm/kg of H_2O. The doses and route of administration are identical to those used in ethylene glycol in toxication (see earlier).

Hemodialysis in methanol toxicity is indicated for the following: serum methanol levels higher than 50 mg/dL, metabolic acidosis (pH < 7.30), visual changes, dose of ingested methanol of more than 30 mL, seizures, deteriorating clinical status despite supportive therapy, renal failure, or electrolyte abnormalities not responsive to standard therapy. Because methanol overdose is associated with an increased frequency of intracerebral hemorrhage, the use of heparin during hemodialysis should be minimized. A methanol concentration of more than 50 mg/dL is no longer an absolute indication for hemodialysis because fomepizole may be used as first-line treatment of methanol poisoning. Hemodialysis is continued until the serum methanol concentration is undetectable or until the methanol level is less than 25 mg/dL and the anion gap metabolic acidosis and osmolal gap are normal. The presence of visual changes is not an indication for continued dialysis. Close monitoring of the serum osmolality and electrolytes should be continued every 2 to 4 hours for 12 to 36 hours after hemodialysis to detect rebound. Fomepizole or ethanol therapy should be continued for several hours after withdrawal of hemodialysis, until methanol levels are undetectable or less than 20 mg/dL with resolution of acidosis and symptoms.

Isopropanol

PHARMACOLOGY Isopropanol (i.e., isopropyl alcohol) is a clear, colorless, bitter liquid commonly found in "rubbing alcohol," skin lotion, hair tonics, aftershave lotion, denatured alcohol, solvents, cements, cleaning products and deicers. Intoxication may occur through ingestion or inhalation of vapors, especially in infants. Isopropanol is rapidly absorbed by the gastrointestinal system and reaches a peak serum concentration 15 to 30 minutes after ingestion with an elimination half-life of 3 to 7 hours. Isopropanol is water soluble, has a molecular weight of 60 g/mol, and has a volume of distribution equivalent to that of water ($V_d = 0.6$ L/kg). Isopropanol is directly responsible for the toxic effects observed, and delaying the metabolism of isopropanol, therefore, is not considered a beneficial method of treatment. It is converted to acetone by alcohol dehydrogenase, which is then excreted in the urine and breath. The lethal dose ranges from 150 to 240 mL, although patients may become symptomatic with doses as low as 20 mL.

CLINICAL PRESENTATION   Clinical symptoms tend to appear within 1 hour of ingestion and include confusion, headache, lethargy, and dizziness progressing to ataxia, coma, and respiratory arrest with severe poisoning. Gastrointestinal effects include nausea, vomiting, and abdominal pain. Hypotension is often severe and is caused by multiple factors, including cardiac depression, arrhythmias from cardiomyopathy (myocyte toxicity), vasodilation, dehydration, and gastrointestinal bleeding. Hypotension is the strongest predictor of death in isopropanol overdose patients.

DIAGNOSIS AND LABORATORY DATA   The diagnosis of isopropanol overdose should be suspected in any patient presenting with altered sensorium, an acetone smell on the breath, an elevated osmolal gap, and acetonemia or acetonuria (i.e., positive sodium nitroprusside reaction in serum or urine) in the absence of hyperglycemia, glycosuria, or acidosis. Acetone is not an organic acid; therefore, there is no elevated anion gap metabolic acidosis unless poor tissue perfusion due to hypotension triggers lactic acid accumulation. Other laboratory abnormalities observed include hypoglycemia and elevated serum creatinine and creatine kinase levels.

TREATMENT   Treatment for isopropanol toxicity focuses on appropriate supportive therapy. Agents that inhibit alcohol dehydrogenase are not used in the treatment of isopropanol poisoning. Intravenous fluids and pressors should be given if hypotension is present. Mechanical ventilation may be indicated for respiratory distress and airway protection. Activated charcoal is highly effective in preventing systemic absorption of isopropanol. Hemodialysis is usually unnecessary, except in severe poisoning.

Indications for hemodialysis include an isopropanol level of more than 400 mg/dL, prolonged coma, hypotension, myocardial depression or tachyarrhythmias, and renal failure.

Lithium

PHARMACOLOGY   Lithium is rapidly and completely absorbed in the upper gastrointestinal tract. After a single oral dose, peak serum levels occur in 1 to 2 hours, and the drug is widely distributed in the body water. It is poorly bound to protein and has a low molecular weight (7 D) and small volume of distribution (0.6 L/kg). Lithium is predominantly located intracellularly and diffuses slowly across cell membranes, making its removal by extracorporeal therapy a slow process.

CLINICAL PRESENTATION   With acute lithium poisoning (e.g., accidental overdose in a child) there is generally less risk of mortality and patients have milder symptoms than those observed in chronic intoxication because the elimination half-life is shorter in lithium-naïve individuals. Chronic intoxication may develop because of inappropriate dose adjustments or in states of sodium retention (e.g., congestive heart failure, cirrhosis, or gastrointestinal losses). The severity of chronic lithium intoxication correlates directly with the serum lithium concentration and may be categorized as mild (1.5 to 2 mEq/L), moderate (2 to 2.5 mEq/L), or severe (> 2.5 mEq/L). The most common manifestation of acute lithium toxicity is altered mental status; other symptoms include nausea, vomiting, and weakness. Severe toxicity, which can be life threatening, is associated with seizures, cardiac arrhythmias, hyperreflexia, coma, and death.

DIAGNOSIS AND TREATMENT   In clinical situations in which lithium excretion is decreased (e.g., volume depletion), the serum lithium concentration should be monitored closely to avoid accumulation to toxic levels. The initial management of acute lithium intoxication involves supportive care, prevention of further absorption, and enhancement of lithium elimination. A nasogastric tube may be placed, followed by gastric lavage. One of the major initial steps in lithium intoxication is volume resuscitation using half-normal saline. Administration of hypotonic fluid is especially important in patients with underlying lithium-induced diabetes insipidus because intravenous administration of normal saline may precipitate hypernatremia. Because lithium is mainly located intracellularly, removal by hemodialysis is inefficient, and dialysis therapy may need to be extended to 8 to 12 hours to prevent postdialysis rebound. Indications for dialysis are as follows: (1) serum lithium level of more than 4 mEq/L regardless of the clinical status; (2) plasma lithium concentration of more than 2.5 mEq/L with neurologic symptoms or renal insufficiency; (3) plasma concentration of more than 2.5 mEq/L in asymptomatic patients with increasing lithium levels after admission; or (4) a plasma concentration of less than 2.5 mEq/L in patients with end-stage renal disease.

Salicylates

PHARMACOLOGY   Salicylates are ubiquitous agents found in many over-the-counter medications and prescription drugs, the most common of which is aspirin (i.e., acetylsalicylic acid). In the liver, acetylsalicylic acid is initially hydrolyzed to salicylic acid and then glycinated to salicyluric acid, which is easily excreted by the kidneys. After intoxication levels rise rapidly as protein-binding sites and renal excretory mechanism become saturated, resulting in an increase in the volume of distribution and drug half-life from 3 to 12 hours up to 15 to 36 hours.

PATHOPHYSIOLOGY OF ACID-BASE ABNORMALITIES   Salicylate is a relatively strong acid and therefore contributes to the development of a high–anion gap metabolic acidosis as does salicylate-induced uncoupling of mitochondrial oxidative phosphorylation, and inhibition of the tricarboxylic acid cycle, which causes an increase in pyruvic acid and lactic acid production. A mixed acid-base disturbance predominates in 40% to 50% of patients because salicylates trigger a respiratory alkalosis by directly stimulating the respiratory center of the brain. An isolated metabolic acidosis is rare in adults but is a common finding in the pediatric population.

CLINICAL PRESENTATION   The clinical manifestations of salicylate toxicity typically occur 3 to 6 hours after ingestion and include disturbances of several organ systems, including the CNS, cardiovascular, pulmonary, hepatic, and renal systems. In severe intoxication, acute CNS abnormalities such as agitation, confusion, seizures, stupor, and coma are common. Patients may also present with nausea, vomiting, fever, tinnitus, and hyperventilation. Noncardiogenic pulmonary edema results from increased capillary permeability and is observed in adult and elderly patients with chronic intoxication. Inhibition of prostaglandin synthesis can cause vasoconstriction within the kidney, resulting in oliguric acute renal failure. The overall severity of salicylate toxicity can be determined using three parameters: dose ingested (< 150 mg/kg portends a benign course), clinical presentation, and serum salicylate concentration. Mild toxicity is seen with serum salicylate levels of 300 to 500 mg/L 6 hours after ingestion, moderate toxicity with 500 to 700 mg/L, and severe toxicity with 750 mg/L or higher.

DIAGNOSIS AND LABORATORY DATA   Salicylate poisoning should be suspected in patients presenting with hyperventilation, diaphoresis, tinnitus, and unexplained acid-base disturbances. Salicylate levels should be monitored every 3 to 4 hours until clinical improvement is observed or until a downward trend in the plasma level is documented. The ingestion of enteric-coated products may delay gastrointestinal absorption, thereby necessitating continuous monitoring of the patient and the plasma salicylate concentrations. The serum Phenistix or urine ferric chloride test may be used to rapidly diagnose salicylate poisoning. The classic mixed acid-base disorder is more common in adults, and the metabolic acidosis tends to be more severe in pediatric patients and in patients with severe toxicity. Hypernatremia results from the insensible loss of free water due to increased metabolism, hyperpyrexia, and hyperventilation. Symptomatic hypokalemia, the consequence of intracellular shifting and urinary potassium wasting, is observed in severe toxicity.

TREATMENT   The use of gastric lavage is controversial, but it may be of benefit if administered within 1 hour of ingestion. Activated charcoal (50 g or 1 g/kg) is effective in reducing gut absorption in mild or moderate toxicity and should be repeated if salicylate levels continue in an upward trend because gut adsorption may be delayed. In mild or moderate toxicity, urinary alkalinization (urine pH > 7.5) enhances renal excretion. An alkaline diuresis can be achieved by adding three ampules of sodium bicarbonate to 1 L of 5% dextrose in water and infusing at a rate of 200 to 250 mL/hr, depending on the patient's volume status. Adequate renal function is necessary for urinary alkalinization to be effective in its elimination of the bicarbonate load. Frequent monitoring of electrolytes, volume status, and urinary pH is mandatory. Hemodialysis is indicated for the clinical signs of severe salicylate toxicity, levels greater than 700 mg/L, or contraindications to conservative management.

Theophylline

PHARMACOLOGY   The therapeutic index of theophylline is very narrow, with a range of 10 to 20 mg/L, and clinical manifestations of theophylline toxicity may be seen at levels as low as 15 mg/L.

CLINICAL PRESENTATION   Mild theophylline intoxication is characterized by nervousness, tremors, tachycardia, abdominal pain, vomiting, and diarrhea. In moderate toxicity, patients are often lethargic and disoriented and exhibit cardiovascular tachyarrhythmias. Severe intoxication is characterized by ventricular tachycardias, seizures, and rhabdomyolysis. The seizures are typically generalized, although focal signs such as lip smacking and ocular deviation may occur. Seizure activity portends a poor prognosis and is often resistant to standard anticonvulsant therapy.

LABORATORY DATA Hypokalemia resulting from a catecholamine-induced intracellular transport of potassium is the most common and although the serum potassium may be profoundly low at the time of presentation, the total body stores of potassium are preserved and return to normal with a reduction in the theophylline concentration. Hyperglycemia, hypomagnesemia, hypophosphatemia, and hypercalcemia are commonly observed. Respiratory alkalosis results from the direct stimulation of the central respiratory center.

TREATMENT Multiple-dose activated charcoal accelerates theophylline clearance and decreases the serum elimination half-life from 7 to 20 hours to 1 to 3 hours. Activated charcoal (50 g or 1 g/kg) should be administered every 4 hours until the serum level is less than 20 mg/L. β-Blockade is a useful adjunct to control tachyarrhythmias. Seizures associated with theophylline toxicity are usually difficult to control and occasionally require general anesthesia. Indications for hemoperfusion are as follows:

- Clinical signs of severe toxicity (cardiac arrhythmias or seizure activity)
- Serum levels greater than 100 mg/L in acute intoxication or 40 mg/L in chronic poisoning

Relative indications include an inability to tolerate activated charcoal, congestive heart failure, and liver disease because metabolism of theophylline is impaired in these situations. If hemoperfusion is not readily available then high-flux hemodialysis should be initiated. Treatment should be continued until clinical signs improve and serum levels are less than 25 mg/L. Special care should be used when sustained-release preparations have been ingested because peak adsorption may be delayed for up to 15 hours.

Valproic Acid

PHARMACOLOGY AND PATHOPHYSIOLOGY Valproic acid (VPA) is an anticonvulsant drug used in several neurologic conditions such as bipolar affective disorder and migraine headaches. Acute VPA intoxication is usually self-limiting, although serious toxicity and deaths have been reported.

CLINICAL PRESENTATION Clinical manifestations of VPA toxicity include coma, severe respiratory depression, hypotension, tachycardia, and death. Common metabolic disorders in acute overdose include hypernatremia, hyperosmolality, hypocalcemia, high–anion gap metabolic acidosis, elevated serum aminotransferase levels, and hyperammonemia.

DIAGNOSIS AND TREATMENT After hemodynamic stabilization, the mainstay of treatment is gastrointestinal tract decontamination with activated charcoal. Charcoal is effective only if it is administered soon after VPA ingestion. Single-dose activated charcoal alone is usually sufficient for most VPA overdoses, and its administration is recommended for all patients. In severe poisoning, removal by extracorporeal therapy may be considered because VPA is a relatively small molecule, is water soluble, and has a low volume of distribution. Severe poisoning should be managed by hemodialysis because this clears the VPA as efficiently as hemoperfusion but also corrects any coincident electrolyte and acid base disorders.

VIII

Renal Transplantation

Clinical Aspects of Renal Transplantation

40

Renal transplantation is the treatment of choice for many patients with end-stage renal disease and is associated with significant improvements in both life expectancy and quality of life for successful transplants. The development of novel immunosuppressive agents allied with improved care for transplant recipients has resulted in significant improvements in both short- and long-term allograft survival rates over the last two decades.

THE RENAL TRANSPLANT PROCEDURE

In adult recipients the donor kidney is transplanted into the extraperitoneal space of the right or left lower abdominal quadrant. Laparoscopic retrieval of kidneys from donors for living donor transplantation is being increasingly used but is associated with an increased incidence of early graft dysfunction. Major surgical complications of renal transplantation are rare but can include major vessel injury. Perinephric lymphoceles occur in up to 15% of transplant recipients and can compress the ureter or the iliac veins or simply cause localized abdominal swelling that may require either percutaneous or internal drainage (marsupialization). The differential diagnosis of a peritransplant fluid collection also includes seroma, hematoma, and urinoma. In a functioning kidney, the fluid creatinine level is higher than the serum level in the presence of a urinoma, distinguishing it from a lymphocele.

CURRENTLY USED IMMUNOSUPPRESSIVE AGENTS IN RENAL TRANSPLANTATION

Overview

The T lymphocyte is the primary target of most immunosuppressive strategies. Currently used agents are classified as follows:

- Mono- or polyclonal anti–T-cell antibodies
- Calcineurin inhibitors (CNIs): cyclosporine and tacrolimus (FK506)
- Glucocorticoids
- Inhibitors of purine synthesis: azathioprine and mycophenolic mofetil (MMF)
- Target of rapamycin (Tor) inhibitors: sirolimus (rapamycin)

The risk of rejection is greatest in the early post-transplant period; hence, maximal immunosuppressive therapy is given at this time and is tapered in the weeks and months thereafter. Combination therapy is used to achieve adequate immunosuppression while drug-related toxicity is minimized. The choice of agents used depends on patient-specific factors such as susceptibility to toxicity and risk of rejection.

Mono- and Poly-clonal Antilymphocyte Antibodies

The available antilymphocyte antibodies include the murine monoclonal antibody OKT3 and polyclonal horse or rabbit antihuman T-cell antibodies, antithymocyte globulin and thymoglobulin, respectively. These are powerful immunosuppressive agents useful in the immediate post-transplant period in patients who have a high risk of acute rejection or who have delayed graft function (DGF). They are also widely used for the reversal of severe acute cellular rejection. Their use results in a rapid and prolonged depletion (months) of circulating T lymphocytes and is associated with a higher incidence of opportunistic infection and post-transplant lymphoproliferative disorder.

Humanized/Chimeric Antiinterleukin-2 Receptor Monoclonal Antibodies

These agents bind to the interleukin-2 receptor on activated T cells, resulting in the clearance of this cell population from the circulation. They are well tolerated with minimal short-term side effects. Randomized, controlled trials have demonstrated a 30% reduction in acute rejection rates with daclizumab or basiliximab compared with placebo. They are indicated only for induction immunosuppression and not for the reversal of acute cellular rejection.

Calcineurin Inhibitors: Cyclosporine

Cyclosporine is a calcineurin inhibitor that prevents T-lymphocyte activation. Important adverse effects include acute and chronic nephrotoxicity, hypertension, hyperlipidemia, glucose intolerance, hirsutism, and gum hypertrophy. The incidence of myositis in cyclosporine-treated patients receiving 3-hydroxy-3 methylglutaryl-coenzyme A reductase inhibitors may be as high as 10% with lovastatin or simvastatin. It appears that pravastatin is associated with a much lower risk of muscle damage and therefore is the lipid-lowering agent of choice in this setting. Trough blood concentrations have traditionally been used to guide dosing and avoid acute nephrotoxicity. Cyclosporine (and tacrolimus) is metabolized by the intestinal and hepatic cytochrome P-450 systems; drugs that induce or inhibit these systems should be used with caution and appropriate therapeutic drug monitoring (Table 40–1).

Tacrolimus (FK-506)

Tacrolimus is structurally distinct from cyclosporine; however, its mechanism of action is similar, and both agents have

---

Table 40–1: Important Cyclosporine/Tacrolimus Drug Interactions

Inhibitors of cyclosporine/tacrolimus metabolism
Antibiotics
  Clarithromycin, erythromycin, norfloxacin
Antifungal agents
  Voriconazole, fluconazole, itraconazole, ketoconazole
Calcium channel blockers
  Diltiazem, nicardipine, verapamil
Others
  Bromocriptine, amiodarone, metoclopramide, cimetidine,
    grapefruit juice, nefazodone, nevirapine, propoxyphene,
    quinupristin-dalfopristin, zafirlukast, zileuton, danazol
Promotors of cyclosporine/tacrolimus metabolism
Antibiotics
  Rifampin, nafcillin
Anticonvulsants
  Carbamazepine, phenobarbital, phenytoin
Others
  Ticlopidine

equivalent nephrotoxicity. Clinically relevant advantages of tacrolimus over cyclosporine include lower rates of acute rejection, better lipid and blood pressure control, and less incidence of hirsutism. Neurotoxicity, alopecia, diarrhea (especially in combination with MMF), and post-transplant diabetes are more common with tacrolimus. In general, treatment with cyclosporine is switched to tacrolimus if patients have an episode of acute rejection or if hyperlipidemia, hypertension, or hirsutism is a concern. There is emerging evidence that medium-term renal allograft survival may be better with tacrolimus than with cyclosporine.

Azathioprine

Azathioprine is a purine analog that inhibits the proliferation of T and B lymphocytes. Leukopenia is the most common side effect, but at doses of 1 or 2 mg/kg/day, azathioprine is usually well tolerated. It has been widely used in clinical transplantation for 30 years, but its role in maintenance therapy is being superseded by MMF. Azathioprine is inactivated by xanthine oxidase, and concomitant use of allopurinol can lead to life-threatening bone marrow suppression and should be avoided.

Mycophenolate Mofetil

MMF is a reversible inhibitor of inosine monophosphate dehydrogenase, the rate-limiting enzyme in de novo purine synthesis. Lymphocytes are uniquely dependent on this pathway for synthesis of guanosine nucleotides and subsequent cell proliferation. The principal adverse effects are nausea, vomiting, and diarrhea that usually respond to dose reduction. Nephrotoxicity is not a concern. The combination of MMF and tacrolimus is highly effective in preventing acute rejection but is associated with a high incidence of diarrhea due to the higher MMF plasma concentrations obtained when the drug is administered with tacrolimus.

Glucocorticoids

Glucocorticoids are widely used in the induction and maintenance of immunosuppression. Their dosage is progressively decreased after transplantation to a maintenance regimen of prednisone 5 to 10 mg/day. Adverse sequelae include hyperlipidemia, hypertension, glucose intolerance, and osteoporosis. Glucocorticoid withdrawal has been associated with increases in the risk of short-term and long-term graft dysfunction. Results from newer "steroid minimization" protocols incorporating various combinations of thymoglobulin, tacrolimus, MMF, and sirolimus are encouraging, but adequate long-term data are not yet available.

Sirolimus

Sirolimus (rapamycin) is a novel immunosuppressive agent that impairs cytokine-induced lymphocyte proliferation. The prolonged half-life of sirolimus means that once-daily dosing is sufficient. It is metabolized via the cytochrome P-450 system; thus, the potential for multiple drug interactions exists. Adverse effects of sirolimus include hyperlipidemia, anemia, thrombocytopenia, diarrhea, and interstitial pneumonitis. Data on long-term outcomes with sirolimus are not yet available.

EVALUATION OF THE RECIPIENT IMMEDIATELY BEFORE TRANSPLANTATION

Medical Status

The potential recipient of a renal transplant should be evaluated to ensure that there are no new contraindications to transplantation or general anesthesia. A key decision is whether or not hemodialysis, with the attendant delay of surgery and prolongation of cold ischemia time, is required. Preoperative hemodialysis is advisable if either a plasma K^+ level higher than 5.5 mmol/L or severe volume overload is present. Patients receiving peritoneal dialysis need only have instilled fluid drained out before surgery; if the patient is hyperkalemic, several rapid exchanges can be performed.

Immunologic Status

A pretransplant crossmatch of a recent recipient serum sample against donor lymphocytes must always be performed to detect preformed antibodies against donor human leukocyte antigens (HLA). The presence of cytotoxic donor immunoglobulin (Ig) G antibodies is a contraindication to transplantation. For immunologically "high-risk" patients (Table 40–2), flow cytometry crossmatching, which can detect low concentrations of antidonor antibodies may be performed. In such patients, a negative antihuman globulin crossmatch but positive flow cytometry crossmatching against donor T cells is a relative contraindication to transplantation. In this setting the decision to proceed with transplantation must be weighed against the higher risk of early acute cellular or antibody-mediated rejection.

Table 40–2: Factors Suggesting That a Recipient Has a High Risk for Acute Rejection

Previous blood transfusions, particularly if recent
Previous pregnancies, particularly if multiple
Previous allograft, particularly if rejected early
History of high panel-reactive antigen
Black race

CLINICAL APPROACH TO ALLOGRAFT DYSFUNCTION

Immediate Post-Transplant Period

Evaluation of the Recipient Immediately after the Transplant

The physician should carefully review the operating room notes with particular emphasis on the following: cold and warm ischemia times, technical difficulties encountered, intraoperative fluid balance, blood pressure, and urine output. Patients can be divided into three groups based on allograft function in the first postoperative week: those with excellent graft function as manifested by a brisk urine output and falling creatinine, those with slow graft function (SGF) (serum creatinine level > 3 mg/dL but dialysis independent at 1 week); and those with DGF (initial failure of allograft function). The causes, management, and outcomes for slow graft function are similar to those for DGF.

Delayed Graft Function

DGF is a clinical diagnosis based on the failure of the renal allograft to function in the first week post-transplant. Risk factors include male sex, black race, a high level of panel reactive antibodies, prolonged cold ischemia time, and nontraumatic death in the donor. The causes of DGF are listed below:

• Ischemic/nephrotoxic acute tubular necrosis (ATN)
• Hyperacute or accelerated acute rejection
• Major surgical complication (vascular thrombosis, ureteric obstruction, or leak)

The diagnosis of the underlying cause of DGF is based on clinical, radiologic, and sometimes histologic findings. Ischemic ATN is the most common cause of DGF in cadaveric kidney transplant recipients. In the absence of a renal biopsy, ischemic ATN can only be diagnosed when radiologic studies have excluded obstruction and confirmed allograft perfusion. ATN is uncommon after living-donor renal transplantation and persistent oliguria despite adequate volume expansion (with or without diuretics) suggests a major surgical complication (renal vein thrombosis or urine leak) that may warrant early surgical re-exploration. Management of ATN is supportive and includes judicious volume management, nutritional support, and renal replacement as required. Calcineurin avoidance with substitution of polyclonal antilymphocyte preparations has been advocated as a means of shortening the clinical course of postoperative ATN. The use of sorbitol-based ion-exchange resins in the management of hyperkalemia should be avoided in the early postoperative period because of the risk of colonic dilation and perforation. Hemodialysis may exacerbate ischemic damage to the allograft and therefore is typically used only if medically imperative. Acute rejection is more common after ATN, and a renal allograft biopsy is often required to exclude untreated acute rejection. Renal function in ischemic ATN typically recovers over 5 to 7 days, but recovery may be delayed for several weeks.

Hyperacute rejection is now a rare cause of primary renal allograft. It is caused by preformed recipient antibodies directed against the ABO blood group or HLA class I antigens. In classic hyperacute rejection, macroscopic changes are seen minutes after vascular anastomosis is established. Clinically, there is cyanosis and mottling of the kidney, anuria, and sometimes disseminated intravascular coagulopathy. Screening for recipient-donor ABO or class I major histocompatibility complex (MHC) incompatibility has ensured that hyperacute rejection is now uncommon. More commonly antibody-mediated acute rejection occurring early in the post-transplant course is triggered by newly synthesized antibodies directed against donor alloantigens (humoral/antibody-mediated rejection). Pretransplant lymphocytotoxicity crossmatch may miss low-level antidonor alloantibodies generated by memory B cells. The diagnosis is made by renal biopsy and a positive repeat donor-recipient crossmatch. Peritubular staining of capillaries for C4d has been proposed as a reliable marker of acute humoral rejection. Early diagnosis of this condition is crucial, and high-risk patients with DGF should have a renal allograft biopsy and repeat crossmatch studies performed 3 to 5 days after transplantation. A regimen of plasmapheresis (to immediately remove donor-specific antibodies) and enhanced immunosuppression including MMF and tacrolimus (to suppress further production of donor-specific antibodies) is now yielding excellent results.

Transplant renal artery or renal vein thrombosis usually occurs within 72 hours after transplantation and is the most common cause of graft loss in the first post-transplant week. Renal artery thrombosis presents with abrupt onset of anuria, a rapidly rising plasma creatinine level, but often little localized graft pain or discomfort. Radiologic studies show absent arterial and venous blood flow, and transplant nephrectomy is indicated. Renal vein thrombosis has a similar presentation but is often accompanied by allograft discomfort. Meticulous surgical technique and avoidance of hypovolemia can minimize the incidence of this devastating complication.

The importance of ischemic injury in cadaveric renal transplantation is emphasized by the impressive graft survival outcomes in living nonrelated donor transplantation for which ischemic times are short but HLA matching is often suboptimal. DGF is an independent predictor of long-term graft loss and lowers the expected graft half-life by one third. Measures to limit the incidence and duration of DGF include optimization of the hemodynamic status of the donor and recipient. Avoidance of postoperative hypotension and minimization of exposure to nephrotoxins, especially radiocontrast material, is essential. No specific intervention, including the administration of dopamine or loop diuretics, has been shown to have a clinical benefit. DGF associated with ATN is likely to remain a significant problem in cadaveric kidney transplantation as the use of marginal donors increases. An algorithm for managing DGF is given in Figure 40–1.

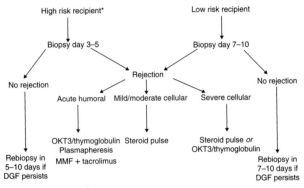

Figure 40–1. Algorithm for diagnostic biopsy of and treatment for persistent delayed graft function (DGF). *The presence of anti-donor HLA antibodies should prompt an immediate biopsy in these patients.

Table 40–3: Causes of Allograft Dysfunction in the Early Postoperative Period

Prerenal
    Hypovolemia/hypotension
    Renal vessel thrombosis
    Drugs: angiotensin-converting enzyme inhibitors, NSAIDs
    Transplant renal artery stenosis
Intrarenal
    Acute rejection
    Acute CNI nephrotoxicity
    CNI-induced thrombotic microangiopathy
    Recurrence of primary disease
    Acute pyelonephritis
    Acute interstitial nephritis
Postrenal
    Urinary tract obstruction/leakage

CNI, calcineurin inhibitor; NSAIDs, nonsteroidal anti-inflammatory drugs.

Prerenal Dysfunction in the Early Post-Transplant Period

Table 40–3 shows the causes of allograft dysfunction during the early (1- to 12-week) post-transplant period.

Hypovolemia

ARF due to hypovolemia may develop from a variety of factors including diminished oral intake, excessive diuresis from the transplanted kidney, or MMF-induced diarrhea. The effects of volume depletion are often compounded by CNI-induced renal vasoconstriction, which further impairs the glomerular filtration rate. Angiotensin-converting enzyme (ACE) inhibitors and non-steroidal anti-inflammatory drugs (NSAIDs) also exacerbate prerenal ARF and should be avoided in the early post-transplant period. Management involves careful reduction of MMF dosage if diarrhea is problematic and oral or intravenous volume expansion.

Acute Calcineurin Inhibitor Nephrotoxicity

CNIs cause an acute reversible decrease in renal plasma flow and glomerular filtration rate mediated by afferent arteriolar vasoconstriction. This is manifested by a blood concentration–dependent increase in plasma creatinine level that responds to dose reduction. On occasion this may occur as a result of the introduction of a medication that interferes with CNI metabolism (see Table 40–1). Conversely, drugs that induce the cytochrome P-450 system can lead to subtherapeutic drug levels with resultant acute rejection episodes. Histologic changes associated with CNI toxicity include tubule and myocyte vacuolization. Clinical findings suggesting acute CNI nephrotoxicity include the following:

- Extrarenal toxicity such as severe tremor
- Moderate increase in plasma creatinine (< 20% over baseline)
- High CNI concentrations (e.g., cyclosporine level > 350 ng/mL or tacrolimus level > 20 ng/mL)

An algorithm for approaching allograft dysfunction in the early post-transplant period is shown in Figure 40–2. The threshold for biopsy should be low in patients with a high risk of rejection, given the risks associated with delayed treatment of undiagnosed acute rejection.

Acute Rejection

Acute rejection is the most common cause of graft dysfunction in the early post-transplant period and is strongly associated with development of chronic rejection and poorer allograft survival rates. An increase in serum creatinine (typically > 20%) is

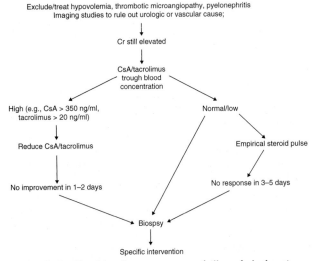

Figure 40–2. Algorithm for management of allograft dysfunction in the early post-transplant period. CR, creatinine; CsA, cyclosporine.

the cardinal sign of acute rejection. With current immunosuppression regimens clinical symptoms (pain, fever, or oliguria) are rare. Definitive diagnosis requires biopsy, but if there is a high likelihood of uncomplicated acute rejection, empirical treatment is sometimes instituted before biopsy. Uncomplicated acute cellular rejection is generally treated with a short course of high-dose intravenous corticosteroid (500 to 1000 mg of methylprednisolone daily for 3 to 5 days). The use of OKT3 or polyclonal antilymphocyte antibody preparations is reserved for steroid-resistant rejection or when there is evidence of severe rejection (endothelialitis) on the initial biopsy (20% to 30% of patients). Treatment of acute rejection with OKT3 may be associated with an increase in plasma creatinine 3 to 4 days into the course due to increased cytokine release. After reversal of rejection, patient compliance with prescribed medications should be reviewed, and if there are no contraindications, baseline immunosuppression should be adjusted. Acute rejection refractory to antibody therapy is associated with very poor allograft outcomes. Uncontrolled studies suggest that tacrolimus and MMF may be beneficial as "rescue" therapy in this setting.

Acute rejection is less common after the first 6 months post-transplantation, and when it occurs it may reflect either patient noncompliance or the inadvertent introduction of an inducer of the cytochrome P-450 system (see Table 40–1). Risk factors for noncompliance include younger age, immunosuppressive-related side effects, lower socioeconomic status, minority status, and psychologic stress or illness. Late acute rejection has a particularly deleterious effect on long-term graft outcome.

Thrombotic Microangiopathy

Thrombotic microangiopathy after renal transplantation is a rare but serious complication. Laboratory findings include a rising plasma creatinine level, thrombocytopenia, anemia, and the presence of schistocytes on the blood film. CNIs and, to a lesser extent, other factors (e.g., OKT3, viral infection, and the antiphospholipid syndrome) are associated with development of this syndrome. Onset usually is seen in the early post-transplant period. The long-term prognosis for graft function is often poor, and early diagnosis and intervention are essential. There have been no prospective controlled trials of therapy in post-transplant thrombotic microangiopathy. Suggested measures include cessation of CNI therapy and tight control of blood pressure. There is no evidence to support the use of plasma exchange. Combination therapy with MMF, corticosteroids, and sirolimus would appear to be the most prudent immunosuppressive regimen in such patients.

Acute Pyelonephritis

Urinary tract infections may occur at any period but are most common shortly after transplantation. Risk factors for urinary tract infections include catheterization, ureteric stenting, and preexisting anatomic or neurologic abnormalities. Urinary tract infections are often heralded by fever, allograft pain and tenderness, and a raised peripheral blood white blood cell count. Diagnosis requires urine culture, but empirical antibiotic treatment should be started immediately if infection is suspected clinically. Renal function usually returns to baseline with antimicrobial therapy and volume expansion. Recurrent pyelonephritis merits investigation to rule out underlying anatomical abnormalities.

Acute Allergic Interstitial Nephritis

Acute interstitial nephritis is occasionally observed in the early postoperative course. Removal of the offending agent (often sulfamethoxazole-trimethoprim [SMX-TMP]) is indicated. A role for augmented steroid therapy is unclear.

Urine Leaks

Urine leaks usually occur within weeks of transplantation. Causes include ureteric infarction due to perioperative disruption of its blood supply and breakdown of the ureterovesical anastomosis. The clinical features include abdominal pain and swelling with rising plasma creatinine levels due to reabsorption of solutes across the peritoneal membrane. If a perirenal drain is being used, a urine leak may present with high-volume drainage. Ultrasound often demonstrates a fluid collection (urinoma). Antegrade pyelography allows precise diagnosis and localization of proximal urinary leaks. Whenever urine leakage is suspected, a bladder catheter should be immediately inserted to decompress the urinary tract, and most leaks require urgent surgical exploration and repair.

Urinary Tract Obstruction

Urinary tract obstruction can cause allograft dysfunction at any time after transplantation but is most common in the early postoperative period. The causes include the following:

- Suboptimal ureterovesical anastomosis
- Ureteric blood clots
- Fibrosis of the ureter due to ischemia or rejection
- Prostatic hypertrophy
- Neurogenic bladder (diabetic neuropathy)
- Lymphocele

Ultrasonography demonstrates hydronephrosis; however, dilation of the transplant urinary collecting system is often seen in the early postoperative period even in the absence of functional obstruction, and serial scans may be required to confirm the diagnosis. Renal scintiscan with diuretic washout may be useful in equivocal obstructions. Open surgical repair is usually required, but endoscopic measures may suffice in certain circumstances. Obstruction in the early postoperative period due to an enlarged prostate should be managed with initial bladder catheter drainage and followed by elective prostatectomy.

Late Allograft Dysfunction

The causes and evaluation of late (>6 months post-transplant) renal allograft dysfunction in the months and years after renal transplantation are listed:

- Chronic allograft nephropathy ("chronic rejection")
- Chronic calcineurin nephrotoxicity
- Recurrent disease in the allograft
- Renal artery stenosis
- Polyoma virus infection
- Chronic allograft nephropathy

Chronic allograft nephropathy is characterized by a slow insidious decline in renal function at least 6 months after renal transplantation. It is typically associated with proteinuria and hypertension and after censoring for death it is the most common cause of late renal allograft loss. Although alloimmune factors are important in the pathogenesis of chronic allograft nephropathy, other etiologic factors include ischemic injury, calcineurin toxicity, hypertension, and glomerular hyperfiltration. There is no specific treatment for chronic allograft nephropathy at this time. Hypertension and hyperlipidemia should be rigorously controlled, the former preferably with either an ACE inhibitor or adrenergic receptor blocker. The use of sirolimus or MMF in place of CNI may lead to a temporary improvement in glomerular filtration rate; however, there are no randomized, controlled trials supporting a long-term benefit from this strategy.

Chronic Calcineurin Nephrotoxicity

Chronic nephrotoxicity associated with CNI is a well-documented phenomenon in both renal and nonrenal organ transplantation. It is caused by chronic exposure to cyclosporine or tacrolimus and can occur even when drug levels are maintained within the normal therapeutic range. It is difficult to distinguish clinically from chronic allograft nephropathy, and often the two may coexist.

The replacement of azathioprine by MMF followed either by elimination or reduction of the CNI is a widespread practice. Many authorities advocate the reduction or removal of CNI-based immunosuppression in all patients; however, with this practice there is a risk of triggering late acute rejection, which is associated with a poor prognosis.

Transplant Renal Artery Stenosis

Transplant renal artery stenosis can arise at any time after transplantation. Retrospective studies report functionally significant stenosis in less than 10% of renal transplant recipients. Suggestive clinical signs include resistant hypertension, acute renal failure after ACE inhibition, an audible renal bruit, and polycythemia. The diagnosis is made by renal angiography, magnetic resnance angiography, or duplex sonography. The clinical response rate to percutaneous angioplasty is approximately 40% to 75%; however, restenosis is common and may require repeat intevention or operative bypass. Particular care must be taken to avoid radiocontrast material–mediated nephrotoxicity in the investigation and management of this condition.

Recurrent Disease in the Allograft

Table 40–4 summarizes the conditions that recur after transplantation. With improvements in short- and long-term renal allograft survival rates, disease recurrence has assumed greater clinical importance. Several diseases such as focal segmental glomerulonephritis, anti–glomerular basement membrane disease, and hemolytic-uremic syndrome/thrombotic thrombocytopenic purpura can occur early in the post-transplant course, but most diseases recur in the months and years after transplantation. The rates of disease recurrence vary, depending on the primary diagnosis. Recurrence rates are highest with focal segmental glomerulonephritis (especially the childhood variant) and membranoproliferative glomerulonephritis for which rates of more than 80% are seen with type II disease and are associated with significant reductions in renal allograft survival. Recurrent diabetic nephropathy is common; however, the poorer outcomes in this patient subpopulation heretofore may have masked the true clinical significance of disease recurrence. Recurrence rates are less common with IgA nephropathy, the rapidly progressive glomerulonephritides, and lupus nephritis. Treatment strategies are broadly similar to those used in native real disease. Notably, whereas less than 5% of all grafts are lost due to recurrent disease, this figure approaches 50% in patients with a second graft loss in whom the first graft was lost due to primary disease recurrence.

Table 40-4: Recurrent Disease after Transplantation

Disease	Approximate Recurrence Rate	Time to Recurrence	Management	Living Donor Transplantation
Primary FSGS	40%–50%	Hours to weeks	ACEI, steroids, ? plasmapheresis	No, if very high risk of recurrence
IgA GN	35%	>2 months	ACEI, ? fish oil	Yes
			Cytotoxics if crescentic GN	
MPGN	30% Type I	Weeks	Type I—? aspirin	Type I—Yes
	80%–100% Type II		Type II—? steroids	Type II—consider (< 50% of grafts lost)
Anti-GBM disease	Rare if antibody negative pretransplant	Immediate	Plasmapheresis, cyclophosphamide	Yes
SLE	<10%	>1 week	Steroids, MMF, cytotoxic drugs	Yes
Wegener granulomatosis	10%	>1 week	Steroids, cytotoxic drugs	Yes
HUS/TTP	Depends on cause: familial > classic HUS	Immediately onward	Plasmapheresis	No if familial HUS/TTP

ACEI, angiotensin-converting enzyme inhibitor; FSGS, focal segmental glomerulosclerosis; GBM, glomerular basement membrane; GN, glomerulonephritis; HUS, hemolytic uremic syndrome; MMF, mycophenolate mofetil; SLE, systemic lupus erythematosus; TTP, thrombotic thrombocytopenic purpura.

Polyomavirus Infection

Reactivation of polyomavirus infection with shedding of infected urothelial cells (decoy cells) is estimated to occur in 10% to 60% of renal transplant recipients. However, clinically significant disease occurs in less than 5%. The clinical features associated with infection in renal transplant recipients include asymptomatic infection (most common), acute and chronic allograft dysfunction, and hemorrhagic cystitis. The acute graft dysfunction usually is due to interstitial nephritis, although ureteric stenosis has been described. The use of more powerful maintenance immunosuppression regimens incorporating MMF and tacrolimus has probably contributed to a rise in the incidence of clinically significant polyoma virus infection. The management of this condition is difficult and primarily involves a progressive reduction in the immunosuppression burden in an attempt to augment host mechanisms of viral clearance. The long-term outlook for graft survival is often poor.

Clinical Outcomes and Allograft Survival Rates in Renal Transplantation

Analysis of survival rates for the general dialysis population and transplant patients is greatly affected by selection bias—in general, patients referred for transplantation are healthier and have better functional status than those patients felt to be unsuitable for transplantation. Comparisons between patients on the waiting list who do or do not receive a transplant demonstrate that for medium- to long-term outcome, transplantation confers a significant survival benefit, particularly in diabetic patients. One year survival rates of more than 90% are now expected for both cadaveric and living-donor transplants. Long-term renal allograft survival rates have also steadily increased over the last 10 years, and the expected graft half-life of a cadaveric transplant is now more than 10 years.

MEDICAL MANAGEMENT OF THE TRANSPLANT RECIPIENT

With the current low acute rejection rates and improvements in long-term graft survival, more emphasis is being placed on the general medical management of transplant recipients. The management of common electrolyte, endocrine, and cardiovascular complications post-transplant is discussed in the following sections.

Electrolyte Disorders

Hypophosphatemia

Hypophosphatemia is common in the early post-transplant period due to residual hyperparathyroidism. Clinical symptoms are uncommon but include muscle weakness and rarely respiratory muscle weakness. The target plasma phosphate level should be 2.5 to 4 mg/dL achieved by increasing dietary phosphate intake and oral phosphate repletion with or without vitamin D.

Hyperkalemia

Mild hyperkalemia due to CNI-mediated impairment of tubule potassium secretion is common after a renal transplant and may be exacerbated by poor allograft function, dietary indiscretion, and medications such as ACE inhibitors or β-blockers. The hyperkalemia is usually not severe and improves with reduction in CNI dosage, treatment is often not required, and exacerbating factors should be minimized.

Metabolic Acidosis

A mild distal (hyperchloremic) renal tubular acidosis is common after transplantation. This reflects tubule dysfunction caused by CNIs, rejection, or residual hyperparathyroidism. Oral bicarbonate replacement is given in severe occurrences.

Other Electrolyte Abnormalities

Hypomagnesemia is common and is due to a magnesuric effect of CNIs. The effectiveness of supplementation is limited and it should only be considered when the serum level is less than 1.5mg/dL.

Bone Disorders after Renal Transplantation

Hyperparathyroidism

Hyperparathyroidism is seen in more than 50% of allograft recipients. Risk factors include the severity of pretransplant hyperparathyroidism and duration of renal replacement therapy. Laboratory findings include hypophosphatemia and mild to moderate hypercalcemia with an inappropriately high parathyroid hormone level. The condition usually resolves spontaneously, and management in the interim consists of repletion of phosphate and the administration of vitamin D analogs if 1,25-vitamin D concentrations are low. Post-transplant subtotal parathyroidectomy is only performed for either severe acute symptomatic hypercalcemia or persistent, moderately severe hypercalcemia (e.g., calcium > 12 mg/dL for 12 months).

Osteoporosis

Osteoporosis, defined as bone density more than 2.5 standard deviations below the mean of sex-matched, young adults, is observed in up to 60% of allograft recipients after transplantation with most of the bone loss occurring in the first 6 months. Pathologic fractures of the appendicular skeleton are common after renal transplantation and diabetic recipients have a particular risk. Corticosteroid use is the primary cause of post-transplant osteoporosis with hyperparathyroidism, hypophosphatemia, and vitamin D resistance acting as contributing factors. The diagnosis can be confirmed by dual x-ray absorptiometry scanning, and all patients thought to have a high risk should be evaluated prospectively. Treatment strategies include administration of 1000 mg/day of elemental calcium and 800 units/day of standard vitamin D (calcitriol if glomerular filtration rate is < 50 mL/min) accompanied by regular weight-bearing exercise. Emerging options include the minimization or elimination of corticosteroid use often in combination with T-cell mono- or polyclonal antibody administration. The use of bisphosphonates or sex hormone repletion is controversial. No prospective data exist to show a reduction in fracture incidence, and these agents should only be used after consultation with an endocrinologist familiar with post-transplant bone disease.

Osteonecrosis

Osteonecrosis (avascular necrosis), the most serious bone complication of renal transplantation, is seen in 5% to 10% of renal transplant recipients. The most commonly affected site is the femoral head, and high-dose corticosteroid use is a risk factor. The principal symptom is pain, and magnetic resonance imaging is diagnostic. Treatment options include rest, core decompression, osteotomy, or joint replacement.

Gout

Most cyclosporine-treated renal transplant recipients develop hyperuricemia, with less than 10% developing clinical symptoms. Acute attacks are treated with colchicine or an oral corticosteroid pulse. The use of nonsteroidal anti-inflammatory drugs should be avoided. The use of azathioprine and allopurinol in combination for the treatment of hyperuricemia can result in severe bone marrow suppression and is best avoided.

Hypertension

Hypertension occurs in up to 80% of kidney transplant recipients and can be attributed to CNIs, weight gain, allograft dysfunction, native kidney disease, and, less commonly, transplant renal artery stenosis. Hypertension should be aggressively managed with a target blood pressure of less than 135/85 mm Hg and less than 125/75 mm Hg in those with proteinuria. ACE inhibitors are typically avoided in the early post-transplantation period. Calcium channel blockers may offer some protection against CNI-mediated nephrotoxicity.

Hyperlipidemia

Hyperlipidemia is seen in 60% to 70% of kidney transplant recipients and may contribute not only to the excess cardiovascular mortality observed but also to chronic allograft nephropathy. The target low-density lipoprotein cholesterol level should be less than 100 mg/dL, and pharmacologic therapy is required to achieve this value in most patients. Other treatment options include steroid minimization and switching from cyclosporine to tacrolimus. Statins are the cholesterol-lowering drug of choice despite concerns about rhabdomyolysis (see earlier). Bile acid sequestrants bind CNIs and should be taken separately.

Post-Transplant Malignancy

The overall incidence of cancer in renal transplant recipients is greater than that in dialysis patients and the general population. For specific "transplant-associated" malignancies, the risk is dramatically increased whereas for common malignancies (lung, breast, and prostate) the risk is broadly similar. The cumulative amount of immunosuppression is the most important factor in the increased risk of malignancy, and the long-term impact of the recent advent of more powerful immunosuppression regimens on cancer incidence is an emerging concern. The common post-transplant malignancies are discussed in the next sections.

Skin and Anogenital Cancers

Squamous cell carcinoma, basal cell carcinoma, and malignant melanoma are more common in renal transplant recipients. Risk factors for skin cancer are the duration and cumulative dose of immunosuppression, exposure to ultraviolet light, and fair skin. Primary and secondary prevention is important: patients should be counseled about minimizing exposure to strong sunlight and self-screening for skin lesions. Cancers of the vulva, uterine cervix, penis, scrotum, anus, and perianal region are more common than in the general population. These tumors tend to be multifocal and more aggressive and are associated with human papillomavirus infection. Prevention measures include yearly physical examination of the anogenital area and, in women, yearly pelvic and cervical histologic examinations. Suspicious lesions should be excised, and patients should be closely followed for recurrence.

Post-Transplant Lymphoproliferative Disorder

Post-transplant lymphoproliferative disorder is not a single disorder but rather represents a spectrum of tumors extending from benign polyclonal lymphoid proliferations to overtly malignant lymphomas. The cumulative incidence in renal transplant recipients is 1% to 5% with most occurring within 2 years of transplantation. More than 90% are non-Hodgkin lymphomas of B-cell origin and most of these are associated with Epstein-Barr virus infection.

Risk factors include the following:

- The combination of Epstein-Barr virus–positive donor and Epstein-Barr virus–negative recipient
- Pediatric recipient (children are more likely to be Epstein-Barr virus negative)
- Degree of immunosuppressive burden (especially use of anti-lymphocyte antibodies)

Thus, the clinical and histologic spectrum of post-transplant lymphoproliferative disorder at presentation and its treatment can vary greatly. Extranodal involvement, including involvement of the renal allograft is more common than in nontransplant-associated lymphomas. Treatment involves reduction of, or with life-threatening disease, elimination of the immunosuppressive burden. Combination therapy involving surgical excision, chemotherapy, and radiotherapy is commonly used.

Infectious Complications of Renal Transplantation

The heightened risk of infection in renal transplant recipients is directly related to the intensity of immunosuppression and exposure to potential pathogens. Given that immunosuppression alters the clinical presentation of life-threatening infections, early and aggressive diagnostic workup followed by empirical antimicrobial therapy is essential if infectious illness is suspected. The spectrum of infection observed in renal transplant recipients change over time. Most infections seen in the first month are related to the operative procedure itself (e.g., wound infection or urinary tract infection). Preventive measures include ensuring that the donor and recipient are free of overt infection before transplantation, good surgical technique, and SMX-TMP prophylaxis to prevent urinary tract infections. After several weeks of intensive immunosuppression, the risk of opportunistic infections with cytomegalovirus (CMV), EBV, *Listeria monocytogenes, Pneumocystis carinii,* and *Nocardia.* Preventive measures include antiviral prophylaxis (for 3 to 6 months after transplant) and SMX-TMP prophylaxis (for 6 to 12 months after transplant). Opportunistic infections after 6 to 12 months are uncommon unless the immunosuppressive burden is increased, for example, after treatment of a late acute rejection. Exceptions include CMV retinitis and colitis, a higher incidence of respiratory syncytial virus and influenza infections, and chronic manifestations of human papilloma virus infections.

Cytomegalovirus

CMV is one of the most important post-transplant pathogens, and disease is typically observed 1 to 6 months post-transplant. CMV infection is seen in 50% to 80% of patients; however, CMV disease implies both laboratory evidence of viral exposure (a rising IgG titer or CMV antigen in body fluids) and symptoms or tissue invasion. The risk of CMV infection or disease is highest in CMV-negative recipients of CMV-positive kidneys. OKT3/polyclonal therapy, particularly when prescribed for treatment of rejection, significantly increases the risk of subsequent CMV disease. Typical clinical features include fever, malaise, leukopenia, pneumonitis, hepatitis, and ulcerating lesions of the gastrointestinal tract. The gold standard diagnostic test is quantitative PCR for CMV DNA. Less sensitive alternatives include conventional and shell vial culture, CMV antigenema assays and hybrid capture CMV DNA assays. Demonstration of shed virus in the urine or sputum correlates poorly with clinical outcomes, and biopsy interpretation is complicated by the focal nature of the infection in many organs. CMV disease should be treated with a reduction in immunosuppression and intravenous ganciclovir therapy for 2 to 4 weeks. Valganciclovir has greatly improved oral bioavailability compared with oral ganciclovir and is emerging as a possible replacement for intravenous ganciclovir in some situations. Foscarnet is reserved for resistant CMV disease. Prevention of CMV disease is of great clinical importance, and patients with the highest risk of CMV disease should routinely receive CMV prophylaxis for up to 6 months; whether all low-risk patients need to receive prophylaxis is controversial.

Pneumocystosis

The incidence of post-transplant *P carinii* infection has declined with the widespread use of SMX-TMP prophylaxis. Alternative agents in patients allergic to sulfa drugs include dapsone and pyrimethamine, atovaquone, and aerosolized pentamidine.

Immunization in Renal Transplant Recipients
Important general rules concerning immunization in renal transplant recipients are the following:

- Immunizations should be completed at least 4 weeks before transplantation.
- Immunization should be avoided in the first 6 months after transplantation.
- Live vaccines are generally contraindicated after transplantation.

Infections are a predictable complication of renal transplantation. Minimizing the risk of infection requires meticulous surgical technique, antiviral prophylaxis for the first 3 to 6 months, SMX-TMP prophylaxis for the first 6 to 12 months, and, of course, avoidance of excessive immunosuppression.

Surgery in the Renal Transplant Recipient

Allograft Nephrectomy
This is an uncommon procedure. Indications for allograft nephrectomy include the following:

- Allograft failure with symptomatic rejection (fever, malaise, and graft pain)
- Allograft infarction due to thrombosis
- Emphysematous pyelonephritis
- Graft rupture

Ongoing rejection in a failed allograft can sometimes be controlled with steroids, but prolonged immunosuppression of the patient with end-stage renal disease is undesirable.

Nontransplant-Related Surgery or Hospitalization
In-patient management of the renal transplant recipient hospitalized for non–transplant-related surgery should focus on the maintenance of adequate volume status, avoidance of nephrotoxic medicines (including nonsteroidal anti-inflammatory drugs and radiocontrast material) and the proper dosing of immunosuppressive drugs. If intravenous administration of a corticosteroid is required then a milligram per milligram dose of intravenous methylprednisolone can be used as maintenance therapy with supplemental stress-dose hydrocortisone prescribed separately. Intravenous cyclosporine should be prescribed in slow infusion form at one third of the total daily oral dose, and intravenous tacrolimus given daily should be prescribed at one fifth of the total oral dose.

The Patient with the Failing Kidney

In patients with a failing allograft, the selection criteria for initiation of dialysis and retransplantation are no different from those for the general end-stage renal disease population. The timely insertion of an access port is essential. The optimal management of immunosuppressive withdrawal is controversial; prolonged tapering of corticosteroids is required to avoid precipitation of Addisonian symptoms. A gradual tapering (weeks to months) of immunosuppressive therapy may help in the avoidance of symptomatic acute rejection or the elaboration of anti-HLA antibodies that can complicate retransplantation.

Pregnancy in the Renal Transplant Recipient

See Chapter 17, The Kidney and Hypertension in Pregnancy.

CONCLUSION

Improvements in renal allograft outcomes have significantly improved the outlook for renal transplant recipients, and transplantation is the treatment of choice for many patients with end-stage renal disease. Given the success in lowering acute rejection rates, the focus of care is shifting toward the management of post-transplant complications such as chronic allograft nephropathy and bone and cardiovascular disease.

Index